"Dr Roni Berger has assembled a large group of authors from around the world to provide an international perspective on posttraumatic growth that demonstrates the universality of this phenomenon. The massive volume will be an invaluable addition to libraries where researchers and students are developing research projects, theses and dissertations. They will relish finding these reviews of virtually any topic of interest in the world of posttraumatic growth."

Richard G. Tedeschi, PhD, *Executive Director, Boulder Crest Institute for Posttraumatic Growth*

"*The Routledge International Handbook of Posttraumatic Growth* is the single most comprehensive volume on posttraumatic growth to date. With contributions from scholars all over the world, it is a unique resource on an important topic. It is indispensable."

Lawrence G. Calhoun, *Professor Emeritus of Psychological Science at UNC Charlotte*

THE ROUTLEDGE INTERNATIONAL HANDBOOK OF POSTTRAUMATIC GROWTH

The Routledge International Handbook of Posttraumatic Growth offers a rich covering of approaches to different traumatic and stressful experiences in relation to posttraumatic growth (PTG).

This handbook explores the benefits that individuals, couples, families, organizations, and communities can experience following the struggle with highly stressful and potentially traumatic events. Split into seven parts and written by a diverse international team of multidisciplinary contributors who provide a comprehensive overview of PTG, topics include religious and spiritual aspects of PTG, gender in PTG, PTG in LGBTQ+, perinatal bereavement, and more.

The Routledge International Handbook of Posttraumatic Growth represents an essential resource for students, researchers, and professionals, including social workers, psychologists, nurses, mental health counselors, and psychiatrists.

Roni Berger, PhD, LCSW, is a professor of social work at Adelphi University in New York, USA. She was born and raised in Israel, and holds a BSW, MSW, and PhD from The Hebrew University of Jerusalem and a Diploma in Psychotherapy from the Tel Aviv University Medical School. Dr. Berger has received several awards and grants and is a recipient of Fulbright Senior Specialist awards.

THE ROUTLEDGE INTERNATIONAL HANDBOOK SERIES

THE ROUTLEDGE INTERNATIONAL HANDBOOK OF PERINATAL MENTAL HEALTH DISORDERS
Edited by Amy Wenzel

THE ROUTLEDGE INTERNATIONAL HANDBOOK OF COMMUNITY PSYCHOLOGY
Facing Global Crises with Hope
Edited by Carolyn Kagan, Jacqui Akhurst, Jaime Alfaro, Rebecca Lawthom, Michael Richards, and Alba Zambrano

THE ROUTLEDGE INTERNATIONAL HANDBOOK OF MORALITY, COGNITION, AND EMOTION IN CHINA
Edited by Ryan Nichols

THE ROUTLEDGE INTERNATIONAL HANDBOOK OF COMPARATIVE PSYCHOLOGY
Edited by Todd M. Freeberg, Amanda R. Ridley and Patrizia d'Ettorre

THE ROUTLEDGE INTERNATIONAL HANDBOOK OF NEUROAESTHETICS
Edited by Martin Skov and Marcos Nadal

THE ROUTLEDGE INTERNATIONAL HANDBOOK OF PSYCHOANALYSIS AND PHILOSOPHY
Edited by Aner Govrin and Tair Caspi

THE ROUTLEDGE INTERNATIONAL HANDBOOK OF PSYCHOLINGUISTIC AND COGNITIVE PROCESSES
Edited by Jackie Guendouzi, Filip Loncke and Mandy J. Williams

THE ROUTLEDGE INTERNATIONAL HANDBOOK OF POSTTRAUMATIC GROWTH
Edited by Roni Berger

THE ROUTLEDGE INTERNATIONAL HANDBOOK OF POSTTRAUMATIC GROWTH

Edited by Roni Berger

Routledge
Taylor & Francis Group
NEW YORK AND LONDON

Designed cover image: © Getty Images

First published 2024
by Routledge
605 Third Avenue, New York, NY 10158

and by Routledge
4 Park Square, Milton Park, Abingdon, Oxon, OX14 4RN

Routledge is an imprint of the Taylor & Francis Group, an informa business

ISBN: 978-1-032-20863-3 (hbk)
ISBN: 978-1-032-20866-4 (pbk)
ISBN: 978-1-032-20868-8 (ebk)

DOI: 10.4324/9781032208688

Typeset in Sabon
by MPS Limited, Dehradun

I am grateful to Marty, Dan, Jen, the chapters' authors, my friends, and colleagues who accompanied and supported me through the journey of conceptualizing and developing this book.

CONTENTS

EDITOR

Dr. Roni Berger, PhD, LCSW, is a professor of social work at Adelphi University in New York, USA. She was born and raised in Israel and holds a BSW, MSW, and PhD from The Hebrew University of Jerusalem and a Diploma in Psychotherapy from Tel Aviv University Medical School. Her fields of expertise are trauma and posttraumatic growth in cultural contexts, immigrants, families, specifically stepfamilies, evidence-based practice, and group work. She dedicated the last two decades of her scholarly and professional activities to trauma-related topics, specifically the cultural context of traumatic experiences, and posttraumatic growth (PTG). She published and presented extensively nationally and internationally. Her books include a co-edited book about PTG across cultures and a textbook about stress, trauma, coping, and PTG, and numerous articles in peer-reviewed reputable journals. Dr. Berger serves on several editorial and advisory boards of professional organizations and consults nationally and internationally (Australia, Hong Kong, Nepal, Ghana, and Israel). She also participated in developing educational and training programs regarding trauma practice in general and PTG in particular. She serves as a consultant to professional organizations domestically and internationally as well as provides mentoring services in developing scholarly publications.

Before she immigrated to the United States in 1990, she worked in Israel in academia, direct practice with individuals, families, and groups in the fields of health and mental health, and held supervisory and administrative positions in diverse social, medical, and educational settings. Dr. Berger received several awards and grants and is a recipient of Fulbright Senior Specialist awards.

CONTRIBUTORS

Victoria Eugenia Acevedo, PsyD, was born and raised in Colombia. She worked in community psychology and violence prevention with women, children, and underserved populations, prior to migrating to the United States to pursue her master's and doctoral degrees. She returned to her homeland, where she has worked as a clinical psychologist serving individuals, couples, and families for the past 25 years. Her professional experiences in Colombia, and the United States, and her personal commitment to working with underserved populations, shaped her interests in human development, recovery from trauma, and family and community resilience. She has published several articles and coauthored three books addressing issues of resilience. She is a Professor at the Universidad Javeriana, Cali in Colombia, and served with distinction as ethics committee magistrate for the Colombian Psychological Association (Colegio Colombiano de Psicólogos). Her work was recognized with the distinguished contribution Award in 2019.

Lauren D'Agostino is a first-year graduate student in the Lewis and Clark Marriage, Couple and Family Therapy program. She received her B.A. in Psychology from the University of San Diego. Her research interests include the human-nature bond, biocentricity, and the wisdom of plant healers.

Amy L. Ai, PhD, MS, MA, MSW, is an interdisciplinary researcher and a Distinguished Research Professor at Florida State University. She received her PhD in psychology and social work and three master's degrees from the University of Michigan, Ann Arbor. Her academic career has focused on cross-disciplinary research on human strengths, spirituality, cardiac health, mental health, existential crisis, gerontology, and well-being. Her studies have been funded by grants from federal, state, international, and private agencies. Dr. Ai has served as a scientific reviewer for grant funders in the United States (e.g., U.S. Department of State, Defense, Health and Human Services; National Institutes of Health) and other Countries (Austria, Canada, Israel, and the United Kingdom). She is a fellow of the Association of Psychological Science, American Psychological Association (Divisions 56, 38, 36, and 20), Gerontological Society of America, and American Academy of Social Work and Social Welfare; a Hartford Geriatric Faculty Scholar and Fulbright Scholar.

Zeynep Akbudak was born and raised in Turkey. She is a candidate for clinical child and adolescent psychology, and a research assistant at the World Human Relief Association where she has been doing voluntary work related to natural and human-caused disasters. She did voluntary and obligatory internships at TED University Corono Virus Pycho-Social Support Team, the Middle East Technical University Child and Adolescent Laboratory and Counseling and Research Center of The Ministry of Education. She is especially interested in preventing child sexual abuse and marriages and believes that a better future is possible with well-raised children, thus she works to help children to shine their lights.

Benjamin N. B. Alexander, PhD, is an associate professor of management at the Orfalea College of Business, California Polytechnic State University. His research focuses on stakeholder management, collective action, and research methods. His interest in how organizations navigate their responsibilities to different stakeholders has motivated projects on social entrepreneurship, family firms, organizational trauma, and business education. His research has been published in outlets such as the Journal of Business Research, The Journal of Applied Behavioral Science, Nonprofit Management & Leadership, Qualitative Research in Organizations and Management, and Research in Organizational Change and Development. He received his PhD from the A.B. Freeman School of Business at Tulane University and his M.A. from George Mason University. Prior to becoming an academic, he worked as a personnel psychologist.

Julien le Jeune d'Allegeershecque is a teaching assistant on both the MSc in Digital Health Interventions and the MSc in Global Mental Health at the University of Glasgow. He conducts and supervises research on gender-based violence, trauma, and positive change following a traumatic experience. He is also involved in research projects aiming to develop Digital Health Interventions for people who have experienced trauma.

Margarida Almeida, MA, is a psychologist, with a master's degree in clinical psychology from ISPA – University Institute and is a doctoral student in clinical psychology at the same institute. She serves as an editorial assistant in the scientific journal Psicologia, Saúde & Doenças of the Health Psychology Portuguese Society.

Pinar Alyagut, a PhD candidate, graduated from philosophy in 2003 at Mersin University and completed her master's program at Akdeniz University, in Antalya, Turkey. Her master's thesis was on characteristics of cosmopolitanism and the possibility of global justice. She is enrolled in a PhD program at Ankara University, where she will complete her dissertation this year entitled "British idealism and self-concept". She is currently a research assistant at the philosophy department at Afyon Kocatepe University in Turkey. Her research interests include metaphysics, idealism, realism, cosmopolitanism, authenticity, human rights, and self-concept.

India Amos is a lecturer in Counselling and Psychotherapy at the University of Salford, United Kingdom, and a Chartered and HCPC-registered Counselling Psychologist. India has worked with people living with HIV in psychological therapy and provides teaching to trainee counselors and psychotherapists on the topic of HIV-related stigma and posttraumatic growth.

Laura Marie Armstrong, PhD, is an associate professor of psychological science and the director of the Child and Family Development lab at the University of North Carolina at Charlotte. She is a licensed psychologist, and she directs the UNC Charlotte Behavioral Health and Resiliency (BeHealthieR) Clinic. She conducts interdisciplinary research at the intersection of developmental and intervention science that focuses on maternal and child health, social-emotional development, and family process to inform intervention, practice, and policies that promote more equitable systems of care for under-served individuals and families. Her work examines the effects of adversity from a life course perspective and the ways that family, social, and educational contexts can foster growth in the aftermath of trauma and protect children and youth from the harmful effects of risk factors and conditions that can undermine well-being.

Pamela Arroyo is an assistant psychologist in the Child and Family Community Psychology Service within the National Health Service (NHS). She obtained an MSc with distinction in Clinical Psychology and Mental Health from Swansea University, in 2020, and undertook a placement year in a community brain injury service within the National Health Service (NHS). One of her contributions to the community brain injury services includes a meta-synthesis about facilitating factors of Posttraumatic Growth (PTG) in survivors of acquired brain injury. Upon this, the team developed a series of interventions in which they tried to build some of those factors to help the service users. Pamela has contributed to other works focused on the promotion of well-being, and is looking forward to continuing her studies towards a doctoral level in the near future.

Anat Ben-Porat, PhD, was born and raised in Israel. She is a clinical social worker and worked at a shelter for women who are victims of domestic violence in Tel Aviv. After pursuing her MSW and PhD, she joined the academy as a faculty member at the Louis and Gabi Weisfeld School of Social Work at Bar-Ilan University. Dr. Ben-Porat is the Head of the BSW Program at Bar-Ilan, and her area of expertise is domestic violence and the implications for therapists of treating trauma victims. For the past two decades, she has practiced, supervised, taught, conducted research, and published numerous articles in the above-mentioned areas. She is an active member of Israel's Ministry of Welfare and Social Affairs professional committees and is an advisor for the Israeli government in regard to shaping policy for the prevention and treatment of domestic violence.

Isabel Berbel graduated in psychology from the University of Seville in 2004. She specialized in psychological intervention with groups at risk of exclusion, especially migrant and refugee populations, the gypsy community, victims of gender violence, and young people in the juvenile justice system. She has also trained in the health sector, in cognitive-behavioral therapy and gestalt therapy, and has developed part of her professional work in private practice. She has been working as a psychologist in the international protection program at the Cepaim Foundation with asylum seekers, refugees, and immigrants since 2016, where she has specialized in the trauma caused by socio-political conflicts and other human rights violations and she works for the psychosocial integration of displaced persons.

Janelle Billingsley, PhD, is an assistant professor in the Department of Psychology at the University of Maryland, Baltimore County. Her research agenda has primarily focused on the study of normative and adaptive processes fostering healthy development among adolescents facing contextual adversity. Specifically, her work has focused on further identifying how adolescents can leverage pre-existing strengths in their lives to promote their social and emotional well-being.

Sabrina Bonichini, PhD, completed her PhD in Developmental and Social Psychology in 2000 at the University of Padua (Italy). She obtained a research fellowship at the Department of Developmental Psychology of Padua from 2000 to 2004. In 2004 she won the title of assistant professor and in 2011 became Associate Professor in Developmental Psychology at the University of Padua, where she teaches assessment of development and pediatric health psychology. Her research interests include pediatric psychoncology, assessment of infant pain, pediatric psychology, research methods, instruments of assessment in infancy and childhood, crying development, cross-cultural differences in sleep rhythms, temperament, individual differences, contextual determinants of development, socio-emotional development, parents' childrearing beliefs and practices, adoption, pet therapy. She wrote books and articles on developmental psychology, is an ad hoc referee for multiple international journals, and is involved in international collaborations.

Sophie Brickman, MA, is a clinical psychology doctoral student at the University of Colorado, Colorado Springs. She earned her bachelor's degree in psychology from Brandeis University. Her research and clinical interests include posttraumatic growth, trauma memory, and the role of creative writing in trauma healing.

Dagmar Bruenig, PhD, is a postdoctoral research fellow in the Stressomics Lab at the School of Biomedical Sciences at the University of Technology, Brisbane, Australia. Dagmar investigated genetic and psychological predisposition of risk and resilience to PTSD in military veterans, being the first researcher to investigate resilience as a psychological construct rather than a disorder absence in molecular research. Dagmar has a keen interest in the broad variations in posttrauma responses with a particular focus on resilience. Having worked in genetics and epigenetics for seven years, she maintains a focus on interdisciplinary research that combines differentiated approaches to understanding psychological constructs.

Susan Cadell, PhD, is a professor in the School of Social Work at Renison University College, affiliated with the University of Waterloo in Waterloo, Ontario, Canada. Susan is a strengths-based social work researcher passionate about grief and end-of-life care. Her research concerns death, dying, and bereavement, with a particular focus on posttraumatic growth and other positive outcomes of caregiving and grief. Some examples of projects concern grief in COVID, after Medical Assistance in Dying (MAiD), and international grief literacy. She has also undertaken studies of growth that are expressed via memorial and healing tattoos. Susan particularly enjoys mentoring students and emerging scholars.

Chih-Tao Cheng, MD, DrPH, is a psychiatrist with a doctorate in public health. After graduating from medical school in Taiwan, he pursued a doctoral degree in public health at the University of California, Berkeley, U.S. His experience includes community mental health and psychosocial health in a variety of populations, including cancer patients and military personnel. He is dedicated to the long-term psychological health of breast cancer survivors. Public mental health, health disparities, and reimbursement systems are also among his research interests. He is the director of the psychiatric department in a cancer hospital and associate professor at the National Defense University in Taiwan.

Elizabeth Counselman-Carpenter, PhD, LCSW, RPT-S, is an associate professor of Social Work at Adelphi University. Her practice and research interests include understanding the role of PTG in decreasing barriers to service provision in social work and medical settings, particularly with the LGBTQIA+ community and with breast cancer survivors. She has co-authored two books and frequently contributes to peer-reviewed journals. Beth has a BA in Sociology from the University of Richmond, an MSW from New York University, and a PhD from Adelphi University. In addition to teaching, she maintains a small private practice and community DEI consultancy practice. She has been using PhotoVoice in her teaching and practice since 2019.

Breda Cullen, PhD, is a senior lecturer in clinical psychology at the University of Glasgow, Scotland, UK. She is professionally registered as a clinical psychologist and neuropsychologist. She conducts research in the field of psychiatric epidemiology, particularly focusing on cognitive function in psychiatric and neurological conditions. She is also involved in intervention development for psychological and cognitive difficulties in people with neurological conditions, including the use of interventions based on positive psychology and mindfulness.

Irene de la Morena graduated in psychology from the Complutense University of Madrid in 2012. She later specialized in the Psychology of Community and Social Intervention through a Master's Degree at the University of Seville and, complementarily, obtained a qualification in General Health Psychology from the UDIMA University of Madrid. She has completed numerous trainings within the field of migration, asylum and refuge, gender violence, human trafficking, and art therapy for social inclusion. In her professional career, she has worked with populations in a situation of vulnerability, such as migrants and refugees, the gypsy community, female victims of gender violence, and survivors of human trafficking, following the values of social justice, equity, and defense of human rights. She has collaborated with different organizations and she currently works as a psychologist at the Association of Women in Conflict Zone (MZC) within the psychological attention service.

Rachel Dekel is a professor at the Louis and Gabi Weisfeld School of Social Work, at Bar-Ilan University in Israel and served as a former head of the school between the years 2012–2016. She currently serves as the academic head of the International School at Bar-Ilan. Prof. Dekel is known for her quantitative and qualitative research on couples and families coping, in the context of trauma, domestic violence, and PTSD. She is the founder and director of the Family Trauma Clinic, which promotes a family-oriented perspective in helping survivors of various traumatic experiences. She has won several Israeli and international grants including the I-CORE grant: Israeli Center of Research Excellence, in the area of mass trauma. She has published more than 150 scientific publications and supervised 60 students.

Whitney Dominick is a professor of psychology at Oakland University and a collaborator with Water Planet, USA. Her specialties include social psychology and animal-assisted therapy, with a focus on posttraumatic growth and social support.

Wenjie Duan, PhD, is a professor at the Department of Social Work, East China University of Science and Technology. He obtained his PhD degree in Applied Social Sciences at the City University of Hong Kong. He served on the Editorial Board for Research on Social Work Practice, the Journal of Evidence-based Social Work, and the Associate Editor for Frontiers in Psychology, as well as the reviewer of more than 30 peer-reviewed journals. He is engaged mainly in evidence-based social work with a strengths perspective, social indicators, and psychometrics, as well as quality of life promotion. His recent publication includes COVID-19-related stigma profiles and risk factors among people who are at high risk of contagion and Interdisciplinary Bridging Response Teams (IBRTs) in the COVID-19 Outbreak Aid Provision in China.

Mithat Durak, PhD, is a clinical psychologist specializing in diagnosing and treating mental, behavioral, and emotional problems via cognitive-behavioral therapy. He is a faculty member at Bolu Abant Izzet Baysal University Department of Psychology. He also studies health psychology, forensic psychology, geropsychology, and positive psychology focusing on psychopathology, trauma psychology, psychological hardiness, and the psychological consequences of forced migration. He developed and adapted various psychometric measurement tools for use in the Turkish culture, published articles in international journals, and has served as an editor, book author, chapter writer, and chapter translator for many national and international books, which are extensively used in psychology Turkish universities. Dr. Durak received the Scientific Incentive Award at the 2nd International Turkish Gerontology (2009) and is a member of the Turkish National Aging Council's founding committee. He served as Turkey's representative to the Geropsychology Task Force of the European Federation of Psychologists' Associations (2012–2014) and is the editor of the *Journal of Aging and Long-Term Care* and the guest editor of *Frontiers in Psychology.*

Pinar Dursun, PhD, graduated in psychology in 2003 and completed her PhD in 2012 at Middle East Technical University (METU) in Turkey. She completed a research fellowship at the Department of Counseling Psychology at Colorado State University in the US (2013–2014). She studied posttraumatic growth and meaning in life in the 2013 Colorado flood survivors supervised by Prof. Michael F. Steger. In addition to multiple internships and training in various hospitals, care centers, and clinical settings, she worked as a visiting scholar with immigrants at the unit of transcultural psychiatry (Transkulturelle Psychiatrie) of the Klinikum Wahrendorff, Hannover, Germany. In 2015, she became an assistant professor at Afyon Kocatepe University, where she teaches introduction to psychology, abnormal psychology, trauma and migration, positive clinical psychology, and family counseling. She conducts research on the relationship between posttraumatic stress, posttraumatic growth, polyvagal theory, neurodevelopmental disorders, and sound therapy, for which she trains at the Listening Center in Toronto, ON, Canada. She currently practices and supervises sound stimulation techniques with neurodevelopmental groups such as ADHD and traumatized clients to increase their executive functions and decrease posttraumatic stress.

Taylor Elam is a research assistant in the Free-Form Posttraumatic Growth (FF-PTG) Lab in the Department of Psychology at Oakland University, where she obtained her Bachelor of Arts degree in psychology in 2020. Throughout her undergraduate and post-Bachelorette studies, Taylor participated in collaborative and independent research projects, including conducting a research study analyzing facial affect recognition, PTG, resiliency, and empathy. She has also collaborated on a project studying attitudes and perceptions of depression subtypes as well as a longitudinal study examining social support, core belief disruption, and PTG throughout the COVID-19 pandemic. Taylor plans to pursue a PhD in social-personality psychology with an interest in studying trauma, emotions, and nonverbal behavior.

Ana Estevez completed her BA in psychology and women's and gender studies from Florida International University. During her undergraduate studies, she assisted in research projects that looked at cyber dating abuse in Latinx samples. She completed her post-baccalaureate certificate at the University of California, Irvine, where she researched trauma, moral injury, and mindfulness. She aims to get a PhD in clinical psychology and ultimately be a clinician and researcher.

Dr. Heather Evans, PhD, is a licensed clinical social worker with a private group counseling practice in Lehigh Valley, Pennsylvania. She has over 20 years of experience providing therapy to children, adolescents, and adults and extensive training and experience with women's issues, particularly sexual trauma, sex trafficking, and aftercare of its victims. Heather received a Doctor of Clinical Social Work degree from the University of Pennsylvania and her dissertation highlighted complex trauma and posttraumatic growth in victims of domestic sex trafficking. Heather is co-founder and chair of VAST (Valley Against Sex Trafficking) Coalition in Lehigh Valley, PA. She is devoted to training and equipping service providers and in 2013, she received the Allied Professional Award from the Crime Victims Council of the Lehigh Valley for outstanding commitment to victims' services. Heather is an adjunct professor of the Global Trauma Recovery Institute at Missio Theological Seminary; she travels and leads trips nationally and internationally, with the goal of partnering with and training trauma-healing caregivers. Heather is the author of two books on complex trauma and posttraumatic growth in sex trafficking survivors and the creator of the Voices of Survivors Project.

Zoe Fisher, PhD, DClinPsych, PGDip, is an associate professor at Health and Wellbeing Academy at Swansea University, Consultant Clinical Psychologist and lead for Community Neuro-rehabilitation Services in Swansea Bay Health Board (National Health Service) and co-founder of the GENIAL science group (www.genialscience.org.uk). She works with people living with acquired brain injury, community providers, and academics at Swansea University to develop and evaluate a range of community-based neuro-rehabilitation programs, which make use of co-production, positive psychology, and task-shifting principles to improve resilience, well-being and facilitate community and social integration. She has contributed to the development of several novel theoretical models of health and well-being. Her works have led to multiple publications and featured in the national media as examples of innovation in clinical practice. In 2021, she received an Advancing Health Care.

Jessica Furtado, MSW, RSW, RECE, is a PhD candidate in the interdisciplinary program of Family Relations and Human Development at the University of Guelph. Her graduate work and clinical fellowship were focused on supporting children and parents through pediatric medical trauma. Jessica's dissertation explores children's experiences of trauma by examining their realities of posttraumatic growth and depreciation with the intention of extending these findings into models of care provided to children and families. She strives to connect her teaching, clinical, and research knowledge in her work as a therapist with children and families, as a sessional instructor, and as a researcher and scholar.

Dana Rose Garfin, PhD, is a Psychologist and faculty in the Department of Community Health Sciences Fielding School of Public Health at the University of California, Los Angeles. Her work explores the impact of individual and collective level negative life events on physical and mental health across the lifespan, and how community-based interventions can alleviate resulting health disparities. Dr. Garfin has studied various collective traumas including 9/11, the Boston Marathon bombings, hurricanes, earthquakes, the Ebola outbreak, and COVID-19. She has expertise in the role of compounding threats, multiple exposures (including media-based exposures), and how individual-level trauma impacts responses to large-scale events. She also studies how individuals make decisions to promote individual and public health and how community and field-based interventions can promote resilience and adaptation. Her work is currently funded by the National Institute of Health and National Science Foundation (NSF) and she is a co-principal investigator of several NSF-funded studies exploring the psychosocial impacts of COVID-19. Her work has been published in high-impact scientific journals and has been covered in numerous domestic and international media outlets, including a 2020 paper on COVID-19 and media exposure that was the 3rd most downloaded article across the American Psychological Association journals.

Bruce E. Greenbaum, PhD, is an associate professor of management at the Orfalea College of Business, California Polytechnic State University. His research focuses on organizational transformation, micro-foundational effects on firm decision-making and corporate strategy, including the influence of CEO personality on firm innovation and new product development. Additional research interests include organizational change and development processes and the influence of leadership on employee commitment and motivation. His work has appeared in journals such as Administrative Science Quarterly, Journal of Change Management, Organization Development Journal, and Strategic Entrepreneurship Journal. He received his PhD in strategic management from the University of Texas at Austin. Prior to his academic career, he spent more than fifteen years as a consultant and investment banker.

Victoria Grinman, PhD, holds a BSW from Adelphi University, MSW from Columbia University, and PhD from Adelphi University. She is a psychotherapist with a background in clinical social work. She holds her private practice in New York and Massachusetts, and speaks internationally at conferences, with professionals, and parents on the topics of trauma and healing, Autism and special needs, parenthood, and best practices for parent engagement and support through the parenthood journey. Having worked with children and families with diverse backgrounds for many years in the community and school settings, Dr. Grinman is passionate about supporting children by nurturing parents to thrive and powerfully navigate their parenthood journey with confidence. Dr. Grinman has served as a lecturer in the Schools of Social Work at Boston College, Adelphi University, and Columbia University.

Along He is a PhD student in the School of Journalism and Communication at Nanjing University. He pursued his Master of Social Work from Wuhan University. He mainly engaged in Health Communication, Media Psychology, and Minority Mental Health.

Liat Helpman, PhD, is a licensed educational and clinical psychologist in Israel and is a senior lecturer at the Counseling and Human Development Department of the Faculty of Education in the University of Haifa, as well as a senior researcher at the Psychiatric Research Unit at Tel Aviv Sourasky Medical Center. Her research focuses on individual differences in stress response, posttraumatic reactions, and the assessment and treatment of trauma-related disorders. She is passionate about employing a bio-psychosocial prism to the investigation of stress responses and related psychopathologies, with the aim of contributing to the tailoring of developmentally- and gender-informed assessment, prevention, and intervention programs.

Pilar Hernandez-Wolfe, PhD, was born and raised in Colombia. She was involved in community psychology prior to migrating to the U.S. to pursue her master's and doctoral degrees. Her professional and political involvement in working with human rights and women's issues shaped her life-long interests in traumatic stress and resilience. As a result of her migration experience, Pilar began exploring her Indigenous ancestry, intergenerational trauma, and the larger social issues involved in colonization and decolonization. She is a Professor at the Lewis and Clark College Graduate School of Counseling and Education, guest faculty at the Universidad Javeriana, Cali in Colombia, and AAMFT-approved supervisor. She pioneered the concept of vicarious resilience in the context of treatment of torture survivors in the U.S. and mental health services addressing politically based violence. She is the author "A Borderlands' view of Latinos, Latin Americans and Decolonization. Rethinking Mental Health," and, co-author of "La resiliencia vicaria en las relaciones de ayuda". She received the Distinguished Contribution to Social Justice Award from the American Family Therapy Academy in 2013.

Shirley Heying, PhD, is an applied sociocultural anthropologist in the government sector and an affiliated faculty member of the University of New Mexico. Her research focuses on the intersections of mental health (particularly genocide-related trauma, resilience, and posttraumatic growth), indigenous identity, race relations, human agency, and state power in Latin America with a particular emphasis on Guatemala. Her cross-disciplinary research has been published in journals such as International Perspectives in Psychology: Research, Practice, Consultation and in her 2022 book entitled *Child Survivors of Genocide: Trauma, Resilience, and Identity in Guatemala*. She received her PhD and MA in anthropology at the University of New Mexico and taught in various capacities for over 10 years at the University of New Mexico where she won several teaching awards and was a visiting professor at Western Oregon University. She volunteers with nonprofit human rights and social justice organizations.

Samuel M.Y. Ho, PhD, FHKPS, is a clinical psychologist with a research and clinical focus on resilience and traumatology. He is the first researcher in Hong Kong to investigate the phenomenon of posttraumatic growth in cancer. Over the past 20 years, he has developed in-depth knowledge about the factors that facilitate adjustments to cancer diagnosis and other traumatic events. He is a fellow of the Hong Kong Psychological Society and is an advisor of many organizations on clinical practices. Professor Ho is the current head of the Department of Social and Behavioural Sciences at the City University of Hong Kong.

Dilwar Hussain, PhD, is an associate professor in the Department of Humanities and Social Sciences at the Indian Institute of Technology Guwahati, Assam, India. His research interests include positive psychology and psychology of stress, trauma, and coping.

Eranda Jayawickreme is the Harold W. Tribble Professor of Psychology at Wake Forest University. He has published extensively on questions of post-traumatic growth, character, and personality. He was formerly the Project Co-Leader for the Pathways to Character Project, an initiative examining the possibilities for the strengthening of character following adversity, challenge, or failure, and the Project Leader for the Growth Initiative, which focused on improving the quality of research on post-traumatic growth. His awards include the 2015 Rising Star award from the Association for Psychological Science, Wake Forest University's Award for Excellence in Research, and a Mellon Refugee Initiative Fund Fellowship.

Zygfryd Juczyński is a professor of psychology at the WSB University in Lodz, Poland, and a specialist in clinical and health psychology. His research interests include issues related to stress management, doctor/therapist-patient/client communication, and the design of tools for measuring stress and coping. He is the author or co-author of many publications, including the monograph: *When the Trauma of Others Becomes Their Own* (PWN, 2020); *Personality, Stress, and Health* (Difin, 2010), Textbooks on Drug Addiction (PZWL, 2008), *Measurement Tools in Health Promotion and Psychology* (PTP, 2009).

Rowan Kemmerly, MA, is a psychology PhD student at Rutgers University. She received her BA from Grinnell College and her MA in Psychology from Wake Forest University. Her current research interests include stress-related growth, the mechanisms of well-being and positive personality change, and the development of scalable well-being interventions.

Andrew H. Kemp, PhD, is a professor in Psychology at Swansea University and co-director of the GENIAL well-being science group. His research spans psychological science, psychiatry, and epidemiology, supported by positions at the University of Sydney in Australia (2004–2012), the University of São Paulo in Brazil (2013–2015), and Swansea University in Wales, United Kingdom (2016-present). The significance of his contributions to the field has been recognized through a fellowship from the British Psychological Society (2019) and the Association for Psychological Science in the United States (2017), as well as a Doctor of Science degree from the University of Melbourne (2019). Driven by the opportunity to have a positive impact on society, he has developed theoretical frameworks of health and well-being (2017, 2019, 2021), leading to significant service redesign and innovation in the healthcare sector in South Wales.

Ryan P. Kilmer, PhD, is a professor of psychology and chair of the Department of Psychological Science at the University of North Carolina at Charlotte. He is also co-editor of the American Journal of Orthopsychiatry. His work has focused on children and families and (1) understanding factors influencing the development of children at risk for emotional, behavioral, and/or academic difficulties, particularly risk and resilience and youngsters' adjustment to trauma; and (2) using evaluation to refine programs, improve service delivery, support organizational development, and guide system change and local policy. His broader professional involvements include his prior service as president of the Global Alliance for Behavioral Health and Social Justice. He is a fellow of the Society for Community Research and Action and the American Psychological Association.

Eyal Klonover, PhD, is a lecturer of social work at the faculty of Ashkelon Academic College in Israel. His fields of interest are social psychology, couple and family studies. His research focuses on power relationships between spouses. He has been part of a research team examining the social aspects of trauma related to psycho-political models and has conducted research on the effects of trauma on Orthodox Jewish groups and the new post-millennial family structures. Dr. Klonover has taught diverse courses related to sociology, social psychology, and family life cycle and played an integral role in creating programs designed to connect the ultra-Orthodox community in Israel with the academic community encouraging their becoming more involved in academic life and more actively contributing members of general society.

Hatice Irem Ozteke Kozan, PhD, received her bachelor's and master's degrees in counseling psychology from Selcuk University and she earned her PhD in counseling psychology from Necmettin Erbakan University, Turkey. She worked as a research assistant at Necmettin Erbakan University during her graduate studies and conducted her PhD research at the University of Kansas. Dr. Ozteke-Kozan is currently an associate professor at Necmettin Erbakan University. She has a number of indexed and high-impact articles, books, and book chapters on the topic of close relationships and the foci of her research are adult attachment, post-traumatic growth, and close relationships.

Michael LaRocca, PhD, is a graduate of the United States Military Academy and a veteran of the U.S. Army. He earned a master's degree in psychology from Pepperdine University and a PhD in clinical psychology from the University of Alabama. A licensed clinical psychologist, he completed his clinical psychology internship at the VA Palo Alto Health Care System, followed by conducting psychological assessment and PTSD research at the War Related Illness & Injury Study Center as a part of a VA Palo Alto postdoctoral fellowship. Dr. LaRocca is interested in interpersonal influences such as leadership and social support, and how they may impact psychological well-being among veterans and other populations. His research interests also extend to positive psychology, including posttraumatic growth and its relation to other measures of well-being. Dr. LaRocca is an assistant professor at Virginia Military Institute, where he teaches a course on leadership. He draws from his prior experience as an army officer, as well as his training in psychology and leadership to contribute to the education and professional development of his students.

Clara López-Torres graduated in psychology from the University of Seville in 2010. After obtaining the qualification of General Health Psychologist, she specialized in social work at the National University of Distance Education in 2017. In her professional career, she focused on caring for refugees and the fight for their rights. Since 2013, she has been part of the team of the Spanish Commission for Refugee Aid (CEAR) where she worked in the Psychological Care Service and, since 2017, has managed a Refugee Reception Center where more than 130 people reside. In her work, she promotes the autonomy, dignity, and psychosocial well-being of refugees.

Sara M. Martínez-Damia is currently pursuing her PhD in Social and Community Psychology at the Catholic University of the Sacred Heart of Milan and the University of Seville. She is a member of the Center for Community Research and Action (CESPYD) at the University of Seville and of the Centre for Research in Community Development and Organizational Quality of Life (CERISVICO) at the University of Sacred Heart of Brescia. Her research interest revolves around the community participation carried out within migrant community-based organizations and its connections with subjective well-being, resilience, and empowerment. She is interested in building useful knowledge and developing projects with community partners to improve social justice and mental health for migrants, refugees, and underprivileged groups.

Allison Marziliano, PhD, is an assistant professor in the Center for Health Innovations and Outcomes Research, in the Feinstein Institutes for Medical Research, at Northwell Health. She obtained her doctorate degree in social and health psychology from Stony Brook University and has several years of experience conducting research on physically ill populations, including patients with or survivors of cancer. Her research interests include a focus on the social impact of physical illness or advanced age, how illness or advanced age affects relationships, and social isolation and loneliness.

Clare McFeely, PhD, is a lecturer in nursing and healthcare at the University of Glasgow, Scotland UK. Before moving to education Clare worked in health services, initially as a midwife and then in research and development roles, latterly focusing on the health service response to survivors of domestic abuse.

Divya Mehta, PhD, is an associate professor in the School of Biomedical Sciences at the Queensland University of Technology, Brisbane, Australia. Since being awarded her PhD in Human Genetics in 2009 from Technical University Munich, Germany, she has had an ever-rising research trajectory through highly prestigious research positions with world-renowned experts at the Max Planck Institute of Psychiatry, Germany, and the University of Queensland, Australia. A geneticist and biostatistician. Prof Mehta's research focuses on understanding why we all respond differently to stress and specifically how genetic and environmental factors interact together to drive the risk for mental health disorders in humans. She has published over 98 articles in international peer-reviewed journals, which have been cited over 9.8k times worldwide, and written 4 book chapters in the area of psychiatric genetics.

Anne Moyer, PhD, is a Professor of Social and Health Psychology in the Department of Psychology at Stony Brook University. Her research interests are in psychosocial issues surrounding cancer and cancer risk, medical decision-making, women's health, research methodology and meta-analysis, and the psychology of research participation. She is a graduate of McMaster University in Ontario Canada and she received her Master's Degree and her PhD in Social/Health Psychology from Yale University. Her current research includes studies of the effectiveness of interventions designed to improve the quality of life of individuals with cancer; the role of optimism in risk perception and treatment decisions and decision-making in veterinary medical contexts; how participant preferences interact with random assignment in clinical trials to affect engagement in treatment; examining the usefulness of including positive psychology exercises in college teaching; and, with systematic review and meta-analytic techniques, examining the relationship between post-traumatic stress and post-traumatic growth in cancer survivors.

Romina Nunes holds an MSc in Health Psychology from ISPA from the Instituto Universitario. She conducts research in the areas of PTG, stress, trauma, and psycho-oncology. She serves as a private clinical and health psychologist, responsible for group psychotherapy of health professionals in primary healthcare, and is a junior member of the Order Portuguese Psychologists.

Dumisani Ngwenya, PhD, is the co-founder and executive director of Grace to Heal, a peacebuilding and community healing organization in Zimbabwe. He sees himself as a peace practitioner first and an academic second. He has been involved in peacebuilding, conflict transformation, and community healing since 2003. His work involves working with the communities in Mathebeleland, which were affected by the 1980s atrocities perpetrated by the Zimbabwean government and left an estimated 20,000 civilians dead and countless others tortured and maimed. This work includes identifying and mapping the mass shallow graves, documenting victims' stories, and creating platforms for victims' families and survivors to confront their past. He has also been involved in peacebuilding efforts in communities torn by political violence. He lectures part-time at a local university and has been a visiting lecturer at the Centre for Peace and Conflict Studies in Cambodia. His current major project is the setting up of an Action Research based Master's program in the Applied Conflict Transformation Studies (ACTS), for peacebuilding and development practitioners in conjunction with the Catholic University of Zimbabwe. His research interests include trauma and memory, historic trauma, transgenerational transmission of trauma, and peacebuilding nexus.

Orit Nuttman-Shwartz, PhD, MSW, GA, is a professor at the School of Social Work at Sapir College in Israel. She was the founder and first head of the school and past chairperson of the Israel National Social Work Council. Her research deals with the effects of continuous and shared exposure to threats on individuals and communities, on clients and social workers. She has published more than 85 articles and book chapters. Nuttman-Shwartz was awarded the Katan Prize and the Israeli Parliament Award for Academic Scholarship in Social Work.

Colin O'Brien is a psychological researcher who holds a bachelor's degree in statistics from the University of Michigan and a master's degree in psychology from Oakland University. He currently serves as a project coordinator in Dr. Kelsie Forbush's Center for the Advancement of Research on Eating Behaviors (CARE lab), focusing on the assessment and diagnosis of eating disorders, where his main research interest lies in the development, maintenance, and treatment of Avoidant/Restrictive Food Intake Disorder (ARFID). He plans to pursue a PhD in clinical psychology.

Nina Ogińska-Bulik is a professor of psychology and the head of the Health Psychology Department at the Institute of Psychology at the University of Lodz, Poland. Her research focuses on posttraumatic stress disorder and posttraumatic growth and their relationship with the cognitive processing of trauma. She is the author of over 300 publications. She is also the author/co-author of many measurement tools used in the psychology of health and stress.

Marilyn (Lyn) Paul, PhD, LCSW, is a clinical associate professor at Adelphi University School of Social Work where she has held a faculty appointment since 2005. In her role at Adelphi, she teaches foundation and advanced year practice, human behavior, and various elective courses. While she largely teaches in the classroom, she has also taught online and in an intensive study-abroad format in Israel. Dr. Paul serves as a faculty field liaison, sits on school and university committees, and is on the Board of the New York State Social Work Education Association. Dr. Paul's research on families conceived with assisted reproductive technology, teaching social work practice along the micro-to-macro continuum, and online pedagogy has been presented throughout the country and published in peer-reviewed journals. Dr. Paul previously worked in hospital inpatient and outpatient settings, and currently maintains a private clinical social work practice in Manhattan, with a specialty practice in women's reproductive health.

Virginia Paloma, PhD, is the director of the Center for Community Research and Action (CESPYD, https://cespyd.es/en) at the University of Seville (US, Spain), where she is a professor of Community Psychology in the Department of Social Psychology. She is also the Coordinator of the US Master Program International Migrations, Health and Wellbeing: Models and Strategies for Intervention and Vice Dean for Community Outreach and Institutional Relations at the US Faculty of Psychology. Her research interests revolve around community participation, subjective well-being, posttraumatic growth, resilience, empowerment, liberation, social change, and social justice in the context of low-income migrants, refugees, and other unprivileged populations. She is committed to knowledge-building that is highly useful for the improvement of unprivileged groups' quality of life and the construction of a fairer society. She has participated in action-research projects where community partners are often allied and has published scientific articles about these issues in top international journals.

Catarina Ramos, PhD, is an assistant professor at the Egas Moniz University Institute and an integrated member of the Egas Moniz Psychology Laboratory, Egas Moniz Interdisciplinary Research Center, Egas Moniz School of Health & Science, Caparica, Portugal. She has been developing research in the areas of PTG, trauma, psycho-oncology, and group psychotherapy intervention for women with breast cancer. Dr. Ramos is a clinical and health psychologist at Clínica ISPA and a candidate member of the Portuguese Society of Existential Psychotherapy. She is responsible for the psychotherapy groups conducted by the Southern Regional Center of the Portuguese League against Cancer, Portugal.

Kenzie Rubens, BBehavSc (Honours), BSc, is a PhD student at the Stressomics Lab, School of Biomedical Sciences, QUT. Kenzie has a decade of counseling experience in the area of trauma from their previous career. Their main research interest is the impact of childhood maltreatment on the body, and how a history of childhood maltreatment influences posttrauma outcomes following adult exposure to trauma. During their honors research, Kenzie investigated the impact of childhood maltreatment on the epigenome and will continue this line of research through their PhD.

Beren Crim Sabuncu, MSW, is a doctoral student at Florida State University. She received her master's degree in clinical social work from New York University. Her research interests include trauma studies, health disparities, intimate partner violence and domestic violence, and queer issues. She has previous experience working with populations in crisis, including victims of sexual assault and violence, at Safe Horizon, Crisis Text Line, Tanzania Development Trust, and Dignified Children International. She works as a research assistant both at the College of Social Work and the Center for Population Sciences and Health Equity, at Florida State University. She is currently serving as the President of the Doctoral Student Organization in her program.

Leia Y. Saltzman, PhD, is an assistant professor in the School of Social Work at Tulane University. She completed her MSW and PhD in Social Work at Boston College. Her research focuses on disaster mental health, bereavement, and the physical health effects of trauma and loss. She is particularly interested in understanding the role of time in the process of coping with loss and trauma and the use of technology when working with trauma-affected communities.

Steven Schmidt, PhD, is an associate professor of psychology at Wilson College. He earned his doctorate degree in Human Development and Family Studies from the University of Connecticut in 2013 (dissertation: *Posttraumatic Growth Reported by Emerging Adults: A Multigroup Analysis of the Roles of Attachment, Support, Coping, and Life Satisfaction*). Dr. Schmidt's interest in psychology began when, following a diagnosis of chronic myelogenous leukemia in 1997 and a bone marrow transplant in 1999, he left his career in information technologies and returned to college. These experiences eventually fostered his research agenda which focuses on adjustment and quality of life in cancer survivors and on adjustment and growth following traumatic events in general from a developmental perspective across the lifespan. Dr. Schmidt is also interested in the development and maintenance of gender-role traits and behaviors and the resulting influence on health behaviors and well-being across the lifespan.

Emre Senol-Durak, PhD, is a faculty member at Bolu Abant Izzet Baysal University, Turkey. Clinical Psychology Program, since 2004. She completed her graduate studies in clinical psychology at the Department of Psychology at Middle East Technical University, a postdoctoral research fellowship at the Department of Psychology at the University of North Carolina at Charlotte (2014–2015), and served as a researcher at the Post-Traumatic Development Laboratory. In addition to her clinical practice and supervision in cognitive-behavioral psychotherapy, she developed psychosocial programs at the units of the Ministry of Justice General Directorate of Prisons and Adult Education (2000–2004) and provided forensic-clinical psychological examination and psychotherapy to the judicial, organized gang, and terrorist convicts, detainees, prison staff, and prisoner families. Since 2010, she is a member of a worldwide research group about internet addiction and problematic use and social networking site addiction. She authored many articles and book chapters about CBT, PTG, depression, anxiety disorders, internet addiction and problematic usage, and subjective well-being published in scientific journals worldwide. She has served as an editor and translator for locally and internationally published books and was the editor-in-chief of the *Journal of Aging and Long-Term Care* and the guest editor of *Frontiers in Psychology*.

Jane Shakespeare-Finch, PhD, is a professor in the School of Psychology and Counselling at Queensland University of Technology, Brisbane, Australia. For more than 25 years professor Shakespeare-Finch has studied trauma, its outcome, correlates, and predictors in a wide range of populations, including first responders and refugees, survivors of sexual assault, and natural disasters. Her research focuses on posttraumatic growth and on ways in which PTG may be facilitated and promoted. Jane works with industry and government in high-risk occupations establishing proactive and reactive interventions to promote mental health. Jane has published more than 130 peer-reviewed works and supervised more than 70 student theses to completion.

Abaraham B. (Rami) Shani, PhD, is a Professor emeritus, of organization development, change, and management, at the Orfalea College of Business, California Polytechnic State University. He also served as a research professor at the School of Management, Politecnico di Milano, Italy, Stockholm School of Economics, Sweden, and the Graduate School of Business, Tel Aviv University, Israel. For the past four decades, he worked with various organizations around the globe in addressing challenges and opportunities for development and change. He is the author, co-author, or co-editor of numerous books, articles, and book chapters; e.g., IDeaLs – Innovation and Design as Leadership: Transformation in the Digital Era (Emerald, 2021 with Press et al); Collaborative Inquiry for Organization Development and Change (Edgar, 2021 with Coghlan); Conducting Action Research (SAGE, 2018 with Coghlan); Learning By Design: Building Sustainable Organizations; (Blackwell, 2003 with Docherty); being the co-editor (with Noumair) of the annual research series Research in Organization Change and Development (Emerald Publications, 2008-present); co-editor of two 4 volume sets Fundamentals of Organization Development and Action Research in Business and Management (SAGE, 2010, 2016 with Coghlan); co-editor of Creating Sustainable Work Systems (Routledge, 2002, 2009 with Docherty et al); co-editor of The Handbook of Collaborative Management Research (SAGE, 2008 with Pasmore et al). His articles have appeared in numerous journals, including the Academy of Management Journal, Action Research, California Management Review, Human Relations, Human Resource Management, Journal of Applied Behavioral Science, Journal of Change Management, Organization Development Journal, Organization Development Review, Organizational Dynamics, Sloan Management Review, Systematic Practice and Action research. He received his PhD in organizational behavior from Case Western Reserve University.

Yael Shoval-Zuckerman, PhD, is a lecturer at Bar-Ilan University, Israel, and a supervisor for individual and group interventions (immediate, focused CBT, long-term dynamic, and

CBT groups). She has a rich clinical experience following many years at the Combat Reaction Unit in the IDF treating soldiers suffering from PTSD and in other trauma populations in different settings, including immediate interventions (group and personal) and treatments of chronic PTSD. In the last six years, she has been involved in the initiation of a unique clinic for conjoint intervention for couples (CBCT) in which one of them suffers from Post-Traumatic Stress Disorder. Her research focuses on assessing the efficacy of PTSD interventions including debriefing group interventions, CBCT, and mindfulness.

Zeynep Simsir Gokalp, PhD, received her bachelor's and master's degrees in guidance and psychological counseling from Necmettin Erbakan University, Turkey. Dr. Simsir Gökalp earned her doctoral degree at Necmettin Erbakan University in 2021, where she served as a research assistant at the Faculty of Eregli Education during her graduate studies. She is currently an assistant professor at Selcuk University, Faculty of Education. She has several indexed and high-impact articles, books, and book chapters on various topics. Her research foci include positive psychology, posttraumatic growth, and self-control/discipline.

Bożena Maria Sztonyk, MA in Political Science, MA, Lecturer at Orchard Hill College in London, UK, while undertaking psychotherapy training with the Viennese School of Existential Analysis and Logotherapy (GLE-UK). Bożena has worked in special education with students with vision impairments and learning difficulties in her homeland Poland, and internationally as a volunteer teacher at Notre Dame Secondary School in Papua New Guinea for three years, as well as in various educational and social care settings in Australia for five years. Upon returning to Europe, she undertook her MA in psychology in Rome, Italy, and is continuing her education in the practice of psychotherapy in existential analysis approaches and the study of grief therapy as meaning reconstruction with Portland Institute, US. She is interested in assisting clients suffering in the aftermath of various traumatic experiences and has a certificate in Stress Traumatic Studies with the Trauma Research Foundation, USA.

Kari Tabag is a licensed clinical social worker with experience in various roles including social work professor, field instructor and field liaison, school social worker, psychotherapist, clinical social work supervisor, college mental health counselor, director of wellness, and dean of student services. Kari received her MSW and PhD from Adelphi University School of Social Work, NY. Her community service extends to leadership and membership within mental health organizations and she founded an Affinity Group for Asian, Asian American, and Native Hawaiian Pacific Islander (AANHPI) social workers. She is an active advocate and reflectivist for racialized, marginalized, and oppressed communities in public and secondary educational settings promoting cultural humility in research, academia, and clinical practice. Kari has published articles and book chapters in scholarly venues, The New York Times, and The FilAm: A magazine for Filipino Americans in New York. Kari's presentations center on microaggressions in micro, mezzo, and macro settings, systemic racism, diversity, inclusion, and equity (DEI), and the promotion of social justice and advocacy among Asian and other racialized, marginalized, and oppressed communities. Kari's research examines experienced gendered racial microaggressions and psychological distress among Filipino American women and reinforces her positionality and agency as a second-generation Filipina/x/o American woman.

Kanako Taku, PhD, is a Professor of the Department of Psychology and the Director of the Free-Form Posttraumatic Growth (FF-PTG) lab at Oakland University, Michigan, where she mentors undergraduate and graduate students who study human experiences of transformative changes in emotions, personality traits, mood, social attitudes, and cognitive judgments. She has conducted a series of cross-national research on how people may change psychologically, cognitively, socially, and spiritually when they struggle with highly stressful life crises. She has authored numerous peer-reviewed articles and published books in both Japan and the US. Dr. Taku has been an editorial board member for the Journal of Loss and Trauma and Personality and Individual Differences. As a clinical psychologist certified in Japan, she has implemented psycho-educational programs focusing on PTG. She also serves as a board member of the Shelby Jane Seyburn Foundation.

Ye Tao is a postgraduate student from the East China University of Science and Technology. She has pursued her bachelor's in social work from Shangqiu Normal University. Currently, she is pursuing her Master's degree in social work. Her area of interest is social psychology.

Howard Tennen, PhD, is a University of Connecticut Board of Trustees Distinguished Professor. He received his doctorate in clinical psychology at the University of Massachusetts. From 1975–1978 he served on the faculty at the University at Albany-SUNY, and since 1978 he has been at the University of Connecticut School of Medicine in the Departments of Public Health Sciences and Psychiatry. Dr. Tennen is the editor of the Journal of Personality. He has received numerous teaching and research awards, including the Clifford M. Clarke Science Award from the National Arthritis Foundation and the Outstanding Contributions to Health Psychology Award from the American Psychological Association. He is a fellow of the American Psychological Association, Association for Psychological Science, Society for Personality Assessment, and The Society of Behavioral Medicine. His research examines stress, coping and adjustment to threatening encounters, the daily dynamics of chronic pain, stress, and alcohol use, and the application of daily process methods in clinical trials.

Olga Thomadaki, PhD, is a chartered counseling psychologist and associate fellow by the British Psychological Society and a licensed psychologist in Greece. She completed her bachelor's in psychology at Deree, The American College of Greece and she then moved to London and earned her MSc, Post-MSc, and a doctorate in counseling psychology at the City University of London with a specialty in trauma, bereavement, and positive psychology. She has worked as a counseling psychologist in various settings in UK and Greece. Currently, she is a privately practicing counseling psychologist and an assistant professor of Psychology at Deree, The American College of Greece, teaching mostly graduate courses in counseling and psychotherapy. Her research interests are qualitative methodologies, psychotherapy, and positive psychology. She has presented papers at various national and international conferences and has published in peer-reviewed journals.

Michal Toporek, PhD, is a clinical social worker specializing in trauma treatment and an adjunct faculty at Tulane University and Tel-Hai College in Israel. She practices in a private clinic and is currently doing her internship in Psychoanalytic Psychotherapy at Haifa University. Michal received her BSW and MSW degrees from Tel Aviv University and her PhD from Tulane University in New Orleans. Her research interests focus on secondary trauma, resilience, and growth among therapists and service providers. She is also interested in relational psychotherapy in trauma treatment and social work practice.

Marta Tremolada, PhD, is a researcher at the Department of Developmental and Social Psychology, University of Padua. She is a psychologist and psychotherapist responsible for the Psychological service at the Pediatric Hematology, Oncology, and Stem Cell Transplant Center, Department of Women and Child's Health, University of Padua. She teaches at the University of Padua Methods and Instruments for the Assessment of Development (School of Psychology), Education and Communication (School of Medicine), and Psychology and Pediatrics (Department of Neurosciences, Audiometric Techniques). Her research interests are principally developmental and social psychology, pediatric psychology, psycho-oncology, well-being, social networking, technology use in children, illness narratives, family functioning, psychological interventions, parenting, and developmental and psychological assessment. She wrote many articles on pediatric health psychology and developmental psychology, is an ad hoc referee for multiple international journals, and is involved in national and international collaborations.

Malwina Tuman, PhD, is a second-year postdoctoral research fellow in psycho-oncology in the Jennifer Hay and Jada Hamilton Genomics, Risk and Health Decision Making Laboratory within the Department of Psychiatry and Behavioral Sciences at Memorial Sloan Kettering Cancer Center (MSK) in New York City, New York. She received her PhD in Social and Health Psychology from Stony Brook University in 2020. Her primary line of research surrounds sociocultural, affective, and cognitive factors that influence how people make health decisions with the goal of leveraging this knowledge to improve behavioral health. Dr. Tuman's second line of research surrounds understanding how patient experiences with health programs, particularly those delivered using eHealth, relate to patient satisfaction, engagement, and program feasibility and efficacy.

Esther van Ginneken, PhD (Cantab), is an assistant professor in criminology at Leiden University, the Netherlands. Her research interests include the experience of imprisonment, prison conditions, and violence in prisons. Her research on posttraumatic growth was conducted as part of a qualitative study on psychological adjustment among adults incarcerated in England and Wales. She has also conducted survey-based research on prison climate and well-being among adults incarcerated in the Netherlands.

Lowri Wilkie (BSc) is a Psychology PhD candidate at Swansea University and assistant psychologist in a Community Neuro-rehabilitation Service within the National Health Service (NHS), where she supports people living with Acquired Brain Injury. Lowri's research involves developing and evaluating community-based interventions, which utilize principles of positive psychology, co-production, and task-shifting to promote well-being and social connectedness. Her research uses a wide range of methodologies, including physiological, qualitative, quantitative, and meta-analytical approaches. Lowri is also a mindfulness teacher and has several years' experience in delivering interventions, workshops, and coaching across a range of healthcare, corporate, and private settings. Lowri has contributed to the development of novel theoretical frameworks of health and well-being and has published several peer-reviewed articles and book chapters on the themes of positive psychology, well-being, post-traumatic growth, and neuro-rehabilitation.

David Witherington, PhD is an associate professor at the University of New Mexico. His empirical work focuses on perception-action, cognitive, and emotional development in infancy and early childhood. His conceptual work focuses on the metatheoretical foundations of developmental science and on delineating, elucidating, and resolving conceptual confusion in the discipline. His research has been published in journals such as Human Development, Developmental Psychology, Child Development, Developmental Review, Infancy, Emotion, and American Psychologist. He received his PhD from the University of California at Berkeley and his B.A. from the University of Iowa. He is also the current president of the Jean Piaget Society.

Ayten Zara, PhD, was born and raised in Turkey. She is a peace and human rights activist and a full-time faculty member at Istanbul Bilgi University, Department of Psychology. She is the founding president of the World Human Relief Association (www.worldhumanrelief.org), which works to improve the living conditions of families, children, and minorities who experience disadvantaged conditions in Africa, Asia, and Turkey. Dr. Zara is the director of the International Trauma Studies and Family Studies Certificate Programs in cooperation with World Human Relief, Istanbul Bilgi University, New York International Trauma Studies Institution, and the City College of the City University of New York. Dr. Zara participates in rights-based civil society activities domestically and internationally and consults efforts for preventing violence and building peace. She has published numerous articles on violence against children, family, and community, gives talks, and offers training to better understand and support people exposed to trauma. Dr. Zara has been working for many years with victims of domestic and sexual violence and their families in Turkey and East Africa and has conducted field studies to prevent collective violence, child sexual abuse, and marriages in Turkey, especially in rural areas.

Claudia Zavala is a mental health counseling student at Teachers College, Columbia University. She is originally from Peru, where she received her undergraduate degree in clinical psychology and completed her training in Gestalt Psychotherapy. With a long-standing passion for social justice and equity, she is committed to researching strengths in multiple marginalized groups (e.g., Latinx sexual and gender minorities) and non-conventional ways of living (e.g., ethical non-monogamy, childfree by choice, living in multiple places). In her private practice, she focuses on leveraging these strengths to promote growth and improve well-being. Claudia hopes to further the field of multicultural psychotherapy, expand community-centered research, and advocate for systems change so that all populations can have equitable access to mental health.

Michelle Zernick graduated from California State University, Long Beach with a bachelor's degree in psychology and American Sign Language. She spent much of her time at the undergraduate level working on projects that were part of an NIH-funded research program. She recently received her post-baccalaureate certificate from the University of California, Irvine where she focused her research on trauma, mindfulness, psychosis, and emotions related to psychological (dys)function. She aims to receive a PhD in clinical psychology, continue her research and teach at the university level.

PART 1

PTG

The Concept, Its Evolving, Components, and Relevant Dimensions of the PTG Model

1
THE GOAL, RATIONALE, AND ORGANIZATION OF THE BOOK

Roni Berger

Conceptualizing Posttraumatic Growth: The Concept, the Model, and Critique

The main tenet of posttraumatic growth (PTG) is the idea that exposure to and struggle with adversity can, in addition to negative outcomes, be a catalyst to changes that generate positive ones and sometimes radical transformation. Highly stressor circumstances that significantly challenge people's life have the potential to create an opportunity for growth, transformation, and thriving. This idea is as old as the Bible. The capacity for human resilience and actualization following the struggle with adversity has been acknowledged throughout history. It is incorporated in the world's major religions (e.g., Christianity, Buddhism, Judaism, Hinduism, and Islam), recognized by leading philosophers (e.g., Nietzsche and Schopenhauer), and in various cultural contexts. The philosophical concept of PTG is rooted in personal construct theory, schema theory, and assumptive world models (Tedeschi et al., 2018). Since the 1970s the idea of traumatic life events as catalysts for positive life change has been increasingly recognized and the fields of helping professions have witnessed mushrooming of studies, articles, books, and training that focus on understanding the nature, processes, and dimensions of PTG as well as offering strategies for facilitating it.

The Concept

The conceptual underpinnings of PTG appear in various disciplines including psychology, sociology, and philosophy, hence calling for an interdisciplinary approach. Multiple theoretical conceptualizations were offered for thinking about post-trauma positive outcomes. They include resilience (Garmezy, 1994; Luthar et al., 2000; Rutter, 2007; Werner & Smith, 1992), sense of coherence (Antonovsky, 1998), hardiness (Kobasa, 1979), ecological resilience (Ungar, 2013), positive psychological change (Aldwin, 1994; Calhoun & Tedeschi, 2006; Weiss & Berger, 2010), stress-related growth (Park et al., 2012), adversarial growth (Linley & Joseph, 2004), perceived benefits (Helgeson et al., 2006; Tennen et al., 1992), thriving (O'Leary & Ickovics, 1995), action-focused growth (Hobfoll et al., 2007), adversity activated development (Papadopoulos, 2007), and redemptive narratives (McAdams et al., 2001). These models employ diverse languages, offer different assumptions about the nature of

DOI: 10.4324/9781032208688-2

positive post-trauma outcomes, identify various mechanisms that generate such outcomes, correlates associated with them (O'Leary & Ickovics, 1995), broader environmental processes that shape them, and interventions to foster them. Many of these theories and models include varied combinations of similar elements (O'Leary et al., 1998). While earlier writers acknowledged that crisis can offer opportunities for transformational change (e.g., Caplan, 1964; Frankl, 1963), recognition of the positive nature of the change became dominant later.

A major development in the field materialized when in the mid-1990s, Tedeschi and Calhoun coined the concept of PTG, developed a model to describe positive cognitive, emotional, and potential behavioral transformations following the struggle with highly stressful events, and developed an instrument (the Posttraumatic Inventory, PTGI, which has several revisions) to measure it (Tedeschi & Calhoun, 1995, 1996). They emphasized that rather than the event itself, it is the struggle following the hardship that leads to PTG. PTG is an experience of improvement above and beyond mere survival, resistance to damage, adaptation, or recovery to the pre-stress baseline. Rather than a goal, PTG is a by-product of the attempt to cope with suffering, which in some people can be profound and significant; further, the pathways to PTG differ from the pathway to recovery from post-stress symptoms (Tedeschi et al., 2018).

The model was originally informed by the authors' experience with adults who had become physically handicapped and with older women who lost their spouses and has been evolving ever since. Concurrent with the advent of positive psychology in the early 2000s, the construct of PTG has been evolving and become increasingly influential in the trauma literature (Jayawickreme & Blackie, 2014). This is evidenced by the numerous citations (Tedeschi et al., 2017), studies informed by it, and translations and employment of the instrument (Weiss & Berger, 2010). A recent special issue of the *Journal of Personality* was dedicated to Post-Traumatic Growth as Positive Personality Change (Volume 89, Issue 1), and a capstone conference at Wake Forest University in 2019 focused on improving the quality of research on PTG.

The Model

PTG has been defined as both a process and an outcome of the attempt to cope with trauma and its aftermath and has been examined via multiple theoretical lenses. Dominant among those are a trauma perspective and a personality viewpoint. The basic components of the model include a potentially seismic event, resulting challenges and emotional distress, rumination, and growth. *The seismic event,* which is the precursor to PTG is disruptive, and can severely shake and threaten many of the schematic structures that have guided understanding, decision-making, and meaningfulness, unsettling people's core beliefs and shuttering their basic assumptions (also called schemas) about the self and the world (e.g., that the world is benevolent, just, and controllable). The seismic event may challenge, contradict, or nullify the way in which people make sense of life, why adverse circumstances happen, and the purpose and meaning of life (Shivali & Dilwar, 2018). The perceived threat that accompanies or follows the exposure is a trigger that creates cognitive and emotional *challenges* potentially causing *distress.* Processing these cognitive and emotional challenges and trying to make meaning of the traumatic experience can help disengage from the shattered assumptions. The process of a shift in core beliefs has been shown to be a catalyst for *rumination*, i.e., processing the traumatic experience and its consequences, which is a main precursor to PTG (Calhoun & Tedeschi, 2013). Rumination can be brooding, i.e., intrusive thoughts that are often automatic, undesired, or deliberate, constructive, and reflective (Matsui & Taku, 2016). Predominately intrusive and unintentional rumination relating to traumatic events is positively associated with distress and a failure to cope. When this type of rumination gives way to deliberate and contemplative rumination there is a potential for PTG to occur (Tedeschi et al., 2017). This process allows people to change their narrative, disengage from prior beliefs and assumptions, develop acceptance of the "changed" world and come to terms with the new reality while rebuilding new beliefs, goals, and identities that incorporate the trauma. The changed perspective may lead to reduced distress and eventually facilitate *growth*. The growth connotes the development of a new meaningful life narrative into which the traumatic event can be incorporated. Indications of PTG may include observable behavioral changes, cognitive elements, changes in personality, and more recently, biological changes (Tedeschi et al., 2018).

Support by people in the social environment who are good listeners, patient, accepting, and humble and who may serve as *expert companions* is critical in processing the trauma as it helps decrease the automatic rumination and consequently the emotional distress. Additionally, self-disclosure to trusted and empathetic others may help people derive meaning from the event and facilitate PTG (Tedeschi et al., 2017). It is important to remember that while PTG has been reported by a considerable number of traumatized people, it does not occur always and its absence does not indicate anything negative about the person. Further, negative trauma reactions and PTG are not mutually exclusive; rather they are two separate processes that can be seen as a double track and may coexist. However, typically, PTG, if it occurs, is reported later in the process of struggling and coping with the traumatizing stressor.

The idea of possible growth post-trauma has been supported by interdisciplinary literature. For example, there is an emerging body of research combining self-report approaches with technology for assessing neural mechanisms (e.g., EEG, MEG, and MRI), and producing evidence for PTG and its impact on cognitive functioning and physical health (Tedeschi et al., 2018). A few studies found a neural basis for psychological growth following adverse experiences. One study reported an association between left frontal brain activity and PTG in survivors of severe motor vehicle accidents (Robe et al., 2006). Another study reported in individuals with higher PTG stronger functional connectivity between brain areas that control memory and social functioning and suggested that they use more memory for mentalizing during their daily social interactions leading to better sociality (Fujisawa et al., 2015).

Applicability of the Model beyond Individuals

Theoretically, the scope of possible growth after trauma can extend to encompass families, communities, organizations, and entire cultural subgroups or societies, impacting collective processes in addition to individuals (Bloom, 1998; Calhoun & Tedeschi, 2006; Waller, 2001). Despite the recognition that human systems of any size may grow in the process of addressing stressful events, a significant part of the knowledge to date has focused on individuals. However, recent years have witnessed a growing body of knowledge about PTG of relational systems of all sizes. Berger and Weiss (2008) presented a conceptual analysis of expanding Calhoun and Tedeschi's model of PTG to the family system level. While originally the family was viewed mostly as providing a context for individual growth, later developments acknowledged the couple, family, organization, or community as the unit that grows.

PTG on the systems level includes changes in collective narratives, attributing meanings by community members to shared traumatic experiences in a process that mirrors schema reconstruction on the individual level (Calhoun & Tedeschi, 2006). Tedeschi and his colleagues (2017) suggested that "There may be a reciprocal relationship where individuals and larger social systems experience PTG by continually influencing each other through the exchange of narratives, reconsideration of social norms, and breaking apart of traditions" (pp. 145–146). However, with a few exceptions, most research to date focused on individuals and to a limited degree on couples. This research has consistently shown that if and when PTG occurs, it is typically later in the process and the journey to achieve it can be long. While there are those whose life change temporarily or permanently for the worse following traumatic exposure, many eventually thrive.

There has been increasing recognition that in addition to PTG in those directly exposed to traumatizing stressors, there is a possibility for vicarious PTG (VPTG) by affiliation. Family members, mental health practitioners, emergency workers, medical personnel, and others who have been in intense contact with survivors of trauma exposure who reported PTG, can experience positive outcomes and growth as a result of this interaction. Witnessing direct survivors overcome adversity can lead to a transformation in those associated with them. VPTG can be manifested in a more positive self-perception, better interpersonal relationships and self-care, higher ability to tolerate negative experiences (Killian et al., 2017).

Critique

The idea of PTG encountered some skepticism. Specifically, concerns were raised regarding the multiple definitions and what some view as limited clarity of the concept (Jayawickreme & Blackie, 2014) as well as regarding methodological issues in studying PTG (Jayawickreme et al., 2021). Most PTG research is cross-sectional and employs retrospective measures of self-reported growth, whereas longitudinal knowledge about PTG over time remains scarce, generating concerns regarding the scientific validity of the construct and ideas for improved methodologies to enhance the study of the phenomenon (Jayawickreme & Blackie, 2014; Tedeschi et al., 2017). "The questions of what posttraumatic growth actually is and what retrospective reports of posttraumatic growth reflect remain undefined and murky" (Jayawickreme & Blackie, 2014, p. 316).

Because it is based mostly (though not exclusively) on subjective reporting, questions have been raised if rather than real "authentic" change, PTG reflects self-deception, wishful thinking, social desirability resulting from the cultural narrative, inaccurate memory, a coping strategy or a positive illusion constructed by theorists, practitioners, and trauma victims. Critiques pointed to the possibility that reports of PTG may represent a self-enhancing cognitive bias optimism, an effort to protect the self against anxiety by creating a favorable self-image, and a desire to restore self-esteem and a sense of control in threatening situations rather than an actual "real" positive change and some have suggested that PTG should only be considered "real" if it involves positive personality change that can be supported by objective evidence (Christiansen et al., 2015; Ho, 2016; Hobfoll et al., 2007; Jayawickreme & Blackie, 2014).

Responding to this critique, studies documented observations of significant beneficial behavioral and psychological changes in those reporting PTG by individuals in their social network. For example, a study by Reynolds and colleagues (2022) has shown that a modest agreement exists between traumatized individuals and close others regarding overall levels of PTG. Additionally, there is evidence that PTG trajectories tend to remain stable over time and are associated with better long-term adjustment following trauma (Tedeschi et al., 2017). Nevertheless, multiple questions requiring further conceptual development and empirical research remain.

Research about PTG

A growing body of interdisciplinary and recently transdisciplinary empirical research offers support to the idea that positive changes may take place after potentially traumatic events (Sleijpen et al., 2016; Tedeschi et al., 2018). A considerable number of people from diverse cultures report viewing their traumatic exposure as an experience by which they were transformed and from which they gained benefits and grew (Weiss & Berger, 2010). While estimates of prevalence vary, probably as a result of methods used, PTG is widely reported with 70% of survivors of various forms of trauma conveying experiencing some positive change in at least one aspect of their life (Jayawickreme & Blackie, 2014). Further, reporting PTG has been found to be correlated with positive outcomes such as reduced revictimization following sexual assault, increased social affiliation and reduced avoidant coping with a diagnosis of breast cancer, better psychological well-being, and reduced distress following a diagnosis of cardiovascular disease, better self-reported physical health in HIV/AIDS and cancer patients, decreased suicide ideation in military personnel post-deployment and increased life satisfaction in a variety of samples (Tedeschi et al., 2017). Thus, PTG may be functioning as a buffer against negative outcomes of traumatic exposure. However, PTG does not and should not be expected to occur in everybody; thus, it may not occur at all or occur in some dimensions but not in others.

In addition to studying the phenomenon of PTG, research indicated multiple interventions as potentially enabling and fostering it. They include psychoeducation about trauma and diverse traditional trauma therapies such as exposure therapy, cognitive restructuring, stress management training, and couples' therapy (Roepke, 2015), as well as a community-based intervention that creates supportive community settings that adopt a mentorship and peer-based approach (Paloma et al., 2020). Such interventions help develop strategies to manage emotional distress and intrusive rumination and encourage written or spoken self-expression and disclosure, which create opportunities to reorganize and reconstruct the system of core beliefs and the life narrative (Berger, 2015; Calhoun & Tedeschi, 2013). Specifically, psychosocial group interventions have been documented as potentially increasing PTG by providing a supportive group environment that may enhance motivation toward growth, fostering emotional disclosure, providing opportunities to process a shared experience, and exposure to modeling behavior that can promote growth (Ramos et al., 2018). Thus, a meta-analysis of 12 studies concluded that group interventions fostered higher levels of PTG, irrespective of whether PTG was a goal of the intervention (Roepke, 2015). For example, participation in a group for cancer survivors promoted significant long-term PTG (Ochoa et al. 2017).

Research regarding PTG left some questions requiring further clarity and yielded some inconsistent findings. For example, the relationships between negative and positive outcomes of exposure to and struggle with traumatic events remain unclear. Some researchers found a significant positive relationship (Hall et al., 2010), others reported a negative relationship (Frazier et al., 2001), and yet others documented no relationship at all (Widows et al., 2005). Similarly, there is no consensus regarding the relationship between PTG and other indications of quality of life. Sleijpen and colleagues (2016) suggested that conflicting findings regarding PTG might imply that a curvilinear relationship exists between PTG and PTSD. A comprehensive review of empirical findings regarding changes in personality following adversity by Jayawickreme and colleagues (2020) provided a critique of current research about PTG, identified challenges and questions that researchers of PTG should consider, and recommended research practices for enhancing and improving it, possibly helping clarify some of the inconsistencies in findings. Specifically, longitudinal or prospective (rather than cross-sectional) research would allow the development of more nuanced knowledge about processes that allow PTG, mechanisms that enable and promote it, and interventions that are effective in fostering it in diverse population groups and contexts.

Correlates of PTG

Multiple factors shape the experience of and reactions to traumatic exposure, including the potential for growing from the struggle with it. Three main factors relate to the WHAT, the WHO, and the WHERE and WHEN of the traumatic event. The WHAT refers to the event that activates the trauma reaction and its nature. This includes whether the source is internal or external and is humane-made or nature made, if the event is developmental or circumstantial, its frequency (one time, recurrent or chronic), duration, valence, predictability, and intensity (Luhmann et al., 2020). "The more 'seismic' an experience is, the more one is caused to question fundamental assumptions and schemas regarding safety, predictability, identity, and meaning." (Calhoun & Tedeschi, 2013, p. 137). Additional relevant dimensions of the traumatic exposure are if it was direct, e.g., the person was actually where the road accident, earthquake, war, homophobic or racist attack occurred, or vicarious, i.e., the impact was generated via intensive affiliation with the direct victim because of family or social ties (e.g., a wife, child, parent, relative or friend of a wounded veteran) or professional role (e.g., therapist, medical personnel, or first responder).

The WHO connotes whether the exposure was by an individual, a couple, a family, a community, or an organization and what were the pre-trauma characteristics and history of those involved. Such characteristics include age, gender, personality traits (e.g., optimism, extraversion, bravery, self-efficacy, fortitude, mindfulness, emotion regulation, religiosity/spirituality, and perseverance), coping and attachment styles, and systemic structural aspects (Gleeson et al., 2021; Schmidt et al., 2019; Wu et al., 2019). For example, younger trauma survivors tend to experience greater PTG as do women, those employing problem (rather than emotion)-focused coping, persons with secure attachment, higher education, and more stable employment. However, these findings vary across types of traumatic exposure (Chan et al., 2016).

The WHERE and WHEN indicate the socio-political-cultural context within which the stressor event occurred including the availability and reception of and satisfaction with social support from different sources (e.g., partners, family members, friends), which is one of the most robust predictors of PTG (Schmidt et al., 2019; Tedeschi et al., 2017). While the universality of the phenomenon of PTG has been recognized and documented, its particular dimensions, meanings, manifestations, and impacts are culture-specific as societal values and narratives color coping with adversity. Both proximal (i.e., immediate primary formal and informal reference groups) and distal (i.e., the community and larger society) socio-cultural political context within which the trauma is experienced impact on whether PTG develops, if it is acceptable to report it and what are its nature, manifestations, and correlates. Consequently, the general experience of growth, its specific features, and predictors vary across cultures and sub-cultures. Later chapters in the book are dedicated to addressing each of these correlates in depth.

How This Book Was Developed

I was first introduced to the concept of PTG in the late 1990s and it had an immediate appeal to me because of its compatibility with my personal and professional tendency to see what IS rather than what IS NOT. I have been involved in researching, teaching, and training in the field domestically and internationally ever since. Thus, the idea of editing a book on PTG was a natural next step. There are multiple developments in the world that make the subject of PTG relevant, including pandemics, life-threatening illnesses, global military conflicts, wars, oppression, human rights abuses, and inequalities. The *Routledge International Handbook of Posttraumatic Growth* has been conceived during one of the most stressful times that the world has known in recent memory, which some described as a world on fire. "Traditional" (hurricanes, earthquakes, technical accidents) and climate-change-caused collective catastrophes (extreme floods, heat, fires, and nature imbalance) as well as the global health crisis due to the COVID-19 pandemic intersected with extensive socio-political protests in multiple countries such as demonstrations to fight racism in the US, speaking out against racial injustice and calling for systemic reform in Hong Kong, France, the Middle East, and other parts of the world increase the need for the multidisciplinary understanding of processes leading to human growth, agency, commitment, and positive developmental trajectories as well as salient and multiple underlying mechanisms enhancing PTG.

I was intrigued by the opportunity to collaborate globally with those who focus on understanding and facilitating PTG following the struggle with such traumatizing stressors. The goal was to make this book as current and as inclusive as possible and to provide readers with a comprehensive reference book that synthesizes cutting-edge knowledge about theoretical perspective, empirical findings, practice and policy implications as well as future directions. The book is intended to equip academics, researchers, postgraduates, and practitioners with the most current culturally-sensitive theoretical and practice knowledge regarding PTG. The knowledge would also be important to professionals in low-income societies, the UN, World Bank, and human rights organizations.

To create a handbook that "casts a broad net," I invited a diverse group of scholars, practitioners, and researchers from across the globe with different affiliations and scholarly foci and who are in different stages of their academic and professional journeys. This generated a choir that includes versatile voices about all aspects of PTG in relation to all types of traumatic exposure in all parts of the world. Contributors to this volume are diverse in multiple ways. They vary in their racial, ethnic, cultural, and personal backgrounds, they are different in their professional disciplines and the theoretical perspectives that guide their approaches to the topic, they are well-established renowned central figures in the field whose work is represented in the citations throughout the literature, mid-career, and emerging authors and they vary in their opinions regarding the construct of PTG. This diversity contributes to the creation of a tapestry that is rich, multifaceted, inclusive, and colorful in understanding PTG. This interdisciplinary collective effort produced a volume that reflects what we know about PTG of human systems big and small that include individuals, couples, families, communities, and organizations in the aftermath of various nature-made and human-made stressors, in different socio-cultural contexts, at all developmental stages.

To make sure that it reflects the state of the art of knowledge in the field of PTG, the book was developed from the ground up. Rather than prescribing specific PTG-related topics, scholars who have published or presented about PTG were contacted and invited to contribute chapters based on the work that they are currently doing or have recently done relative to PTG. This open approach generated a rich fabric of current conceptual, empirical, and clinical knowledge. Further, it allows providing access to content that is often not accessible to readers, especially those in the North-Western culture. For example, by relying heavily on non-English resources, Zara and Akbudak present and illustrate PTG in survivors of child, early, and forced marriages.

The Structure of the Book

This book includes chapters that reflect the aforementioned aspects of PTG and their impact on the probability and the nature of PTG as well as its outcomes. The first section introduces issues related to illusory versus constructive PTG, the role of gender, race, and ethnicity in PTG, and some of the critiques regarding the concept and directions for necessary future research. The following sections include chapters that analyze PTG through individual and relational lenses in those who are impacted directly or vicariously due to personal or professional relationships. For example, chapters are dedicated to direct PTG in various age groups and following different stressors as well as to vicarious PTG in those affiliated with them personally or professionally. Regarding the WHAT is PTG, authors discuss the process following the struggle with stressors such as life-threatening and chronic diseases, the COVID-19 pandemic, racial and sexual discrimination, war related-traumas, genocide, infertility, traumatic loss, parenting a child diagnosed with Autism Spectrum Disorder, domestic violence, earthquake, and other natural disasters. Relative to the WHO grows following the struggle with traumatic exposure, chapters address PTG in individuals as well as relational systems of all sizes including couples, families, communities, and organizations. Consistent with the theoretical conceptualizing of trauma and its impact on child development and resilience by life span developmental theories (e.g., Masten & Wright, 2010), authors discuss PTG in diverse stages of the developmental cycle, i.e., unique age-specific characteristics, processes, preconditions, and outcomes in different ages including childhood, youth, emerging adulthood, adults and older adults.

That the discussion of PTG occurs in various ages and in diverse cultural contexts, adds a dimension of intersectionality to the examination of the role of multi-dimensional positioning in PTG. From the WHERE and WHEN perspectives, cultural representativeness is reflected in three ways. First, by global authorship. Authors from Australia, Canada, China, England, Greece, Hong Kong, India, Israel, Japan, New Zealand, Poland, Scotland, South Africa, Turkey, the USA, and Zimbabwe wrote about PTG in their unique contexts. Second, a specific chapter is dedicated to understanding and illustrating how and why cultural scripts impact the conceptualization of PTG, its correlates, and strategies to enable/foster it. Finally, four chapters are focused on discussing PTG in diverse cultural contexts while understanding cultural aspects is embedded in additional chapters in various parts of the book.

Chapters also vary in their nature. Some emphasize conceptual issues related to PTG, others concentrate on research and reporting empirical findings, and yet others focus on practice and policy implications. For example, Whitney and Taku discuss PTG and illusory growth, Ogińska-Bulik and Juczyński highlight issues of measuring VPTG and present an innovative scale to asses it, Ai and Sabuncu provide a critical review of studies about PTG in cardiac patients and Paul presents a case example of PTG in the context of infertility. While they vary, all authors provide the reader with a rich picture and highlight aspects of PTG relevant to the population, context, and types of events based on contemporary theoretical, empirical, and practical knowledge regarding PTG.

The process of developing this volume was both a pleasure and an educational journey. While I thought that after two decades of researching, writing, teaching, and training on PTG, I know a lot, authors were able to expand my understanding and illuminate for me new and intriguing corners of the field and for this, I am humbled and extremely grateful. I hope that readers will find the book as informative, interesting, and helpful as I experienced while developing it.

Clusters and Gasps in the Current Knowledge about PTG

The structure of the book reflects the state of knowledge about PTG as well as the gaps in it. The process of mapping the knowledge and seeking to identify authors and the analysis of a recent comprehensive book by pillars in the field who summarized the theory, research, and practice implications of PTG (Tedeschi et al., 2018) revealed three major areas, which require further development. They are additional traumatic stressors, socio-cultural contexts, and effective interventions for enabling and fostering PTG. *Additional traumatic stressors.* In spite of a deliberate effort to identify and recruit chapters that are diverse and although PTG has increasingly been acknowledged, addressed, and studied, knowledge about PTG in relation to diverse stressors is uneven. Thus, a disproportionate body of currently available research about PTG is in relation to diseases and medical conditions (specifically cancer) whereas knowledge about PTG in immigrants, veterans, prison guards, survivors of rape, sexual assault, torture, and additional stressors is relatively skim and sometimes absent. *Socio-cultural context.* Most chapters were written by North Western authors whereas information about the conceptualization, meaning, applicability, characteristics, and correlates of PTG in other cultures is limited at best or totally absent. An intensive search for writers about PTG in Africa, South America, Eastern Europe, and the Arab world yielded a thin body of knowledge and a limited response to the invitation to contribute chapters. Knowledge about PTG in first nations people around the globe and in the context of different religions is also limited. Although the book includes chapters about the religious and spiritual aspects of PTG (Chapter 6) and about the importance of culture in PTG (Chapter 9), more specific knowledge in this field is very much needed. *Interventions.* Knowledge is relatively sparse regarding effective strategies for enabling and fostering PTG. The field could benefit greatly from more knowledge about micro and macro programs and policies designed to enable and possibly enhance PTG. To the degree that it exists, authors tend to discuss this topic within the context of addressing other issues rather than focusing exclusively on interventions. Thus, while Part 7 that addresses interventions for facilitating PTG may appear to be rather meager, content regarding effective strategies to enable and facilitate PTG as they apply to the particular respective traumas is interwoven in multiple chapters throughout the book. For example, in her chapter about perinatal bereavement, Thomadaki introduces and illustrates the expert companion; similarly, in his discussion of serving survivors of the Gukurahundi genocide in Matabeleland, Zimbabwe, Dumisani Maqeda Ngwenya explains and illustrates the application of the Tree of Life (TOL) workshop; Zara and Akbudak point to therapies that can help survivors change trauma-related negative schemas, Hussain and Bhushan discuss cognitive-emotional regulation strategies in facilitating growth in Tibetan refugees, and LaRocca discusses potentially effective interventions with veterans. However, to the degree that such content is addressed, it is mostly encapsulated in the discussion of PTG following specific traumatic experiences rather than independently. The aforementioned gaps in the existing knowledge as manifested in the chapters of the current book point to topics that require further development and suggest directions where scholars should focus future research.

References

Aldwin, C. M. (1994). *Stress, coping and development: An integrative perspective*. New York, NY: Guilford Press.

Antonovsky, A. (1998). The sense of coherence: An historical and future perspective. In H. I. McCubbin, E. A. Thompson, A. I. Thompson, & J. E. Fromer (Eds.), *Stress, coping, and health in families: Sense of coherence and resiliency* (pp. 3–21). Thousand Oaks, CA: Sage.

Berger, R. (2015). *Stress, trauma, and posttraumatic growth: Social context, environment, and identities*. New York, NY: Routledge.

Berger, R., & Weiss, T. (2008). The posttraumatic growth model: An expansion to the family system. *Traumatology*, *15*, 63–74. doi:10.1177/1534765608323499

Bloom, S. (1998). By the crowd they have been broken, by the crowd they shall be healed: The social transformation of trauma. In R. G. Tedeschi, C. L. Park, & L. G. Calhoun (Eds.), *Posttraumatic growth: Positive changes in the aftermath of crisis* (pp. 179–213). Mahwah, NJ: Lawrence Erlbaum.

Calhoun, L. G., & Tedeschi, R. G. (Eds.) (2006). *Handbook of posttraumatic growth: Research and practice*. Mahwah, NJ: Erlbaum.

Calhoun, L. G., & Tedeschi, R. G. (2013). *Posttraumatic growth in clinical practice*. New York, NY: Routledge.

Caplan, G. (1964). *Principles of preventive psychiatry*. New York, NY: Basic Books.

Chan, K. J., Young, M. Y., & Sharif, N. (2016). Well-being after trauma: A review of posttraumatic growth among refugees. *Canadian Psychology*, *57*(4), 291–299. doi: 10.1037/cap0000065

Christiansen, D. M., Iversen, T. N., Ambrosi, S. L., & Elklit, A. (2015). Posttraumatic growth: A *critical review of problems with the current measurement of the term*. In C. Martin, V. Preedy, & V. Patel (Eds.), *Comprehensive guide to post-traumatic stress disorder*. Cham: Springer. 10.1007/978-3-319-08613-2_5-1

Frankl, V. E. (1963). *Man's search for meaning: An introduction to logotherapy*. New York, NY: Pocket Books.

Frazier, P., Conlon, A., & Glaser, T. (2001). Positive and negative life changes following sexual assault. *Journal of Consulting and Clinical Psychology*, *69*(6), 1048–1055. doi: 10.1037//0022-006X.69.6.1048

Fujisawa, T. X., Jung, M., Kojima, M., Saito, D. N., Kosaka, H., & Tomoda, A. (2015). Neural basis of psychological growth following adverse experiences: A resting-state functional MRI study. *PLoS One*, *10*(8), e0136427. doi:10.1371/journal.pone.0136427

Garmezy, N. (1994). Reflections and commentary on risk, resilience, and development. In R. J. Haggerty, L. R. Sherrod, N. Garmezy, & M. Rutter (Eds.), *Stress, risk and resilience in children and adolescents: Processes, mechanisms and interventions*. New York.

Gleeson, A., Curran, D., Reeves, R., Dorahy, M. J., & Hanna, D. (2021). A meta-analytic review of the relationship between attachment styles and posttraumatic growth. *Journal of Clinical Psychology*, *77*(7), 1521–1536.

Hall, B. J., Hobfoll, S. E., Canetti, D., Johnson, R., Palmieri, P., & Galea, S. (2010). Exploring the association between posttraumatic growth and PTSD: A national study of Jews and Arabs during the 2006 Israeli-Hezbollah War. *Journal of Nervous and Mental Disease, 198*(3), 180–186. doi: 10.1097/NMD.0b013e3181d1411b

Helgeson, V. S., Reynolds, K. A., & Tomich, P. L. (2006). A meta-analytic review of benefit finding and growth. *Journal of Consulting and Clinical Psychology, 74*(5), 797–816. doi:10.1037/0022-006X.74.5.797

Ho, S. M. Y. (2016) Post-traumatic growth: Focus on concepts and cross-cultural measurement issues. In C. Martin, V. Preedy, & V. Patel (Eds.), *Comprehensive guide to post-traumatic stress disorders*. Cham: Springer.

Hobfoll, S. E., Hall, B. J., Canetti-Nisim, D., Galea, S., Johnson, R. J., & Palmieri, P. A. (2007). Refining our understanding of traumatic growth in the face of terrorism: Moving from meaning cognitions to doing what is meaningful. *Applied Psychology: An International Review, 56*(3), 345–366. doi:10.1111/j.1464-0597.2007.00292.x

Jayawickreme, E., & Blackie, L. E. (2014). Post-traumatic growth as positive personality change: Evidence, controversies and future directions. *European Journal of Personality, 28*(4), 312–331.

Jayawickreme, E., Infurna, F. J., Alajak, K., Blackie, L. E., Chopik, W. J., Chung, J. M., Dorfman, A., Fleeson, W., Forgeard, M. J. C., Frazier, P., Furr, R. M., Grossmann, I., Heller, A. S., Laceulle, O. M., Lucas, R. E., Luhmann, M., Luong, G., Meijer, L., McLean, K. C., Park, C. L., Roepke, A. M., al Sawaf, Z., Tennen, H., White, R. M. B., & Zonneveld, R. (2021). Post-traumatic growth as positive personality change: Challenges, opportunities, and recommendations. *Journal of Personality, 89*(1), 145–165.

Killian, K., Hernandez-Wolfe, P., Engstrom, D., & Gangsei, D. (2017). Development of the vicarious resilience scale (VRS): A measure of positive effects of working with trauma survivors. *Psychological Trauma: Theory, Research, Practice, and Policy, 9*(1), 23–31.

Kobasa, S. C. (1979). Stressful life events, personality and health: An inquiry into hardiness. *Journal of Personality and Social Psychology, 37*(1), 1–11.

Linley, P. A., & Joseph, S. (2004). Positive change following trauma and adversity. *Journal of Traumatic Stress, 17*, 11–21.

Luhmann, M., Fassbender, I., Alcock, M., & Haehner, P. (2020). A dimensional taxonomy of perceived characteristics of major life events. *Journal of Personality and Social Psychology*. doi:10.1 037/pspp0000291

Luthar, S. S., Cicchetti, D., & Becker, B. (2000). The construct of resilience: A critical evaluation and guidelines for future work. *Child Development, 71*(3), 543–562.g25.

Masten, A. S., & Wright, M. O'D. (2010). Resilience over the lifespan: Developmental perspectives on resistance, recovery, and transformation. In J. W. Reich, A. J. Zautra, & J. S. Hall (Eds.), *Handbook of adult resilience* (pp. 213–237). New York, NY: Guilford Press.

Matsui, T., & Taku, K. (2016). A review of posttraumatic growth and help-seeking behavior in cancer survivors: Effects of distal and proximate culture. *Japanese Psychological Research, 58*(1), 142–162.

McAdams, D. P., Reynolds, J., Lewis, M., Patten, A. H., & Bowman, P. J. (2001). When bad things turn good and good things turn bad: Sequences of redemption and contamination in life narrative and their relation to psychosocial adaptation in midlife adults and in students. *Personality and Social Psychology Bulletin, 27*(4), 474–485.

Ochoa, C., Casellas-Grau, A., Vives, J., Font, A., & Borràs, J. M. (2017). Positive psychotherapy for distressed cancer survivors: Posttraumatic growth facilitation reduces posttraumatic stress. *International Journal of Clinical and Health Psychology, 17*(1), 28–37. doi:10.1016/j.ijchp.201 6.09.002

O'Leary, V. E., Alday, C. S., & Ickovics, J. R. (1998). Models of life change and posttraumatic growth. In R. G. Tedeschi, C. L. Park, & L. G. Calhoun (Eds.), *Posttraumatic growth: Positive changes in the aftermath of crisis* (pp. 127–151). Mahwah, NJ: Lawrence Erlbaum Associates.

O'Leary , V. E., & Ickovics , J. R. (1995). Resilience and thriving in response to challenge: an opportunity for a paradigm shift in women's health. *Womens Health, 1*(2), 121–42. PMID: 9373376.

Paloma, V., de la Morena, I., & Clara López-Torres (2020). Promoting posttraumatic growth among the refugee population in Spain: A community-based pilot intervention. *Health & Social Care in the Community, 28*(1), 127–136.

Papadopoulos, R. K. (2007). Refugees, trauma and adversity-activated development. *European Journal of Psychology and Counselling*, *9*(3), 301–312.
Park, C. L., Riley, K. E., & Snyder, L. B. (2012). Meaning making coping, making sense, and posttraumatic growth following the 9/11 terrorist attacks. *Journal of Positive Psychology*, *7*(3), 198–207.
Rabe, S., Zöllner, T., Maercker, A., & Karl, A. (2006). Neural correlates of posttraumatic growth after severe motor vehicle accidents. *Journal of Consulting Clinical Psychology*, *74*(5), 880–886. doi:10.1037/0022-006X.74.5.880
Ramos, C., Costa, P. A., Rudnicki, T., Maroco, A. L., Leal, I., Guimaraes, R., Fougo, J. L., & Tedeschi, R. G. (2018). The effectiveness of a group intervention to facilitate posttraumatic growth among women with breast cancer. *Psycho Oncology*, *27*(1), 258–264.
Reynolds, C. J., Blackie, L. E. R., Furr, R. M., Demaske, A., Roepke, A. M., Forgeard, M., & Jayawickreme, E. (2022). Investigating corroboration of self-perceived posttraumatic growth among Sri Lankan Tamil survivors of ethnopolitical warfare through trait, domain, and profile agreement approaches. *Psychological Assessment*. doi:10.1037/pas0001172
Roepke, A. M. (2015). Psychosocial interventions and posttraumatic growth: A meta-analysis. *Journal of Consulting and Clinical Psychology*, *83*(1), 129–142. doi:10.1037/a0036872129.
Rutter, M. (2007). Resilience, competence, and coping. *Child Abuse & Neglect*, *31*(3), 205–209.
Schmidt, S. D., Blank, T. O., Bellizzi, K. M., & Park, C. L. (2019). Posttraumatic growth reported by emerging adults: A multigroup analysis of the roles of attachment, support, and coping. *Current Psychology*, *38*(5), 1225–1234.
Shivali, K., & Dilwar, H. (2018). Cross-cultural challenges to the construct "Posttraumatic Growth". *Journal of Loss & Trauma*, *23*(1), 51–69.
Sleijpen, M., Haagen, J., Mooren, T., & Kleber, R. (2016). Growing from experience: An exploratory study of posttraumatic growth in adolescent refugees. *European Journal of Psychotraumatology*, *7*(1), 28698. doi:10.3402/ejpt.v7.28698
Tedeschi, R. G., & Calhoun, L. G. (1995). *Trauma and transformation: Growing in the aftermath of suffering*. Thousand Oaks, CA: Sage.
Tedeschi, R. G., & Calhoun, L. G. (1996). The posttraumatic growth inventory: Measuring the positive legacy of trauma. *Journal of Traumatic Stress*, *9*(3), 455–471. doi:10.1007/BF02103658.
Tedeschi, R. G., Blevins, C. L., & Riffle, O. M. (2017). Posttraumatic growth: A brief history and evaluation. In M. A. Warren, & S. I. Donaldson (Eds.), *Scientific advances in positive psychology* (pp. 131–163). Praeger/ABC-CLIO.
Tedeschi, R. G., Shakespeare-Finch, J., Taku, K., & Calhoun, L. G. (2018). *Posttraumatic growth: Theory, research, and applications*. New York, NY: Routledge.
Tennen, H., Affleck, G., Urrows, S., Higgins, P., & Mendola, R. (1992). Perceiving control, construing benefits, and daily processes in rheumatoid arthritis. *Canadian Journal of Behavioural Science/Revue canadienne des sciences du comportement*, *24*(2), 186–203. doi:10.1037/h0078709
Ungar, M. (2013). Resilience, trauma, context, and culture. *Trauma, Violence, & Abuse* *14*(3), 255–266.
Waller, M. A. (2001). Resilience in ecosystemic context: Evolution of the concept. *American Journal of Orthopsychiatry*, *71*, 290–297.
Weiss, T., & Berger, R., Eds. (2010). *Posttraumatic growth and culturally competent practice: Lessons learned from around the globe*. Hoboken, NJ: Wiley.
Werner, E. E., & Smith, R. S. (1992). *Overcoming the odds: High risk children from birth to adulthood*. Ithaca, NY: Cornell University Press.
Widows, M. R., Jacobsen, P. B., Booth-Jones, M., & Fields, K. K. (2005). Predictors of posttraumatic growth following bone marrow transplantation for cancer. *Health Psychology*, *24*(3), 266–273. doi: 10.1037/0278-6133.24.3.266
Wu, X., Kaminga, A. C., Dai, W., Deng, J., Wang, Z., Pan, X., & Liu A. (2019). The prevalence of moderate-to-high posttraumatic growth: A systematic review and meta-analysis. *Journal of Affective Disorders*, *243*(15), 408–415. doi:10.1016/j.jad.2018.09.023

2

EPIGENETIC MARKERS OF POSTTRAUMATIC GROWTH

Kenzie Rubens, Jane Shakespeare-Finch, Divya Mehta, and Dagmar Bruenig

Why individuals differ in their response to trauma exposure has been a long-standing question. A pathogenic focus within molecular biology research has limited the scope of biomarker discovery in trauma research. With a recent move towards longitudinal and prospective research designs, new profound insights into the drivers of trauma exposure and subsequent health trajectories will provide a more holistic picture of posttraumatic outcomes.

The nature and severity of trauma exposure can result in different psychological outcomes, which is reflected in neurobiology. Varied changes in neuroendocrinology and gene activity have been associated with trauma exposure. This exposure releases chemicals, including cortisol and enhanced production of inflammatory cells, as part of the body's biological response to stress (McFarlane et al., 2011). These biological changes can indirectly influence the brain and cause both immediate and long-term changes to an individual's physical and mental health. The level of response is, in part, determined by the underlying genetics that informs the reactivity of the stress response (Gillespie et al., 2009).

Genetics

Human DNA is made up of over 30,000 genes. Each gene has multiple alleles, i.e., alternative forms that can alter the structure of the proteins that the gene produces. These alleles can be seen physically, such as in eye color, or have more subtle effects, such as the cortisol concentration required to self-regulate the biological stress response. Individuals typically carry two copies of a gene, one inherited from each of their biological parents, which are stable over their lifetime. The effect of trauma on the individual cannot be isolated from the impact of a single gene. Multiple gene pathways have been associated with posttraumatic outcomes, including the genes responsible for the body's inflammation response, stress response, and learning and memory. The genes responsible for regulating the Hypothalamic-Pituitary-Adrenal Axis (HPA axis) have been a primary focus of researchers in studies of genetics and trauma. The HPA axis is the neurological area responsible for the body's response to stress. When a threat is perceived in the environment, the hypothalamus signals the pituitary gland for hormonal activation throughout the body. Hormones travel from the pituitary to the

DOI: 10.4324/9781032208688-3

adrenal gland via the bloodstream. Upon activation, the adrenal glands produce cortisol, the primary mechanism by which the HPA axis activates the sympathetic nervous system and prepares the body to respond to environmental threats. Many genes are related to this process and modify the individual components, such as the production of the signaling hormones and the receptors for these signals. Different alleles of these genes can influence the likelihood of different posttraumatic outcomes (e.g., Bruenig et al., 2017). Due to their pleiotropic nature, most genes contribute only minutely to phenotypes with small effect sizes leading to the combined genetic variance in complex human traits.

As the effects of trauma are dynamic and varied across individuals, genetics alone does not sufficiently explain differences in posttraumatic outcomes. Hence, studies investigating how the environment and genes (gene-by-environment [GxE] studies) interact have shown promise in uncovering consequent health trajectories. The FK506 binding protein 5 (*FKBP5*) gene influences the sensitivity of receptors to cortisol within the body, resulting in higher levels of cortisol required for effect. Different alleles of the *FKBP5* gene interact with childhood trauma exposure to produce different levels of risk for the development of posttrauma outcomes such as Posttraumatic Stress Disorder (PTSD; Binder et al., 2008). The Regulator of G Protein Signaling 2 (*RGS2)* gene is responsible for protein signaling and has been implicated in anxiety disorders. In a study with African American survivors of Hurricane Katrina in New Orleans, the allele type of RGS2 interacted with the severity of trauma exposure during the hurricane to predict the level of posttraumatic growth (PTG) 9–18 months after the hurricane (Dunn et al., 2013).

Epigenetics

"Epi" is a Greek prefix meaning "on top of." Therefore, epigenetics is the study of chemical modifications to DNA in response to environmental factors. Epigenetic processes, such as DNA methylation (DNAm), acetylation, and histone modification, alter the accessibility of DNA without changing the underlying DNA sequence of genes. The modifications affect how the DNA is expressed and the level at which it is transcribed. As such, epigenetic processes can be conceptualized as a dimmer switch attached to our DNA where the good and bad experiences throughout our life change the amount by which each of our genes is turned on. DNAm is the most common and widely studied epigenetic process within trauma research (Klengel et al., 2014). The methylation process involves the addition of a methyl molecule to specific sites within the DNA. This addition alters the degree to which the gene at that site is expressed. GxE studies in traumatized populations have shown distinct DNAm changes in the *FKBP5* gene that lead to differences in how the DNA folds (Klengel et al., 2013). The difference in folding shape altered the access to the machinery that translates DNA into proteins. This led to a cascade of downstream effects in the protein encoded by FKBP5 and thousands of other stress-associated genes.

While DNAm is a powerful indicator of biological change, the epigenetic approach to studying trauma outcomes has been mired by a bias towards pathological consequences such as PTSD. Additionally, though positive and negative posttraumatic outcomes can co-occur (Shakespeare-Finch & Lurie-Beck, 2014), this has rarely been reflected in methylation data analysis (Mehta et al., 2020). An additional assessment of epigenetic change is the measurement of epigenetic aging. The epigenetic age is a statistical calculation of how environmental factors can impact biological processes for more rapid tissue degeneration than expected based on a person's chronological age. The implications of this observed disparity suggest that healthy aging is associated with the integrity of the methylome (Seale et al., 2022).

Paramedic Pilot Project

A pilot study broke ground by investigating the epigenetic changes associated with PTG within a cohort of first-year paramedicine students (Miller et al., 2020). The study was longitudinal with two timepoints. The first timepoint occurred in the first semester of the participants' studies. The second was 12 months later when the participants completed a 6-week practical placement in ambulances. At each timepoint, psychological and social data was assessed via self-report questionnaires, and saliva samples were collected for extraction of DNA to measure methylation. The psychosocial data included assessments of PTSD symptoms, resilience, giving and receiving social support, organizational belongingness, general feelings of stress, and PTG. Additionally, at timepoint 1, participants described traumatic event(s) they had before commencing their studies, assessing severity and associated level of distress. This allowed for control of potentially traumatic experiences outside of the experience in the workplace. At timepoint 2, participants were asked to describe traumatic experiences they may have had during the placement, with the accompanying assessment of severity and level of distress. The DNA from saliva samples was run on microarrays to generate genome-wide DNA methylation profiles across each individual.

A cross-sectional analysis of the data found that considering PTG, resilience, and PTSD symptom severity, each had distinct methylation profiles on the same HPA axis-related genes (Miller et al., 2020). An additional longitudinal analysis was conducted of the candidate genes Nuclear Receptor Subfamily 3 Group C Member (*NR3C1)* and *FKBP5* with respect to their influence on trauma outcomes. Results revealed that organizational belongingness and receiving social support from peers positively mediated the impact of traumatic experiences on the epigenome and mental health outcomes (Pierce, 2022). When assessing epigenetic aging, results suggested that organizational belongingness and receiving social support had moderating effects across the entire genome. The study's longitudinal design allowed for identifying cause-and-effect in the relationship between DNAm and trauma exposure. This was a world first, as no previous research had examined the association of PTG with DNAm in a longitudinal, prospective design.

Intergenerational Transmission of Trauma Exposure

Molecular research into posttraumatic outcomes has primarily focused on individual-level experiences. Events that affect entire cultural groups, such as genocides, may pose a different challenge. The trauma transcends a single incident and instead continuously challenges the position of the individual within their potentially dispersed community (Yehuda & Lehrner, 2018). The recent discovery that these culture-wide experiences are heritable intergenerationally opens a new field of investigation of the lasting biological imprint in following generations of trauma-exposed populations. Similar patterns of dysfunction in the HPA axis were identified in survivors of the Holocaust and their offspring (Yehuda, 1998). The addition of epigenetic methods has yielded further insight into how traumatic experiences are transmitted intergenerationally.

Differential DNAm at the *FKBP5* gene was found in another population of Holocaust survivors and their offspring (Yehuda et al., 2016). Research conducted with mothers from the Tutsi ethnic group who had been pregnant during the genocide and their offspring found similar profiles of DNAm in another gene related to the HPA axis: *NR3C1* (Perroud et al., 2014). These findings represent a potential biological mechanism by which the experience of trauma can be passed from one generation to the next, despite the subsequent generation having no exposure to the traumatizing event itself. These epigenetic markers have phenotypic effects that can affect offspring throughout their lifespan. A study investigating intergenerational transmission of methylation marks on sperm cells in veterans of the Vietnam War showed a significant association of DNAm with the mental health symptomology of the veterans' offspring (Mehta et al., 2019). These findings add to the growing body of evidence for the impact that individual and collective trauma can have on subsequent generations. While the bulk of this research has been conducted on the pathogenic outcomes of trauma, these discoveries also open the door for similar research on the transmission of PTG and resilience.

Considerations in Epigenetic Research

While epigenetics offers strong evidence for distinct physiological profiles between different posttrauma outcomes, there are limiting factors to consider when analyzing epigenetic research. Findings from studies examining DNAm can be difficult to compare as they draw the epigenetic sample from different biological tissues. Tissue from the brain is the most useful in trauma research that examines psychological factors, as this tissue is responsible for regulating the stress response and learning pathways. Extracting neural tissue for methylation analysis is not an option in research with living people, and the use of neural tissue is more common in studies employing post-mortem populations (e.g., Fujisawa et al., 2019; McGowan et al., 2008). However, methylation levels can vary between tissue types within the body, questioning the validity of research drawing methylation data from tissue outside the brain. Blood and saliva samples are commonly used in lieu of neural tissue due to ease of collection while presenting minimal risk to participants. Recent research has found that methylation sites from neural tissue were replicable in a blood sample (Logue et al., 2020), and a combination of saliva and buccal-epithelial cells (skin from the inside of the cheek) has the most significant correlation to brain tissue regarding methylation when assessed across the genome (Braun et al., 2019) and are suitable to use in investigating methylation levels in the context of posttrauma outcomes.

Epigenetic mechanisms are dynamic. Just as traumatic experiences can result in epigenetic modifications that result in worse health outcomes, therapeutic and prosocial experiences can be restorative. With much of the epigenetic research on posttrauma outcomes conducted on clinical populations, the effect of therapeutic and pharmaceutical interventions on DNAm cannot be completely disentangled from the effect of trauma. Contemporary studies employ prospective research designs in non-clinical populations to highlight the methylation markers specifically associated with trauma exposure. Additionally, pharmaceuticals are undergoing development that specifically targets the process of DNAm and prevents or reverses methylation at targeted genes (Karsli-Ceppioglu, 2016). These pharmaceuticals, termed DNMT Inhibitors, have successfully been used to treat schizophrenia (Kundakovic et al., 2007) and have shown promising results in animal studies on treating stress-induced DNAm (Sales et al., 2011). A holistic understanding of the epigenetic mechanisms that underlie the posttraumatic response would allow for the development of more intervention strategies from various approaches.

Conclusion

Novel projects extending the longitudinal prospective design used in the paramedic student study described above are underway. Employing more robust assessments of relevant psychosocial factors, expanding the sample size, and drawing participants from professional populations that face a heightened risk of trauma exposure could deepen the epigenetic insights provided by research in the trauma field. Knowledge of which psychological interventions are effective at a biological level can inform treatment for individuals. Finally, as was demonstrated in the paramedic pilot study, epigenetic research can identify protective psychosocial factors to promote positive mental health at the organizational level (Mehta et al., 2022). The esoteric benefit of epigenetic research in the trauma field is that DNAm is biological evidence in support of a theoretical model that had previously been derived from clinical practice and observation.

Acknowledgment

The authors acknowledge that Kenzie Rubens, Divya Mehta, and Dagmar Bruenig are funded by a grant from the National Health and Medical Research Council (#20045360).

References

Binder, E. B., Bradley, R. G., Liu, W., Epstein, M. P., Deveau, T. C., Mercer, K. B., Tang, Y., Gillespie, C. F., Heim, C. M., & Nemeroff, C. B. (2008). Association of FKBP5 polymorphisms and childhood abuse with risk of posttraumatic stress disorder symptoms in adults. *JAMA*, *299*(11), 1291–1305. doi:10.1001/jama.299.11.1291

Braun, P. R., Han, S., Hing, B., Nagahama, Y., Gaul, L. N., Heinzman, J. T., Grossbach A. J., Close, L., Dlouhy, B. J., HowardIII, M. A., Kawasaki, H., Potash, J. B., & Shinozaki, G. (2019). Genome-wide DNA methylation comparison between live human brain and peripheral tissues within individuals. *Translational Psychiatry*, *9*(1), 1–10. doi:10.1038/s41398-019-0376-y

Bruenig, D., Mehta, D., Morris, C. P., Harvey, W., Lawford, B., Young, R. M., & Voisey, J. (2017). Genetic and serum biomarker evidence for a relationship between TNF[alpha] and PTSD in Vietnam war combat veterans. *Comprehensive Psychiatry*, *74*, 125–133. doi:10.1016/j.comppsych.2017.01.015

Dunn, E. C., Solovieff, N., Lowe, S. R., Gallagher, P. J., Chaponis, J., Rosand, J., Koenen, K. C., Waters, M. C., Rhodes, J. E., & Smoller, J. W. (2013). Interaction between genetic variants and exposure to Hurricane Katrina on post-traumatic stress and post-traumatic growth: A prospective analysis of low income adults. *Journal of Affective Disorders*, *152-154*, 243–249. doi:10.1016/j.jad.2013.09.018

Fujisawa, T. X., Nishitani, S., Takiguchi, S., Shimada, K., Smith, A. K., & Tomoda, A. (2019). Oxytocin receptor DNA methylation and alterations of brain volumes in maltreated children. *Neuropsychopharmacology*, *44*(12), 2045–2053. doi:10.1038/s41386-019-0414-8

Gillespie, C. F., Phifer, J., Bradley, B., & Ressler, K. J. (2009). Risk and resilience: Genetic and environmental influences on development of the stress response. *Depression and Anxiety*, *26*(11), 984–992.

Karsli-Ceppioglu, S. (2016). Epigenetic mechanisms in psychiatric diseases and epigenetic therapy. *Drug Development Research*, *77*(7), 407–413.

Klengel, T., Mehta, D., Anacker, C., Rex-Haffner, M., Pruessner, J. C., Pariante, C. M., Pace, T. W., Mercer, K. B., Mayberg, H. S., & Bradley, B. (2013). Allele-specific FKBP5 DNA demethylation mediates gene–childhood trauma interactions. *Nature Neuroscience*, *16*(1), 33–41.

Klengel, T., Pape, J., Binder, E. B., & Mehta, D. (2014). The role of DNA methylation in stress-related psychiatric disorders. *Neuropharmacology*, *80*, 115–132. doi:10.1016/j.neuropharm.2014.01.013

Kundakovic, M., Chen, Y., Costa, E., & Grayson, D. R. (2007). DNA methyltransferase inhibitors coordinately induce expression of the human reelin and glutamic acid decarboxylase 67 genes. *Molecular Pharmacology*, *71*(3), 644–653. doi:10.1124/mol.106.030635

Logue, M. W., Miller, M. W., Wolf, E. J., Huber, B. R., Morrison, F. G., Zhou, Z., & Verfaellie, M. (2020). An epigenome-wide association study of posttraumatic stress disorder in US veterans implicates several new DNA methylation loci. *Clinical Epigenetics*, *12*(1), 46–46. doi:10.1186/s13148-020-0820-0

McFarlane, A. C., Barton, C. A., Yehuda, R., & Wittert, G. (2011). Cortisol response to acute trauma and risk of posttraumatic stress disorder. *Psychoneuroendocrinology*, *36*(5), 720–727.

McGowan, P. O., Sasaki, A., Huang, T. C., Unterberger, A., Suderman, M., Ernst, C., Meaney, M. J., Turecki, G., & Szyf, M. (2008). Promoter-wide hypermethylation of the ribosomal RNA gene promoter in the suicide brain. *PLoS One*, *3*(5), e2085.

Mehta, D., Bruenig, D., Pierce, J., Sathyanarayanan, A., Stringfellow, R., Miller, O., Mullens, A. B., & Shakespeare-Finch, J. (2022). Recalibrating the epigenetic clock after exposure to trauma: The role of risk and protective psychosocial factors. *Journal of Psychiatric Research*, *149*, 374–381. doi:10.1016/j.jpsychires.2021.11.026. Epub 2021 Nov 19. PMID: 34823878.

Mehta, D., Miller, O., Bruenig, D., David, G., & Shakespeare-Finch, J. (2020). A systematic review of DNA methylation and gene expression studies in posttraumatic stress disorder, posttraumatic growth, and resilience. *Journal of Traumatic Stress*, *33*(2), 171–180.

Mehta, D., Pelzer, E. S., Bruenig, D., Lawford, B., McLeay, S., Morris, C. P., Gibson, J. N., Young, R. M., Voisey, J., & Harvey, W. (2019). DNA methylation from germline cells in veterans with PTSD. *Journal of Psychiatric Research*, *116*, 42–50.

Miller, O., Shakespeare-Finch, J., Bruenig, D., & Mehta, D. (2020). DNA methylation of NR3C1 and FKBP5 is associated with posttraumatic stress disorder, posttraumatic growth, and resilience. *Psychological Trauma: Theory, Research, Practice, and Policy*, *12*(7), 750–755. doi:10.1037/tra0000574

Perroud, N., Rutembesa, E., Paoloni-Giacobino, A., Mutabaruka, J., Mutesa, L., Stenz, L., Malafosse, A., & Karege, F. (2014). The Tutsi genocide and transgenerational transmission of maternal stress: Epigenetics and biology of the HPA axis. *The World Journal of Biological Psychiatry*, *15*(4), 334–345. doi:10.3109/15622975.2013.866693. Epub 2014 Apr 1. PMID: 24690014

Pierce, J. (2022). *The moderating effect of social support and belongingness on the interaction of trauma, DNA expression, and trauma outcomes: A longitudinal study* [Unpublished Master's Thesis]. Brisbane, Australia: Queensland University of Technology.

Sales, A. J., Biojone, C., Terceti, M. S., Guimarães, F. S., Gomes, M. V., & Joca, S. R. (2011). The antidepressant-like effect induced by systemic and intra-hippocampal administration of DNA methylation inhibitors. *British Journal of Pharmacology*, *164*(6), 1711–1721. doi:10.1111/j.1476-5381.2011.01489.x

Seale, K., Horvath, S., Teschendorff, A. M., Eynon, N., & Voisin, S. (2022). Making sense of the ageing methylome. *Nature Reviews Genetics*, 1–21. doi:10.1038/s41576-022-00477-6

Shakespeare-Finch, J., & Lurie-Beck, J. (2014). A meta-analytic clarification of the relationship between posttraumatic growth and symptoms of posttraumatic distress disorder. *Journal of Anxiety Disorders*, *28*(2), 223–229. doi:10.1016/j.janxdis.2013.10.005

Yehuda, R. (1998). Psychoneuroendocrinology of post-traumatic stress disorder. *Psychiatric Clinics of North America*, *21*(2), 359–379. doi:10.1016/s0193-953x(05)70010-1

Yehuda, R., Daskalakis, N. P., Bierer, L. M., Bader, H. N., Klengel, T., Holsboer, F., & Binder, E. B. (2016). Holocaust exposure induced intergenerational effects on FKBP5 methylation. *Biological Psychiatry*, *80*(5), 372–380. doi:10.1016/j.biopsych.2015.08.005

Yehuda, R., & Lehrner, A. (2018). Intergenerational transmission of trauma effects: Putative role of epigenetic mechanisms. *World Psychiatry*, *17*(3), 243–257. doi:10.1002/wps.20568

3

ILLUSORY VERSUS CONSTRUCTIVE POSTTRAUMATIC GROWTH IN CANCER

Samuel M.Y. Ho and Chih-Tao Cheng

In clinical settings, it has been well-known that many cancer survivors report positive changes following their disease experience and that posttraumatic growth (PTG) (Tedeschi & Calhoun, 2004; Tedeschi et al., 1998a, 1998b) is a common phenomenon in oncology. Evidence shows that more than half of breast cancer survivors reported PTG (Collins et al., 1990) and that PTG is even more common than posttraumatic stress disorder (PTSD) in oncology. A systematic review of 24 studies conducted among breast cancer survivors found that most participants reported PTG, whereas only a minority exhibited PTSD (Koutrouli et al., 2012). Thus, both anecdotal clinical experience and systematic research findings show that PTG is a common experience reported by patients with cancer making it indispensable to investigate the phenomenon of PTG among cancer patients to inform clinical practices.

In their original account, Ho and Bai (2010) reported that cancer survivors could exhibit four dimensions of PTG: Self, Interpersonal, Spiritual, and Intrapersonal. These dimensions echo the dimensions of PTG proposed by Tedeschi, Calhoun, and their colleagues in the USA (Tedeschi & Calhoun, 1996; Tedeschi et al., 1998b). Similar dimensions were reported in studies conducted among other populations, such as bereaved individuals (Epel et al., 1998; Lehman et al., 1993). The authors argued that there are universal dimensions of PTG shared among people in different cultures and types of traumatic events (Ho & Bai, 2010). The authors later proposed that cancer survivors who have an optimistic explanatory style, i.e., explain positive events as internal, stable, and global, are more inclined to exhibit PTG (Ho et al., 2011). This chapter builds on research conducted during the last decade to examine further constructive versus illusory PTG and PTG versus posttraumatic depreciation (PTD) in cancer patients.

Constructive versus Illusory PTG

PTG as a common phenomenon in oncology settings is an undeniable fact. Whether PTG represents an adaptive adjustment to cancer is a different question and must be subject to careful investigation. Studies among breast cancer patients have reported a non-significant

DOI: 10.4324/9781032208688-4

relationship between PTG and PTSD symptoms (Chan et al., 2011; Cordova et al., 2001). A more recent critical review of 72 PTG studies on cancer patients concluded that no consistent relationship exists between PTG and psychiatric symptoms (Casellas-Grau et al., 2017). These findings suggest that there may be different types of PTG. Some PTG types are related to adaptive outcomes, whereas others may have no or even negative relationships with adaptive psychological adjustment.

One of the most famous models to delineate the above proposition is the Janus-face model of PTG proposed by Zoellner and Maercker (Maercker & Zoellner, 2004; Zoellner & Maercker, 2006). According to this model, PTG consists of two components: constructive PTG and illusory PTG. *Constructive PTG* represents a real and positive transformation, relating to good psychological adjustments; *Illusory PTG* represents a mechanism adopted by an individual for coping with the traumatic experience and does not represent genuine positive changes, and its beneficial effect, if any, is short-lived (Ho, 2016; Pat-Horenczyk et al., 2016).

Almost at the same time when Ho and Bai (2010) were preparing their report on PTG, Cheng and colleagues (2018) started a seven-year longitudinal study to investigate different types of PTG among breast cancer survivors. The study was conducted at the Koo Foundation Sun Yat-Sen Cancer Center (KFSYSC) in Taipei, Taiwan's only specialty cancer hospital at that time. Eighty-four breast cancer survivors completed the Chinese Posttraumatic Growth Inventory (CPTGI) (Ho et al., 2013) and other inventories, including the Mini Mental Adjustment to Cancer Scale (Mini-MAC) (Ho et al., 2003; Watson et al., 1988), three times over seven years in 2009, 2012, and 2016. Latent class growth analysis (LCGA) on the CPTGI Total score revealed three types of PTG.

Constructive PTG

Cancer survivors with this PTG pattern tend to report a high level of PTG and use less maladaptive coping mechanisms.

Illusory PTG

Cancer survivors with this PTG pattern tend to report a high level of PTG but exhibit more maladaptive coping mechanisms.

Distressed PTG

Cancer survivors with this PTG pattern report a low level of PTG and use more maladaptive coping mechanisms.

The research team conducted a follow-up study on the 10th Anniversary of the commencement of the above project and assessed the same group of breast cancer survivors again in 2019 (Cheng et al., 2020). Consistent with their hypothesis, breast cancer survivors with an illusory PTG trajectory in 2016 exhibited more anxiety and depressive symptoms and more maladaptive mechanisms (hopelessness/helplessness and anxious preoccupation) in 2019 than those with a constructive PTG trajectory. The Distressed PTG group was excluded from the analysis because of the small number of individuals with this pattern. Hence, Illusory PTG may represent an individual attempt to cope with post-cancer adjustment by creating a positive illusion of the experience whereas Constructive PTG shows a genuine positive transformation of an individual after the diagnosis and treatment of cancer.

Posttraumatic Growth versus Posttraumatic Depreciation

While many cancer survivors report PTG, only a minority of them exhibit PTSD (Koutrouli et al., 2012). Since PTSD is a psychiatric disorder, whereas PTG is a subjective report of personal experience, it is not surprising that the prevalence of PTG is higher than that of PTSD. Thus, it should be more meaningful to compare self-reported positive changes with self-reported negative changes to better understand the phenomenological world of cancer survivors. Baker et al. (2008) attempted to address the issue by adding 21 negatively worded items to the original 21-item PTGI (Tedeschi & Calhoun, 1996) to represent negative changes and called the negatively worded items posttraumatic depreciation (PTD) items. For example, "I am more likely to try to change things that need changing (a growth item)" versus "I am less likely to try to change things that need changing (a depreciation item)." The growth and depreciation items are presented in pairs to encourage the participants to consider both types of change, i.e., growth and depreciation, at the same time (Cann et al., 2010). Later, Taku et al. (2020) added four spiritual–existential change (SEC) items to Baker's et al. (2008) aforementioned inventory and developed a 50-item (25 growth items and 25 paired depreciation items) Posttraumatic Growth and Depreciation Inventory - Expanded version (PTGDI-X). Taku and colleagues (2020) then administered the PTGDI-X to heterogeneous samples consisting of undergraduate students, firefighters, community adults, and others from 10 countries. Results showed that PTG scores were higher than PTD scores in all countries. Moreover, PTD had a positive correlation with PTSD symptoms in all countries, but the relationship between PTG and PTSD symptoms was inconsistent across countries; no correlation was reported in five countries, while in the other five countries, a curvilinear correlation was reported.

In 2020, Ho et al. (2021) translated the English version of PTGDI-X into Chinese and administered it to 265 cancer survivors who had completed their treatment at the Koo Foundation Sun Yat-Sen Cancer Center in Taiwan, together with the Chinese version of the PTSD Checklist for DSM-5 (PCL-5) (Fung et al., 2019). The results showed that PTG and PTD have five parallel domains similar to the original PTGI. These five domains are shown in Table 3.1.

Ho et al.'s (2021) study further yielded several key findings. First, in corroboration of the results of other studies (Baker et al., 2008; Cann et al., 2010; Taku et al., 2020), all five domains of PTG scores were significantly higher than the corresponding PTD scores. It seems that cancer survivors, on average, experience more positive changes than negative changes related to their illness experience. Second, a significant positive correlation was observed between the PTD total scores and PTSD symptoms. Consistent with the cognitive model, negative (and distorted) appraisals are always related to higher distress among cancer patients (Moorey & Greer, 2012). Third, more PTG was related to more PTSD symptoms until it reached a threshold, and beyond this level, more PTG was related to fewer PTSD symptoms (Figure 3.1). The same inverted U-shape relationship occurred in a previous meta-analysis of 42 studies (Shakespeare-Finch & Lurie-Beck, 2013). Finally, PTG and PTD show a similar inverted U-shape relationship as above, i.e., more

Table 3.1 Domains of Posttraumatic Growth and Posttraumatic Depreciation in Cancer

Posttraumatic Growth	*Posttraumatic Depreciation*
Relating to Others – positive changes in the quality of relationships after a cancer diagnosis	*Relating to Others* – negative changes in the quality of relationships after a cancer diagnosis
New Possibility – more effort to find a new path in life after a cancer diagnosis	*New Possibility* – less effort to find a new path in life after a cancer diagnosis
Personal Strength – an increase in the sense of self-reliance or strength after a cancer diagnosis	*Personal Strength* – a decrease in the sense of self-reliance or strength after a cancer diagnosis
Spiritual and Existential Changes – positive spiritual and existential changes after a cancer diagnosis	*Spiritual and Existential Changes* – negative spiritual and existential changes after a cancer diagnosis
Appreciation of Life – an increased understanding of the meaning and priority of life after a cancer diagnosis	*Appreciation of Life* – a decreased understanding of the meaning and priority of life after a cancer diagnosis

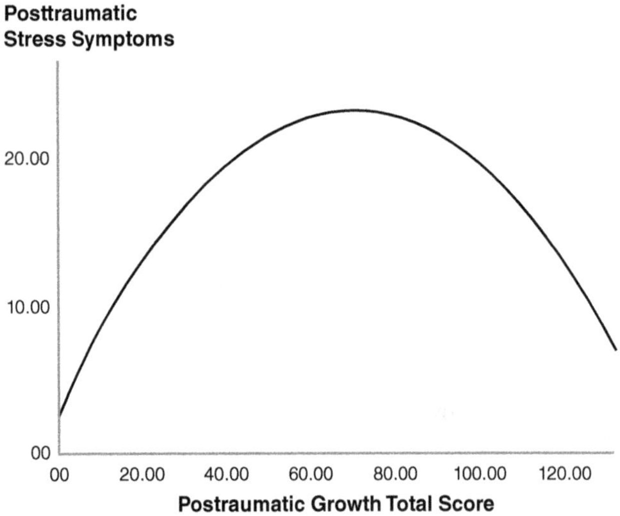

Figure 3.1 Posttraumatic stress symptoms as a function of posttraumatic growth.

self-perceived positive change will lead to less post-cancer depreciation appraisal only among cancer survivors with a high level of PTG.

The above relationships could be explained by the model of PTG proposed by Calhoun and Tedeschi (2012). The researchers argue that a traumatic encounter challenges one's existing assumptive world, and an individual must conduct deliberate cognitive processing to rebuild it before PTG can occur (Henson et al., 2021). Cancer survivors would discover both PTG and PTD in the cognitive processing stage. More cognitive processing would probably lead them to recall more PTG and PTD experiences. If the level of PTG is not sufficient to offset the effect of PTD, more PTSD may result (i.e., the linear relationship between PTD and PTSD mentioned above). Above a certain PTG level, when the discovery of PTG outweighs the effect of PTD, less PTSD may result, and the individual would pay less attention to the PTD experience. This situation may be similar to house cleaning. When we start tidying up our house, we discover both trashed and valuable items. When the valuable items cannot offset the trashed items, we feel distressed whereas if we find more valuable articles, we would pay less attention to the trashed items and have a more positive feeling.

Practice Implications for Cancer Care

Several clinical implications can be derived from the above studies. First, some cancer patients may adopt an illusory pattern of PTG to cope with the disease. These patients should be distinguished from those exhibiting a constructive pattern of PTG. Coping should inform whether the PTG experiences reported by patients are illusory or constructive. Those with an adaptive coping mechanism are more likely to exhibit a constructive PTG pattern whereas PTG experienced by patients with a maladaptive coping mechanism (e.g., hopelessness–helplessness) is more likely to be illusory. Table 3.2 summarizes the coping characteristics of these PTG patterns.

Second, PTG is a genuine phenomenon in oncology. Clinicians and mental health providers should not invalidate PTG reported by cancer survivors as doing so may deprive the coping effort of the patients and lead to more severe psychological symptoms. However, a small percentage of survivors (probably under 10%) cannot experience PTG because of other factors like deprived social support and financial difficulty. It is not appropriate to expect that all cancer survivors exhibit PTG.

PTG needs to exceed a certain level before it can positively affect psychological adjustment. However, intervention to increase the PTG of cancer patients and survivors should be avoided as doing so may generate illusory PTG among them, leading to undesirable outcomes. We recommend interventions to facilitate adaptive coping and reduce maladaptive coping to enable them to generate constructive PTG.

PTG and PTD should be regarded as related but separate constructs that exert differential effects on the psychological adjustment of cancer patients and survivors. PTD provides valuable information on potential cognitive distortion to inform cognitive therapy (CT) intervention for symptom reduction (Moorey & Greer, 2012). PTG experiences of cancer patients and survivors give a more comprehensive picture of the phenomenological world of the patients to guide other modalities of intervention, such as supportive-expressive therapy (SET) (Ho et al., 2004). Both CT and SET are evidence-based interventions in psycho-oncology (Ho, 2017).

Table 3.2 Coping Characteristics and Patterns of PTG

	PTG Level	
Maladaptive Coping Strategies	High	Low
High	Illusory PTG	Distressed PTG
Low	Constructive PTG	–

Conclusion and the Way Forward

Since the first study to establish the Posttraumatic Growth Inventory for cancer patients (Ho et al., 2004), our team has been conducting research on the topic in the past decades. Our research has gone through several stages, from the development of assessment tools to investigate the underlying mechanisms of PTG to dismantling different types of PTG and to examining the relationships between PTG and the psychological outcomes of cancer patients. We witness a change in attitude among oncology professionals toward PTG as well. In the early days, many healthcare workers in oncology viewed PTG with skepticism. They either denied the existence of PTG or considered it irrelevant to clinical care. However, the concept of PTG gradually received attention from oncology healthcare workers. There has been a sudden increase in PTG interventions for cancer patients about ten years ago in Hong Kong and we are glad to see that there has been a growing trend towards a more objective and scientific approach to the phenomenon of PTG in recent years.

Some unresolved puzzles to be worked on in the future remain. First, it would be helpful to study PTG and PTD among patients in their early phase of cancer diagnosis since all studies thus far focus on survivors. The findings may give important insight into the phenomenological world of cancer patients to inform cancer care. Second, strategies to integrate the concept of PTG into conventional psycho-oncology interventions could be developed. For instance, traditional coping skills intervention may include adaptive coping strategies to enhance PTG and examine whether it could increase treatment efficacy. Third, whether there are different types of PTD (e.g., distorted PTD, genuine PTD) similar to PTG could be established to inform interventions. Finally, it would be interesting to examine if the same relationships among PTG, PTD, and PTSD documented in our studies would hold for individuals with multiple exposures to different types of traumatic events.

Acknowledgment

We express sincere gratitude to our patients and colleagues for their support in the past 20+ years for the projects mentioned in this chapter.

References

Baker, J. M., Kelly, C., Calhoun, L. G., Cann, A., & Tedeschi, R. G. (2008). An examination of posttraumatic growth and posttraumatic depreciation: Two exploratory studies. *Journal of Loss and Trauma*, *13*(5), 450–465. doi:10.1080/15325020802171367

Calhoun, L. G., & Tedeschi, R. G. (2012). *Posttraumatic growth in clinical practice*(1ed.). Routledge. 10.4324/9780203629048

Cann, A., Calhoun, L. G., Tedeschi, R. G., & Solomon, D. T. (2010). Posttraumatic growth and depreciation as independent experiences and predictors of well-being. *Journal of Loss and Trauma*, *15*(3), 151–166. doi:10.1080/15325020903375826

Casellas-Grau, A., Ochoa, C., & Ruini, C. (2017). Psychological and clinical correlates of post-traumatic growth in cancer: A systematic and critical review. *Psycho-Oncology*, *26*(12), 2007–2018. doi:10.1002/pon.4426

Chan, M. W. C., Ho, S. M. Y., Tedeschi, R. G., & Leung, C. W. L. (2011). The valence of attentional bias and cancer-related rumination in posttraumatic stress and posttraumatic growth among women with breast cancer. *Psycho-Oncology*, *20*, 544–552. doi:10.1002/pon.1761

Cheng, C.-T., Wang, G. L., & Ho, S. M. Y. (2020). The relationship between types of posttraumatic growth and prospective psychological adjustment in women with breast cancer: A follow-up study. *Psycho-Oncology*, *29*(3), 586–588. doi:10.1002/pon.5312

Cheng, C. T., Ho, S. M. Y., Hou, Y. C., Lai, Y., & Wang, G. L. (2018). Constructive, illusory, and distressed posttraumatic growth among survivors of breast cancer: A 7-year growth trajectory study. *Journal of Health Psychology, 25*(1), 1359105318793199. doi:10.1177/1359105318793199

Collins, R. L., Taylor, S. E., & Skokan, L. A. (1990). A better world or a shattered vision? Changes in life perspectives following victimization. *Social Cognition, 8*(3), 263–285. doi:10.1521/soco.1990.8.3.263

Cordova, M. J., Cunningham, L. L. C., Carlson, C. R., & Andrykowski, M. A. (2001). Posttraumatic growth following breast cancer: A controlled comparison study. *Health Psychology, 20*(3), 176–185.

Epel, E. S., McEwen, B. S., & Ickovics, J. R. (1998). Embodying psychological thriving: Physical thriving in response to stress. *Journal of Social Issues, 54*(2), 301–322.

Fung, H. W., Chan, C., Lee, C. Y., & Ross, C. A. (2019). Using the post-traumatic stress disorder (PTSD) checklist for DSM-5 to screen for PTSD in the Chinese context: A pilot study in a psychiatric sample. *Journal of Evidence-Based Social Work, 16*(6), 643–651. doi:10.1080/26408066.2019.1676858

Henson, C., Truchot, D., & Canevello, A. (2021). What promotes post traumatic growth? A systematic review. *European Journal of Trauma & Dissociation, 5*(4), 100195. doi:10.1016/j.ejtd.2020.100195

Ho, S. M. Y. (2016). Posttraumatic growth: Focus on concepts and cross-cultural measurement issues. In C. Martin, V. Preedy, & V. Patel (Eds.), *Comprehensive guide to post-traumatic stress disorder* (pp. 1831–1848). Springer.

Ho, S. M. Y. (2017). Empirically supported psycho-oncology practices: Reflection based on some research findings in Hong Kong. *Psycho-Oncology, 26*(10), 1704–1706. doi:10.1002/pon.4345

Ho, S. M. Y., & Bai, Y. (2010). Posttraumatic growth in Chinese culture. In T. Weiss & R. Berger (Eds.), (pp. 147–156). John Wiley & Sons Inc.

Ho, S. M. Y., Chan, C. L. W., & Ho, R. T. H. (2004). Post-traumatic growth in Chinese cancer Survivors. *Psycho-Oncology, 13*(6), 377–389.

Ho, S. M. Y., Chan, M. W. Y., Yau, T. K., & Yeung, R. M. W. (2011). Relationships between explanatory style, posttraumatic growth, and posttraumatic stress disorder symptoms among Chinese breast cancer patients. *Psychology & Health, 26*(3), 269–285. doi:10.1080/08870440903287926

Ho, S. M. Y., Cheng, C.-T., Shih, S.-M., Taku, K., & Tedeschi, R. G. (2021). The Chinese version of posttraumatic growth and depreciation inventory—Expanded version (PTGDI-X) for cancer survivors. *Supportive Care in Cancer*. Advance online publication. doi:10.1007/s00520-021-06223-8

Ho, S. M. Y., Law, L. S. C., Wang, G.-L., Shih, S.-M., Hsu, S.-H., & Hou, Y.-C. (2013). Psychometric analysis of the Chinese version of the posttraumatic growth inventory with cancer patients in Hong Kong and Taiwan. *Psycho-Oncology, 22*(3), 175–179. doi:10.1002/pon.3024

Ho, S. M. Y., Saltel, P., Machavoine, J.-L., Rapoport-Hubschman, N., & Spiegal, D. (2004). Cross-cultural aspects of cancer care. In R. J. Moore & D. Spiegal (Eds.), *Cancer, culture, and communication* (pp. 157–183). Kluwer Academic/Plenum Publishers.

Ho, S. M. Y., Wong, K. F., Chan, C. L.-W., Watson, M., & Tsui, Y. K. Y. (2003). Psychometric properties of the Chinese version of the mini mental adjustment to cancer (Mini-MAC) scale. *Psycho-Oncology, 12*(6), 547–556.

Koutrouli, N., Anagnostopoulos, F., & Potamianos, G. (2012). Posttraumatic stress disorder and posttraumatic growth in breast cancer patients: A systematic review. *Women Health, 52*(5), 503–516. doi:10.1080/03630242.2012.679337

Lehman, D. R., Davis, C. G., DeLongis, A., Wortman, C. B., Bluck, S., Mandel, D. R., & Ellard, J. H. (1993). Positive and negative life changes following bereavement and their relations to adjustment. *Journal of Social and Clinical Psychology, 12*(1), 90–112.

Maercker, A., & Zoellner, T. (2004). The Janus face of self-perceived growth: Toward a two-component model of posttraumatic growth. *Psychological Inquiry, 15*(1), 41–48.

Moorey, S., & Greer, S. (2012). *Oxford guide to CBT for people with cancer*. Oxford University Press.

Pat-Horenczyk, R., Saltzman, L. Y., Hamama-Raz, Y., Perry, S., Ziv, Y., Ginat-Frolich, R., & Stemmer, S. M. (2016). Stability and transitions in posttraumatic growth trajectories among cancer patients: LCA and LTA analyses. *Psychological Trauma*, *8*(5), 541–549. doi:10.1037/tra0000094

Shakespeare-Finch, J., & Lurie-Beck, J. K. (2013). A meta-analytic clarification of the relationship between posttraumatic growth and symptoms of posttraumatic distress disorder. *Journal of Anxiety Disorders*, *28*(2), 223–229.

Taku, K., Tedeschi, R. G., Shakespeare-Finch, J., Krosch, D., David, G., Kehl, D., Grunwald, S., Romeo, A., Di Tella, M., Kamibeppu, K., Soejima, T., Hiraki, K., Volgin, R., Dhakal, S., Zięba, M., Ramos, C., Nunes, R., Leal, I., Gouveia, P., Silva, C. C., Chaves, P. N. D. P., Zavala, C., Paz, A., Senol-Durak, E., Oshio, A., Canevello, A., Cann, A., & Calhoun, L. G. (2020). Posttraumatic growth (PTG) and posttraumatic depreciation (PTD) across ten countries: Global validation of the PTG-PTD theoretical model. *Personality and Individual Differences*, 110222. doi:10.1016/j.paid.2020.110222

Tedeschi, R. G., & Calhoun, L. G. (1996). The posttraumatic growth inventory: Measuring the positive legacy of trauma. *Journal of Traumatic Stress*, *9*(3), 455–471.

Tedeschi, R. G., & Calhoun, L. G. (2004). Posttraumatic growth: Conceptual foundations and empirical evidence. *Psychological Inquiry*, *15*(1), 1–18.

Tedeschi, R. G., Park, C. L., & Calhoun, L. G. (1998a). Posttraumatic growth: Conceptual issues. In R. G. Tedeschi, C. L. Park, & L. G. Calhoun (Eds.), *Posttraumatic growth: Positive changes in the aftermath of crisis* (pp. 1–22). Lawrence Erlbaum Associates.

Tedeschi, R. G., Park, C. L., & Calhoun, L. G. (Eds.). (1998b). *Posttraumatic growth: Positive changes in the aftermath of crisis*. Lawrence Erlbaum Associates.

Watson, M., Greer, S., Young, J., Inayat, Q., Burgess, C., & Robertson, B. (1988). Development of a questionnaire measure of adjustment to cancer: The MAC scale. *Psychological Medicine*, *18*, 203–209.

Zoellner, T., & Maercker, A. (2006). Posttraumatic growth in clinical psychology – A critical review and introduction of a two component model. *Clinical Psychology Review*, *26*(5), 626–653. doi:10.1016/j.cpr.2006.01.008

4

APPLICATION OF A THEORETICAL MODEL OF POSTTRAUMATIC GROWTH TO DISTINGUISH BETWEEN POSTTRAUMATIC GROWTH AND ILLUSORY GROWTH

Whitney Dominick and Kanako Taku

Background of Posttraumatic Growth

Sometimes people change in a positive way after experiencing a painful and stressful psychological struggle with traumatic life events, known as posttraumatic growth or PTG (Tedeschi & Calhoun, 1996). PTG involves positive, transformative changes in cognitive and emotional life occurring after the trauma. PTG refers to both the whole bio-psycho-social-spiritual processes initiated by encountering the trauma, and the outcome that may be observed as a self-awareness of the "here and now" fostered by reflecting on what happened, what one has been going through, and connecting the past with the present. PTG can take various forms, from the simple but strong sense of "I've changed" to more complex changes in the form of altered life narratives.

Qualitative (Hefferon et al., 2009; Kissil et al., 2010) and quantitative studies (Linley et al., 2007; Taku et al., 2008; Tedeschi & Calhoun, 1996) have revealed that people often experience PTG in five primary domains, namely, new possibilities, personal strength, appreciation of life, relating to others, and existential/spiritual changes. PTG in other areas, such as an increased sense of the importance of the body and health, known as corporal growth or physical growth (Walsh et al., 2018), has also been suggested. Although the precise number of PTG domains varies from culture to culture (e.g., a higher order two-factor structure found in Chinese cancer survivors; Ho et al., 2004), the five PTG domains have been well observed around the globe (Taku et al., 2021).

These positive changes are deeply personal and can result from events perceived as highly stressful and impactful, regardless of whether those events meet the Diagnostic and Statistical Manual of Mental Disorders or DSM criteria of "trauma" (Tedeschi & Calhoun, 1996). As such, PTG has been found in many different children and adult populations, with diverse cultural backgrounds (Bostock et al., 2009; Kilmer et al., 2014;

DOI: 10.4324/9781032208688-5

Meyerson et al., 2011; Shaw et al., 2005). The same expressions of PTG, such as noticing truly special and precious things that used to be taken for granted, like small flowers, birds, or people's mere existence, have been observed in people around the world regardless of demographic and cultural differences (Tedeschi et al., 2018). Still, the important thing is that PTG is a process, rather than an end goal, and may continue for the rest of the lives after the trauma. Therefore, it cannot be the same for everyone even though thin-sliced one-time self-reports of PTG may appear so similar within the five major domains.

PTG Theoretical Model

The researchers who coined the term PTG proposed a theoretical model (Tedeschi & Calhoun, 2004), which they later refined to outline the general psychological processes of PTG (Tedeschi et al., 2018). One major component in both versions is the challenged worldviews or assumptive core beliefs triggered by a trauma. The assumptive worldviews or core beliefs are fundamental ideas that help people to structure their inner world. According to the theoretical model, PTG occurs because people struggle to re-establish worldviews or core beliefs that are disrupted by experiencing a life crisis, and thus need to be rebuilt (Cann et al., 2010; Taku et al., 2015). In the model, a stressful event challenges and disrupts a person's previously held values, core beliefs, and assumptions about the world, such as "the world is safe," "bad things should only happen to bad people," "all humans will die but she is not going to die in the near future." The PTG process starts when the trauma forces people to reexamine these assumptions and beliefs. People then begin to experience PTG by rebuilding new perspectives or reconstructing their sense of the world. However, PTG is unlikely to occur for people who find no need to reexamine or re-question their core beliefs, who resist doing so, or who are in denial (Seyburn et al., 2020). If one's values are not shaken and the assumptive world is not collapsed because the trauma is not severe enough or because they know how to cope with stressful situations in a flexible and adaptive way, there is no need to rebuild and PTG may not occur.

The disturbance in assumptions then facilitates cognitive and emotional processing, leading to rumination about the world, themselves, and the event. Initially, most of this rumination is automatic or intrusive, such as when memories of the stressful event pop into the mind unintentionally. Eventually, often with the assistance of self-disclosure, narratives, and social support, a person may start deliberately and purposefully ruminating about what had happened, trying to make meaning of it and developing new schemas about the world, while attempting to accept a new normal. This complex cognitive process may lead to the recognition of PTG, typically observed in the aforementioned five domains. However, perceiving positive changes without the accompanying struggle or any cognitive elements outlined in the model implies "illusory growth," or at least something different from PTG.

Self-Reported PTG and Illusory Growth

Although PTG is both a process and an outcome, researchers often focus on the outcome by measuring the five domains of PTG in a self-report form, partly because reflecting on the past is critical for PTG (e.g., "The world is no longer the same without her, but I know I've changed into a different person since and now I look at the things from a different angle that I'd never imagined before"). As PTG has been reported in various populations, especially by using standardized inventories that are designed to capture PTG experiences, such as the PTG Inventory (PTGI; Tedeschi & Calhoun, 1996), it becomes clear that the prevalence rates, the expression, and the conceptualization of PTG vary across groups. Group differences in the levels of PTG are occasionally attributed to the self-reporting method often used to assess it and call into question whether reports of growth, manifested as a score on the self-report inventories, reflect actual experiences of PTG. Self-report methods are potentially subject to self-defense mechanisms, whereby a person reports positive changes following a highly stressful life event to avoid a painful reality and reduce distress, without experiencing actual changes or personal growth (Zoellner & Maercker, 2006). Another potential problem is the use of retrospective measurement techniques, where participants' report of positive changes may reflect an inaccurate memory of how they were prior to the traumatic experience (Fraiser et al., 2009). This inaccurate memory, known as a "downward comparison," may lead to reporting higher growth than actually occurred.

The aforementioned issues concerning using self-report to assess PTG lead to the possible existence of "illusory growth," i.e., inaccurate perceptions of growth or positive psychological changes. Given that illusory growth is considered a self-protection mechanism rather than true positive change (Tedeschi & Calhoun, 2004), those reporting illusory growth believe they have changed in a positive manner even though they did not experience any changes after exposure to a highly stressful life event. Identifying the differences between PTG and illusory growth is necessary to help understand better the defense mechanisms people may use to cope with adversity and to design interventions to help people experience PTG rather than illusory growth.

While, unlike PTG, there is no consensus among researchers regarding what constitutes illusory growth, five different ways of looking at it have been suggested. These approaches are not mutually exclusive. The first defines illusory growth as an inconsistency between chronological numeric changes in a person's perceptions and reflective reports of PTG and relies on longitudinal research designs. For example, a prospective study by Fraiser et al. (2009) found that changes in five areas of PTG (i.e., positive relationship, life satisfaction, gratitude, meaning in life, and religious commitment) between pre- (Time 1) and post-trauma (Time 2) scores, were inconsistent with reflective growth measured by the PTG Inventory at Time 2. Although some participants reported noticeable differences (i.e., "actual changes") between Time 1 and Time 2, these changes had little correlation with their self-perceived growth at Time 2, providing evidence for the presence of illusory growth.

A second approach looks at the relationship between perceived growth and changes in distress. According to this approach, if self-reported growth is not associated with heightened well-being or improved quality of life, it may reflect illusory growth. For example, the aforementioned Frazier (2009) study indicates that participants who reported significant changes in perceptions between Time 1 and Time 2 also reported decreased distress indicating "real" or "actual" growth, whereas those reporting *perceived* growth at Time 2 and increased distress, were endorsing the "illusory" nature of reflected growth.

The third commonly used approach to illusory growth focuses on the relationship between self-reported PTG and coping strategies, assuming that if self-reported PTG is used as a method to avoid coping, it reflects illusory growth, whereas if self-reported PTG is correlated with the use of more active coping mechanisms such as problem-solving, it reflects PTG. For instance, the Janus-Face model (Zoellner & Maercker, 2006) argues that illusory growth is a self-protective mechanism whereby a person may report positive changes as avoidant coping. Thus, a person may state having experienced some benefit from the stressful situation to protect themselves from the psychological distress of the experience, without going through the rumination needed to experience PTG. By combining these first three approaches, Pat-Horenczyk and her colleagues (2015) define illusory growth as a rise in PTG but no improvement in coping, as opposed to constructive growth (i.e., a rise in PTG and improved coping).

The fourth approach addresses the duration of reported growth, such that illusory growth is conceived of as a temporary sense of growth that occurs shortly after the stressful event and is short-lived, without the time needed to fully process the stressful event. In contrast, PTG is thought of as long-lasting change. If an individual says, "I've found a new opportunity because of what happened to me," researchers are unlikely to expect them to say "I changed my mind. I had a bad day today. I don't think I found a new opportunity after all" in the following days, because if the remarks truly reflect PTG, it should not be affected by mood or context.

The fifth commonly used definition of illusory growth focuses on behavioral changes. In this approach, illusory growth is observed when people report having experienced positive changes without demonstrating the corresponding behavioral changes. For example, reporting "becoming more compassionate and having a better understanding of others' pain as a result of life crises," while not acting any differently towards other people. According to this view, PTG is "authentic" if it corresponds to chronological behavior changes, perhaps even verified by a third person, whereas illusory growth is experienced if it does not (Tallman et al., 2014).

Challenges in the Current Approaches to Defining Illusory Growth

Despite the multiple interrelated conceptualizations of illusory growth that have been proposed and investigated, the aforementioned approaches to illusory growth present challenges. The first approach, i.e., focusing on the consistency between chronological differences and reflective changes to assess prospective longitudinal changes, requires extensive resources and presents uncontrollable large "noises" in the data due to the time intervals needed to allow for a significant number of participants to experience a traumatic event that is impactful enough to result in a psychological and cognitive struggle and eventually possible PTG. A very large sample size would be required to compare those who did not experience trauma between the two-time points, those who are experiencing illusory growth, and those experiencing PTG. Fraiser et al.'s (2009) study was one of the first to examine the inconsistency between prospective changes and reflective growth by gathering longitudinal data among college students. However, it was conducted over the course of one semester, which arguably, is not enough time for students who have experienced a stressful event to fully process it and be able to recognize growth. More importantly, studies that use this approach, such as Fraiser et al. (2009), expect all "actual" changes to occur in a linear manner (i.e., decrease or increase), by relying on the differences in scores from Time 1 to Time 2. However, not all changes are linear, and some, such as the meanings of "psychological states (e.g., compassion, self-reliance, appreciation)" can occur in an oscillating way, which requires a more sophisticated measurement strategy. During reflection, a person may undergo a transformational change, reevaluate their prior definitions, or experience changes in meaning. For example, a person may originally think of 'compassion' as a willingness to do something for someone else, but upon reflection after experiencing a traumatic event, may expand their definition of compassion to include non-judgmental listening. This more nuanced definition of compassion would likely not be captured by simply comparing self-report scores over time. Furthermore, this approach does not allow those who are at a higher end (e.g., highly compassionate) at Time 1 to demonstrate their growth at Time 2 due to the ceiling effect.

The second approach that actual growth should increase psychological functioning may reflect a cognitive bias that to be truly positive, changes should corroborate with "positive" outcomes (e.g., decreased distress, increased satisfaction, heightened wellbeing). However, studies demonstrating a curvilinear relationship between PTG and PTSD symptoms indicate that the experiences of personal growth following trauma are paradoxical in nature and can co-exist (Shakespeare-Finch & Lurie-Beck, 2014). PTG is not synonymous with recovery and could often occur when some parts of psychological functioning seem to be deteriorating. For example, philosophical shifts are part of PTG (Tedeschi et al., 2018). When people experience PTG, they change the way they make sense of the world and themselves, sometimes involving a philosophical shift from the view that they held before a trauma happened, which does not necessarily lead to increased well-being or decreased pain. Thus, the differences between PTG and illusory growth cannot boil down to the levels of psychological functioning or distress.

The third approach that looks at coping strategies presents fewer challenges, especially when the opposite of illusory growth is defined as constructive growth rather than actual or authentic growth. According to the most updated PTG theoretical model (Tedeschi et al., 2018), the direct path to self-recognized PTG is acceptance of a changed world. Thus, it is plausible to define self-recognized growth as "illusory" if it is expressed and used as a means of an avoidant coping mechanism. However, once illusory growth is viewed as a self-protective mechanism or lack of effective coping strategies, the distinction between PTG and illusory growth becomes blurry because some types of defense mechanisms, such as sublimation or rationalization, may overlap with PTG.

The fourth approach, focusing on the duration of the change, is also less problematic, especially if illusory growth is defined as the self-reported positive changes that vary daily according to one's mood. However, the opposite may not be true. PTG may or may not last, depending on later experiences. While individuals may know in the here and now how they changed as a result of what had happened, in the future, they may experience something different that impacts their perception of growth. For example, researchers may observe people who claim they changed at Time 1 but no longer claim the same at Time 2 because new experiences or self-analyses occurring between Time 1 and Time 2 led them to change their perception of growth; however, this should not automatically cancel their PTG experiences at the past (Time 1).

Finally, the approach that expects behavioral changes to correspond with PTG requires objective data supporting the existence of such changes. While behavioral change reflecting some domains of PTG can be measured through observation (e.g., "putting more effort into one's own relationship"), others may not. For instance, experiencing a greater sense of harmony or being better able to accept the way things work out, are unlikely to correspond with specific behavioral changes. Moreover, seemingly non-PTG behaviors (e.g., quitting a job and starting a business) may in fact indicate PTG (Roepke et al., 2014). This approach would also require many resources to gather large enough objective data, given that some behaviors rarely happen in daily lives and others may not be objectively identifiable.

Applying the PTG model (Tedeschi et al., 2018) offers an alternative method for conceptualizing illusory growth that may overcome some of the aforementioned problems.

Because according to the model, PTG occurs only when the event is stressful and severe enough to shake established worldviews or when an individual admits to being forced by the trauma to reexamine their own core beliefs without being in denial, growth reported in the absence of the key cognitive components of shattered core beliefs, rumination, and self-disclosure, can be conceptualized as illusory growth (Taku et al., 2015). This method of distinguishing between PTG and illusory growth focuses on the importance of the cognitive struggle to come to terms with shattered core beliefs, without which self-growth is not likely to be PTG (Orille et al., 2019).

Empirical Findings

To demonstrate the practical utility of using the elements of the theoretical model to distinguish between PTG and illusory growth, a study of adolescents living in the United States and Japan is presented. This study measured PTG, levels of stress and disrupted core beliefs by life crises, and perceptions of personal growth were assessed qualitatively. It was hypothesized that those reporting illusory growth and those experiencing PTG would conceptualize personal growth differently, as personal growth is a value-laden concept that is likely influenced by the experience of growth per se. Therefore, assessing perceptions of what personal growth means or constitutes in those who report PTG compared to those who report illusory growth is useful in further supporting the importance of the theoretical model of PTG. Moreover, linking a subjective image of personal growth to PTG or illusory growth can help illustrate whether experiencing PTG may help to change perceptions about the world or concepts. For example, if those experiencing illusory growth have a qualitatively different perception of personal growth than those experiencing PTG, it is reasonable to assume that the experience of PTG itself has contributed to a more nuanced conception of personal growth.

Assessing the perceptions of adolescents from two different cultures is particularly useful. The experience of PTG varies among cultures, thus methods that accurately differentiate between PTG and illusory growth in multiple cultures can be assumed to be more easily generalizable. Additionally, adolescents are in the process of maturing and discovering their individual identities and may struggle to understand more abstract concepts with which they have little experience (Kuhn, 1993). However, adolescents who have experienced a traumatic or highly stressful life event need to integrate the experience into their worldview, which can help them mature and emerge with a deeper understanding of themselves and the world, and in turn, affect conceptual shifts of what personal growth means to them.

To assess differences in growth, 439 high school students (165 from the United States and 274 from Japan) were asked to complete a survey assessing their definitions of personal growth, their experiences with stressful life events and the level of stress of these events, how much it shook their beliefs about the world, and how much growth they experienced. Based on the level of shaken beliefs and stress at the time of the event, these adolescents were grouped into those who scored in the top quartile for stress and shaken beliefs and thus were considered as reporting PTG ($n = 85$), those who scored in the bottom quartile for stress and shaken beliefs and thus were considered as reporting illusory growth ($n = 56$), and those who scored in the middle ($n = 298$). Comparisons were made between the two groups of those supposedly reporting PTG and illusory growth. In addition to the PTG Inventory, participants were asked to use open-ended questions to generate words they associate with personal growth, yielding a total of 443 distinct words. Informed by a study by Dominick and Taku (2018), these words were clustered into 16 overarching categories, in addition to a category of "other." The categories included: physical change, social connection, behavior, maturity, change, independent accomplishments, overcoming, spirituality, acceptance, knowledge, flexibility, compassion, adult, duty, positives, negatives, and others.

Results suggested that Japanese adolescents were more likely than those from the United States and males were more likely than females to report illusory growth. Although both groups reported a moderate level of PTG, those experiencing high stress and a high level of shaken beliefs (classified in the PTG group) reported higher scores both overall and on each of the domains encompassing PTG than those who did not experience high levels of stress or shaken beliefs and thus were classified in the illusory growth group. Additionally, there were qualitatively different perceptions of personal growth between both the different cultures and the PTG and illusory growth groups. Japanese adolescents conceptualize personal growth in terms of social connections, whereas participants from the United States conceptualize it as change (Dominick & Taku, 2018). Those who have experienced significant stress and struggled to rebuild their shaken worldviews (the PTG group) conceptualize their process as one of overcoming the odds and ultimately viewed their struggle as worthwhile, helping them to assess the process as positive. Further, those reporting PTG recognized that personal growth is a process that takes time and effort. On the other hand, those experiencing illusory growth have a perspective of personal growth as a physical rather than psychological change. Counterintuitively, they were also more likely to report compassion when thinking of personal growth. This is surprising given that one of the domains of PTG is "Relating to Others," which includes connections with other people, and theoretically would include increased compassion. However, it is possible that those experiencing illusory growth were more likely to think of personal growth as an increased appreciation, love, and gentleness because they did not have to endure high stress levels or need to rebuild their worldviews, perhaps due to strong social support or available personal resources, which allowed them to report positive changes following a specific stressful life event without cognitive disturbance. It is also possible that those who are experiencing illusory growth are being compassionate to themselves, allowing themselves to feel as if they are better off after the event than they were before it and leading to the conceptualization of compassion as representative of personal growth. However, these speculations require further investigation.

The results of this study indicate that focusing on the key cognitive components of the PTG theoretical model is a fruitful and simple way to distinguish between PTG and illusory growth. The usefulness of the PTG theoretical model in identifying types of growth is strengthened by the different conceptualizations of growth by each group. These different perceptions and processes can be used to help identify those who are experiencing illusory growth rather than PTG, providing an area of focus for further research and possible psycho-educational interventions aimed at helping foster PTG rather than illusory growth. Additionally, these results help demonstrate that the process of experiencing PTG can change adolescents' perceptions, giving them a more complete, mature, perspective of personal growth.

While using the PTG theoretical model to distinguish experiencing PTG from illusory growth appears to be effective, there are some limitations to this study. First, PTG and illusory growth were determined by examining the level of stress and reported shaken beliefs at the time of the event. However, these aspects were assessed by a single item. It is possible that using standardized scales with more items would fully represent the degree to which an event is perceived to be stressful and would capture the degree of shaken worldviews in more detail. Second, not all of the key elements of the theoretical model were utilized to create the groups of PTG and illusory growth. For example, intrusive and deliberate rumination, as well as self-disclosure and acceptance, which are key elements in the PTG process were not included. Additional scales that fully cover the PTG theoretical model might have increased reliability in distinguishing between the two concepts. Thirdly, perceptions of personal growth were examined in adolescents only. While this provides valuable information, the results cannot be generalized to adults, who may have a more developed conceptualization of personal growth regardless of their personal experiences. Finally, since personal growth is a value-laden term and participants were asked to report their personal adversity, social desirability bias might have been a contributing factor.

Conclusion

While no single method is the best to characterize illusory growth as opposed to PTG, applying the PTG theoretical model has the potential to effectively distinguish those who have experienced PTG from those reporting illusory growth. This method presents fewer drawbacks than other methods, is simple to implement, and can be used cross-culturally. Defining and examining illusory growth as self-reflected personal growth occurring in the absence of key cognitive features of the PTG theoretical model has theoretical and clinical implications. Theoretically, it allows increased integration of past research that has found differing levels of PTG across populations. It may also provide some clarity regarding the ongoing debate about the relationship between PTG and distress. Inconsistent results found in previous studies may be due to confounds of classifying illusory growth as PTG rather than distinguishing between the two. In addition, this provides further support for the validity of the PTG model and the phenomenon of PTG in general. Clinically, being able to distinguish between those experiencing PTG and those experiencing illusory growth can allow therapists to help identify which of their clients has experienced PTG and focus on helping clients who are experiencing illusory growth continue their journey triggered by the stressful event. Additionally, this information can be used for psycho-education designed to help elucidate the possibility of PTG and the importance of allowing oneself to fully experience and process the event and its impact on own worldviews in order to begin experiencing PTG.

Future studies should continue to evaluate the differences between those who are experiencing PTG and those who are experiencing illusory growth as well as examine the full theoretical model, including rumination and self-disclosure, to continue to clarify the key cognitive components that differentiate between illusory growth and PTG.

References

Bostock, L., Sheikh, A. I., & Barton, S. (2009). Posttraumatic growth and optimism in health-related trauma: A systematic review. *Journal of Clinical Psychology in Medical Settings*, *16*, 281–296. doi:10.1007/s10880-009-9175-6

Cann, A., Calhoun, L. G., Tedeschi, R. G., Kilmer, R. P., Gil-Rivas, V., Vishnevsky, T., & Danhauer, S. C. (2010). The core beliefs inventory: A brief measure of disruption in the assumptive world. *Anxiety, Stress, & Coping*, *23*, 19–34. doi:10.1080/10615800802573013

Dominick, W., & Taku, K. (2018). Cultural differences in the perception of personal growth among adolescents. *Cross-Cultural Research*. doi:10.1177/1069397118815111

Fraiser, P., Tennen, H., Gavian, M., Park, C., Tomich, P., & Tashiro, T. (2009). Does self-reported posttraumatic growth reflect genuine positive change? *Psychological Science*, *20*, 912–919. doi:10.1111/j.1467-9280.2009.02381.x

Hefferon, K., Grealy, M., & Mutrie, N. (2009). Post-traumatic growth and life threatening physical illness: A systematic review of the qualitative literature. *British Journal of Health Psychology*, *14*, 343–378. doi:10.1348/135910708X332936

Ho, S. M. Y., Chan, C. L. W., & Ho, R. T. H. (2004). Posttraumatic growth in Chinese cancer survivors. *Psychological-Oncology*, *13*, 377–389. doi:10.1002/pon.758

Kilmer, R. P., Gil-Rivas, V., Griese, B., Hardy, S. J., Hafstad, G. S., & Alisic, E. (2014). Posttraumatic growth in children and youth: Clinical implications of an emerging research literature. *American Journal of Orthopsychology*, *84*, 506–518. doi:10.1037/ort0000016

Kissil, K., Nino, A., Jacobs, S., Davey, M., & Tubbs, C. Y. (2010). "It has been a good growing experience for me": Growth experiences among African American youth coping with parental cancer. *Families, Systems, & Health*, *28*, 274–289. doi:10.1037/a0020001

Kuhn, D. (1993). Connecting scientific and informal reasoning. *Merril-Palmer Quarterly*, *39*, 74–103.

Linley, P. A., Andrews, L., & Joseph, S. (2007). Confirmatory factor analysis of the posttraumatic growth inventory. *Journal of Loss and Trauma*, *12*, 321–332. doi:10.1080/15325020601162823

Meyerson, D. A., Grant, K. E., Carter, J. S., & Kilmer, R. P. (2011). Posttraumatic growth among children and adolescents: A systematic review. *Clinical Psychological Review*. doi:10.1016/j.cpr.2011.06.003

Orille, A., Harrison, L., & Taku, K. (2019). Individual differences in attitudes and perceptions toward posttraumatic growth and illusory growth. *Personality and Individual Differences*, *142*, 153–158. doi:10.1016/j.paid/2019.02.002

Pat-Horenczyk, R., Perry, S., Hamama-Raz, Y., Ziv, Y., Schramm-Yavin, S., & Stemmer, S. M. (2015). Posttraumatic growth in breast cancer survivors: Constructive and illusory aspects. *Journal of Traumatic Stress*, *28*, 214–222. doi:10.1002/jts.22014

Roepke, A. M., Forgeard, M. J. C., & Elstein, J. G. (2014). Providing context for behavior: Cognitive change matters for post-traumatic growth. *European Journal of Personality*, *28*, 347–348. doi:10.1002/per.1970

Seyburn, S. J., LaLonde, L., & Taku, K. (2020). A sense of growth among teenagers after hurting others: A potential application of posttraumatic growth theory. *Journal of Loss and Trauma*, *25*(1), 22–33. doi:10.1080/15325024.2019.1645449

Shakespeare-Finch, J., & Lurie-Beck, J. (2014). A meta-analytic clarification of the relationship between posttraumatic growth and symptoms of posttraumatic distress disorder. *Journal of Anxiety Disorders*, *28*, 223–229. doi:10.1016/j.janxdis.2013.10.005

Shaw, A., Joseph, S., & Linley, P. A. (2005). Religion, spirituality, and posttraumatic growth: A systematic review. *Mental Health, Religion & Culture*, *8*, 1–11. doi:10.0/1367467032000157981

Taku, K., Cann, A., Calhoun, L. G., & Tedeschi, R. G. (2008). The factor structure of the posttraumatic growth inventory: A comparison of five models using confirmatory factor analysis. *Journal of Traumatic Stress*, *21*, 158–164. doi:10.1002/jts.20305

Taku, K., Cann, A., Tedeschi, R. G., & Calhoun L. G. (2015). Core beliefs shaken by an earthquake correlate with posttraumatic growth. *Psychological Trauma: Theory, Research, Practice, & Policy*, *7*, 563–569. doi:10.1037/tra0000054

Taku, K., Tedeschi, R. G., Shakespeare-Finch, J., Krosch, D., David, G., Kehl, D., Grunwald, S., Romeo, A., Di Tella, M., Kamibeppu, K., Soejima, T., Hiraki, K., Volgin, R., Dhakal, S., Zieba, M., Ramos, C., Nunes, R., Leal, I., Gouveia, P. … , & Calhoun, L. G. (2021). Posttraumatic growth (PTG) and posttraumatic depreciation (PTG) across ten countries: Global validation of the PTG-PTD theoretical model. *Personality and Individual Differences*, *169*. doi:10.1016/j.paid.2020.110222

Tallman, B. A., Lohnberg, J., Yamada, T. H., Halfdanarson, T. R., & Altmaier, E. M. (2014). Anticipating posttraumatic growth from cancer: Patients' and collaterals' experiences. *Journal of Psychosocial Oncology*, *32*, 342–358. doi:10.1080/07347332.2014.897291

Tedeschi, R. G., & Calhoun, L. G. (1996). The posttraumatic growth inventory: Measuring the positive legacy of trauma. *Journal of Traumatic Stress*, *9*, 455–472. doi:10.1002/jts.2490090305
Tedeschi, R. G., & Calhoun, L. G. (2004). Posttraumatic growth: Conceptual foundations and empirical evidence. *Psychological Inquiry*, *15*, 1–18. doi:141.210.2.69
Tedeschi, R. G., Shakespeare-Finch, J., Taku, K., & Calhoun, L. G. (2018). *Posttraumatic growth: Theory, research, and applications*. NY and London: Routledge.
Walsh, D. M. J., Morrison, T. G., Conway, R. J., Rogers, E., Sullivan, F. J., & Groarke, A. (2018). A model to predict psychological- and health-related adjustment in men with prostate cancer: The role of post traumatic growth, physical post traumatic growth, resilience and mindfulness. *Frontiers in Psychology*, *9*, 136. doi:10.3389/fpsyg.2018.00136
Zoellner, T., & Maercker, A. (2006). Posttraumatic growth in clinical psychology. A critical review and introduction of a two component model. *Clinical Psychological Review*, *26*, 626–653.

5

SEX, GENDER, AND THEIR ROLE IN POSTTRAUMATIC GROWTH

Liat Helpman

Sex and Gender-Related Patterns in Posttraumatic Reactions

Both sex, as a biological variable, and gender, as a psychosocial variable, have been repeatedly implicated in the unfolding of posttraumatic reactions (see Christiansen & Berke, 2020 for a review). Women have been consistently documented as being exposed to traumatic events less frequently than men, but suffer posttraumatic reactions such as depression, anxiety, and PTSD at a rate twice as high as men (Sayed et al., 2015). This disparity has been tied to both psychological mechanisms, such as gendered coping strategies (Tolin & Foa, 2006), and to biological mechanisms, such as sex-related patterns in stress response and recovery (Juster et al., 2011). More recently, similar disparities were identified in PTG such that women were found to be more likely than men to respond to stress both with PTSD and with PTG (Tedeschi et al., 2018). Although research on this pattern is still scarce, accumulating evidence suggests that the very same mechanisms that contribute to the increased risk of adverse outcomes following trauma may also contribute to the increased likelihood of PTG. This chapter reviews the evidence for such linkage between the psychological and biological mechanisms purportedly underlying sex and gender differences in PTG and those underlying such differences in posttraumatic psychopathology. Within psychological mechanisms, intrapersonal, interpersonal, and contextual factors are discussed, and within biological mechanisms, endocrine, neural, and genetic mechanisms are reviewed. Finally, the possible interplay between these mechanisms is addressed.

Psychological Correlates of Gender Differences in PTG

Psychological correlates of gender differences in PTG include intrapersonal, interpersonal, and contextual mechanisms.

Intrapersonal Mechanisms

Coping mechanisms are leading contenders for explaining gender differences in both adverse outcomes of traumatic exposure and PTG. High use of avoidant coping mechanisms, such as

DOI: 10.4324/9781032208688-6

distraction and disengagement, may put women at increased risk of PTSD as compared to their male counterparts (Tolin & Foa, 2006). However, other coping mechanisms such as deliberate thought have been directly linked to mediating the relationship between PTG and gender among survivors of natural disasters (Akbar & Witruk, 2016).

One coping mechanism associated with PTG is rumination, which includes both passive and active components (Nolen-Hoeksema & Morrow, 1991). The brooding (passive) component has been tied to internalizing psychopathologies such as anxiety, depression, and PTSD (Smith & Alloy, 2009). However, other, more active, components of rumination may promote processing and meaning-making that is more prevalent among women (Vishnevsky et al., 2010). For example, following a university shooting, deliberate, but not intrusive rumination, predicted PTG (Wozniak et al., 2019).

In addition to cognitive coping strategies, emotional regulation strategies also have been found to be differentially beneficial for men and women; specifically, the avoidance strategy of emotional suppression has been found to be associated with more dire consequences for women than men (Rogier et al., 2017). The use of reappraisal, an active regulation strategy, has been shown to be positively associated with PTG (Kira et al., 2020); however, gender patterns in this relationship have yet to be examined. More research is needed about the relationship between PTG and the interaction between gender and type of emotional regulation strategy.

Cognitive and emotional coping strategies such as rumination and emotional regulation may provide a nuanced array of both protective and risk factors in a gendered fashion. However, such mechanisms may contribute to positive changes both in one's intrapersonal, subjective coping, and in coping behaviors.

Interpersonal Mechanisms

Social ties play an important role in the unfolding of posttraumatic sequelae. Social support has been tied both to lower risk of PTSD and to higher rates of PTG (Schubert et al., 2016). However, this role of social support may be gender-specific as social support explained PTG among women, but not men who survived Sweol ferry disaster (Han et al., 2019). In an additional study, both empathy and social support coping were found to be significant mediators in the relationship between gender and stress-related growth, with empathy evincing a stronger mediational effect (Swickert et al., 2012). The interpersonal, gendered correlates of PTG may extend to coping strategies in the wake of trauma. Particularly, posttraumatic changes in relationships with others were tied to social support (Wolfe & Ray, 2015). This appears to be gendered, such that women utilize interpersonal coping styles more than men do (Dekel et al., 2016). Jin and colleagues (2014) have also noted that women consistently report higher improved relationships with others than men. This may support the notion that rather than "fight or flight," women respond to stressful experiences with "tend and befriend" (Taylor et al., 2000), a response which may support PTG.

The interpersonal aspects of posttraumatic sequelae may have an additive effect to those of intrapersonal ones on PTG; indeed, changes both in appreciation of life (intrapersonal) and in relationships with others (interpersonal), were documented to be associated with PTG among women who lost a loved one (Ogińska-Bulik, 2015). In another study, social support (interpersonal) was a positive predictor of PTG, with event centrality (intrapersonal) negatively predicting resilience in women, but not in men (Wolfe & Ray, 2015). This suggests a gendered interplay between inter-and intrapersonal factors in their relationship with PTG.

Contextual Mechanisms

The gendered patterns in PTG may be grounded in addition to intra- and interpersonal factors, also in the broader context in which women exist, the roles they play, and the culture in which they live. For example, professional roles, albeit in similar workplaces, may impact PTG in a gendered manner; among health professionals, higher PTG was associated with the female gender, consistent with previous findings. When broken down further by professional role, an interaction between gender and role appears such that for men, there was no difference in PTG between nurses and physicians, whereas for women, nurses reported higher levels of PTG than did physicians (Hamama-Raz et al., 2020). This interaction may be taken as evidence of the importance of gender roles and the sociocultural context they create for women. Research on gender role adherence and PTG has demonstrated that gender itself did not significantly predict PTG; however, both masculine and feminine role adherence significantly and positively did (Barlow & Hetzel-Riggin, 2018). It has been argued that women's participation in the workforce, particularly engaging in more traditionally "masculine" roles, has added to their overall strain (Mayor, 2015). Therefore, perhaps the strain of deviating from a role detracted from a sense of social connectedness or added to overall strain, minimizing PTG among women who deviate from said role, personally (gender role) and professionally (physicians vs. nurses). However, these findings do not appear to converge with research suggesting a connection between androgyny and well-being (Juster et al., 2016). Clearly, more research is needed.

Correlates of PTG also appeared to interact with gender, depending on community features. While for women, both high community resources and a positive attitude towards seeking psychological help correlated positively with PTG (and only the latter with PTS), for men, attitudes toward help-seeking positively associated with both PTSD and PTG only for those with low community resources (Shigemoto et al., 2020).

The gendered patterns of PTG also appear to depend on culture. While gender significantly correlated with all PTG domains except New Possibilities and Spiritual Change in an American sample, gender differences emerged only in the Personal Strength domain in a comparable Japanese sample (Taku & Cann, 2014). This may be attributed to gender roles and their culturally-bound aspects.

In sum, that PTG appears to associate with gender as dependent on intrapersonal processes such as rumination, coping, and emotional regulation, on interpersonal processes such as garnering and offering support, and on socio-contextual factors such as gender roles, as well as their professional and cultural correlates, suggests an interaction of environmental aspects and individual differences in determining one's PTG.

Biological Correlates of Sex-Related Patterns in PTG

When discussing individual differences, we would be remiss in overlooking possible biological substrates that include endocrine, neural, and genetic aspects.

Endocrine

Post Traumatic responses have been closely tied to endocrine correlates of stress systems such as the hypothalamic-pituitary axis (HPA; Lucassen et al., 2014) and, more recently, the hypothalamic-pituitary gonadal axis (HPG; Ravi et al., 2019). Similarly, PTG has been tied to these mechanisms as documented in the only study to date that explicitly examined the relationship between HPA and PTG (Diaz et al., 2014). This study found that healthy diurnal cortisol patterns (e.g., reactive and not blunted) were positively associated with PTG in women with metastatic breast cancer. While no extant literature addresses the role of sex in this relationship, a significant body of research indicated sex-related heterogeneity in cortisol response to stress (Uhart et al., 2006). Future research should explore this more directly as such information may be critical in understanding processes of immune functioning following trauma, particularly the positive relationship between immune function and PTG, which may be associated with HPA function (Dunigan et al., 2007).

PTG has been examined extensively among women who are breast cancer survivors (Diaz et al., 2014; Morris & Shakespeare-Finch, 2011). Many of these women take hormone therapy, and these effects are usually controlled for but remain unexamined, despite the long-established relationship between sex steroids, particularly estrogen, and stress responses (Nagaya & Maren, 2015). As a relationship between PTG and HPA has been demonstrated in breast cancer patients (Diaz et al., 2014), and HPA and steroid hormones appear to interact in response to stress, the role of sex steroids in sex-specific patterns PTG offers a promising avenue of research.

Neural

PTG has been found to associate with the down-modulation of global synchronous neural interactions, particularly in the mPFC (Anders et al., 2015). This region has been associated with the modulation of limbic function (i.e., emotional processing and response; see Etkin et al., 2011). Specifically, the synchronicity of mPFC and prefrontal regions of the central executive network (CEN), associated with memory and with mentalization, have been tied to PTG (Fujisawa et al., 2015). Taken together, these findings suggest that individuals with higher PTG may have stronger functional connectivity between memory functions within the CEN and mentalization regions, as well as better modulation of emotional response, which may contribute to better retention of social ties. Additionally, PTG, and particularly its aspect of relating to others, were associated with structural changes in the DLPFC (Nakagawa et al., 2016), a part of the CEN. Functional changes in DLPFC were also observed in PTG, but not PTSD, during emotional regulation (Wei et al., 2017). Therefore, it may be concluded that PTG associates with patterns of executive function, which may indicate better top-down control, perhaps similar to that of active emotional regulation strategies such as reappraisal (Morawetz et al., 2016). It appears that some executive functions such as visual memory, categorization, and fluency relate to the personal rather than the relational growth aspect of PTG (Eren-Koçak & Kiliç, 2014). Therefore, relational growth may be associated with executive functions relating to mentalization and memory, while personal growth is associated with more traditional executive functions.

Neurobiology of executive functions has been repeatedly tied to sex, and to HPG in particular; in fact, DLPFC activity during the downregulation of negative emotion using reappraisal was positively associated with estrogen levels in females (Chung et al., 2019). Therefore, it appears that the relationship between DLPFC, executive function during emotional regulation, and PTG may be further complicated by sex-specific patterns, not yet explored.

Genetic

While many studies have examined the genetic underpinnings of distress following trauma, few have examined resilience and PTG, precluding substantiation of genetic mechanisms of growth (Mehta et al., 2020). The mechanisms identified as associated with PTG correspond to those associated with PTSD: namely, genes involved in HPA function.

Low PTG was significantly associated with both FKBP5 and NR3C1 methylation (Bakusic et al., 2017; Dudley et al., 2011), i.e., methylation of sites associated with HPA function, and were previously found to associate with distress following trauma (Watkeys et al., 2018). Therefore, methylation of NR3C1 may result in heightened gene expression, reduced PTG, and dysfunctional HPA-axis function, and thus be associated with growth-mitigating mechanisms rather than growth promotion (Miller et al., 2017). It is apparent that more research is needed to identify the genetic underpinnings involved in PTG.

To date, no direct evidence for the involvement of sex in the relationship between PTG and these genetic substrates appears to exist. However, sex-dependent patterns in the relationship between posttraumatic psychopathology and HPA-related genetics have previously been identified (Binder et al., 2008), suggesting relevant sex-dependent patterns here as well.

In sum, PTG has been associated with genetic, endocrine, and neural underpinnings previously identified to correspond to posttraumatic sequelae. Some of these underpinnings have already been identified as contributing to posttraumatic responses in a sex-specific manner; however, at this time, there are more questions than empirical findings regarding such patterns in the biological foundations of PTG.

Summary, Conclusions, and Future Directions

To date, much of the focus in exploring the aftermath of traumatic events has been on the pathological, rather than on the salutogenic. This is slowly shifting, with more and more research on resilience and PTG. However, there is still a substantial gap in understanding the intricate relationship between biological, psychological, and contextual factors underlying PTG. Even more so, the understanding of how sex as a biological construct and gender as a psychosocial one may be involved in this relationship is still very much a preliminary endeavor. Still, from the literature reviewed, we can conclude that several underlying mechanisms may be delineated.

First, endocrine and neural underpinnings of response to trauma appear to shape both pathological outcomes and PTG in a sex-dependent manner, with possible genetic components underlying these changes. Genetics underlying HPA-response, subsequent HPA-response, and its interaction with gonadal steroids appear to differentially shape neural responses in a sex-dependent manner. The literature to date may thus be taken to infer that genetics underlying stress response, which in turn, holds endocrine correlates that interact with other endocrine systems, may underly some of the sex-specific patterns in both salubrious (e.g., PTG, resilience) and pathological (e.g., PTSD, depression) responses. Neural pathways similarly confer risk or PTG by virtue of bolstering, or disrupting, regulatory pathways that may take control of what may become a runaway stress response. These pathways may be associated with PTG-related intrapersonal (e.g., active coping, reappraisal, active rumination) and interpersonal (e.g., seeking connection and support) processes.

Both the biological factors and socially constructed factors such as gender roles may contribute to interpersonal behavior following traumatic events and the ability to garner social support, an important predictor of PTG, and to engage in prosocial behaviors such as "tend and befriend" (Taylor et al., 2000). Such empathetic exchanges may contribute to higher PTG (Swickert et al., 2012). The gendered relationship between PTG and interpersonal propensities may also manifest itself in the ability to benefit from help-seeking, which appears associated with PTG consistently among women only (Shigemoto et al., 2020). Gender roles appear to associate with PTG and adherence to them appears to be beneficial for both genders, as greater cis-gendered role adherence was found to be associated with PTG (Barlow & Hetzel-Riggin, 2018), perhaps reflecting the impact of role-congruent behavior on either social responsiveness of others or the tendency to garner social support. Cultural factors, which may also impact gendered expectations, appear to play a part in the relationship between gender and specific subtypes of PTG (Taku & Cann, 2014).

Taken together, it may be concluded that interpersonal, contextual, and intrapersonal processes mitigate risk, and promote PTG and adaptation, in a gendered manner. Much as women's adverse responses to stress may be exacerbated by biological (e.g., naturally occurring hormonal fluctuations) and psychosocial (e.g., role strain, socialization towards internalizing blame) factors, aspects of these same biological (e.g., enhanced plasticity) and psychosocial (e.g., tend-and-befriend responses, active rumination) factors may also encourage PTG. Therefore, it may be (carefully) deduced that trauma has a more pronounced impact on women.

Future research must further disentangle these mechanisms and chart out the complex interactions among them, providing a bio-psycho-social model of the impact of trauma, considering both sexes as a biological variable and gender as a psychosocial one. Such research may inquire into the relationship between inter- and intra-personal attitudes and behaviors, coping mechanisms, HPA, and HPG, as well as underlying neural and genetic substrates.

By answering these questions, we may come closer to designing sex- and gender-informed interventions, which may utilize both preventative measures in policy and ameliorative interventions in response to trauma, targeting sex- and gender-informed mechanisms to increase individual fit and facilitating growth in the wake of trauma.

References

Akbar, Z., & Witruk, E. (2016). Coping mediates the relationship between gender and posttraumatic growth. *Procedia - Social and Behavioral Sciences*, *217*, 1036–1043.

Anders, S. L., Peterson, C. K., James, L. M., Engdahl, B., Leuthold, A. C., & Georgopoulos, A. P. (2015). Neural communication in posttraumatic growth. *Experimental Brain Research*, *233*(7), 2013–2020. 10.1007/s00221-015-4272-2

Bakusic, J., Schaufeli, W., Claes, S., & Godderis, L. (2017). Stress, burnout and depression: A systematic review on DNA methylation mechanisms. *Journal of Psychosomatic Research*, *92*, 34–44. 10.1016/J.JPSYCHORES.2016.11.005

Barlow, M. R., & Hetzel-Riggin, M. D. (2018). Predicting posttraumatic growth in survivors of interpersonal trauma: Gender role adherence is more important than gender. *Psychology of Men and Masculinity*, *19*(3), 446–456. 10.1037/men0000128

Binder, E. B., Bradley, R. G., Liu, W., Epstein, M. P., Deveau, T. C., Mercer, K. B., Tang, Y., Gillespie, C. F., Heim, C. M., Nemeroff, C. B., Schwartz, A. C., Cubells, J. F., & Ressler, K. J., (2008). Association of FKBP5 Polymorphisms and childhood abuse with risk of posttraumatic stress disorder symptoms in adults. *JAMA*, *299*(11), 1291–1305. 10.1001/JAMA.299.11.1291

Christiansen, D. M., & Berke, E. T. (2020). Gender- and sex-based contributors to sex differences in PTSD. *Current Psychiatry Reports*, 22(4), 1–9. 10.1007/s11920-020-1140-y

Chung, Y. S., Poppe, A., Novotny, S., Epperson, C. N., Kober, H., Granger, D. A., Blumberg, H. P., Ochsner, K., Gross, J. J., Pearlson, G., & Stevens, M. C. (2019). A preliminary study of association between adolescent estradiol level and dorsolateral prefrontal cortex activity during emotion regulation. *Psychoneuroendocrinology*, *109*, 104398. 10.1016/j.psyneuen.2019.104398

Dekel, S., Hankin, I. T., Pratt, J. A., Hackler, D. R., & Lanman, O. N. (2016). Posttraumatic growth in trauma recollections of 9/11 survivors: A narrative approach. *Journal of Loss and Trauma*, *21*(4), 315–324. 10.1080/15325024.2015.1108791

Diaz, M., Aldridge-Gerry, A., & Spiegel, D. (2014). Posttraumatic growth and diurnal cortisol slope among women with metastatic breast cancer. *Psychoneuroendocrinology*, *44*, 83–87. 10.1016/J.PSYNEUEN.2014.03.001

Dudley, K. J., Li, X., Kobor, M. S., Kippin, T. E., & Bredy, T. W. (2011). Epigenetic mechanisms mediating vulnerability and resilience to psychiatric disorders. *Neuroscience & Biobehavioral Reviews*, *35*(7), 1544–1551. 10.1016/J.NEUBIOREV.2010.12.016

Dunigan, J. T., Carr, B. I., & Steel, J. L. (2007). Posttraumatic growth, immunity and survival in patients with hepatoma. *Digestive Diseases and Sciences*, *52*(9), 2452–2459. 10.1007/s10620-006-9477-6

Etkin, A., Egner, T., & Kalisch, R. (2011). Emotional processing in anterior cingulate and medial prefrontal cortex. *Trends in Cognitive Sciences*, *15*(2), 85–93. 10.1016/j.tics.2010.11.004

Eren-Koçak, E., & Kiliç, C. (2014). Posttraumatic growth after earthquake trauma is predicted by executive functions: A pilot study. *Journal of Nervous & Mental Disease*, *202*(12), 859–863. 10.1097/NMD.0000000000000211

Fujisawa, T. X., Jung, M., Kojima, M., Saito, D. N., Kosaka, H., & Tomoda, A. (2015). Neural basis of psychological growth following adverse experiences: A resting-state functional MRI study. *PLoS One*, *10*(8), e0136427. 10.1371/journal.pone.0136427

Hamama-Raz, Y., Ben-Ezra, M., Bibi, H., Swarka, M., Gelernter, R., & Abu-Kishk, I. (2020). The interaction effect between gender and profession in posttraumatic growth among hospital personnel. *Primary Health Care Research & Development*, *21*, 1–8. 10.1017/S1463423620000377

Han, K. M., Park, J. Y., Park, H. E., An, S. R., Lee, E. H., Yoon, H. K., & Ko, Y. H. (2019). Social support moderates association between posttraumatic growth and trauma-related psychopathologies among victims of the Sewol Ferry Disaster. *Psychiatry Research*, *272*, 507–514. 10.1016/j.psychres.2018.12.168

Jin, Y., Xu, J., & Liu, D. (2014). The relationship between post-traumatic stress disorder and posttraumatic growth: Gender differences in PTG and PTSD subgroups. *Social Psychiatry and Psychiatric Epidemiology*, *49*(12), 1903–1910. 10.1007/s00127-014-0865-5

Juster, R. P., Bizik, G., Picard, M., Arsenault-Lapierre, G., Sindi, S., Trepanier, L., Marin, M. F., Wan, N., Sekerovic, Z., Lord, C., Fiocco, A. J., Plusquellec, P., McEwen, B. S., & Lupien, S. J. (2011). A transdisciplinary perspective of chronic stress in relation to psychopathology throughout life span development. *Development and Psychopathology*, *23*(3), 725–776. 10.1017/S0954579411000289

Juster, R. P., Pruessner, J. C., Desrochers, A. B., Bourdon, O., Durand, N., Wan, N., Tourjman, V., Kouassi, E., Lesage, A., & Lupien, S. J. (2016). Sex and gender roles in relation to mental health and allostatic load. *Psychosomatic Medicine*, *78*(7), 788–804. 10.1097/PSY.0000000000000351

Kira, I. A., Arıcı Özcan, N., Shuwiekh, H., Kucharska, J., Al-Huwailah, A. H., & Kanaan, A., (2020). The compelling dynamics of "will to exist, live, and survive" on effecting posttraumatic growth upon exposure to adversities: Is it mediated, in part, by emotional regulation, resilience, and spirituality? *Traumatology*, *26*(4), 405–419. 10.1037/trm0000263

Lucassen, P. J., Pruessner, J., Sousa, N., Almeida, O. F. X., Van Dam, A. M., Rajkowska, G., Swaab, D. F., & Czéh, B. (2014). Neuropathology of stress. *Acta Neuropathology*, *127*(1), 109–135. 10.1007/s00401-013-1223-5

Mayor, E. (2015). Gender roles and traits in stress and health. *Frontiers in Psychology*, *6*(JUN). 10.3389/FPSYG.2015.00779

Mehta, D., Miller, O., Bruenig, D., David, G., & Shakespeare-Finch, J. (2020). A systematic review of DNA methylation and gene expression studies in posttraumatic stress disorder, posttraumatic growth, and resilience. *Journal Traumatic Stress*, *33*(2), 171–180. 10.1002/jts.22472

Miller, M. W., Maniates, H., Wolf, E. J., Logue, M. W., Schichman, S. A., Stone, A., Milberg, W., & McGlinchey, R. (2017). CRP polymorphisms and DNA methylation of the AIM2 gene influence associations between trauma exposure, PTSD, and C-reactive protein. *Brain Behavior and Immunity*, *67*(Suppl. 1). 10.1016/j.bbi.2017.08.022

Morawetz, C., Bode, S., Baudewig, J., Kirilina, E., & Heekeren, H. R. (2016). Changes in effective connectivity between dorsal and ventral prefrontal regions moderate emotion regulation. *Cerebral Cortex*, *26*(5), 1923–1937. 10.1093/cercor/bhv005

Morris, B. A., & Shakespeare-Finch, J., (2011). Cancer diagnostic group differences in posttraumatic Growth: Accounting for age, gender, trauma severity, and distress. *Journal of Loss and Trauma*, *16*(3), 229–242. 10.1080/15325024.2010.519292

Nagaya, N., & Maren, S. (2015). Sex, steroids, and fear. *Biological Psychiatry*, *78*(3), 152–153. 10.1016/j.biopsych.2015.06.010

Nakagawa, S., Sugiura, M., Sekiguchi, A., Kotozaki, Y., Miyauchi, C. M., Hanawa, S., Araki, T., Takeuchi, H., Sakuma, A., Taki, Y., & Kawashima, R. (2016). Effects of post-traumatic growth on the dorsolateral prefrontal cortex after a disaster. *Scientific Reports*, *6*(1), 34364. 10.1038/srep34364

Nolen-Hoeksema, S., & Morrow, J. (1991). A prospective study of depression and posttraumatic stress symptoms after a natural disaster: The 1989 Loma Prieta Earthquake. *Journal of Personality and Social Psychology*, *61*(1), 115–121. 10.1037/0022-3514.61.1.115

Ogińska-Bulik, N. (2015). The relationship between resiliency and posttraumatic growth following the death of someone close. *OMEGA – Journal of Death Dying*, *71*(3), 233–244. 10.1177/0030222815575502

Ravi, M., Stevens, J. S., & Michopoulos, V. (2019). Neuroendocrine pathways underlying risk and resilience to PTSD in women. *Frontiers in Neuroendocrinology*, *55*, 100790. 10.1016/j.yfrne.2019.100790

Rogier, G., Garofalo, C., & Velotti, P. (2017). Is emotional suppression always bad? A matter of flexibility and gender differences. *Current Psychology*, *38*, 411–420. 10.1007/S12144-017-9623-7

Sayed, S., Iacoviello, B. M., & Charney, D. S. (2015). Risk factors for the development of psychopathology following trauma. *Current Psychiatry Reports*, *17*(10), 1–7. 10.1007/s11920-015-0612-y

Schubert, C. F., Schmidt, U., & Rosner, R. (2016). Posttraumatic growth in populations with posttraumatic stress disorder—A systematic review on growth-related psychological constructs and biological variables. *Clinical Psychology and Psychotherapy*, *23*(6), 469–486. 10.1002/CPP.1985

Shigemoto, Y., Banks, A., & Boxley, B. (2020). Gender differences in the interaction effect of community resources and attitudes toward seeking professional help on posttraumatic stress, depression, and posttraumatic growth. *Journal of Community Psychology*, *48*(3), 693–708. 10.1002/jcop.22287

Smith, J. M., & Alloy, L. B. (2009). A roadmap to rumination: A review of the definition, assessment, and conceptualization of this multifaceted construct. *Clinical Psychology Review*, *29*(2), 116–128. 10.1016/j.cpr.2008.10.003

Swickert, R. J., Hittner, J. B., & Foster, A. (2012). A proposed mediated path between gender and posttraumatic growth: The roles of empathy and social support in a mixed-age sample. *Scientific Research*, *3*(12A), 1142–1147. 10.4236/psych.2012.312A168

Taku, K., & Cann, A. (2014). Cross-national and religious relationships with posttraumatic growth: The role of individual differences and perceptions of the triggering event. *Journal of Cross-Cultural Psychology*, *45*(4), 601–617. 10.1177/0022022113520074

Taylor, S. E., Klein, L. C., Lewis, B. P., Gruenewald, T. L., Gurung, R. A. R., & Updegraff, J. (2000). Biobehavioral responses to stress in females: Tend-and-befriend, not fight-or-flight. *Psychological Review*, *107*(3), 411–429. 10.1037//0033-295X.107.3.411

Tedeschi, R. G., Shakespeare-Finch, J., Taku, K., & Calhoun, L. G. (2018). *Posttraumatic growth: Theory, research, and applications*. 10.4324/9781315527451

Tolin, D. F., & Foa, E. B. (2006). Sex differences in trauma and posttraumatic stress disorder: A quantitative review of 25 years of research. *Psychological Bulletin*, *132*(6), 959–992. 10.1037/0033-2909.132.6.959

Uhart, M., Chong, R. Y., Oswald, L., Lin, P.-I., & Wand, G. S. (2006). Gender differences in hypothalamic-pituitary-adrenal (HPA) axis reactivity. *Psychoneuroendocrinology*, *31*, 642–652. 10.1016/j.psyneuen.2006.02.003

Vishnevsky, T., Cann, A., Calhoun, L. G., Tedeschi, R. G., & Demakis, G. J. (2010). Gender differences in self-reported posttraumatic growth: A meta-analysis. *Psychology of Women Quarterly*, *34*(1), 110–120. 10.1111/j.1471-6402.2009.01546.x

Watkeys, O. J., Kremerskothen, K., Quidé, Y., Fullerton, J. M., & Green, M. J. (2018). Glucocorticoid receptor gene (NR3C1) DNA methylation in association with trauma, psychopathology, transcript expression, or genotypic variation: A systematic review. *Neuroscience & Biobehavioral Reviews*, *95*, 85–122. 10.1016/J.NEUBIOREV.2018.08.017

Wei, C., Han, J., Zhang, Y., Hannak, W., Dai, Y., & Liu, Z. (2017). Affective emotion increases heart rate variability and activates left dorsolateral prefrontal cortex in post-traumatic growth. *Scientific Reports*, *7*(1), 16667. 10.1038/s41598-017-16890-5

Wolfe, T., & Ray, S. (2015). The role of event centrality, coping and social support in resilience and posttraumatic growth among women and men. *International Journal of Mental Health Promotion*, *17*(2), 78–96. 10.1080/13642529.2015.1008799

Wozniak, J. D. S., Caudle, H. E., Harding, K., Vieselmeyer, J., & Mezulis, A. H. (2019). The effect of trauma proximity and ruminative response styles on posttraumatic stress and posttraumatic growth following a university shooting. *Psychological Trauma: Theory, Research, Practice, and Policy*, *12*(3), 227–234. 10.1037/tra0000505

6

PTG JOURNEY WITH HEIDEGGER'S "AUTHENTIC" SELF AND YUNUS EMRE'S "MISKIN" (FULFILLED/ GROUNDED) SELF

Pinar Dursun and Pinar Alyagut

Although not conceptualizing it as PTG, both the Turkish poet Yunus Emre and the German philosopher Martin Heidegger presented the idea that from the struggle with suffering, people can grow, i.e., achieve PTG.

Yunus Emre and the "Miskin" Self

Yunus Emre (Jonah) (1238–1328) was a distinguished Turkish folk poet and Sufi mystic who significantly influenced Turkish culture and was greatly appreciated due to his incredible talent, influence, and writing in spoken Turkish rather than Persian or Arabic (Özçelik, 2013).

Similar to his contemporaneous Rumi (1207–1273) and Ibn Muhiddin-i Arabi (1165–1240), Yunus Emre held a perspective of "the unity of existence" (*Wahdat-i vujud*). As far as is known, all his life, he produced two main works, i.e., *Risaletun Nushiyye* and *Divan* (Tatçı, 1990). In his poems, Yunus usually used a didactic method to call for people to wake up, remember and love their God (Başkal, 2004). He used humble and self-critic language such as *Poor Yunus*, *Dervish Yunus*, or *Miskin Yunus*, *Destitute*, or *Ignorant Yunus* to describe himself and the distress of his path, always emphasizing that he needs only God in every work or issue, and always presenting all his needs to God (Özçelik, 2013).

For Sufis, poetry is the main channel for expressing and inspiring ideas and feelings, facilitating the sensational experience such as visual and auditory imagination like *Sema* (mystic dance). With the sophisticated and enthusiastic language in his poems, many scholars agree that Yunus Emre acted as a spiritual counselor in the chaotic period he lived in due to continuous attacks by the Mongols, the Crusades, and several civil wars (Özçelik, 2013). With his inspiring expressions, he helped many traumatized people heal. He wandered across Anatolia, interacted with traumatized people and helped to make sense of traumatic events by providing support, offering acceptance and positive reinterpretation to reframe these events from a Sufism outlook.

 DOI: 10.4324/9781032208688-7

Sufism

At its deepest, Islam is a religion that teaches people how they can transform themselves and achieve harmony, which is the foundation of all existence. When activity, heart, and understanding are combined, this union brings goodness and excellence, which lies above all, in the original human disposition, i.e., the selves or souls (*nafs*) created in Allah's (God's) image (*fitrah*). God is viewed as one *(tawhid)*, and He is believed to have created human beings in His image by distributing His names, characters, and attributes in an infinite universe. The primary duty of a human being is to discover His reflection and actualize this latent divine attribution of character and eventually become united with God (Chittick, 2007; Schimmel, 1975, 2018a). This effort to become one with God is a continuum of degree rather than a dichotomic all-or-none process because, like breath (*nefes*), the self (*nafs*) is an entity that can grow, expand, weaken or decrease at any moment, depending on one's experience and relationship with God. The genuine Sufi is constantly aware of the importance of the moment and their own "no-self" position (Schimmel, 1975, 2018b), similar to mindfulness skills.

Sufism does not have a definite description even though it is used interchangeably with Tasawwuf (Arabic for equivalent), Islamic mysticism, esotericism, or spirituality. Scholars agree that Sufis (literally meaning "one who wears the wools") are the ones "to see the things with their hearts" rather than pure logic, thoughts, and behaviors. They emphasize opening or unveiling their hearts to establish a union with God via poetry, art, music, and dance to express divine love, compassion, mercy, beauty, kindness, and the immanence side of God. Nevertheless, some Sufi schools criticize this "drunken" style for losing the ability to prioritize the transcendence character of God, asserting more manners and rules followed by Sunnah and Sharia. Modern Sufis generally try to balance these two styles, indicating that God is both immanence and transcendence. Thus, Sufism contains all the principles of Islam, including the ways to God such as knowledge, activity, and love, and Sufis who adopt all styles emphasize the "love" part suggesting deepening the understanding, purifying the hearts, and doing what is beautiful.

The Miskin Self of Yunus Emre

The most famous expression of Yunus Emre is "Know Yourself," indicating that one should be self-aware to become fully aware of God. In Sufism, *Gnosis* refers to self-knowledge and God-knowledge (Chittick, 2007) or wisdom of the heart (Schimmel, 1975). The goal of gnostic Sufis is to remove inner barriers to the knowledge of God. The ultimate aim is to discover or actualize the true self (full actualization of self-knowledge) and experience the joy of being united with God. Yunus Emre stated in his poems that "Knowledge is knowing knowledge, and knowledge is but knowing oneself" (Balcı, 2018, p.28). This knowledge of self and God is already in people's hearts but it is hidden because of being forgotten or lost in daily life. Yunus Emre argued that ordinary life is full of egocentrism, hatred, resentment, arrogance, envy, or greed, "Arrogance is self, knows not the King, Eternally rebellious toward the King is the self" (Sezer, 1967, p.52) and "see those rich people, what happened to them all? Finally, they had to wear a sleeveless robe (i.e., are dead)" (Balcı, 2018, p.36). Because mortals are constructed by social classes, status, titles, or money, the real solution is to get rid of these "worldly" attitudes by killing the greedy self, as Yunus posits "Your self (nafs) is your enemy, kill (it), selves must always be dead" (Sezer, 1967, p.53). He further declared "I have been enveloped with flesh and bone and been seen as Yunus" (Balcı, 2018, p.18), indicating a body is just the guest of the soul/self (Kaval, 2013).

According to Yunus Emre, a human being is a guest, seeker, or traveler in this temporary world, and eventually is condemned to go to his real home, i.e., the home of God. He emphasizes that "I have no intention [of staying] in this world, I have come here in order to go, changing my duality, I came in order to arrive at oneness" (Sezer, 1967, p.29), or "Come to this lifeless door that you may find an everlasting life" (p.38).

Since the ultimate aim is to become engaged with God entirely or to the degree possible, the process of seeking never ends. Every traveler is allowed to stop wherever he wants or is capable of since all travelers do not carry the exact character of God's names and attributions. Nevertheless, Yunus Emre did not explain Miskin's stage in the Sufi path, perhaps due to his modesty reflected in his calling himself *Miskin,* referring to one full of divine love and grounded, fulfilled, or peaceful self. Nevertheless, like a breath, the self is temporary; *Miskin self* is the one who succeeds in entering this path and keeps walking on the challenging and long road; i.e., like PTG, *Miskin self* can refer to both process, a long-term effort and an outcome.

The Miskin Self and PTG

To understand the relationship between PTG and the perspective of Yunus Emre, it is important to understand the conceptualization of self (*nafs*) in Sufi philosophy. Rather than stable concepts, Sufism views the self and soul as constantly changing because every choice or decision makes the self grow and ascend or shrink and descend like climbing or falling off a ladder. The Qur'an does not ascribe to the self-inherited qualities of good or evil, but views it as needing to be nurtured, cultivated, and self-regulated through thoughts, emotions, and primarily actions, in order to become "good" and "meaningful" (Schimmel, 1975). Specifically, with free will, people become a new self with decisions they make at every moment, and cannot foresee what they will be and into what kind of self they turn at the end. One has to face one's unknown and dimensions of self at every moment and the self needs to be continuously trained and retrained. This training process is only possible with the deconstruction of an old self and the cultivation or purification of a new self. Because human beings have the potential to be higher beings than angels or lower creatures than animals or monsters via their conscious choices, this authentic path is called in Sufism *Seyru Suluk* on which Yunus Emre succeeded in walking as a *Miskin.*

There are at least seven stages or degrees for the self (*maqam*) in this *seyru suluk* process of which three are crucial turning points. The first self called "*nafs-i emmare,* (the inciting self)" is the lowest, narcissistic, darkest, evil, or animal-driven, most primitive or inauthentic one that includes all the possessive, ambitious, addictive, and egocentric motives and feelings such as pride, greed, jealousy, lust, stinginess, malice, and backbiting. The next stage and essential turning point is the *nafs-i levvame,* which refers to questioning, criticizing, or condemning one's self, especially the materialistic self. At this stage, self-awareness, conscience, and mindfulness skills are developed or awakened. After this second critical point, a self can get inspiration from God and start to ascend gradually with continuous efforts such as prayer, faith, love, and awareness of God to the highest, authentic, and most harmonic with nature self and be at peace with God (*nafs-i mutmaine*). These stages continue until the self transforms into "selflessness" (*tazkiyat an-nafs*), which refers to the stage of *Insan-i Kamil,* or *Fanafillah,* i.e., union, absorbing into or disappearing in God (Schimmel, 1975). Yunus Emre described this path as the death of an animal or evil part inside a human, "they announce that Lover died, He who dies is animal, Lovers die not" (Sezer, 1967, p.90).

Hence, the Sufi path is an authentic journey similar to the PTG process that can be a gate to leave the primitive or inauthentic self (*nafs-i emmare)* via self-critic and self-awareness stage (*nafs-i levvame*). Like PTG enables opening to construct new selves, Yunus Emre defined this process as *re-birth, suggesting* that "each moment, we are born anew, who could satiate with us" (Sezer, 1967, p.25).

Sufism, including Yunus Emre, assigns to a traumatic event different meanings than modern psychology does. Rather than punishments and misfortunes, traumatic events are seen as a gift from God, offering an opportunity for care and purification, a possibility for change and growth. Thus, even when a person is in great distress and experiences tremendous pain, it is a test of his ability to grow and elevate. Because God only tests his beloved servants, a traumatic event is a form of God's love, care, and concern for His servants for their ascendings. Accordingly, Yunus Emre said "I had been sighing from Affliction, I found that my affliction was itself my remedy" (Balcı, 2018, p.61). This reframing of traumatic events instills hope for the survivors and facilitates the widening of the new narratives.

Psychological traumas are viewed as God-given events that can trigger the spiritual journey in which the self must be purified and cultivated to become a *Miskin self*. These events are opportunities for being tested to determine which stage a self can reach. Hence, one can infer that from the perspectives of Yunus Emre, when a traumatic event happens, the narcissistic, primitive, or inauthentic self (*nafs-i emmare*) is broken by the seismic effect of the event. Because of having a narcissistic or inauthentic self, one cannot believe what happened. The narcissistic self feels shocked, upset, finally opening, awakening, and questioning their daily lost life. Yunus Emre defined this shock as gaining sobriety and awakening via unveiling and purifying the heart, "I did away with my I-ness (myself), I opened the veil of my eyes, I reached the Friend [God], let my doubts be sacked, My I-ness moved out of me and all my existence the Friend invaded" (Sezer, 1967, p.43).

Similar to the PTG process, this path can be painful. Yunus Emre characterized this struggle as drinking poison, "Putting aside the Sharbat (soft drink), he should drink poison, he should be disciplined, should abandon all that he knows, let him abandon his form, he should forget what he knows" (Sezer, 1967, p.66). One needs to examine everything, including himself, "I assumed the title of *Miskin*, I am decked with the attire of the dervish, I looked at the road [examined myself], I was ashamed, all I did is wrong" (Sezer, 1967, p.26). This resonates with the need for deliberate rumination using self-disclosure, self-analysis, and social support in the PTG model (Dursun & Söylemez, 2020; Tedeschi et al., 2018).

At this point of self-transformation, Yunus Emre recommended in his poems hope, faith, love, patience, forgiveness, and continuous religious practices with trustworthy guidance from his master Tapduk. Yunus Emre himself completed many stages as a *Miskin* with the help of writing poems, the themes and metaphoric meanings of which vary, reflecting his multiple stages on the Sufi path. Yunus Emre's own ascension agrees with the importance of self-disclosure in the PTG model.

Yunus Emre believed that a purified heart filled with true divine love is the only medium to relieve the spiritual pain of the journey. In his poems, he was screaming his divine love after giving up materialistic love and life, "O, wine-offerer bring that cup [of wine] that drinking we be drunk; Annihilate us with love that we be existent" (Sezer, 1967, p.31); "Your love has intoxicated me, I am in need of You; I am burning night and day, I am in need of You (Balcı, 2018, p.25), and "My self has been annihilated; All my possessions by the Friend [God] are owned/I have become placeless/Let my place be plundered now" (Balcı, 2018, p.33).

In addition to divine love, to purify the heart, Yunus Emre strongly recommended forgiveness, solidarity, tolerance, and having faith in God and His order rather than "dark" feelings of revenge, anger, or hatred, (Kaval, 2013), "We pray even to those who are hostile to us" (Tatçı, 1990, p.307); "We love the created, because of the Creator" (Sezer, 1967, p.94).

The aforementioned spiritual self-transformation is challenging as Yunus Emre stated, "These sons of self are nine persons; Hypocrisy and polytheism are their task" (Sezer, 1967, p.52) and "This way is too long; it has many way-stations; and there are impassable; deep waters on its path" (Balcı, 2018, p.128). Similar to the expert companionship in the PTG model, an empathic friend, companion, or guide is critical. For Yunus Emre, this was Tapduk, his master, teacher, and dedicated support, for whom he always announced his respect and love, "We are in the presence of Tapduk; As servants at his door; O poor Yunus once raw; Now you are cooked-praise to be God" (Balcı, 2018, p.56). Tapduk provided guidance to different dervishes individually or in a group. Indeed, the gathering of friends (*Sohbet*) is essential to Dervish culture as Yunus Emre stated, "In sohbet, Let Yunus always be remembered" (Balcı, 2018, p.103). Similar to group therapy, in these groups, dervishes can get support from each other or from their masters when they feel confused or would like to share. This togetherness can help to accept the stressor event, expand coping strategies, change the narratives, and increase wisdom as an outcome parallel to PTG.

In sum, both the *Seyru Suluk* and PTG represent one's processing of their experiences to reach a grounded, calm, or fulfill selfves and use social support in the struggle to help in the journey.

Heidegger's Authentic Self

German philosopher Martin Heidegger (1889–1976) was a radical thinker who, despite his ambivalent political affinity and relationship with Hannah Arendt, provided a point of reference for many existential philosophers in the twentieth century and postmodern approaches. Heidegger first studied theology at the University of Freiburg and later turned to studying philosophy. His work reflects ideas from the theological school and from the views of the German poet Hölderlin, of whom he was a big admirer. The ontological foundation of Descartes's cogito ergo sum, i.e., I think therefore I am has been deconstructed by Heidegger and his followers, and a new paradigm has emerged: I am therefore I think (Bracken, 2002). This non-Cartesian approach offers a different perspective for comprehending the influence of trauma since traumatic events can transform people's caring styles or relational modes with the self, the environment, and the world. Even though Heidegger never mentioned the word "trauma" or "posttraumatic stress" in his famous 1927 book *Being and Time, h*is definition of anxiety (angst) seems to have a similar meaning and impact (Bracken, 2002; Stolorow, 2011). To understand his perspective on the relationship between anxiety, posttraumatic stress, and authenticity, it is important to discuss Heidegger's basic philosophical arguments and distinct terminology.

Dasein: The Human Self

In his seminal book *Being and Time*, Heidegger (1953) described a human being or the self as *Dasein* (i.e., to-be-there). Dasein is an entity or a being capable of questioning its own self and being open to all changes and possibilities, including growth (Haugeland, 2005; Sheehan, 2001). This self must establish a daily routine and worldly relations to survive and needs to realize its own meaning (because it has the capacity to search for meaning in life) through relating to others, *being with* them, and *taking care of* the world, conceptualized as *being-in-the-world* (Dreyfus, 1990; Vallega-Neu, 2003). For Heidegger, Dasein practically inhabits and starts to display in everyday activities within a network of intelligibility totality of involvements with being in the world; thus, the world opens itself to Dasein as a pre-reflective, pre-conscious, pre-ontological, and meaningful but inauthentic way (Heidegger, 1993). Dasein engages with "worldliness" through encountering a particular awareness of space and time. For Heidegger, unlike Cartesian Cognito, time is not linear or a collection of a series of moments in which past (throwness, humans' individual existences as being 'thrown' into the world), present (fallenness, being degraded), and future subsequently flow.

Dasein can lose its own self to the public self, i.e., the "they" (Heidegger, 1993), which can be manifested by *idle* (i.e., lazy and shallow) *talk*, *curiosity* (constant novelty-seeking), and *ambiguity* (inability to show sensitivity to anything). This over-involvement of Dasein with "the they" and the being of everydayness (i.e., everyone is the other and no one is himself) refers to the *inauthentic* mode or *unownedness* of Dasein. According to Heidegger (1953), the inauthenticity of Dasein does not signify a "lesser" being or a "lower" degree of being. Authenticity and non-authenticity refer to two modes of being, with a different emphasis on the degree of "mine-ness" or "essence." While some people can remain inauthentic and never transform into an authentic version of themselves, Dasein's ultimate aim or destiny is to find meaning in its own potential being, true nature, and authentic self (Dreyfus, 1990).

To explain the entangled inauthentic relationship of Dasein to its world, Heidegger (1953, 1993) used a metaphor of the skilled carpenter who keeps working every day and does not consciously recognize the tools such as hammer, nail, or workbench he is using in his routine working day or question what he is really doing until he is distracted and the tools he uses automatically become phenomenologically transparent to him. Similarly, the world is "ready-to-hand" for this Dasein that is a skilled problem-solver to restore smoothness or disruptions (Schalow & Denker, 2010). Dasein attempts to preserve or protect its routineness and inauthentic way of being under all circumstances until a shocking trauma or *angst* happens.

Posttraumatic Stress, Authentic Self, and PTG

Heidegger (1953) *argued that anxiety (angst)* originates from the Dasein of which it has always been a part that was latent. When Dasein realizes the inevitability of death for everyone, including itself, it becomes enormously anxious. This anxiety as defined by Heidegger is similar to posttraumatic stress that leads to feelings of "indefiniteness," "groundlessness," or "unhomelike" (Bracken, 2002, p.136), "not-being-at-home" or "nothing and nowhere" (Heidegger, 1953, p.176) as if the world splits and time freezes. With the loss of the referential system and disruption in time perception, Dasein becomes silent, loses its connection with "regular" life, and feels lonely although it remains surrounded by "the they." Consequently, Dasein begins to self-question who it is and where it belongs; it also explores the possibility of its non-being and of coming into its own and re-consider the possibility of its "not-fallen" mode into everydayness. Thus, Dasein starts to individualize.

However, it is challenging for Dasein to decide "who," "what," or "which Dasein" it should be as it had adjusted and was lost in "the they" since birth (Reuther, 2014). Dasein ought to find a way to solve this dilemma, either by choosing to remain an inauthentic way of being or by allowing itself to transform into an *authentic* being while resolutely anticipating its reality of death and the responsibility of living. Since inauthentic, pre-ontological, pre-reflective Dasein becomes dysfunctional, Dasein must first overcome the feeling of alienation and start over, such as finding something or someone to re-attach and re-socialize with, like re-birth and re-grow oneself. Thus, death anxiety helps individualize Dasein to reach its *authentic* self (Bracken, 2002; Stolorow, 2011).

Authenticity and the PTG Model

Heidegger (1993) argued that rather than found outside himself, a person builds or rebuilds meaning continuously through mental structures such as assumptions, beliefs, and core schemas. When a traumatic event occurs, it is not the person's mental meaning system that is broken; rather, traumatized individuals "jump" into a different version of reality and temporality, time perception changes, and future, past, and present become entangled, or united as anxiety or traumatic stress ruptures the entire ontology and Dasein is initiated into authenticity.

The authenticity path is challenging, similar to the PTG process. It requires a considerable psychological effort of Dasein to find resoluteness and adapt to the new model of caring for the world, its own new self, and future projections. Because Dasein does not know clearly what it could become, it is reasonable to infer that the process of authenticity is similar to intrusive and deliberate rumination in PTG. This process consists mainly of self-awareness, self-examination, or self-criticism, an effort to make accurate decisions through listening to one's conscience and being open to all possibilities of oneself, accepting the reality of death for everyone and self.

In the rumination stages, Dasein needs to examine its own old versions and relational modes (i.e., being lost in "the they") from past (throwness) and present (fallenness) times and modify them. Dasein should finally notice that it has free will to choose what kind it will be and how to respond to any self-calls. Additionally, an authentic being should confront existential anxiety with resoluteness and anticipate the indefiniteness of being mortal. This openness, tolerance of uncertainty, and flexibility are essential to expanding new narratives or authentic selves. With this maturity and wisdom, Dasein should be ready to "make possible, first and foremost choices for its authentic potentiality-of-being and project itself essentially upon possibilities" (Heidegger, 1953, p.248). While Dasein should make appropriate choices, according to Heidegger, these should not be conscious cognitive decisions as in the Cartesian view; Dasein should make the "right" but not "rational" choices. Even though Heidegger did not explain what the "right choices" are or how they function, he stated that through a *call of conscience* and *existential guilt*, Dasein needs to focus on its inner voice rather than listening to the external sound of "the they." Dasein was once entangled with "being-with-others" and surrounded by the noise of "the they"; if it succeeds in silencing this surrounding discourse, it can finally hear its own voice, namely its conscience and guilt and for the first time, be available to answer the calls of its true self. This self-focus provides the opportunity for own actions and decisions.

Heidegger emphasized the loneliness of Dasein in reaching its own deepness, rather than proximate cultural factors such as a social network or support described in the PTG process. Instead, he argued that an inauthentic self has already had surroundings and now it is the time to listen only to itself and make decisions with his heart. This over-emphasis on loneliness may be due to the fascist environment in which Heidegger lived. Nevertheless, an authentic self is not "a state detached from the they" (p.122) or refers to an isolated being, as it requires a harmonic ability to establish new interactions with others in different ways without a threat of losing the self for the sake of "they-self." Authenticity requires a balance among dilemmas related to the past (throwness), presence (falling/worldliness), and future (death anxiety). Dasein needs to integrate the characteristics of temporality, be open to all possibilities of itself, and learn to relate to the world with a new caring style, including the voice of conscience and existential guilt while facing the indefinite certainty of death.

Thus, anxiety, particularly related to death, offers Dasein an opportunity to transform its authentic being in a new relational context. Similar to PTG, this unique self-transformation is not an all-or-none process; rather it is a matter of degrees. In each traumatic experience, one can gradually feel less overwhelmed and dissociative, and thus more bearable, fulfilled, and integrated with the world, leading to disclosure and being open to many projections and possibilities of his existences, i.e., the authentic self.

Summary and Conclusion

Similar to the PTG process, several Western and Eastern mythological, literature, theological, and philosophical sources suggested that shattering traumatic events could lead to a path that becomes an ascending experience if one contextualizes these traumas and integrates them into a new self. The Sufi tradition of Yunus Emre and Heidegger's phenomenological approach manifest common themes related to this process. Both saw life as a difficult journey that offers the possibility to become an *authentic* or *miskin* self if one succeeds in making certain sacrifices. At birth, all people have a raw, egocentric, pre-reflective version of themselves, then gradually adapting to "worldly" habits and practices without knowing their true self and denying their essence, i.e., their primitive or inauthentic self (*nafs-i emmare*). For Heidegger, change starts when a person encounters the reality of death and the resulting anxiety enlightens, individualizes, and liberates him. Like trauma, anxiety shatters intertwined relationships, resulting in singularity and desperation. If the person can review his past, listen to himself, especially to his conscience, and take responsibility for his actions with resoluteness while accepting the indefiniteness of death, he has an opportunity to reach the highest possibilities of himself, his authentic self. Similarly, for Yunus Emre, life is characterized by many challenges because God constantly tests His servants, primarily the beloved ones to see their ascending potential, including following traumatic events. It is expected that with self-knowledge and self-examination, everyone rises as high as his potential allows and attempts to leave his basic, arrogant, and primitive self with a purified heart full of divine love. This gradual purification effort that leads to the grounded, calm, or fulfilled self is the *Miskin* self.

Traumatic experiences are painful and no one wants to undergo them, even if it helps lead to wisdom and maturity. Nevertheless, when these traumatic experiences are well processed and reframed, a new understanding as in the PTG process, can offer an opportunity for a person to reach their newly fulfilled self with an entirely different vision and outlook for life. Yunus Emre, one of the greatest Sufi figures, characterized this change as a Miskin self-having the wisdom of the heart with the help of divine love; Heidegger argued that the authentic self includes a discovery of essence or mine-ness in one's existence with anticipatory resoluteness.

References

Balcı, E. (2018). *Journey to the Beloved: Sufi poems by Yunus Emre*. Kopernik Yayınları.

Başkal, Z. (2004). *Claiming Yunus Emre: Historical contexts and the politics of reception* (Unpublished dissertation). Languages and Cultures of Asia, University of Wisconsin, Madison. 3128100

Bracken, P. (2002). *Trauma: Culture, meaning and philosophy*. London: Whurr Publishers.

Chittick, W. C. (2007). *Sufism: A beginner's guide*. London: Oneworld publications.

Dreyfus, H. L. (1990). *Being-in-the-world: A commentary on Heidegger's being and time*. Cambridge: MIT Press.

Dursun, P., & Söylemez, İ. (2020). Posttraumatic growth: A comprehensive evaluation of the recently revised model. *Turkish Journal of Psychiatry*, *31*(1), 59–69. 10.5080/u23694

Haugeland, J. (2005). Reading Brandom reading Heidegger. *European Journal of Philosophy*, *13*(3), 421–428. 10.1111/j.1468-0378.2005.00237.xCitati

Heidegger, M. (1953). *Being and time*. (Ed. D. Schmidt; Trans. by J. Stambaugh). SUNY series in contemporary continental philosophy. State University of New York Press.

Heidegger, M. (1993). *Basic writings: Ten key essays, plus the introduction to being and time*. New York: Harper Press.

Kaval, M. (2013). Yunus Emre ve Mevlâna'nın eserlerinde insan ve tekâmülü. [Human and his evaluation in Yunus Emre's and Rumi's works of art]. *Uşak Üniversitesi Sosyal Bilimler Dergisi*, *6*(2), 101–122.

Özçelik, M. (2013). *Bizim Yunus*. [Our Yunus]. Nar Yayıncılık.

Reuther, B. T. (2014). On our everyday being: Heidegger and attachment theory. *Journal of Theoretical and Philosophical Psychology*, *34*(2), 101–115. 10.1037/a0033040

Schalow, F., & Denker, A. (2010). *Historical dictionary of Heidegger's philosophy*. Lanham, MD: The Scarecrow Press.

Schimmel, A. (1975). *Mystical dimensions of Islam*. University of North Carolina Press.

Schimmel, A. (2018a). *Tasavvuf Notları*. [Tasawwuf notes] (Translated by D. Yabul). Sufi Yayıncılık.

Schimmel, A. (2018b). *İslamın Mistik Boyutları* [Mystical dimensions of Islam] (Translated by E. Kocabıyık). Alfa Yayıncılık.

Sezer, R. A. (1967). *A concept of love in Yunus Emre's thoughts*. (Unpublished dissertation). Montreal, Canada: McGill University, Institute of Islamic Studies.

Sheehan, T. A. (2001). A paradigm shift in Heidegger research. *Continental Philosophy Review*, *34*(2), 183–202. 10.1023/A:1017568025461

Stolorow, R. D. (2011). *World, affectivity, trauma: Heidegger and post-Cartesianpsychoanalysis*. New York: Routledge.

Tatçı, M. (1990). *Yunus Emre Divanı* [Divan of Yunus Emre]. Kültür Bakanlığı Yayınları.

Tedeschi, R. G., Shakespeare-Finch, J., Taku, K., & Calhoun, L. G. (2018). *Posttraumatic growth: Theory, research, and applications*. NY and London: Routledge.

Vallega-Neu, D. (2003). *Heidegger's contributions to philosophy: An introduction*. Bloomington, Indiana: Indiana University Press.

7
POSTTRAUMATIC GROWTH AND RESILIENCE

Taylor Elam, Colin O'Brien, and Kanako Taku

Resilience: Background and Definitions

The concept of resilience originated in the early 1970s when trying to understand how ecological systems are able to withstand disastrous events (Holling, 1973). This quickly intrigued researchers from other disciplines, such as psychology and psychiatry, to study this phenomenon and apply it to early childhood development (Masten & Garmezy, 1985; Rutter, 1979; Werner & Smith, 1977; Werner et al., 1971). Early studies focused on understanding how children and adolescents who experienced prolonged adversities were able to maintain an average or above average level in educational competence, psychological health and relationships, job performance, and various other domains (DiRago & Vaillant, 2007; Gralinski-Bakker et al., 2004; Sampson & Laub, 1992; Vaillant & Davis, 2000). For example, Werner (2000, 2002) conducted multiple longitudinal studies on school-aged children of various races and ethnicities who had been experiencing several psychological and social risk factors including chronic poverty, living in a negative neighborhood environment, exposure to child abuse, chronic familial conflict, and discordance, having parents with mental illnesses or struggling with substance abuse, and having experienced parental divorce. She found that these at-risk children utilized external sources of support to adapt to their circumstances and exhibited inner protective factors, such as being intellectually competent, having an internal locus of control, a positive self-concept, an ability to plan ahead, and an optimistic personality with a good sense of humor – in other words, resilience.

Today, definitions of resilience vary. One definition focuses on a dynamic process that explains the development of positively adapting and maintaining one's psychological health after facing adversity (Egeland et al., 1993; Norris et al., 2008). Another definition refers to a positive outcome following adversity or stressful life experiences that lead to varying benefits (e.g., Bonanno, 2004; Masten, 2007; Norris et al., 2008; Rutter, 2000). Yet others consider resilience to be an aspect of one's personality or a characteristic, such as trait resilience or ego-resilience (Block, 2002; Block & Turula, 1963; Connor & Davidson, 2003; Ong et al., 2006; Smith et al., 2008; Wagnild & Young, 1993), or an all-encompassing cluster of resources, characteristics, and capacities that allow for swift recovery during hard times (Aldrich, 2012; Norris et al., 2008). Overall, resilience can be

DOI: 10.4324/9781032208688-8

understood as the dynamic processes, traits, and outcomes involved in recovering from traumatic or stressful chronic or acute life events, experienced by an individual or in the context of families, organizations, societies, and cultures (Bonanno & Diminich, 2013; Oshio et al., 2018; Southwick et al., 2014).

One main distinction between PTG and resilience is that resilience explains *adaptation* and *adjustment* with or without experiencing psychological struggle in the face of adversity (i.e., "bouncing back"), whereas PTG focuses on *advancement* or *growth* as a result of experiencing psychological struggle due to one's core values being shaken following significant trauma or stressful life events.

The Relationship between PTG and Resilience

While PTG has received less attention than resilience in literature, the two constructs are often confused with, compared to, or mentioned alongside each other. Depending on how each construct is defined operationally, both PTG and resilience often involve dynamic processes that share positive post-trauma outcomes. However, despite their similarities, PTG and resilience are markedly different constructs that should not be conflated.

The relationship between PTG and resilience has been analyzed, but the results are equivocal. Some studies have found a positive relationship between PTG and resilience, implying that the more PTG someone has experienced, the more resilient they are and vice versa (Bensimon, 2012; Duan et al., 2015; Ikizer & Ozel, 2021; Yu et al., 2014). This could mean that the individual characteristics that aid in the ability to recover from adversity may also help promote growth. It is also plausible that an experience of PTG can make people more resilient or that other characteristics, such as extraversion, may explain why resilience and PTG are sometimes positively correlated since they have both been found to be positively associated with this specific trait (Balgiu, 2017; Fayombo, 2010; Jia et al., 2015; Panjikidze et al., 2020).

On the other hand, at least two studies have found a negative relationship between PTG and resilience (Levine et al., 2009; Zerach et al., 2013), implying that these psychological constructs are inversely related. It is possible that highly resilient people are less influenced by "traumatic" experiences, and therefore, their need for growth is withheld, perhaps due to a ceiling effect (Taku et al., 2018). An experience of PTG may also influence one's self-perceptions and cause the realization that a human can be vulnerable and acceptance of needing help, which, in turn, may make the individual more aware and willing to admit that they are not highly resilient. Alternatively, sorrow or deep pain caused by a triggering event may lead people to experience PTG concurrently with a decline in resilience.

Although several studies have found no linear relationship between PTG and resilience (e.g., DeViva et al., 2016; Vieselmeyer et al., 2017), some researchers have found a curvilinear relationship (Kaye-Tzadok & Davidson-Arad, 2016; Li et al., 2015). These findings suggest the possibility of a threshold, or "tipping point," in the relationship between PTG and resilience, i.e., that resilience and PTG show a positive relationship up to a certain point, at which the individual becomes too resilient to experience growth or be influenced by traumatic events, perhaps explaining why results in literature have been equivocal.

Nonetheless, literature has sufficiently demonstrated that PTG and resilience are different. Distinguishing the specific ways in which they are different from one another will help clarify them, as well as aid in the improvement of education about them and subsequently improve intervention programs aimed at fostering PTG and/or resilience on a clinical level.

PTG and Resilience: Empirical Findings Regarding Similarities and Differences

Conceptually, PTG is a process that involves rumination and reflection upon the shattering of one's core beliefs that provokes an individual to reshape the way in which they perceive themselves, their lives, and their world. This process requires a change of outlook on both internal and external factors. Similarly, resilience involves undergoing an internal process, using certain characteristics (e.g., flexibility, optimism, adaptive coping strategies, and self-esteem) and/or external resources (e.g., social support, environment) in order to readily adjust to distressful circumstances. However, the experience of a life crisis that is impactful enough to shake one's core beliefs is irrelevant to resilience due to its flexible nature. Furthermore, unlike PTG, being or becoming more resilient does not involve a transformational change in perception. It was hypothesized early on that there is a need to assess whether there is a capacity or threshold associated with the construct of resilience over the lifespan that "caps" one's ability to continue to adapt, adjust, or be influenced by change (Staudinger et al., 1993; Werner, 2005).

Therefore, the primary difference between PTG and resilience is that PTG requires transformational changes, whereas resilience involves adaptive processes. Additionally, resilience does not require the experience of the seismic events that challenge one's worldview that engender PTG. To enhance the understanding of PTG versus resilience, the authors conducted two studies that examined PTG and resilience as they relate to emotion recognition ability and empathy, as well as to attitudes toward mental disorders.

Emotion Recognition Ability and Empathy

Empathy and emotion recognition ability have been utilized to demonstrate empirical differences between PTG and resilience by displaying the intra- and inter-personal nature of PTG vs. the intrapersonal nature of resilience. The authors of this chapter investigated the relationship between PTG, resilience, empathy, and emotion recognition ability (ERA) in 420 undergraduate students at a Midwestern university in the US (mean age of 21.04 years; SD = 5.15) and expected that the patterns of the relationships with empathy and ERA would differ between PTG and resilience (Elam & Taku, 2022). Participants were first asked to identify emotions based on photographs of facial expressions (JACFEE; Ekman & Matsumoto, 1993; Matsumoto & Ekman, 1988) and then to complete a questionnaire to assess their level of emotional empathy (Questionnaire of Emotional Empathy; QMEE; Mehrabian & Epstein, 1972), report if they experienced a potentially traumatic event (Taku, 2011, 2013), and complete measures evaluating levels of PTG (PTGI-SF; Cann et al., 2010) and resilience (Brief Resilience Scale; BRS; Smith et al., 2008).

The results showed a weak, positive relationship between PTG and resilience such that the more PTG was reported by individuals following their most impactful traumatic event, the more resilient they were, and vice versa. On the other hand, emotional empathy was not related to PTG and negatively associated with resilience, indicating that the more empathetic the individuals were, the less they demonstrated resilient characteristics. Regarding emotion recognition ability, because on average the majority of participants were good at recognizing emotions, two groups were created representing high and low emotion recognition ability (ERA-high and ERA-low respectively). Higher perceived PTG was more likely to be associated with high ERA, but such relationships were not found between resilience and ERA groups, suggesting that higher PTG, but not higher resilience, is more likely to be connected with increased emotion recognition.

These findings demonstrate that PTG and resilience have different associations with constructs related to interpersonal aspects such as empathy and the cognitive ability to "read" others' emotions. People who have experienced PTG may be better able to recognize facial expressions potentially as a result of the psychological struggle they have experienced as well as positive changes following their struggle with trauma, such as appreciating life, having more compassion, being able to do better things in life, and/or the ability to understand how others feel. On the other hand, highly resilient individuals may rate themselves as less empathetic – not necessarily making them depreciate the cognitive ability that aids in their perception of people, but perhaps decreasing their susceptibility to being impacted or influenced by the emotional states of others.

Attitudes Toward Mental Disorders

A second study investigated the differences between PTG and resilience in regard to one's perceptions of and attitudes toward mental disorders, particularly depression (O'Brien & Taku, 2022). Two subtypes of depression were analyzed: traditional-type depression (TTD) and modern-type depression (MTD). Although these two depression subtypes are still understudied in most Western cultures, both have been recognized specifically in Japan and the United States (Kashihara et al., 2019; Kato et al., 2011).

TTD is known as the "typical" type of depression associated with melancholic feelings and symptoms of anxiety, mood swings, poor sleeping habits, and a loss of interest in daily activities and responsibilities. In the workplace, those who suffer from TTD are often perceived as being loyal and diligent due to trying not to inconvenience or cause any trouble to their colleagues. These individuals often prefer forgoing diagnosis and finding solutions independently rather than seeking professional help, as well as often blaming their inner characteristics (Kato et al., 2016; Sakamoto et al., 2016).

On the other hand, those who suffer from MTD have difficulty carrying out their work-related tasks and responsibilities but are reprieved of their negative psychological symptoms during leisure time. They put less effort into their work, are less concerned about helping their coworkers, and are reluctant to follow social norms. They are also readily accepting of a diagnosis for their depression or may self-diagnose. Due to these factors, their colleagues often perceive them as selfish, and their depression and symptoms as illegitimate, even though they suffer from the same degree of symptoms (Kato et al., 2016; Sakamoto et al., 2016).

The researchers hypothesized that individuals with high levels of PTG would show more understanding attitudes toward both types of depression (e.g., that the cause must be lack of support), whereas those with high levels of resilience would look at internal causal attribution, such as taking individual responsibility (e.g., that the cause must be lack of motivation), and show different attitudes toward each type of depression (e.g., more negative view for MTD because they put less effort into work).

A sample of 300 college students at a Midwestern university completed a survey that assessed their perceived PTG (PTGI-SF; Cann et al., 2010) and resilience (Brief Resilience Scale; BRS; Smith et al., 2008). The participants were also asked to read stories describing an individual with either traditional-type or modern-type depression and report their reactions to the stories. Overall, the results showed differences in perceptions and attitudes associated with the levels of PTG and resilience. Participants who were high in resilience were less likely to relate to the depressed individuals or found them less familiar, especially those with MTD. Highly resilient individuals were more likely to attribute the cause of depression to lack of effort and were less likely to think that therapy and pharmacotherapy would serve as effective treatments. On the other hand, those who exhibited high PTG showed high familiarity with the TTD and MTD individuals, and, unlike the highly resilient individuals, were more likely to attribute the cause of depression to external factors, such as lack of support. They also were more willing to support those suffering from TTD or MTD.

In sum, these findings demonstrate that the nature of resilience is mainly intrapersonal, focusing more on development within the individual, while the nature of PTG can be both intra- and inter-personal, focusing both on development within the individual and within relationships and communication with others. As such the findings suggest that interpersonal development may be less relevant to resilience but more relevant to PTG following adversity.

Resilience and PTG Intervention Programs: Benefits and Challenges

Resilience intervention programs have existed since the late 1970s and have continued to develop over time (Luthar et al., 2000). Forbes and Fikretoglu (2018) reviewed 92 articles to conduct an analysis of resilience interventions. Although programs took slightly different approaches and spent varying amounts of time on certain tasks, all programs began with some form of psychoeducation where participants had an opportunity to learn about trauma, stress, mental health, and well-being. The programs also taught coping skills or relaxation techniques such as positive self-talk, cognitive restructuring, goal-setting, and arousal regulation. Some of the interventions focused specifically on a technique known as an "inoculation intervention" where participants are asked to focus on practicing the skills they have learned and acquired throughout the program while in the presence of images of stressful or traumatic situations that one may experience in the real world (Andersen et al., 2015; Arnetz et al., 2008; Sarason et al., 1979).

Almost all intervention programs (90%) took place over multiple sessions and identified a theoretical basis. About 22% were based on Cognitive Behavioral Theory (CBT), 16.1% on resilience theory, 16.1% on stress management theory, and 11.8% on mindfulness theory; the remaining programs used previous research to support their intervention activities. The majority of the intervention studies measured resilience by accounting for a change in protective factors (such as self-esteem and social support), which was thought to lead to an improvement in well-being. Although studies varied in their subject populations, methodology, and outcome measures, all the programs were found to be effective in increasing the protective factors associated with resilience and there were consistent increases in self-reported well-being or health across all studies.

However, the aforementioned intervention studies may have some limitations. The majority of the programs consisted of psychologically healthy individuals (83%) who were not currently undergoing disruptive circumstances, partly because resilience programs are often designed as part of life skills training programs rather than a part of treatment for those who experienced trauma and struggle with symptoms. Even though resilience training programs promote improvement in protective factors, it is difficult to know whether these factors or skills will take effect when a traumatic experience occurs. To expand programs to be more comprehensive rather than just assisting people to be more resilient, the aforementioned findings that showed distinctions between PTG and resilience could imply that it would be beneficial for programs to include interpersonal components to foster empathy and cultivate understanding toward those who are struggling, which does not seem to be the focus of highly resilient individuals.

PTG intervention programs have also been introduced, refined, and developed (Roepke, 2015). For example, Ramos et al. (2016) created a PTG eight-week psychotherapeutic group intervention program for nonmetastatic breast cancer patients. Women were randomly assigned to an intervention group or a control group and completed a baseline assessment measuring their PTG and related variables, such as stressfulness and rumination. These variables were measured again 6 months after the interventions and 12 months following the baseline assessment. Each of the eight 90-minute weekly sessions included a topic related to breast cancer and education (e.g., fears or concerns surrounding breast cancer) and CBT psychological strategies (e.g., emotional regulation skills and redefining life goals). PTG was never mentioned directly but was used as a theoretical basis for the discussions (e.g., developing new values and priorities in life). The results showed that women in the intervention group reported higher levels of PTG than women in the control group (Ramos et al., 2018), suggesting that the intervention program was effective in fostering PTG.

More psychotherapies and educational programs that involve PTG (e.g., Moore et al., 2021; Roepke et al., 2018; Taku et al., 2017) and are based on Calhoun et al.'s (2010) PTG theoretical model, exist. While resilience programs can assume that an increase of resilience (e.g., increased self-esteem, increased coping skills, and a more positive outlook on life) is a valid indicator of its effectiveness, PTG programs deal with integration as a whole person, acceptance of a new normal after trauma, and developing new perspectives – all of which may take time. Therefore, heightened self-reported PTG may not be a valid measure to assess PTG interventions; rather, based on the aforementioned empirical findings, the effectiveness of a program is likely to be shown in one's interpersonal relationships and attitudes toward other people, especially those who are suffering. Questions regarding the kind of evaluations or assessments that can capture the effectiveness of PTG programs, when the transformative changes like PTG should be observed, and whether or not PTG itself must be expected as a result of an intervention following trauma, require further discussion.

Conclusion

Both a theoretical analysis of PTG and resilience intervention programs and empirical findings, suggest that these two concepts are not exactly the same. On one hand, it may be helpful to consider an integrative approach for educating about and fostering both processes in those who have suffered traumatic life experiences. Not many intervention programs exist that incorporate a way to foster PTG and display long-lasting positive effects and outcomes. By incorporating aspects of resilience intervention programs in addition to taking on a PTG theoretical approach, PTG may be easier to access. On the other hand, it may be helpful to keep the two separate to allow people the flexibility of choosing their preferred approach, depending on situations, conditions, and personal needs or values. Most importantly, despite their overlapping complexion, resilience and PTG should never be assumed to be identical in nature.

References

Aldrich, D. P. (2012). *Building resilience: Social capital in post-disaster recovery*. The University of Chicago Press.

Andersen, J. P., Papazoglou, K., Koskelainen, M., Nyman, M., Gustafsberg, H., & Arnetz, B. B. (2015). Applying resilience promotion training among special forces police officers. *SAGE Open*, *5*(2). Advanced online publication. 10.1177/2158244015590446

Arnetz, B. B., Nevedal, D. C., Lumley, M. A., Backman, L., & Lublin, A. (2008). Trauma resilience training for police: Psychophysiological and performance effects. *Journal of Police and Criminal Psychology*, *24*(1), 1–9. 10.1007/s11896-008-9030-y

Balgiu, B. A. (2017). Self-esteem, personality and resilience. Study of a students emerging adults group. *Journal of Educational Sciences and Psychology*, *7*(1), 93–99.

Bensimon, M. (2012). Elaboration on the association between trauma, PTSD and posttraumatic growth: The role of trait resilience. *Personality and Individual Differences*, *52*(7), 782–787. 10.1016/j.paid.2012.01.011

Block, J. (2002). *Personality as an affect-processing system: Toward an integrative theory* (1st ed.). Psychology Press. 10.4324/9781410602466

Block, J., & Turula, E. (1963). Identification, ego control, and adjustment. *Child Development*, *34*(4), 945–953. 10.2307/1126537

Bonanno, G. A. (2004). Loss, trauma, and human resilience: Have we underestimated the human capacity to thrive after extremely aversive events?. *American Psychologist*, *59*(1), 20–28. 10.1037/0003-066X.59.1.20

Bonanno, G. A., & Diminich, E. D. (2013). Annual research review: Positive adjustment to adversity–trajectories of minimal–impact resilience and emergent resilience. *Journal of Child Psychology and Psychiatry*, *54*(4), 378–401. 10.1111/jcpp.12021

Cann, A., Calhoun, L. G., Tedeschi, R. G., Taku, K., Vishnevsky, T., Triplett, K. N., & Danhauer, S. C. (2010). A short form of the posttraumatic growth inventory. *Anxiety, Stress, & Coping*, *23*(2), 127–137. 10.1080/10615800903094273

Calhoun, L. G., Cann, A., & Tedeschi, R. G. (2010). The posttraumatic growth model: Sociocultural considerations. In T. Weiss, & R. Berger (Eds.), *Posttraumatic growth and culturally competent practice: Lessons learned from around the globe* (pp. 1–14). John Wiley & Sons Inc. 10.1002/9781118270028.ch1

Connor, K. M., & Davidson, J. R. (2003). Development of a new resilience scale: The Connor-Davidson resilience scale (CD-RISC). *Depression and Anxiety*, *18*(2), 76–82. 10.1002/da.10113

DeViva, J. C., Sheerin, C. M., Southwick, S. M., Roy, A. M., Pietrzak, R. H., & Harpaz-Rotem, I. (2016). Correlates of VA mental health treatment utilization among OEF/OIF/OND veterans: Resilience, stigma, social support, personality, and beliefs about treatment. *Psychological Trauma: Theory, Research, Practice, and Policy*, *8*(3), 310–318. 10.1037/tra0000075

DiRago, A. C., & Vaillant, G. E. (2007). Resilience in inner city youth: Childhood predictors of occupational status across the lifespan. *Journal of Youth and Adolescence*, *36*(1), 61–70. 10.1007/s10964-006-9132-8

Duan, W., Guo, P., & Gan, P. (2015). Relationships among trait resilience, virtues, post-traumatic stress disorder, and post-traumatic growth. *PLoS One*, *10*(5), e0125707. 10.1371/journal.pone.0125707

Egeland, B., Carlson, E., & Sroufe, L. A. (1993). Resilience as process. *Development and Psychopathology*, *5*(4), 517–528. 10.1017/S0954579400006131

Ekman, P., & Matsumoto, D. (1993). *Japanese and Caucasian facial expressions of emotion (JACFEE). Department of Psychiatry*. San Francisco, CA: University of California.

Elam, T., & Taku, K. (2022). Differences between posttraumatic growth and resiliency: Their distinctive relationships with empathy and emotion recognition ability. *Frontiers in Psychology*, *13*, 825161. 10.3389/fpsyg.2022.825161

Fayombo, G. A. (2010). The relationship between personality traits and psychological resilience among the Caribbean adolescents. *International Journal of Psychological Studies*, *2*(2), 105–116. 10.5539/ijps.v2n2p105

Forbes, S., & Fikretoglu, D. (2018). Building resilience: The conceptual basis and research evidence for resilience training programs. *Review of General Psychology*, *22*(4), 452–468. 10.1037/gpr0000152

Gralinski-Bakker, J. H., Hauser, S. T., Stott, C., Billings, R. L., & Allen, J. P. (2004). Markers of resilience and risk: Adult lives in a vulnerable population. *Research in Human Development*, *1*(4), 291–326. 10.1207/s15427617rhd0104_4

Holling, C. S. (1973). Resilience and stability of ecological systems. *Annual Review of Ecology and Systematics*, *4*(1), 1–23. 10.1146/annurev.es.04.110173.000245

Ikizer, G., & Ozel, E. P. (2021). Examining psychological resilience and posttraumatic growth following terrorist attacks in Turkey. *Traumatology*, *27*(2), 236–243. 10.1037/trm0000255

Jia, X., Ying, L., Zhou, X., Wu, X., & Lin, C. (2015). The effects of extraversion, social support on the posttraumatic stress disorder and posttraumatic growth of adolescent survivors of the Wenchuan earthquake. *PLoS One*, *10*(3), e0121480. 10.1371/journal.pone.0121480

Kato, T. A., Hashimoto, R., Hayakawa, K., Kubo, H., Watabe, M., Teo, A. R., & Kanba, S. (2016). Multidimensional anatomy of 'modern type depression' in Japan: A proposal for a different diagnostic approach to depression beyond the DSM-5. *Psychiatry and Clinical Neurosciences*, *70*(1), 7–23. http://dx.doi.org.huaryu.kl.oakland.edu/10.1111/pcn.12360

Kato, T. A., Shinfuku, N., Fujisawa, D., Tateno, M., Ishida, T., Akiyama, T., Sartorius, N., Teo, A. R., Choi, T. Y., Wand, A. P. F., Balhara, Y. P. S., Chang, J. P., Chang, R. Y., Shadloo, B., Ahmed, H. U., Lerthattasilp, T., Umene-Nakano, W., Horikawa, H., Matsumoto, R., Kuga, H., Tanaka, M., & Kanba, S. (2011). Introducing the concept of modern depression in Japan; an international case vignette survey. *Journal of Affective Disorders*, *135*(1), 66–76. 10.1016/j.jad.2011.06.030

Kashihara, J., Yamakawa, I., Kameyama, A., Muranaka, M., Taku, K., & Sakamoto, S. (2019). Perceptions of traditional and modern types of depression: A cross-cultural vignette survey comparing Japanese and American undergraduate students. *Psychiatry and Clinical Neurosciences*, *73*(8), 441–447. 10.1111/pcn.12838

Kaye-Tzadok, A., & Davidson-Arad, B. (2016). Posttraumatic growth among women survivors of childhood sexual abuse: Its relation to cognitive strategies, posttraumatic symptoms, and resilience. *Psychological Trauma: Theory, Research, Practice, and Policy*, *8*(5), 550–558. 10.1037/tra0000103

Levine, S. Z., Laufer, A., Stein, E., Hamama-Raz, Y., & Solomon, Z. (2009). Examining the relationship between resilience and posttraumatic growth. *Journal of Traumatic Stress: Official Publication of the International Society for Traumatic Stress Studies*, 22(4), 282–286. 10.1002/jts.20409

Li, Y., Cao, F., Cao, D., & Liu, J. (2015). Nursing students' post-traumatic growth, emotional intelligence and psychological resilience. *Journal of Psychiatric and Mental Health Nursing*, *22*(5), 326–332. 10.1111/jpm.12192

Luthar, S. S., Cicchetti, D., & Becker, B. (2000). Research on resilience: Response to commentaries. *Child Development*, *71*(3), 573–575. 10.1111/1467-8624.00168

Masten, A. S. (2007). Resilience in developing systems: Progress and promise as the fourth wave rises. *Development and Psychopathology*, *19*(3), 921–930. 10.1017/S0954579407000442

Masten, A. S., & Garmezy, N. (1985). Risk, vulnerability, and protective factors in developmental psychopathology. In *Advances in clinical child psychology* (pp. 1–52). Boston, MA: Springer.

Matsumoto, D., & Ekman, P. (1988). *Japanese and Caucasian facial expressions of emotion (JACFEE) and neutral faces. Department of Psychiatry*. San Francisco, CA: University of California.

Mehrabian, A., & Epstein, N. (1972). A measure of emotional empathy. *Journal of Personality*, *40*(4), 525–543. 10.1111/j.1467-6494.1972.tb00078.x

Moore, B. A., Tedeschi, R. G., & Greene, T. C. (2021). A preliminary examination of posttraumatic growth-based program for veteran mental health. *Practice Innovations*, 6(1), 42–54. 10.1037/pri0000136

Norris, F. H., Stevens, S. P., Pfefferbaum, B., Wyche, K. F., & Pfefferbaum, R. L. (2008). Community resilience as a metaphor, theory, set of capacities, and strategy for disaster readiness. *American Journal of Community Psychology*, *41*(1), 127–150. 10.1007/s10464-007-9156-6

O'Brien, C., & Taku, K. (2022). Distinguishing between resilience and posttraumatic growth: Perceptions and attitudes toward depression. *Psychology, Health & Medicine*(CPHM). 10.1080/13548506.2022.2064521

Ong, A. D., Bergeman, C. S., Bisconti, T. L., & Wallace, K. A. (2006). Psychological resilience, positive emotions, and successful adaptation to stress in later life. *Journal of Personality and Social Psychology*, *91*(4), 730–749. 10.1037/0022-3514.91.4.730

Oshio, A., Taku, K., Hirano, M., & Saeed, G. (2018). Resilience and big five personality traits: A meta-analysis. *Personality and Individual Differences*, *127*, 54–60. 10.1016/j.paid.2018.01.048
Panjikidze, M., Beelmann, A., Martskvishvili, K., & Chitashvili, M. (2020). Posttraumatic growth, personality factors, and social support among war-experienced young Georgians. *Psychological Reports*, *123*(3), 687–709. 10.1177/0033294118823177
Ramos, C., Costa, P. A., Rudnicki, T., Marôco, A. L., Leal, I., Guimarães, R., Fougo, J. L., & Tedeschi, R. G. (2018). The effectiveness of a group intervention to facilitate posttraumatic growth among women with breast cancer. *Psycho-Oncology*, *27*(1), 258–264. 10.1002/pon.4501
Ramos, C., Leal, I., & Tedeschi, R. G. (2016). Protocol for the psychotherapeutic group intervention for facilitating posttraumatic growth in nonmetastatic breast cancer patients. *BMC Women's Health*, *16*(1), 1–9. 10.1186/s12905-016-0302-x
Roepke, A. M. (2015). Psychosocial interventions and posttraumatic growth: A meta-analysis. *Journal of Consulting and Clinical Psychology*, *83*(1), 129–142. 10.1037/a0036872
Roepke, A. M., Tsukayama, E., Forgeard, M., Blackie, L., & Jayawickreme, E. (2018). Randomized controlled trial of SecondStory, an intervention targeting posttraumatic growth, with bereaved adults. *Journal of Consulting and Clinical Psychology*, *86*(6), 518–532. 10.1037/ccp0000307
Rutter, M. (1979). Protective factors in children's responses to stress and disadvantage. *Annals of the Academy of Medicine, Singapore*, *8*(3), 324–338.
Rutter, M. (2000). Resilience reconsidered: Conceptual considerations, empirical findings, and policy implications. In J. P. Shonkoff, & S. J. Meisels (Eds.), *Handbook of early childhood intervention* (pp. 651–682). Cambridge University Press. 10.1017/CBO9780511529320.030
Sakamoto, S., Yamakawa, I., & Muranaka, M. (2016). A comparison of perceptions of 'modern-type' and melancholic depression in Japan. *International Journal of Social Psychiatry*, *62*(7), 627–634. 10.1177/0020764016665410
Sampson, R. J., & Laub, J. H. (1992). Crime and deviance in the life course. *Annual Review of Sociology*, *18*(1), 63–84. 10.1146/annurev.so.18.080192.000431
Sarason, I. G., Johnson, J. H., Berberich, J. P., & Siegel, J. M. (1979). Helping police officers to cope with stress: A cognitive-behavioral approach. *American Journal of Community Psychology*, *7*(6), 593–603.
Smith, B. W., Dalen, J., Wiggins, K., Tooley, E., Christopher, P., & Bernard, J. (2008). The brief resilience scale: Assessing the ability to bounce back. *International Journal of Behavioral Medicine*, *15*(3), 194–200. 10.1080/10705500802222972
Southwick, S. M., Bonanno, G. A., Masten, A. S., Panter-Brick, C., & Yehuda, R. (2014). Resilience definitions, theory, and challenges: Interdisciplinary perspectives. *European Journal of Psychotraumatology*, *5*(1), 25338. 10.3402/ejpt.v5.25338
Staudinger, U. M., Marsiske, M., & Baltes, P. B. (1993). Resilience and levels of reserve capacity in later adulthood: Perspectives from life-span theory. *Development and Psychopathology*, *5*(4), 541–566. 10.1017/S0954579400006155
Taku, K. (2011). Commonly-defined and individually-defined posttraumatic growth in the US and Japan. *Personality and Individual Differences*, *51*(2), 188–193. 10.1016/j.paid.2011.04.002
Taku, K. (2013). Posttraumatic growth in American and Japanese men: Comparing levels of growth and perceptions of indicators of growth. *Psychology of Men & Masculinity*, *14*(4), 423–432. 10. 1037/a0029582
Taku, K., Cann, A., Tedeschi, R. G., & Calhoun, L. G. (2017). Psychoeducational intervention program about posttraumatic growth for Japanese high school students. *Journal of Loss and Trauma*, *22*(4), 271–282. 10.1080/15325024.2017.1284504
Taku, K., Limura, S., & McDiarmid, K. (2018). Ceiling effects and floor effects of the posttraumatic growth inventory. *Journal of Child and Family Studies*, *27*, 387–397. 10.1007/s10826-017-0915-1
Vaillant, G. E., & Davis, J. T. (2000). Social/emotional intelligence and midlife resilience in schoolboys with low tested intelligence. *American Journal of Orthopsychiatry*, *70*(2), 215–222. 10.1037/h0087783
Vieselmeyer, J., Holguin, J., & Mezulis, A. (2017). The role of resilience and gratitude in posttraumatic stress and growth following a campus shooting. *Psychological Trauma: Theory, Research, Practice, and Policy*, *9*(1), 62–69. 10.1037/tra0000149

Wagnild, G. M., & Young, H. M. (1993). Development and psychometric evaluation of the Resilience Scale. *Journal of Nursing Measurement*, *1*(2), 165–178.
Werner, E. E. (2000). Protective factors and individual resilience. In E. Zigler, J. Shonkoff, & S. Meisels (Eds.), *Handbook of early childhood intervention* (pp. 115–132). Cambridge, CA: Cambridge University Press. 10.1017/CBO9780511529320.008
Werner, E. E. (2002). Looking for trouble in paradise: Some lessons learned from the Kauai longitudinal study. In E. Phelps, F. F. Furstenberg, & A. Colby (Eds.), *Looking at lives: American longitudinal studies in the twentieth century* (pp. 297–314). New York, NY: Russell Sage.
Werner, E. E. (2005). Resilience research. In R. D. Peters, B. Leadbeater, & R. J. McMahon, (Eds.), *Resilience in children, families, and communities* (pp. 3–11). Boston, MA: Springer. 10.1007/0-387-23824-7_1
Werner, E. E., Bierman, J. M., & Fresnch, F. E. (1971). *The children of Kauai: A longitudinal study from the prenatal period to age ten*. Honolulu, HI: University of Hawaii Press.
Werner, E. E., & Smith, R. S. (1977). *Kauai's children come of age*. Honolulu, HI: University Press of Hawaii.
Yu, Y., Peng, L., Chen, L., Long, L., He, W., Li, M., & Wang, T. (2014). Resilience and social support promote posttraumatic growth of women with infertility: The mediating role of positive coping. *Psychiatry Research*, *215*(2), 401–405. 10.1016/j.psychres.2013.10.032
Zerach, G., Solomon, Z., Cohen, A., & Ein-Dor, T. (2013). PTSD, resilience and posttraumatic growth among ex-prisoners of war and combat veterans. *The Israel Journal of Psychiatry and Related Sciences*, *50*(2), 91–98.

8

AN AGENDA FOR THE NEXT GENERATION OF POSTTRAUMATIC GROWTH RESEARCH

Rowan Kemmerly, Howard Tennen, and Eranda Jayawickreme

The idea that it is possible to change in positive ways after experiencing adversity—for example, to experience new insights about the world and oneself, for life to become more meaningful, and to change one's thoughts, feelings, and behaviors—is intuitively appealing to many, and furthermore constitutes a key feature of cultural scripts of redemption and heroism in North America (e.g., Rogers et al., 2023). Perhaps consequently, scientific interest in the idea of *post-traumatic growth* (PTG) has increased greatly over the past 30 years (Jayawickreme & Blackie, 2014). However, PTG is a challenging concept to study empirically, because of the pervasive cultural narrative that something good must come out of bad experiences (Jayawickreme et al., 2021) and long-standing concerns about the methodological limitations of assessments used to measure PTG (e.g., Tennen & Affleck, 1998; 2009).

PTG is typically assessed by scales such as the Post-Traumatic Growth Inventory (PTGI; Tedeschi & Calhoun, 1996) that ask participants to retrospectively recall how they were before the adversity, estimate how much they have changed since the adversity, and ascertain the extent to which this change can be attributed to the adversity (Infurna & Jayawickreme, 2019). As noted by Ford and colleagues (2008), completing this process accurately would involve (a) deducing one's current standing on a particular growth-relevant dimension, (b) recalling one's prior standing pre-adversity, (c) comparing those standings, (d) computing the degree of change, and (e) deciding how much of the change was due to the adversity. It is unlikely that most participants can accurately complete this metacognitive process successfully. Furthermore, self-reported perceptions of change have been found across multiple studies to be only weakly related to observed pre- to post-change (e.g., Bossert et al., 2022), and people may not be able to consistently identify key adverse life events that caused growth retrospectively (Jayawickreme et al., 2018).

Some 15 years ago, Tennen and Affleck (2009) warned that PTG as a topic of study would become increasingly marginalized as a result of concerns over the methodological limitations inherent in much of the research. Despite this warning, work on PTG utilizing measures of perceived growth has continued to grow. Two recent reviews (Boals et al., 2022; Jayawickreme et al., 2018) revealed that the vast majority of research on PTG

DOI: 10.4324/9781032208688-9

continues to use retrospective assessments of perceived growth. For example, recent reviews found that 66 of 70 articles published in 2016 and 2017, and 23 of 33 articles on PTG published in 2018 and 2019, utilized the PTGI (Tedeschi & Calhoun, 1996), despite the fact that this measure assesses retrospective self-perceived growth rather than observed change pre-to post-adversity (Ford et al., 2008).

This continued reliance on measures such as the PTGI is unfortunate. The evidence is clear from multiple studies that measures of perceived growth lack validity as measures of change (e.g., Frazier et al., 2009; Owenz & Fowers, 2019), and predictors of mental health (e.g., Engelhard et al., 2015; Park et al., 2022; Zalta et al., 2017). Despite the increasing number of research studies on PTG, the lack of construct validity of these measures has obscured rather than clarified our understanding of how positive changes do occur following the experience of adversity.

However, we are also heartened that many PTG scholars are somewhat cognizant of these limitations and an increasing number of researchers have been striving to improve the methods utilized in PTG research (e.g., Frazier et al., 2009; Infurna et al., 2023; Jayawickreme et al., 2022; see reviews in Infurna & Jayawickreme, 2019; Jayawickreme & Blackie, 2014; Jayawickreme et al., 2021). This chapter aims to summarize some of this research and sketch out some recommendations for a "mature" science of PTG.

Do People Grow from Adversity? Examining the Evidence for Positive Change

Tennen and Affleck (2009) provided initial guidelines for examining positive life change following adversity with scientific rigor through strategies that allow for the assessment of pre- to post-event change. Building on similar insights from Tennen and Affleck (1998), Weststrate and colleagues (2022) further argued that researchers can study PTG in a methodologically rigorous and theoretically sound manner by making use of the three-level model of personality (e.g., McAdams & Pals, 2006). This approach allows investigators to examine PTG either in terms of dispositional traits, characteristic adaptations (e.g., goals, values, motives) or one's subjectively construed sense of identity (e.g., narrative identity). Utilizing this framework opens up the opportunity for addressing a host of novel questions regarding PTG, including identifying the level of personality at which PTG is most likely to occur (e.g., Blackie et al., 2023), whether changes in one level subsequently translate into changes in the other levels, and what the implications of differential (or "misaligned" change) are for the person. The following sections summarize research examining change in personality in each of the three levels following the experience of adversity.

Changes in Traits

Dispositional traits reflect relatively stable patterns of thinking, feeling, and behaving. Such traits are typically (although not always) identified within the Big Five framework (i.e., open-mindedness, conscientiousness, extraversion, agreeableness, and neuroticism/emotional stability; John & Srivastava, 1999; McCrae & John, 1992; Soto & John, 2017). There is evidence of normative personality change across the lifespan, with individuals becoming more emotionally stable, agreeable, conscientious, and socially dominant (Atherton et al., 2021; Damian et al., 2019). In studying change at the trait level, it is therefore important that personality "growth" in the wake of adversity be shown to exceed normative personality trait development, i.e., "maturation" (Weststrate et al., 2022).

Research on Big Five trait change associated with negative life events has mostly focused on events including unemployment, divorce, bereavement, or major illnesses (Bleidorn et al., 2018; Denissen et al., 2019) and has shown changes in personality traits. For example, a recent examination has shown that experiencing major negative life events leads to subsequent increases in the experience of negative social events in the following weeks (Jayawickreme et al., 2023) and increases in neuroticism (Jayawickreme et al., 2021). However, no consistent increases in agreeableness, extraversion, openness, or conscientiousness have been observed after experiencing a range of major life events (Denissen et al., 2019; Forgeard et al., 2022; Lüdtke et al., 2011; Specht et al., 2011). Consistent with the notion that PTG is a relatively rare phenomenon, individuals can vary substantially in their behavioral responses to such events (Neyer et al., 2014). For example, one study found that young adults showed small increases in open-mindedness when the adverse event was rated as central to their lives (Boals et al., 2015), whereas another study reported that providing care to a spouse living with terminal lung cancer was associated with positive changes in facets of extraversion, agreeableness, and conscientiousness (Hoerger et al., 2014). One interesting future direction for research highlighted by this study involves focusing on facets of specific personality traits, as well as more conceptual work linking specific life events with specific personality trait facets.

Changes in Characteristic Adaptations

Characteristic adaptations refer to motivational and social-cognitive individual differences. They include values, self-efficacy, coping strategies, or cognitive schemas (McAdams, 2015; McAdams & Pals, 2006). Tedeschi and Calhoun's (1996) five domains of PTG—improved relations with others, identification of new possibilities for one's life, increased personal strength, spiritual change, and enhanced appreciation of life—arguably constitute examples of such adaptations (Jayawickreme et al., 2021; Linley & Joseph, 2004).

There is some evidence that the experience of adversity across the course of one's life may be associated with both increased resilience and changes in prosocial values. Moderate levels of cumulative lifetime adversity have been associated with increased life satisfaction and lower levels of impaired daily functioning in a representative U.S. sample (Seery et al., 2010). In addition, cumulative lifetime adversity has been found to be associated with increases in prosocial behavior, empathy, and compassion (Lim & DeSteno, 2016). However, as these studies were cross-sectional in nature, other explanations for this observed difference cannot be ruled out.

The link between adversity and wisdom has been the focus of multiple studies (Jayawickreme et al., 2018). However, while people subjectively perceive themselves to have grown in wisdom through adverse life experiences (Weststrate et al., 2018), recent research suggests that, at least in the immediate wake of adversity, there is little evidence for increases in reasoning processes associated with wisdom (Dorfmann et al., 2021). Similarly, there is limited evidence for changes in other character traits in the immediate aftermath of adversity (Blackie & McLean, 2022; Infurna & Jayawickreme, 2019). For example, a longitudinal study found no evidence that the experience of health adversities predicted positive changes in character strengths over a period of three and a half years (Gander et al., 2020), and no relationship was observed between interpersonal loss and subsequent changes in character strengths (Blanchard et al., 2021). A recent two-year longitudinal study found that experiencing an increasing number of adverse life events was associated with an increase in depressive symptoms, lower life satisfaction, and lower levels of meaning, while high levels of concurrent adversity were associated with higher levels of depressive symptoms, as well as lower levels of life satisfaction generativity, gratitude, and meaning (Infurna et al., 2023).

Changes in Narrative Identity

Narrative identity refers to a person's life story characterized by a series of central self-defining autobiographical memories integrating the person's past, present, and anticipated future (Adler et al., 2016; McAdams & McLean, 2013; McLean et al., 2020). The experience of PTG can be coded by examining themes in high and low points in life as described in life narratives (Lilgendahl & McAdams, 2011). These themes may include clarifying self-knowledge, goals, beliefs, and values, conceptual shifts in thinking that deepen or broaden one's perspective on self, others, or life in general, and forming or repairing meaningful, healthy relationships (Lilgendahl & McAdams, 2011). Meaning-making—the extent to which people report learning lessons or gleaning insights from life experiences in their narratives (McLean & Pratt, 2006)—represents another potential indicator of PTG. Meaning-making in response to low-point memories has been observed to predict emotional maturity two years later (Cox & McAdams, 2014), and narrative meaning-making was found to be positively associated with wisdom (Webster et al., 2018). While there is also evidence that structural and linguistic features of meaning-making are correlated with self-reported PTG in trauma narratives (Booker et al., 2020; Waters et al., 2013), many of these studies are limited by their retrospective and cross-sectional nature.

How Ubiquitous Is Positive Change Following Adversity?

Overall, studies show limited evidence for the ubiquity of positive change following the experience of major negative life events. One possible reason for these findings is that current measures of traits and characteristic adaptations may lack the sensitivity required to capture such changes (Jayawickreme et al., 2021). For example, it is possible that people may experience positive changes following adversity in one or two domains of their life (e.g., with their romantic partner or parents). In addition, it is possible that observing positive personality change at the trait and characteristic adaptation levels may require a clearer understanding of the contextual and intrapersonal moderators that may promote or forestall growth, as well as more conceptual work linking specific life events with specific personality characteristics.

Recommendations for Future Work

While "PTG-as-usual" research continues apace (Boals et al., 2022; Jayawickreme et al., 2018), we are somewhat encouraged by increased awareness of the importance of using more valid methods for examining PTG. An increasing number of researchers examining PTG using standard measures of PTG now acknowledge the limitations of these methods (e.g., Park et al., 2022), which compared to 15 years ago, represents a modest degree of improvement. Hopefully, more and more PTG researchers will move on from "traditional" assessments, and with that goal in mind, this section provides recommendations for future work. Interested readers may also review the nine recommendations for credible research on PTG discussed by Jayawickreme and colleagues (2021).

Acknowledge the Limited Validity of Perceived PTG

Even in the early days of research on PTG, psychologists were mindful of the unique methodological challenges in assessing positive change following adversity. For example, in their article describing the development of the Stress-Related Growth Scale (SRGS), Park and colleagues (1996) explicitly acknowledge that the instrument measures self-reported, perceived growth and that the scores may not necessarily reflect a veridical change. Similarly, in their early review of how change may occur in the face of adversity, Tennen and Affleck (1998) highlighted the limitations of retrospective measures of growth.

Given that the distinction between perceived and observed growth has been well-established and increasingly acknowledged by many (but not all) PTG researchers, does perceived growth have value as a distinct construct in its own right? Even research that recognizes the difference between perceived and veridical growth often suggests that believing that one has changed for the better differs from finding positive outcomes in a bad situation (Park & Boals, 2021). Unlike forms of coping, perceived PTG is purported to involve a change in one's sense of self and overall perspective on the world. Appraisals such as perceived PTG may have a positive "self-fulfilling" effect (Calhoun & Tedeschi, 2014; Park & Boals, 2021; Tedeschi et al., 2018). However, multiple studies suggest that scores on the PTGI are associated with increased distress (e.g., Engelhard et al., 2015; Zalta et al., 2017), and a perceived growth in the wake of a major negative life event did not predict subsequent changes in PTG-relevant thoughts, feelings, and behaviors measured through both "current-standing" and aggregated experience-sampling assessments of behavior (Gangel et al., in revision).

As Tennen and Affleck (2009) noted, perceived growth may reflect a form of coping, and some studies suggest a strong relationship between positive reinterpretation coping and perceived growth (Hamama-Raz et al., 2019; Shand et al., 2015). Additionally, some researchers have worked on revised measures of perceived growth that reduce the likelihood of socially desirable responses (e.g., by replacing unidirectional scales that assume growth with a bidirectional scale; Boals & Schuler, 2018). However, even with such methodological adjustments, it remains unclear whether these scales have discriminant validity compared to assessments of related constructs, such as positive reappraisal coping (Boals et al., 2022). In light of the evidence reviewed above, PTG researchers should rethink the value of perceived growth assessments, given that they do not closely track measured change over time, have limited utility as predictors of positive mental health outcomes, and may not reflect a distinct construct when compared with measures of coping and secondary control (Jayawickreme et al., 2018).

Reconsider the Term "Post-Traumatic Growth"

Researchers should reconsider the term "post-traumatic growth," which may obscure the understanding of positive changes that can occur following adversity. There are two reasons for this recommendation. First, the term implies that traumatic events are a condition for change. The PTG model assumes that the process of PTG begins with a seismic event (Tedeschi & Calhoun, 2004) that may create a shift in people's identity and "shatter" one's assumptions about the world (Janoff-Bulman, 1992). However, it is likely that a wider range of events may have short- or long-term impacts on one's personality and functioning (Seery et al., 2010), and that characteristics of the event beyond its traumatic nature, e.g., a sense of control over the event may be predictive of change (Luhmann et al., 2021). Second, "growth" may indicate to some people that the person is better off overall for having experienced the trauma. PTG theories have acknowledged that experiencing PTG may be accompanied by challenges and distress (Calhoun & Tedeschi, 2014). This acknowledgment is exactly the reason why "growth" may not be an appropriate term for labeling the experience of survivors of adversity. As noted by multiple philosophers who have written critically of psychologists' use of the term "growth," the term is a "thick" concept that indicates a meaningful and positive shift in an individual's character that is clearly good for that person (Brady & Jayawickreme, 2023; Miller, 2014; Tiberius, 2021). Given that the experience of adversity may lead to both positive and negative changes, ascribing the term "growth" would require a clear understanding of how both types of changes should be weighed against each other (Miller, 2014). Without this clear understanding, labeling someone's experience as "growth" may have the unintended consequence of misrepresenting someone's experience following adversity (Zachry & Jayawickreme, 2022).

Commit to Prospective Designs

Tennen and Affleck (2009) called for the norming of prospective and quasi-prospective designs in PTG research. We reiterate this call, as estimating whether and how people change in positive ways following adversity necessitates such designs. Such studies should ideally track a large sample over time, allowing for the selection of those who have experienced specific major life events, as well as comparing their measured change to the normative change observed in a matched sample from the non-adversity condition (Weststrate et al., 2022). For example, one study examining changes in life satisfaction before and after major life events found that changes in groups who experienced these events were distinct from those in the control group, suggesting a causal role for adversity (Anusic et al., 2014).

Such designs would also allow researchers to examine multi-phase changes that may occur before the adverse event, at the onset of the event, or after the event (Lucas, 2007). Relatedly, utilizing analytic approaches such as multilevel modeling can afford the opportunity to examine between-person differences in degrees and rates of change in the outcome of interest and, importantly, between-person predictors of these differences. For example, Infurna et al. (2017) found that younger age at a spousal loss was associated with a stronger initial decline in life satisfaction at the time of the loss, but stronger improvements in the years thereafter. Additionally, both social participation and health status were associated with better adaptation following spousal loss.

An additional analytic strategy of possible interest to PTG researchers is growth mixture modeling, which is used to determine whether there are multiple distinct trajectories in the sample based on between-person differences in change (e.g., resilient, recovery, or growth trajectories; Infurna & Jayawickreme, 2019). However, there are important questions regarding model specification and the methodological assumptions underlying each trajectory that should be considered (Infurna & Luthar, 2018). While a few studies have identified growth trajectories (e.g., Mancini et al., 2016), it is possible that this trajectory may constitute a methodological artifact (Infurna & Luthar, 2018; Jayawickreme et al., 2021; Sher et al., 2011).

Make Use of Secondary Data Analysis (But Be Mindful of Its Limitations)

Given the challenge in conducting longitudinal research on PTG, researchers may consider using secondary data sources, such as panel studies, to capitalize on prospective assessments of multiple psychological constructs. Panel studies have the added benefit of tracking large samples, a proportion of whom will eventually experience an adversity event such as a disability or unemployment (Infurna & Luthar, 2016, 2018). Such data have been useful for characterizing how and why personality changes following adverse life events occur (Bleidorn et al., 2018). For example, optimism was found to increase in response to positive life events but remain stable in the wake of adverse events (Schwaba et al., 2019). These datasets have become increasingly more accessible and convenient for researchers to use (see https://www.personalitydevelopmentcollaborative.org for existing datasets).

Despite the multiple benefits that they provide, the aforementioned data sources present several challenges. Reported studies are typically initiated to answer research questions unrelated to PTG, alterations to the questionnaires and assessment protocol are typically very difficult or impossible and often use a checklist focused on events that occurred since the last assessment, which complicates the ability to examine the effects of adversity (Jayawickreme et al., 2021). Assessments of how life events are interpreted are typically absent and assessments of psychological constructs that may be sensitive to change (beyond the Big Five) may not be included. Finally, the nature of the dataset may oblige researchers to measure change at a particular time scale even if there is good reason to think that positive change may only be detectable across a different timespan (Hopwood et al., 2022). Nevertheless, these datasets provide unique opportunities for PTG researchers, and given the challenges that many will have in collecting longitudinal data, secondary datasets should be the focus of more PTG research going forward.

Aspects Requiring Attention in Future Research

While many of the reviewed studies found little evidence of meaning change, these findings hide the fact that people's individual trajectories of change might be very different. Some might experience sharp increases immediately after the event, but end up changing for the worse over time, while others may experience long-term stability with considerable short-term variability (Infurna & Jayawickreme, 2019). Future research should examine idiosyncratic resilience, growth, and decline trajectories for different participants, as well as individual differences that may predict these trajectories. In addition, it is important to allow facet-level (Soto & John, 2017; see the aforementioned Hoerger et al., 2014 findings), or even item-level (Mõttus et al., 2017) analyses, as well as assessments of domain-specific manifestations of traits (Bühler et al., 2021), because these data can afford opportunities for identifying positive life change at a more granular level (Lamarche, 2022; Weststrate et al., 2022).

Additionally, a critical challenge for further theorizing on PTG is providing far greater clarity on the length of time needed following the adverse experience for long- or short-term change to occur, and a clear understanding of the characteristics of the adverse event (e.g., affective valence; controllability over the event) that may predict change (Weststrate et al., 2022). While such considerations have hitherto been impossible to test with existing instruments assessing PTG (Tennen & Affleck, 2009) this knowledge is critical for planning the length of studies, the number of assessments needed to test theoretical predictions, and the frequency of administering them to capture short-term versus long-term change (Gangel et al., in revision; Hopwood et al., 2022).

Given the U.S.-centric dominance of the master narrative of redemption (McAdams, 2015), future work on the cross-cultural validity of the idea of PTG is important. For example, a recent study found that recuperation rather than redemption was the dominant narrative in a U.K. sample suggesting that the cultural master narrative of redemption is not necessarily present in non-North American contexts, (Blackie 2020). Further, positive changes people report may vary as a function of both cultural and contextual differences, e.g., reports of positive changes in life opportunities rather than psychological change (Zapffe et al., 2023).

Beware of Rushing to Intervene Too Quickly

Multiple intervention techniques have been developed with the goal of promoting PTG (Roepke et al., 2021). Given the sincere motivation of PTG researchers for using research for promoting well-being in society, it is not surprising that there has been increasing interest in developing such protocols (Boals et al., 2022). However, given evidence that perceived PTG is frequently associated with increased distress, concerns were raised that such interventions may be ineffective, or even harmful (Coyne & Tennen, 2010; Lilienfeld, 2007).

Recent work in personality science suggests that interventions focused on self-regulated change may be effective and work on volitional personality change and has highlighted how people may be motivated to intentionally change specific personality traits (Hudson & Fraley, 2015). Such interventions work in part by shaping people's goals and habits, and the experience of an adverse life event may possibly provide a distinctive opportunity for personality change through goal shifts and habit formation. For example, if the adverse event both disrupts individuals' habits and forces them into new contexts, especially those that reinforce new ways of acting (Blackie 2015, Adler 2016), the formation of new and long-lasting habits may be facilitated. In such contexts, an adverse event may impact the person by first changing their context, available reinforcers, and contingencies between behaviors and outcomes, which consistent with current dynamic personality theories, subsequently lead to behavior change (Fleeson & Jayawickreme, 2021). Such environmental and behavioral changes may lead to subsequent changes in perspective/worldview as individuals make sense of their new habits and incorporate them into their identity. In these scenarios, change may be initially observed at the behavioral level, and only later at the level of narrative identity.

Empirical support for the utility of such interventions for promoting change is limited. A recent investigation examined whether people who had recently experienced a major negative life event (compared to a no-trauma control condition) were able to successfully change personality traits they had selected in a 16-week study (Blackie & Hudson, 2022) and found that agreeableness *declined* in the trauma relative to the control group who did not want to change that trait. Additionally, conscientiousness declined for individuals who had experienced life events high in event centrality. Another study similarly found that utilizing goal-setting strategies and future-minded thinking to promote observed change among a sample of recently bereaved individuals was ineffective at promoting "current-standing" PTG

(Roepke et al., 2018). This intervention incorporated components of Narrative Exposure Therapy (NET), which following PTG theory, may have utility in fostering adaptive changes in one's subjective identity in the wake of adversity. Evidence for "narrative-as-process" as a facilitator of growth in the realm of personality psychology is mixed (Blackie & McLean, 2022) though generally, the consensus in clinical fields is that Narrative Exposure Therapy (NET) is helpful (see Lely et al., 2019, for meta-analytic evidence). On balance, it may be that focusing on intervention development to directly engineer PTG is premature, given the current status of research on PTG, and in particular the limited evidence for positive change.

Conclusion

The years since Tennen and Affleck's (2009) recommendation that PTG researchers work on improving their methods present a mixed picture. On one hand, standard "PTG-as-usual" research has continued apace (as perhaps reflected in many of the chapters in this volume) despite long-standing criticism of its methods. However, there has been increasing interest by multiple researchers in personality and clinical psychology in striving towards more "meticulous methods" for studying PTG (Tennen & Affleck, 2009). In summarizing this research and providing some insights for future directions, we hope that more PTG researchers will move towards adopting methods that allow us to build together a robust science concerned with clarifying the compelling and controversial question of whether adversity can spur positive change.

References

Adler, J. M., Lodi-Smith, J., Philippe, F. L., & Houle, I. (2016). The incremental validity of narrative identity in predicting well-being: A review of the field and recommendations for the future. *Personality and Social Psychology Review*, *20*(2), 142–175. doi:10.1177/1088868315585068

Anusic, I., Yap, S. C., & Lucas, R. E. (2014). Does personality moderate reaction and adaptation to major life events? Analysis of life satisfaction and affect in an Australian national sample. *Journal of Research in Personality*, *5*, 69–77. doi:10.1016/j.jrp.2014.04.009

Atherton, O. E., Grijalva, E., Roberts, B. W., & Robins, R. W. (2021). Stability and change in personality traits and major life goals from college to midlife. *Personality and Social Psychology Bulletin*, *47*(5), 841–858. doi:10.1177/0146167220949362

Blackie, L. E. R., Colgan, J. E. V., McDonald, S., & McLean, K. C. (2020). A qualitative investigation into the cultural master narrative for overcoming trauma and adversity in the United Kingdom. *Qualitative Psychology*. Advanced online publication. doi:10.1037/qup0000163

Blackie, L. E., & Hudson, N. W. (2022). Trauma exposure and short-term volitional personality trait change. *Journal of Personality*. doi:10.1111/jopy.12759

Blackie, L. E. R., & Jayawickreme, E. (2015). The example of adverse life experiences as unique situations. *European Journal of Personality*, *29*(3), 385–386.

Blackie, L. E., & McLean, K. C. (2022). Examining the longitudinal associations between repeated narration of recent transgressions within individuals' romantic relationships and character growth in empathy, humility, and compassion. *European Journal of Personality*, *36*(4), 507–528. doi:10.1177/08902070211028696

Blackie, L. E., Weststrate, N. M., Turner, K., Adler, J. M., & McLean, K. C. (2023). Broadening our understanding of adversarial growth: The contribution of narrative methods. *Journal of Research in Personality*. doi:10.1016/j.jrp.2023.104359

Blanchard, T., McGrath, R. E., & Jayawickreme, E. (2021). Resilience in the face of interpersonal loss: The role of character strengths. *Applied Psychology: Health and Well-Being*, *13*(4), 817–834. doi:10.1111/aphw.12273

Bleidorn, W., Hopwood, C. J., & Lucas, R. E. (2018). Life events and personality trait change. *Journal of Personality*, *86*(1), 83–96. doi:10.1111/jopy.12286

Boals, A., Jayawickreme, E., & Park, C. L. (2022). Advantages of distinguishing perceived and veridical growth: Recommendations for future research on both constructs. *The Journal of Positive Psychology*, 1–11. doi:10.1080/15427609.2018.1495515

Boals, A., & Schuler, K. L. (2018). Reducing reports of illusory posttraumatic growth: A revised version of the stress-related growth scale (SRGS-R). *Psychological Trauma: Theory, Research, Practice, and Policy*, *10*(2), 190–198. doi:10.1037/tra0000267

Boals, A., Southard-Dobbs, S., & Blumenthal, H. (2015). Adverse events in emerging adulthood are associated with increases in neuroticism. *Journal of Personality*, *83*(2), 202–211. doi:10.1111/jopy.12095

Booker, J. A., Fivush, R., Graci, M. E., Heitz, H., Hudak, L. A., Jovanovic, T., Rothbaum, B. O., & Stevens, J. S. (2020). Longitudinal changes in trauma narratives over the first year and associations with coping and mental health. *Journal of Affective Disorders*, *272*, 116–124. doi:10.1016/j.jad.2020.04.009

Bossert, S. A., Tsukayama, E., Blackie, L. E., Cole, V. T., & Jayawickreme, E. (2022). Do we know whether we're happier? Corroborating perceived retrospective assessments of improvements in well-being. *Journal of Personality Assessment*, *104*(4), 458–466. doi:10.1080/00223891.2022.2039167

Brady, M., & Jayawickreme, E. (2023) Can philosophical theorizing on the value of adversity improve research on posttraumatic growth?

Bühler, J. L., Krauss, S., & Orth, U. (2021). Development of relationship satisfaction across the life span: A systematic review and meta-analysis. *Psychological Bulletin*, *147*(10), 1012–1053. doi:10.1037/bul0000342

Calhoun, L. G., & Tedeschi, R. G. (Eds.). (2014). *Handbook of posttraumatic growth: Research and practice*. Routledge.

Cox, K., & McAdams, D. P. (2014). Meaning making during high and low point life story episodes predicts emotion regulation two years later: How the past informs the future. *Journal of Research in Personality*, *50*, 66–70. doi:10.1016/j.jrp.2014.03.004

Coyne, J. C., & Tennen, H. (2010). Positive psychology in cancer care: Bad science, exaggerated claims, and unproven medicine. *Annals of Behavioral Medicine*, *39*(1), 16–26. doi:10.1007/s12160-009-9154-z

Damian, R. I., Spengler, M., Sutu, A., & Roberts, B. W. (2019). Sixteen going on sixty-six: A longitudinal study of personality stability and change across 50 years. *Journal of Personality and Social Psychology*, *117*(3), 674–695. doi:10.1037/pspp0000210

Denissen, J. J., Luhmann, M., Chung, J. M., & Bleidorn, W. (2019). Transactions between life events and personality traits across the adult lifespan. *Journal of Personality and Social Psychology*, *116*(4), 612–633. doi:10.1037/pspp0000196

Dorfman, A., Moscovitch, D. A., & Grossmann, I. (2021). Pathways from adversity to wisdom. In F. J. Infurna, & E. Jayawickreme (Eds.), *Redesigning research on post-traumatic growth: Challenges, pitfalls, and new directions* (pp. 259–279). Oxford University Press. 10.1093/med-psych/9780197507407.003.0015

Engelhard, I. M., Lommen, M. J. J., & Sijbrandij, M. (2015). Changing for better or worse? Posttraumatic growth reported by soldiers deployed to Iraq. *Clinical Psychological Science*, *3*(5), 789–796. doi:10.1177/2167702614549800

Fleeson, W., & Jayawickreme, E. (2021). Whole traits: Revealing the social-cognitive mechanisms constituting personality's central variable. In B. Gawronski (Ed.), *Advances in experimental social psychology* (pp. 69–128). Elsevier Academic Press. 10.1016/bs.aesp.2020.11.002

Ford, J. D., Tennen, H., & Albert, D. (2008). A contrarian view of growth following adversity. In S. Joseph., & P. A. Linley (Eds.), *Trauma, recovery, and growth: Positive psychological perspectives on posttraumatic stress* (pp. 297–324). Hoboken, NJ: John Wiley & Sons.

Forgeard, M., Roepke, A. M., Atlas, S., Bayer-Pacht, E., Björgvinsson, T., & Silvia, P. J. (2022). Openness to experience is stable following adversity: A case-control longitudinal investigation. *European Journal of Personality*, *36*(4), 483–506. doi:10.1177/0890207022107690

Frazier, P., Tennen, H., Gavian, M., Park, C., Tomich, P., & Tashiro, T. (2009). Does self-reported posttraumatic growth reflect genuine positive change? *Psychological Science*, *20*(7), 912–919. doi:10.1111/j.1467-9280.2009.02381.x

Gander, F., Hofmann, J., Proyer, R. T., & Ruch, W. (2020). Character strengths–Stability, change, and relationships with well-being changes. *Applied Research in Quality of Life*, *15*, 349–367. doi:10.1007/s11482-018-9690-4

Gangel, M., Kemmerly, R., Wilson, L., Glickson, S., Frazier, P. A., Tennen, H., & Jayawickreme, E. (in revision). Does perceived posttraumatic growth predict observed changes in current-standing and state posttraumatic growth?

Hamama-Raz, Y., Pat-Horenczyk, R., Roziner, I., Perry, S., & Stemmer, S. M. (2019). Can posttraumatic growth after breast cancer promote positive coping?—A cross-lagged study. *Psycho-Oncology*, *28*(4), 767–774. doi:10.1002/pon.5017

Hoerger, M., Chapman, B. P., Prigerson, H. G., Fagerlin, A., Mohile, S. G., Epstein, R. M., Lyness, J. M., & Duberstein, P. R. (2014). Personality change pre- to post-Loss in spousal caregivers of patients with terminal lung cancer. *Social Psychological and Personality Science*, *5*(6), 722–729. doi:10.1177/1948550614524448

Hopwood, C. J., Bleidorn, W., & Wright, A. G. (2022). Connecting theory to methods in longitudinal research. *Perspectives on Psychological Science*, *17*(3), 884–894. doi:10.1177/17456916211008407

Hudson, N. W., & Fraley, R. C. (2015). Volitional personality trait change: Can people choose to change their personality traits? *Journal of Personality and Social Psychology*, *109*(3), 490507. doi:10.1037/pspp0000021

Infurna, F. J., & Jayawickreme, E. (2019). Fixing the growth illusion: New directions for research in resilience and posttraumatic growth. *Current Directions in Psychological Science*, *28*(2), 152–158. doi:10.1177/0963721419827017

Infurna, F. J., & Luthar, S. S. (2016). Resilience to major life stressors is not as common as thought. *Perspectives on Psychological Science*, *11*(2), 175–194. doi:10.1177/1745691615621271

Infurna, F. J., & Luthar, S. S. (2017). The multidimensional nature of resilience to spousal loss. *Journal of Personality and Social Psychology*, *112*(6), 926–947. doi:10.1037/pspp0000095

Infurna, F. J., & Luthar, S. S. (2018). Re-evaluating the notion that resilience is commonplace: A review and distillation of directions for future research, practice, and policy. *Clinical Psychology Review*, *65*, 43–56. doi:10.1016/j.cpr.2018.07.003

Infurna, F. J., Staben, O. E., Gardner, M. J., Grimm, K. J., & Luthar, S. S. (2023). The accumulation of adversity in midlife: Effects on depressive symptoms, life satisfaction, and character strengths. *Psychology and Aging*. Advanced online publication. doi:10.1037/pag0000725

Janoff-Bulman, R. (1992). *Shattered assumptions: Towards a new psychology of trauma*. New York, NY: Free Press.

Jayawickreme, E., & Blackie, L. E. (2014). Post–traumatic growth as positive personality change: Evidence, controversies and future directions. *European Journal of Personality*, *28*(4), 312–331. doi:10.1002/per.1963

Jayawickreme, E., Rivers, J., & Rauthmann, J. M. (2018). Do we know how adversity impacts human development?. *Research in Human Development*, *15*(3-4), 294–316. doi:10.1080/15427609.2018.1495515

Jayawickreme, E., Tsukayama, E., & Blackie, L. E. (2023). Examining the impact of major life events on the frequency and experience of daily social events. *Journal of Personality*. Online first publication. doi:10.1111/jopy.12819

Jayawickreme, E., Blackie, L. E. R., Forgeard, M., Roepke, A. M., & Tsukayama, E. (2022). Examining associations between major negative life events, changes in weekly reports of post-traumatic growth and global reports of eudaimonic well-being. *Social Psychological and Personality Science*, *13*(4), 827–838. 194855062110433. doi:10.1177/19485506211043381

Jayawickreme, E., Infurna, F. J., Alajak, K., Blackie, L. E., Chopik, W. J., Chung, J. M., ... & Zonneveld, R. (2021). Post-traumatic growth as positive personality change: Challenges, opportunities, and recommendations. *Journal of Personality*, *89*(1), 145–165. doi:10.1111/jopy.12591

John, O. P., & Srivastava, S. (1999). The big five trait taxonomy: History, measurement, and theoretical perspectives. In L. A. Pervin, & O. P. John (Eds.), *Handbook of personality: Theory and research* (pp. 102–138). Guilford Press.

Lamarche, V. M. (2022). Interdependent transformations: Integrating insights from relationship science to advance post-traumatic growth and personality change research. *European Journal of Personality*, *36*(4), 640–652. doi:10.1177/08902070211022119

Lely, J. C., Smid, G. E., Jongedijk, R. A., W. Knipscheer, J., & Kleber, R. J. (2019). The effectiveness of narrative exposure therapy: a review, meta-analysis and meta-regression analysis. *European Journal of Psychotraumatology*, *10*(1). doi:10.1080/20008198.2018.1550344

Lilgendahl, J. P., & McAdams, D. P. (2011). Constructing stories of self-growth: How individual differences in patterns of autobiographical reasoning relate to well-being in midlife. *Journal of Personality*, *79*(2), 391–428. doi:10.1111/j.1467-6494.2010.00688.x

Lilienfeld, S. O. (2007). Psychological treatments that cause harm. *Perspectives on Psychological Science*, *2*(1), 53–70. doi:10.1111/j.1745-6916.2007.00029.x

Lim, D., & DeSteno, D. (2016). Suffering and compassion: The links among adverse life experiences, empathy, compassion, and prosocial behavior. *Emotion*, *16*(2), 175–182. doi:10.1037/emo0000144

Linley, P. A., & Joseph, S. (2004). Positive change following trauma and adversity: A review. *Journal of Traumatic Stress*, *17*(1), 11–21. doi:10.1023/B:JOTS.0000014671.27856.7e

Lucas, R. E. (2007). Adaptation and the set-point model of subjective well-being: Does happiness change after major life events?. *Current Directions in Psychological Science*, *16*(2), 75–79. doi:10.1111/j.1467-8721.2007.00479.x

Lüdtke, O., Roberts, B. W., Trautwein, U., & Nagy, G. (2011). A random walk down university avenue: Life paths, life events, and personality trait change at the transition to university life. *Journal of Personality and Social Psychology*, *101*(3), 620–637. doi:10.1037/a0023743

Luhmann, M., Fassbender, I., Alcock, M., & Haehner, P. (2021). A dimensional taxonomy of perceived characteristics of major life events. *Journal of Personality and Social Psychology*, *121*(3), 633–668. doi:10.1037/pspp0000291

Mancini, A. D., Littleton, H. L., & Grills, A. E. (2016). Can people benefit from acute stress? Social support, psychological improvement, and resilience after the Virginia Tech campus shootings. *Clinical Psychological Science*, *4*(3), 401–417. doi:10.1177/2167702615601001

McAdams, D. P. (2015). *The redemptive self: Generativity and the stories Americans live by*. Psychology Press.

McAdams, D. P., & McLean, K. C. (2013). Narrative identity. *Current Directions in Psychological Science*, *22*(3), 233–238. doi:10.1177/096372141347562

McAdams, D. P., & Pals, J. L. (2006). A new big five: Fundamental principles for an integrative science of personality. *American Psychologist*, *61*(3), 204–217. doi:10.1037/0003-066X.61.3.204

McCrae, R. R., & John, O. P. (1992). An introduction to the five-factor model and its applications. *Journal of Personality*, *60*(2), 175–215. doi:10.1111/j.1467-6494.1992.tb00970.x

McLean, K. C., & Pratt, M. W. (2006). Life's little (and big) lessons: Identity statuses and meaning-making in the turning point narratives of emerging adults. *Developmental Psychology*, *42*(4), 714–722. doi:10.1037/0012-1649.42.4.714

McLean, K. C., Syed, M., Pasupathi, M., Adler, J. M., Dunlop, W. L., Drustrup, D., Fivush, R., Graci, M. E., Lilgendahl, J. P., Lodi-Smith, J., McAdams, D. P., & McCoy, T. P. (2020). The empirical structure of narrative identity: The initial big three. *Journal of Personality and Social Psychology*, *119*(4), 920–944. doi:10.1037/pspp0000247

Miller, C. B. (2014). A satisfactory definition of 'post-traumatic growth' still remains elusive. *European Journal of Personality*, *28*(4), 344–346.

Mõttus, R., Bates, T. C., Condon, D. M., Mroczek, D., & Revelle, W. (2017). Your personality data can do more: Items provide leverage for explaining the variance and co-variance of life outcomes. *Retrieved from psyarxiv. com/4q9gv*

Neyer, F. J., Mund, M., Zimmermann, J., & Wrzus, C. (2014). Personality-relationship transactions revisited. *Journal of Personality*, *82*(6), 539–550. doi:10.1111/jopy.12063

Owenz, M., & Fowers, B. J. (2019). Perceived post-traumatic growth may not reflect actual positive change: A short-term prospective study of relationship dissolution. *Journal of Social and Personal Relationships*, *36*(10), 3098–3116. doi:10.1177/0265407518811662

Park, C. L., & Boals, A. (2021). Current assessment and interpretation of perceived post-traumatic growth. In F. J. Infurna, & E. Jayawickreme (Eds.), *Redesigning research on post-traumatic growth: Challenges, pitfalls, and new directions* (pp. 12–27). New York, NY: Oxford University Press.

Park, C. L., Cohen, L. H., & Murch, R. L. (1996). Assessment and prediction of stress-related growth. *Journal of Personality*, *64*(1), 71–105. doi:10.1111/j.1467-6494.1996.tb00815.x

Park, C. L., Wilt, J. A., Russell, B. S., & Fendrich, M. R. (2022). Does perceived post-traumatic growth predict better psychological adjustment during the COVID-19 pandemic? Results from a national longitudinal survey in the USA. *Journal of Psychiatric Research, 146*, 179–185. doi:10.1016/j.jpsychires.2021.12.040

Roepke, A. M., Tsukayama, E., Forgeard, M., Blackie, L., & Jayawickreme, E. (2018). Randomized controlled trial of SecondStory, an intervention targeting posttraumatic growth, with bereaved adults. *Journal of Consulting and Clinical Psychology, 86*(6), 518–532. doi:10.1037/ccp0000307

Roepke, A. M., Zikopoulos, A., & Forgeard, M. (2021). Post-traumatic growth interventions. In F. J. Infurna, & E. Jayawickreme (Eds.), *Redesigning research on post-traumatic growth: Challenges, pitfalls, and new directions* (pp. 28–46). New York, NY: Oxford University Press.

Rogers, B. A., Chicas, H., Kelly, J. M., Kubin, E., Christian, M. S., Kachanoff, F. J., Berger, J., Puryear, C., Mcadams, D., & Gray, K. (2023). Seeing your life story as a Hero's Journey increases meaning in life. *Journal of Personality and Social Psychology*. doi:10.1037/pspa0000341

Schwaba, T., Robins, R. W., Sanghavi, P. H., & Bleidorn, W. (2019). Optimism development across adulthood and associations with positive and negative life events. *Social Psychological and Personality Science, 10*(8), 1092–1101. doi:10.1177/1948550619832023

Seery, M. D., Holman, E. A., & Silver, R. C. (2010). Whatever does not kill us: Cumulative lifetime adversity, vulnerability, and resilience. *Journal of Personality and Social Psychology, 99*(6), 1025–1041. doi:10.1037/a0021344

Shand, L. K., Cowlishaw, S., Brooker, J. E., Burney, S., & Ricciardelli, L. A. (2015). Correlates of post-traumatic stress symptoms and growth in cancer patients: A systematic review and meta-analysis. *Psycho-Oncology, 24*(6), 624–634. doi:10.1002/pon.3719

Sher, K. J., Jackson, K. M., & Steinley, D. (2011). Alcohol use trajectories and the ubiquitous cat's cradle: Cause for concern? *Journal of Abnormal Psychology, 120*(2), 322–335. doi:10.1037/a0021813

Specht, J., Egloff, B., & Schmukle, S. C. (2011). Stability and change of personality across the life course: The impact of age and major life events on mean-level and rank-order stability of the Big Five. *Journal of Personality and Social Psychology*, 101(4), 862–882. doi:10.1037/a0024950

Soto, C. J., & John, O. P. (2017). Short and extra-short forms of the big five inventory–2: The BFI-2-S and BFI-2-XS. *Journal of Research in Personality, 68*, 69–81.

Tedeschi, R. G., & Calhoun, L. G. (1996). The posttraumatic growth inventory: Measuring the positive legacy of trauma. *Journal of Traumatic Stress, 9*(3), 455–472. doi:10.1002/jts.2490090305

Tedeschi, R. G., & Calhoun, L. G. (2004). Posttraumatic growth: Conceptual foundations and empirical evidence. *Psychological Inquiry, 15*(1), 1–18. doi:10.1207/s15327965pli1501_01

Tedeschi, R. G., Shakespeare-Finch, J., Taku, K., & Calhoun, L. G. (2018). *Posttraumatic growth: Theory, research, and applications*. Routledge.

Tennen, H., & Affleck, G. (1998). Personality and transformation in the face of adversity. In R. G. Tedeschi, C. Park, & L. G. Calhoun (Eds.), *Posttraumatic growth: Positive changes in the aftermath of crisis* (pp. 65–98). Mahwah, NJ: Lawrence Erlbaum Associates Publishers.

Tennen, H., & Affleck, G. (2009). Assessing positive life change: In search of meticulous methods. In *Medical illness and positive life change: Can crisis lead to personal transformation?* (pp. 31–49). American Psychological Association. doi:10.1037/11854-002

Tiberius, V. (2021). Growth and the multiple dimensions of well-being. In F. J. Infurna, & E. Jayawickreme (Eds.), *Redesigning research on post-traumatic growth: Challenges, pitfalls, and new directions* (pp. 1–11). New York, NY: Oxford University Press.

Waters, T. E., Shallcross, J. F., & Fivush, R. (2013). The many facets of meaning making: Comparing multiple measures of meaning making and their relations to psychological distress. *Memory, 21*(1), 111–124. doi:10.1080/09658211.2012.705300

Webster, J. D., Weststrate, N. M., Ferrari, M., Munroe, M., & Pierce, T. W. (2018). Wisdom and meaning in emerging adulthood. *Emerging Adulthood, 6*(2), 118–136.

Weststrate, N. M., Ferrari, M., Fournier, M. A., & McLean, K. C. (2018). "It was the best worst day of my life": Narrative content, structure, and process in wisdom-fostering life event memories. *The Journals of Gerontology: Series B, 73*(8), 1359–1373. doi:10.1093/geronb/gby005

Weststrate, N. M., Jayawickreme, E., & Wrzus, C. (2022). Advancing a three-tier personality framework for posttraumatic growth. *European Journal of Personality*, *36*(4), 704–725. doi:10.1177/08902070211062

Zachry, C. E., & Jayawickreme, E. (2022). Unbelieving wisdom: Does critiquing reports of perceived growth following adversity constitute an epistemic injustice? In M. Monore, & M. Ferrari (Eds.), *Post-traumatic growth to psychological well-being: Coping wisely with adversity*. New York, NY: Springer.

Zalta, A. K., Gerhart, J., Hall, B. J., Rajan, K. B., Vechiu, C., Canetti, D., & Hobfoll, S. E. (2017). Self-reported posttraumatic growth predicts greater subsequent posttraumatic stress amidst war and terrorism. *Anxiety, Stress, & Coping*, *30*(2), 176–187. doi:10.1080/10615806.2016.1229467

Zapffe, L., Hennig, K., Jayawickreme, N., & Jayawickreme, E. (2023). What does it mean to be resilient and grow in the face of adversity? A qualitative analysis of civilian interviews from survivors of the 1994 Rwandan genocide.

PART 2

Cultural Contexts of PTG

How the Environment Shapes the Phenomenon

9

THE ROLE OF CULTURE IN PTG

How Socio-Political Context Shapes the Process, Dynamics, and Outcomes

Roni Berger and Eyal Klonover

Culture is a determinant in all human experiences (Pedrotti & Edwards, 2017). The physical, ecological, and social environment impacts diverse intrapersonal and interpersonal aspects of human development such as cognitions, behaviors, values, attitudes, worldviews moral reasoning, and social relationships (Ellis & Solms, 2017; Kagitcibasi, 2017; López-Pérez et al., 2015). Trauma is no exception. Cultural contexts play a major role in shaping diverse aspects of the struggle with traumatic events. The fact that self and culture are inseparable makes it imperative to use a cultural lens in understanding all trauma-related issues including PTG (Shivali & Dilwar, 2018).

Culture includes a "socially constructed constellation consisting of practices, competencies, ideas, schemas, symbols, values, norms, institutions, goals, constitutive rules, artifacts, and modifications of the physical environment" (Fiske, 2002, 85). It includes the totality of norms and values held by individuals, families, social systems and institutions, systems of knowledge, concepts, rules, and practices (APA, 2013), and is transmitted through environmental influences and social interactions.

Cultural contexts may comprise race, age (e.g., youth culture), ethnicity, gender, sexual orientation, religiosity and spirituality, disability, and social class (Hays, 2016). In addition to the culture of the broad social groups with which they are affiliated (such as nation and community), people are also members of sub-groups (e.g., workplace, a sports team, a gang) whose cultures too may impact people's approach and attitudes to PTG. Cultural norms regarding these contexts shape the worldview of individuals and groups and provide lenses through which people perceive and attribute meanings to their experiences.

That cultural context shapes the experience and determinants of stress, influencing the types of events that an individual might perceive as traumatic or stressful and the coping mechanisms employed to deal with it has long been recognized (Pérez-Sales, 2008). Hence, there has been increasing recognition of the importance of applying cultural lens to understanding individuals, families, and communities affected by trauma. The DSM-V (American Psychiatric Association, 2013) emphasized the importance of including culture in assessing trauma reactions. Impacted aspects of trauma include the definition of what constitutes trauma, the exposure to, appraisal of, and response to traumatizing events (Marques et al., 2016). Culture determines which stressful life events are likely to

DOI: 10.4324/9781032208688-11

befall people in which frequency, form, and intensity, what are norms regarding what is perceived as stressful and traumatic, appropriate language for addressing the experience, and suitable coping strategies and outcomes (Lemelson et al., 2007; Pals & McAdams, 2004). For example, there is greater predictability of certain traumatic exposures among certain groups. Thus, gay youth are more likely to encounter trauma related to bullying (Mitchum & Moodie-Mills, 2014) and inner-city inhabitants are more likely to encounter trauma related to community violence (Gillikin et al., 2016). A meta-analysis reported great heterogeneity among countries, geographical regions, and population groups in the prevalence of post-pandemic PTSD (Yuan et al., 2021). Outcomes for members of an indigenous or otherwise historically minority group may be rooted in historically situated collective traumatic events (Ortega-Williams et al., 2021) and differ for those that are of other racial ethnic affiliation. Oakley and colleagues (2021) reported a meta-analysis designed to compare the PTSD prevalence across different trauma exposures and cultural contexts. They concluded that refugees displaced outside their culture suffer from less negative trauma reactions than those displaced in other cultural contexts supporting the importance of culture in coping with traumatic exposure.

That culture may shape the perception of and reaction to traumatic experiences of individuals and communities was clearly illustrated during the COVID-19 pandemic as morbidity and mortality rates, governmental responses to the situation and policies regarding measures to contain the spread of the virus (e.g., shutdowns, mask-wearing, vaccination, and mandated isolation) as well as public attitudes and level of compliance with them vary across cultures.

Most of the literature to date has focused on the impact of culture on pathogenic outcomes of trauma exposure whereas knowledge regarding the extent to which cultural contexts influence growth following trauma has remained limited. Further, while theoretically, the concept appears to be valid cross-culturally, the prominent theoretical conceptualization and most empirical studies of PTG to date have been from a Western perspective whereas there has been a fundamental deficiency in operationalizing the concept in regard to cultures that are non-Western (Shivali & Dilwar, 2018). Application of PTG theories and measurement strategies and instruments developed in the West may reflect a cultural bias, impose Western assumptions about the potential salutogenic aftermath of trauma and fail to reflect relevant cultural context when applied in other cultures (Splevins et al., 2010). Finally, a major part of the knowledge about PTG comes from etic (outsiders' perspective) studies rather than generated by those who are members of the relevant culture and thus, have an insider's (emic) deep understanding of the nuances in viewing and addressing PTG within the context of particular cultures. This chapter discusses how cultural context influences salutogenic outcomes, specifically PTG.

Culture and PTG

Compatible with the aforementioned aspects of trauma reaction, PTG and the associated processes are impacted by socio-political cultural context and thus, should be understood with the framework of culture. Diversity and culture have been recognized as having a vital role in the creation of resilience in individuals, families, and communities. Informed by a review of literature, Tedeschi and colleagues (2018, p. 31) posit that "PTG is not tied to one specific culture, but is observed in many cultures, albeit with subtle differences".

Research has demonstrated that cultural origin influences resilience capacity, i.e., the ability to buffer effects of adversity, which is a protective factor and a potential predictor of

PTG (Zheng et al., 2020). Sawyer and colleagues (2010) concluded from a meta-analysis of findings from 38 studies of PTG following cancer or HIV/AIDS that "growth in ethnic minority samples may reflect more fundamental and existential changes resulting in enhanced wellbeing. In comparison, growth in predominantly white samples may be used more as a strategy to reduce distress" (p. 444).

The recognition that culture impacts PTG was manifested by the expansion of the PTGI (Posttraumatic Growth Inventory), the most widely used scale in PTG research, to include more extensive and cross-culturally applicable items (Tedeschi et al., 2018). In 2010, Weiss and Berger cross-analyzed a dozen studies about PTG from around the globe including Japanese, German, Israeli, Australian, Chinese, the Spanish speaking world, Turkish, Palestinian, Kosovar, and Dutch and concluded that PTG is a universal phenomenon, which was reported by researchers and practitioners from diverse cultures and subcultures; however, it has unique culture-specific aspects. Since then, translations of the PTGI to additional languages mushroomed (e.g., Albanian, Czech, French, Georgian, Urdu, and many more), sometimes including multiple versions in some languages (Tedeschi et al., 2018), allowing to conduct PTG research in numerous diverse cultural contexts. The rich and evolving international research of PTG has shown that to fully understand its cultural aspects, it is important to look at the characteristics of the culture that impacts PTG and its dimensions.

Characteristics of Culture That Impact PTG

Cultural influences on PTG include proximal and distal factors. *Proximal* influences come from immediate primary formal and informal reference groups to which individuals belong and with whom they interact directly such as friends, family, teams, and social and religious groups. Thus, knowing somebody with an experience of PTG following a similar traumatic exposure to one's own may provide a role model and support PTG. *Distal* influences are broad socio-cultural political narratives, values from the community and larger society and are typically transmitted through impersonal media such as movies, books, television, and social media (Calhoun et al., 2010). For example, the narrative of progress as desirable and the assumption that people have the ability to bring about positive changes, which is integral to the US culture, is compatible with the basic assumptions of PTG more than narratives of more fatalistic and deterministic cultures.

Multiple dimensions of both proximate and distal cultural contexts and people's cultural identities determine and shape PTG. They include traditions, goals, symbols, norms, ideas, beliefs, legacies, institutions, values, constitutive rules, and practices (Bryant-Davis, 2019). Values underlying the idea of PTG vary across cultures as some societies value change, self-examination, self-criticism, and self-correction, whereas others value constancy and minimizing interpersonal conflict (Vázquez et al., 2014). Whether a culture is deterministic, fatalistic or hope cultivating impacts on PTG. Thus, cultures that emphasize an expectation for a positive outlook on life may be more receptive to PTG and generate social pressure to become positive (Shigemoto & Poyrazli, 2013) than a culture where suffering is expected and the emphasis is on acceptance and continuity (Vázquez et al., 2014). Similarly, emphasis on values of privacy, refraining from burdening others and modesty can impact on cultural depiction of PTG. For example, cultures that put high value on modesty may not welcome viewing own post-trauma self as better than the pre-trauma. Meili and Maercker (2019) identified metaphors used in various cultures to describe positive responses to extreme adversity, demonstrated that metaphorical expressions related to positive responses to extreme adversity vary widely across cultures and discussed cultural values that shape them. For example, the Euro-American emphasis on values of self-actualization and self-expression is consistent with the PTG element of deliberate rumination.

Research in a variety of cultural settings identified culture-specific factors facilitating PTG though relatively limited research has focused on the mechanism by which adversity-related resilience capacity affects the development of positive outcomes among trauma survivors (Zheng et al., 2020).

Dimensions of PTG Impacted by Culture

While studies have shown the universality of PTG experiences and people in different cultural contexts report growth after trauma (Weiss & Berger, 2010), Tedeschi et al. (2018) posit that "culture affects what constitutes growth and its processes" (p. 114) and hence cultural context should be considered in understanding PTG. Culture may impact the overall level of growth as well as perceptions of its sub-domains (Matsui & Taku, 2016). Specifically, cultural factors impact the nature of rumination, cognitive strategies, and the process of growth (Shivali & Dilwar, 2018).

Some aspects of PTG are universal across cultures (Weiss & Berger, 2010). For example, similar positive changes after a diagnosis of COVID-19 were documented in Chinese (Wenxiu Chile et al., 2021), Turkish (Arslan & Yıldırım, 2021), Israeli (Hisham Abu-Raiya et al., 2021), Portuguese and British (Stallard et al., 2021) studies. In all these cultural contexts reported positive changes included reevaluation of life priorities, improved relationships within social circles, personal growth, and greater awareness of the significance of own health. Further, similar variables, notably social support, reframing, problem-solving coping, and rumination, have been identified to correlate with PTG across cultures as diverse as the US, Chile, and Nigeria (Eze et al., 2020; García et al., 2016; Tedeschi et al., 2018), although no uniform mechanism seems to apply in this process across the domains of PTG in various cultures.

Other aspects are similar across cultures with nuanced differences. For example, variations were reported in greater appreciation for life, discovery and embracing of new possibilities, positive spiritual change, and being forced to slow down the pace of life in the UK and Portugal (Stallard et al., 2021). However, some cultural differences also exist. For example, Khatib et al. (2021) examined the contribution of ethnic group status and social support to PTG among Jewish, Muslim, and Druze Israeli widows after sudden spousal loss and found differences among the ethnic groups in levels of reported PTG and the degree to which social support contributed to it. These differences may reflect cultural permission to express growth rather than differences in the experience itself.

Culture affects the conceptualization and meaning of PTG, its prevalence, dimensions and manifestations, the PTG process, and correlates (Berger, 2015; Clauss-Ehlers, 2008; Zheng & Maercker, 2021).

Conceptualization and Meaning

In different cultures, growth may mean different things and include varying aspects impacting on the degree of change reported in specific domains of PTG. Thus, what constitutes resilience in traditional societies such as Latino and Bosnian cultures differs from its meaning in modern, individualistic societies such as Australia and Germany. For example, in some north-western cultures feeling more pride is part of what is conceived as PTG whereas in other cultures (e.g., Japan), PTG is conceptualized as increased self-awareness of one's weaknesses and limitations and loss of desire for possessions (Weiss & Berger, 2010). For the indigenous South American Mapuche community, PTG means progression toward the correct way of living and gaining an ideal identity and wisdom through tradition (Shivali & Dilwar, 2018). The East vs. North-West cultural differences and similarities in understanding PTG were reported in a comparative study of participants from the US, Hong Kong (which is characterized by a combination of Eastern and British cultural traditions), and Mainland China (Zheng et al., 2020).

Cultural differences in conceptualizing PTG are also reflected in the translations and adaptations of the PTGI, which is the most commonly used scale to measure PTG. The original PTG model conceptualized it as composed of three domains: the perception of self, the experience of relationships with others, and a philosophy of life (Tedeschi & Calhoun, 1996). However, empirical studies yielded different PTG dimensions depending on the socio-cultural context. In a US sample, five dimensions have been identified (personal strength, new possibilities, relating to others, appreciation of life, and spiritual change; (Tedeschi & Calhoun 1996). International research identified between two and five domains of growth, some of which mirrored those originally identified whereas multiple variations also emerged. For example, studies in North-Western cultures such as Germany and Australia found a dimension structure similar to those in the US; studies in some familistic societies such as Latino, Kosovar, and Palestinian, PTG emerged as three-dimensional and studies in Chinese and Israelis found two dimensions (Weiss & Berger, 2010).

Prevalence

Because certain cultures welcome and support the idea of PTG whereas others embrace it to a more limited degree, cultures and sub-cultures vary in the total level of reported PTG. Vázquez et al. (2014) posit that "The idea of perpetual possibilities of change underlying concepts such as PTG and flourishing is probably not universal despite being common in modern Western societies, or if universal, its magnitude and relative importance in our cultural scripts can be very different" (p. 69). For example, a significantly lower level of PTG was documented among Japanese than in other countries, a finding that was interpreted as associated with the tendency of Western people to seek positives while the Japanese accept negatives as a part of life, exercise humility, and refrain from putting themselves at the center of attention (Matsui & Taku, 2016; Taku & Cann, 2014). Latinos in the US reported higher levels of PTG, Guatemalans scored higher than participants in the US and in Spain (Weiss & Berger, 2010) and higher levels of PTG have been reported in the US than in Australia (Morris et al., 2005) and in Spain (Steger et al., 2008) as well as in Colombia and Chile more than in Spain (Wlodarczyk et al., 2016). Zhunzhun and colleagues (2021) reported 25% of breast cancer survivors in a German sample, compared to 60–73% in a Chinese sample, 66% in a Polish sample, and 56% in a Portuguese sample (Wu et al., 2018). In addition to internationally, differences in the prevalence of PTG were reported also in sub-cultures. For example, in racially diverse cohorts of breath cancer survivors in the US, African American breast cancer survivors reported higher levels of posttraumatic growth than White women (Bellizzi et al., 2010).

Dimensions and Manifestations

Just like culture impacts on the presentation of psychological disorders in general and trauma reactions in particular (APA, 2013), the same is true for PTG. Specifically, qualitative studies yielded in-depth understanding of aspects of PTG that are unique to particular cultures. For example, in a study of Tibetan refugees, Hussain and Bhushan (2013) documented, in addition to PTG dimensions similar to those reported in North-Western samples such as increased empathy and compassion, also unique dimensions rooted in Tibetan cultural narratives and Buddhism such as acceptance of events that are beyond one's control.

In some Anglo-Saxon cultures (e.g., Australia, US), reported manifestations of PTG differed from those in more traditional, familistic, or collectivistic societies like Latino, Palestinians, Israelis, Spanish and Chinese. Similarly, changes in religiosity and spirituality were less frequent in atheistic societies such as East Germany, the Netherlands, and Australia (Weiss & Berger, 2010). In familistic societies, aspects related to the family role and responsibilities in PTG were highlighted, compatible with the cultural value of familismo (i.e., the strong ties to immediate and extended family members as a determining feature of life in Latino cultures). In highly communal societies (e.g., Spain, Kosovo) a prominent aspect of PTG was greater social cohesion and growth (Weiss & Berger, 2010).

However, even within collectivistic societies, studies documented differences. For instance, Tedeschi and colleagues (2018) indicated that collectivistic societies in East Asia emphasize harmony and suppress emotional expressivity whereas collectivistic societies in South America emphasize expressiveness and social sharing of positive emotions. Zheng and colleagues (2020) found different manifestations of resilience capacity following traumatic events in Americans and Chinese from Hong Kong and mainland China. While the American manifestation of resilience focused on successful coping ability, progressive self-development, and endeavor, the Chinese manifestation stressed pursuing the dynamic relationship between human and nature. Li and colleagues (2016) posited that the social demand in the collectivistic Chinese culture is for individuals to be resilient when coping with stress as a demonstration of concern for others. In the Netherlands, part of what people conceived as PTG was feeling more pride, whereas in Japanese culture, which glorifies modesty, PTG increased self-awareness of one's weaknesses and limitations and loss of desire for possessions were emphasized. In a series of studies of PTG in Japan, Taku (2011) documented more intrapersonal manifestations of PTG, reflecting the cultural norm that emphasizes the centrality of the collective over the individual as compared to the opposite emphasis in Western cultures on individual dimensions in agreement with the greater self-enhancing tendencies in these cultures.

Culture-specific manifestations of PTG have been highlighted, in addition to the individual level, also at the broader societal level. For example, in a study of PTG in post-genocide Rwanda, Williamson (2014) concluded that while PTG on the individual level is mostly cognitive, collective PTG is a manifestation of socially shared ideological changes as "survivors can use their religious ideology to inspire positive change at the group level through the collective pursuit of communion (via reconciliation) and agency (via empowerment and autonomy)." (p. 953).

The PTG Process and Correlates

Cultures differ in the nature of the process that leads to PTG. For example, self-disclosure is an important aspect of the process in the PTG model as it allows moving on after a trauma to develop new ideas, build a new narrative and eventually achieve growth. However, in some cultures, self-disclosure is discouraged especially as it relates to topics of intra-family abuse (which is viewed as sharing "dirty laundry" in public badmouthing the family), suicide (Levi-Belz, 2016), and certain diseases. For example, the Ultra-Orthodox Jewish community has traditionally refrained from using direct terms for physical and mental health issues because of a belief in the strength of the spoken word and the risk of attention from the "evil eye"; experiences with cancer are instead referencing the Yiddish term of yenneh machlah, i.e., that disease (Tkatch et al., 2014). Similarly, the assumption of cognitive processing, which is central to the PTG model, is rooted more in North-Western cultures whereas Eastern cultures emphasize the effect of the trauma on people's ability to maintain their social roles and on how they are perceived by the community (Shivali & Dilwar, 2018).

While some correlates of PTG are similar across cultures, others are not. For example, generally, women report higher levels of PTG; however, this gender-based difference varies across cultural contexts (Tedeschi et al., 2018). Similarly, event centrality, which is a predictor of PTG, was only supported in some cultural contexts but not in others (Taku et al., 2021). Stress reactions and posttraumatic stress disorder (PTSD) have been documented as correlates of PTG in multiple cultures. For example, a recent cross-cultural study (Taku et al., 2021) showed the impact of positive and negative disclosure on PTG and PTD in all countries studied (Australia, Germany, Italy, Japan, Nepal, Peru, Poland, Portugal, Turkey, and the US) while negative disclosure did not preclude PTG experience across cultures. The same study also reported culture-specific aspects of the relationships between PTG and PTD and different patterns of cognitive predictors for PTG such as reexamination of core beliefs, deliberate rumination. Research regarding cultural uniqueness of correlates of PTG is limited and would benefit from further investigations.

Discussion

Because of the critical role that culture plays in understanding and facilitating PTG, it is of utmost importance that practitioners become familiar with the social rules and norms, religious faith and rituals by which those encountering trauma abide, and the relevant linguistic idioms in their cultural milieu (Calhoun et al., 2010). Culture-specific trauma-informed interventions have been found to be effective in helping those whose lives were touched by trauma (Hahm et al., 2019).

It is critical to acknowledge that people belong to multiple cultural groups and have multiple identities, some of which can be potentially hidden (e.g., sexual orientation, some disabilities).

Thus a full understanding of the complexity of the role of culture in PTG requires moving away from a "cultural competence" perspective to adopting an intersectional lens. For example, PTG following the exposure to the Covid-19 virus of a black transgender individual will be impacted by the person's racial, gender, and sexual orientation cultural affiliations. Cárdenas et al. (2018) illustrated the impacts of such multiple cultural affiliations in a study of direct and indirect effects of perceived stigma on PTG in gay men and lesbian women in Chile, reflecting the combination of racial/ethnic and sexual orientation cultures in shaping the experience of PTG.

Although the role of culture has been acknowledged, the development of culture-specific models for both treatment and assessment has been recent and slow (Berger, 2015). Yet,

Bryant-Davis (2019) represents a current position that it is critical that "culturally responsive trauma models expand their frame to include the cultural context and the socio-political history of the survivor and their community" (p. 400). Such models should be acknowledged and integrated into all interventions designed to facilitate growth.

References

American Psychiatric Association (2013). *Diagnostic and statistical manual of mental disorders.* Washington, DC: APA.

Arslan, G., & Yıldırım, M. (2021). Coronavirus stress, meaningful living, optimism, and depressive symptoms: A study of moderated mediation model. *Australian Journal of Psychology, 73*(2), 113–124. 10.1080/00049530.2021.1882273

Bellizzi, K. M., Smith, A. W., Reeve, B. B., Alfano, C. M., Bernstein, L., Meeske, K., Baumgartner, K. B., & Ballard-Barbash, R. R. (2010). Posttraumatic growth and health-related quality of life in a racially diverse cohort of breast cancer survivors. *Journal of Health Psychology, 15*(4), 615–626. 10.1177/1359105309356364.

Berger, R. (2015). *Stress, trauma and posttruamtic growth: Social context, environment and identities.* New York, NY: Routledge.

Bryant-Davis, T. (2019). The cultural context of trauma recovery: Considering the posttraumatic stress disorder practice guideline and intersectionality. *Psychotherapy, 56*(3), 400–408. 10.1037/pst0000241

Calhoun, L. G., Cann, A., & Tedeschi, R. G. (2010). The posttraumatic growth model sociocultural considerations. In T. Weiss, & R. Berger (Eds.), *Posttraumatic growth and culturally competent practice: Lessons learned from around the globe* (pp. 1–14). Hoboken, NJ: Wiley. 10.1002/9781118270028.ch1

Cárdenas, M., Barrientos, J., Meyer, I., Gómez, F., Guzmán, M., & Bahamondes, J. (2018). Direct and indirect effects of perceived stigma on posttraumatic growth in gay men and lesbian women in Chile. *Journal of Traumatic Stress, 31*(1), 5–13.

Clauss-Ehlers, C. S. (2008). Sociocultural factors, resilience, and coping: Support for a culturally sensitive measure of resilience. *Journal of Applied Developmental Psychology, 29*(3), 197–212. 10.1016/j.appdev.2008.02.004

Ellis, G., & Solms, M. (2017). *Beyond evolutionary psychology.* Cambridge University Press.

Eze, J. E., Ifeagwazi, C. M., & Chukwuorji, J. C. (2020). Core beliefs challenge and posttraumatic growth: Mediating role of rumination among internally displaced survivors of terror attacks. *Journal of Happiness Studies, 21*(2), 659–676. 10.1007/s10902-019-00105-x

Fiske, A. P. (2002). Using individualism and collectivism to compare cultures--a critique of the validity and measurement of the constructs: Comment on Oyserman et al. (2002). *Psychological Bulletin, 128*(1), 78–88. 10.1037//0033-2909.128.1.78

García, F. E., Cova, F., Rincón, P., Vázquez, C., & Páez, D. (2016). Coping, rumination and post-traumatic growth in people affected by an earthquake. *Psicothema, 28*(1), 59–65. 10.7334/psicothema2015.100

Gillikin, C., Habib, L., Evces, M., Bradley, B., Ressler, K. J., & Sanders, J. (2016). Trauma exposure and PTSD symptoms associate with violence in inner city civilians. *Journal of Psychiatric Research, 83*, 1–7. 10.1016/j.jpsychires.2016.07.027

Hahm, H. C., Zhou, L., Lee, C., Maru, M., Petersen, J. M., & Kolaczyk, E. D. (2019). Feasibility, preliminary efficacy, and safety of a randomized clinical trial for Asian women's action for resilience and empowerment (AWARE) intervention. *American Journal of Orthopsychiatry, 89*(4), 462–474. 10.1037/ort0000383

Hays, P. A. (2016). *Addressing cultural competencies in practice: Assessment, diagnosis, and therapy.* Washington, DC: American Psychological Association.

Hisham Abu-Raiya Sasson, T., & Russo-Netzer, P. (2021). Presence of meaning, search for meaning, religiousness, satisfaction with life and depressive symptoms among a diverse Israeli sample. *International Journal of Psychology, 56*(2), 276–285. 10.1002/ijop.12709

Hussain, D., & Bhushan, B. (2013). Posttraumatic growth experiences among Tibetan refugees: A qualitative investigation. *Qualitative Research in Psychology, 10*(2), 204–216. 10.1080/14780887.2011.616623

Kagitcibasi, C. (2017). Doing psychology with a cultural lens: A half-century journey. *Perspectives on Psychological Science, 12*(5), 824–832. 10.1177/1745691617700932

Khatib, A., Ben-David, V. Gelkopf, M., & Levine, S. Z. (2021). Ethnic group and social support contribution to posttraumatic growth after sudden spousal loss among Jewish, Muslim, and Druze widows in Israel. *Journal of Community Psychology, 49*(5), 1010–1023. 10.1002/jcop.22565

Lemelson, R., Kirmayer, L. J., & Barad, M. (2007). Trauma in context: Integrating cultural, clinical and biological perspectives. In R. Lemelson, L. Kirmayer, & A. Tobin (Eds.), *Inscribing trauma: Cultural, psychological, and biological perspectives on terror and its aftermath* (pp. 451–474). Cambridge: Cambridge University Press. 10.1017/CBO9780511500008.024

Levi-Belz, Y. (2016). To share or not to share? The contribution of self-disclosure to stress-related growth among suicide survivors. *Death Studies, 40*(7), 405–413. 10.1080/07481187.2016.1160164

Li, W. J., Miao, M., Gan, Y. Q., Zhang, Z. J., & Cheng, G. (2016). The relationship between meaning discrepancy and emotional distress among patients with cancer: The role of posttraumatic growth in a collectivistic culture. *European Journal of Cancer Care, 25*(3), 491–501. 10.1111/ecc.12298

López-Pérez, B., Gummerum, M., Keller, M., Filippova, E., & Gordillo, M. V. (2015). Sociomoral reasoning in children and adolescents from two collectivistic cultures. *European Journal of Developmental Psychology, 12*(2), 204–219. 10.1080/17405629.2014.989985

Marques, L., Eustis, E. H., Dixon, L., Valentine, S. E., Borba, C. P. C., Simon, N., Kaysen, D., & Wiltsey-Stirman, S. (2016). Delivering cognitive processing therapy in a community health setting: The influence of Latino culture and community violence on posttraumatic cognitions. *Psychological Trauma: Theory, Research, Practice and Policy, 8*(1), 98–106. 10.1037/tra0000044

Matsui, T., & Taku, K. (2016). A review of posttraumatic growth and help-seeking behavior in cancer survivors: Effects of distal and proximate culture. *Japanese Psychological Research, 58*(1), 142–162. 10.1111/jpr.12105

Meili, I., & Maercker, A. (2019). Cultural perspectives on positive responses to extreme adversity: A playing field for metaphors. *Transcultural Psychiatry, 56*(5), 1056–1075. 10.1177/1363461519844355

Mitchum, P., & Moodie-Mills, A. C. (2014). *Beyond bullying: How hostile school climate perpetuates the school-to-prison pipeline for LGBT youth.* Washington, DC: Center for American Progress.

Morris, B. A., Shakespeare-Finch, J., Rieck, M., & Newbery, J. (2005). Multidimensional nature of posttraumatic growth in an Australian population. *Journal of Traumatic Stress, 18*(5), 575–585. 10.1002/jts.20067

Oakley, L. D., Wan-chin, K., Kowalkowski, J. A., & Wanju, P. (2021). Meta-analysis of cultural influences in trauma exposure and PTSD prevalence rates. *Journal of Transcultural Nursing, 32*(4), 412–424. 10.1177/1043659621993909

Ortega-Williams, A., Beltrán, R., Schultz, K., Ru-Glo Henderson, Z., Colón, L., & Teyra, C. (2021). An integrated historical trauma and posttraumatic growth framework: A cross-cultural exploration. *Journal of Trauma Dissociation, 22*(2), 220–240. 10.1080/15299732.2020.1869106

Pals, J. L., & McAdams, D. P. (2004). The transformed self: A narrative understanding of posttraumatic growth. *Psychological Inquiry, 15*(1), 65–69.

Pedrotti, J. T., & Edwards, L. M. (2017). Scientific advances in positive psychology. In M. Warren, & S. I. Donaldson (Eds.), *Cultural context in positive psychology: History, research, and opportunities for growth* (pp. 257–287). Santa Barbara, CA: Praeger.

Pérez-Sales, P. (2008). Positive psychotherapy in adverse situations. In C. Vázquez, & G. Hervás (Eds.), *Applied positive psychology* (pp. 155–190). Bilbao: Desclée De Brouwer.

Sawyer, A., Ayers, S., & Field, A. P. (2010). Posttraumatic growth and adjustment among individuals with cancer or HIV/AIDS: A meta-analysis. *Clinical Psychology Review, 30*(4), 436–447. 10.1016/j.cpr.2010.02.004.

Shigemoto, Y., & Poyrazli, S. (2013). Factors related to posttraumatic growth in US and Japanese college students. *Psychological Trauma: Theory, Research, Practice, and Policy, 5*(2), 128–134. 10.1037/a0026647

Shivali, K., & Dilwar, H. (2018). Cross-cultural challenges to the construct "Posttraumatic Growth". *Journal of Loss & Trauma, 23* (1), 51–69.

Splevins, K., Cohen, K., Bowley, J., & Joseph, S. (2010). Theories of posttraumatic growth: Cross-cultural perspectives. *Journal of Loss and Trauma, 15*(3), 259–277. 10.1080/15325020903382111

Stallard, P., Pereira, A. I., & Barros, L. (2021). Post-traumatic growth during the COVID-19 pandemic in carers of children in Portugal and the UK: Cross-sectional online survey. *British Journal of Psychiatry Open, 7*(1).10.1192 /bjo.2021.1

Steger, M. F., Frazier, P. A., & Jose Luis Zacchanini, J. (2008). Terrorism in two cultures: Stress and growth following September 11 and the Madrid train bombings. *Journal of Loss and Trauma, 13*(6), 511–527. 10.1080/15325020802173660

Taku, K. (2011). Commonly-defined and individually-defined posttraumatic growth in the US and Japan. *Personality and Individual Differences, 51*(2), 188–193. 10.1016/j.paid.2011.04.002

Taku, K., & Cann, A. (2014). Cross-national and religious relationships with posttraumatic growth: The role of individual differences and perceptions of the triggering event. *Journal of Cross-Cultural Psychology, 45*(4), 601–617. 10.1177/0022022113520074

Taku, K., Tedeschi, R. G., Shakespeare-Finchc, J., Krosch, D., David, G., Kehl, D., Grunwald, S., Romeo, A., Di Tella, M., Kamibeppu, K., Soejima, T., Hiraki, K., Volgin, R., Dhakal, S., Zięba, M., Ramos, C., Nunes, R., Leal, I., Gouveia, P., Silva, C. C., Núñez Del Prado Chavesn, P., Zavala, C., Paz, A., Senol-Durak, E., Oshio, A., Canevello, A., Cann, A., & Calhoun, L. G. (2021). Posttraumatic growth (PTG) and posttraumatic depreciation (PTD) across ten countries: Global validation of the PTG-PTD theoretical model. *Personality and Individual Differences, 169*, article 110222. 10.1016/j.paid.2020.110222

Tedeschi, R. G., & Calhoun, L. G. (1996). The posttraumatic growth inventory: Measuring the positive legacy of trauma. *Journal of Traumatic Stress, 9*(3), 455–471. 10.1007/BF02103658

Tedeschi, R. G., Shakespeare-Finch, J., Taku, K., & Calhoun, L. G. (2018). *Posttraumatic growth: Theory, research, and applications*. New York, NY: Routledge.

Tkatch, R., Hudson, J., Katz, A., Berry-Bobovski, L., Vichich, J., Eggly, S., Penner, L. A., & Albrecht, T. L. (2014). Barriers to cancer screening among orthodox Jewish women. *Journal of Community Health, 39*(6), 1200–1208. 10.1007/s10900-014-9879-x

Vázquez, C., Pérez-Sales, P., & Ochoa, C. (2014). Posttraumatic growth: Challenges from a cross-cultural viewpoint. In G. A. Fava, & C. Ruini (Eds.), *Increasing psychological well-being in clinical and educational settings: Interventions and cultural contexts* (pp. 57–74). Springer Science + Business Media. 10.1007/978-94-017-8669-0_4

Weiss, T., & Berger, R. (2010). *Posttraumatic growth and culturally competent practice: Lessons learned from around the globe.* NJ: Wiley & Sons.

Wenxiu, S., Chen, W., Zhang, Q., Siyue, M., Huang, F., Zhang, L., & Hongzhou, L. (2021). Posttraumatic growth experiences among COVID-19 confirmed cases in China: A qualitative study. *Clinical Nursing Research, 30*(7), 1079–1087. 10.1177/10547738211016951

Williamson, C. (2014). Posttraumatic growth and religion in Rwanda: Individual well-being vs. collective false consciousness. *Mental Health, Religion & Culture, 17*(9), 946–955.

Wlodarczyk, A., Basabe, N., Páez, D., Reyes, C., Villagrán, L., Madariaga, C., Palacio, J., & Martínez, F. (2016). Communal coping and posttraumatic growth in a context of natural disasters in Spain, Chile, and Colombia. *Cross-Cultural Research: The Journal of Comparative Social Science, 50*(4), 325–355. 10.1177/1069397116663857

Wu, X., Kaminga, A. C., Dai, W., Deng, J., Wang, Z., Pan, X., & Liu, A. (2018). The prevalence of moderate-to-high posttraumatic growth: A systematic review and meta-analysis. *Journal of Affective Disorders, 15*(243), 408–415. 10.1016/j.jad.2018.09.023

Yuan, K., Gong, Y.-M., Liu, L., Sun, Y.-K., Tian, S.-S., Wang, Y.-J., Zhong, Y., Zhang, A.-Y., Su, S.-Z., Liu, X.-X., Zhang, Y.-X., Lin, X., Shi, L., Yan, W., Fazel, S., Vitiello, M. V., Bryant, R. A., Zhou, X.-Y., Ran, M.-S., Bao, Y.-P., Shi, J., & Lu, L. (2021). Prevalence of posttraumatic stress disorder after infectious disease pandemics in the twenty-first century, including COVID-19: A meta-analysis and systematic review. *Molecular Psychiatry, 26*(9), 4982–4998. 10.1038/s41380-021-01036-x

Zheng, P., Gray, M. J., Duan, W. J., Ho, S. M., Xia, M., & Clapp, J. D. (2020). Cultural variations in resilience capacity and posttraumatic stress: A tri-cultural comparison. *Cross-Cultural Research, 54*(2-3), 273–295. 10.1177/1069397119887669

Zheng, P., & Maercker, A. (2021). Resiliency and posttraumatic growth: Cultural implications for psychiatrists. *Psychiatric Times*, *38*(7). https://www.psychiatrictimes.com/view/ resiliency-and-posttraumatic-growth-cultural-implications-for-psychiatrists

Zhunzhun, L., Thong, M., Doege, D., Koch-Gallenkamp, L., Bertman, H., Eberle, A., Hollczek, B., Waldman, A., Zeissig, S., Pritzkuleit, R., Brenner, H., & Arndt, V. (2021). Prevalence of benefit finding and posttraumatic growth in long-term cancer survivors: Results from a multi-regional population-based survey in Germany. *The British Journal of Cancer*, *125*(6), 877–883. 10.1038/s41416-021-01473-z

10

CULTURE, TRAUMA, AND PTG

Insights from Tibetan Refugees

Hussain Dilwar

Introduction

Understanding traumatic experiences and their aftermath necessitates an understanding of the cultural factors that shape one's viewpoint. Culture has a significant influence on people's minds, and gaining a better understanding of its various aspects could have far-reaching ramifications for psychological theories and models. Accordingly, some scholars have cautioned against portraying findings in the context of Western culture as universal (Sue & Sue, 1990), arguing that doing so risks pathologizing people of other cultures who do not comply with Western cultural norms (Castillo, 1997). According to Wilson (2007), "the relationship between trauma and culture is an important one because traumatic experiences are part of the life cycle, universal in manifestation and occurrence, and typically demand a response from culture in terms of healing, treatment, interventions, counseling, and medical care" (p. 3). Even under extreme traumatic situations, community ideology, beliefs, and value systems have been shown to give meaning to stressor events and support adaptive functioning in everyday life (Baker & Shalhoub-Kevorkian, 1999). For example, Kinsie (1988, 1993) reported that Cambodian refugees who had experienced several traumatic occurrences understood their experiences using Buddhist ideas about karma and fate.

Calhoun et al. (2010) revised their original functional descriptive model of PTG to include the influence of both distal and proximal cultural influences on PTG, based on newer research. They posited that cultural influences can have a substantial impact on the assumptive beliefs that shape how people perceive events. Proximal cultural influence comes from people with whom the person interacts (i.e., the primary reference groups such as close friends and families, teams, and religious groups), whereas distal cultural influence is transmitted through impersonal media such as movies, books, television, and podcasts, among others (Kashyap & Hussain, 2018). The primary reference groups' social norms and rules also have a significant proximate influence (Argyle et al., 1981) as they impact the predicted coping behavior, the desirability of disclosure, and the individual's growth in the aftermath of a trauma. Distal cultural influences, on the other hand, are based on societal narratives and broad cultural perspectives such as

 DOI: 10.4324/9781032208688-12

individualism or collectivism (Kashyap & Hussain, 2018). In the context of cultural influences on PTG, Calhoun et al. (2010) stated,

> Our general assumption is that the idioms of trauma, coping, and growth, the social norms and rules about trauma, its aftermath, and the views about what helps, in both proximate and distal forms, are likely to play a role in the kinds and degree of growth that is experienced and acknowledged. A major challenge is the development of methodologies that allow for specific testing in systematic and quantitative ways of the impact of these various *sociocultural elements on PTG (p. 5).*

Therefore, examining the role of different cultural factors in relation to PTG requires attention to broaden our understanding of cross-cultural aspects of trauma and its outcomes. This chapter strives to offer a few insights in this direction by providing evidence from studies conducted on Tibetan refugees.

Tibetan Refugees: Historical and Cultural Background

The story of Tibetan refugees started with the escape of the Dalai Lama from Tibet after it was annexed as a province to China in 1959. He was followed by about 80,000 Tibetan refugees. The Indian prime minister at the time Pandit Jawahar Lal Nehru provided land and support to the refugees to settle in various states of India and Dalai Lama established his exile government in the state of Himachal Pradesh (Dharamasala) of India. Since then, thousands of Tibetan refugees have fled to India and other neighboring countries. Based on a census conducted in 2009, the Central Tibetan Administration (n.d.) reported that approximately 128,014 refugees are living in exile mostly in India (https://tibet.net/), Nepal, and Bhutan. Tibetan refugees include monastics (monks and nuns), students, farmers, and nomads.

The majority of Tibetan refugees have accumulated violent, terrorizing, and devastating experiences as a result of multiple traumatic events in their recent past and such events are frequently accompanied by ongoing uncertainties about the future (Elsass & Phuntsok, 2009). One study (Hussain & Bhushan, 2009) found three major categories of traumatic aspects related to the experience of Tibetan refugees:

a Survival-related traumatic events such as scarcity of food, medical facilities, unemployment, and overcrowding at the place of stay;
b Ethnic concerns related to traumatic events such as ethnic discrimination, concern about the loss of own unique culture and identity, and destruction of the place of worship;
c Deprivation and uncertainty-related traumatic events such as feelings of deprivation, injustice, and uncertainties of the future.

Another study (Terheggen et al., 2001) reported that the major traumatic factors of Tibetan refugees include the destruction of religious signs, torture of relatives, prohibition to speak one's own language, and lack of cultural and religious freedom.

Tibet's most cherished possession has historically been its religion and distinctive religion and culture and a substantial number of Tibetans have dedicated their lives to religion. The Bon religion, the indigenous religion of Tibet, got fused with Buddhism in the eighth century. Consequently, Tibetans have been practicing a specific branch of Buddhism called Mahayana Buddhism with its distinctive characteristics such as reincarnating Lamas; therefore, it is also known as Lamaism or Tibetan Buddhism. Tibetan Buddhism was developed under the influence of neighboring countries such as India and China. It has two dominant schools of thought, i.e., Madhyamika, which is characterized by meditation and spiritual experiences, and Yogacara, which is characterized by philosophical and theoretical discussion (Gelek, 2002).

In Tibetan Buddhism, large numbers of deities are worshiped and there are many Lamas who hold a critical role. Therefore, understanding Lamaism is critical to understand Tibetan culture and religion. A Lama is a superior accomplished spiritual master who has attained exalted mental states and spiritual development. Lamas of the highest order include Dalai Lama, Karmapa Lama, and Panchen Lama, each representing different sects within Tibetan Buddhism. Lamas have a very high position in Tibetan society and they influence all the institutions and lifestyles of Tibetans (Gelek, 2002) as reflected in a Tibetan proverb, "there is no approach to god, unless a lama leads the way" (Gelek, 2002; p. 24). It is customary for Tibetans to seek advice from Lamas regarding all decisions from mundane to profound. Further, Tibetan culture has highly developed indigenous music, painting, literature, and handicrafts, which are also shaped by Buddhist worldviews and beliefs.

The aforementioned traditions have been maintained by Tibetan refugees. Studies indicated that Buddhist culture provides diverse coping resources to Tibetan in exile (Elsass & Phuntsok, 2009). Tibetan Buddhist religious coping mediates the psychological effects of trauma and could be responsible for low psychological distress symptoms found among Tibetan refugees (Sachs et al., 2008). Studies have also indicated that Tibetan refugees manifest successful coping with refugee life as they have adapted well and preserved their cultural identity in exile (Mahmoudi, 1992). Their strong religious affinity appears to have influenced all parts of their lives, distinguishing them as a separate refugee group that requires special consideration in order to comprehend the interplay of culture and traumatic experiences (Hussain & Bhushan, 2011a). As Tibetans in exile continue to fight for their religion and culture's survival, cultural factors play a critical role in influencing their traumatic experiences and outcomes, including PTG.

PTG among Tibetan Refugees

A few studies explored traumatic experiences and outcomes among the Tibetan refugees and most of them focused on negative outcomes of trauma exclusively. For example, Servan-Schreiber et al. (1998) reported that 11.5% of the children who escaped Tibet met the criteria of PTSD; Mills et al. (2005) reported 11%–23% prevalence of PTSD among Tibetan refugees in a review of five studies; Sachs and colleagues (2008) reported an extremely low level of psychological distress among Tibetan refugees.

Very little is known about the positive outcomes such as PTG among Tibetan refugees. Hussain and Bhushan (2011b) conducted a study of 226 (113 males and 113 females) Tibetan refugees across two generations. They found that Tibetan refugees reported both negative impact (a mean score of 40.56, SD = 7.05 out of a possible range of 15 to 60 on the impact of events scale IES measuring PTS) and growth (mean score on PTGI 76.68, SD = 9.36 out of a potential range of 0 to 105) relative to multiple traumatic events associated with refugee life. Tibetan refugees reported growth in all five dimensions of PTGI, i.e., *relating to others* (mean = 27.09, SD = 3.22; range 0 to 35), *new possibilities* (mean = 17.07, SD = 3.39;

range 0 to 25), *personal strength* (mean = 15.74, SD = 2.38; range 0 to 20), *spiritual change* (mean = 7.20, SD = 1.73; range 0 to 10) and *appreciation of life* (mean = 9.68, SD = 2.05, range 0 to 15). The study also showed a positive association between posttraumatic stress and growth supporting the notion of the coexistence of distress and growth. Furthermore, cognitive coping strategies such as positive refocusing, specifically on planning and putting into perspective partially mediated the relationship between traumatic experiences and PTG indicating that positive cognitive coping may act as a catalyst in promoting PTG.

Culture, Coping, and PTG: Insights from Qualitative Case Studies

While quantitative studies using PTG inventories have contributed to the advancement of PTG research, qualitative data may offer valuable insights into culture-specific dimensions of PTG not covered by measures such as PTGI. According to Pals and McAdams (2004), PTG inventory captures the view of culturally sanctioned outsiders rather than the inside voice of the individual. Smith and Cook (2004) argued that measures of PTG may actually underestimate it to a small but significant degree. In addition, most studies from other cultures are based on quantitative assessment of PTG using standardized measures and therefore, it is inconclusive to what degree PTG and its domains are universal (Shakespear-Finch & Copping, 2006). Qualitative methods, especially narrative assessment of traumatic accounts, can serve as a promising complementary approach to assessment.

Hussain and Bhushan (2013) conducted a qualitative inquiry to understand how despite multiple traumatic experiences, Tibetan refugees continue to survive with the endeavor to heal through reconnecting with their heritage. They used semi-structured interviews with 12 Tibetan refugees (8 males and 4 females) to gain better insight into the effect of culture-specific dimensions of PTG, the unique cultural features of Tibetan refugees impacting their responses to traumatic situations and the role that cultural factors play in coping with trauma and promoting PTG in this population group. They identified themes that can be characterized as culture-specific dimensions of PTG in addition to the findings from quantitative research using PTGI that showed that Tibetan refugees reported PTG experiences in all the domains that the instrument measures. These themes include acceptance of traumatic events, development of a sense of compassion and responsibility, perception of self as a survivor, and community bonding.

Acceptance of Traumatic Events

The narratives of some participants indicated that multiple and recurrent traumatic experiences led them to acceptance of such events as they understood that things happen that are beyond their control. Many participants, particularly older ones, expressed a lack of resistance to traumatic events. The combination of their personal struggle with Buddhist wisdom appears to have taught them humility and acceptance of suffering as part of a larger existential scheme. The strong imprint of Buddhist cultural worldviews such as *the law of karma* (loosely meaning that present circumstances and consequences are caused by past actions including in past lives) made many adversities simpler to accept. Furthermore, according to Buddhist philosophy, "life is suffering". So, for Tibetan refugees who are ardent followers of Buddhism, sufferings in life is a rule rather than an exception. It appears that for some, the interpretation of traumatic events in terms of these Buddhist ideas and philosophies has served as a useful approach for finding purpose and peace of mind throughout traumatic encounters and helped them grow and transcend suffering. For example, one man remarked that by following Buddhist teachings he has learned to cope with the traumas of refugee life and that Buddhism teaches that everything happens as a result of past actions. Thus, it is critical that we accept our current situation and make the best of it in order to improve our future lives.

Development of Sense of Compassion and Responsibility

Compassion is a very important quality cherished by Tibetans as they considered it a very noble spiritual attribute. One of the most recurrent themes in the Dalai Lama's teachings is the development of compassion for all people because sometimes personal suffering sensitizes people toward the suffering of others. Some participants in the study considered it an important realization and their personal sufferings helped them become more inclusive in their compassion and empathy. For example, one ex-prisoner who had been subjected to tremendous pain and torture stated that his own experiences with great suffering made him more aware of human suffering and as a result, he developed greater empathy and compassion for other people who were suffering.

A few participants also expressed that certain traumatic events in their life taught them the lesson of responsibility. They felt more responsible regarding their life and tried to change in a positive direction. For example, one individual expressed his frustration with being unable to do anything to improve his living conditions; however, he is now working to protect the rights and well-being of Tibetan refugees. This positive transition occurred after he realized that as a refugee, he needed to survive in addition to his personal sake but also for the welfare of the community.

Some shared their experience of gloomy periods, where they felt hopelessness and even contemplated committing suicide. However, these gloomy periods were short-lived and they regained their optimism and appreciation for life. In Buddhism, human life is considered very precious as it provides opportunities for spiritual growth. This fundamental belief had a very deep impact on many and helped their survival during trying situations.

Changes in Self-Perception from Victim to Survivor

Some participants' narratives revealed a shift in their perception of themselves from victim to survivor, which can be indicating a positive shift and growth. Specifically, participants who had been persecuted in their home countries and fled to India, perceived themselves as survivors. This sense of survival gave them the courage to navigate life's bumpy roads. For example, one individual who fled persecution in Tibet and now lives in exile, revealed that he had considered suicide several times. He went on to say that he is grateful for his survival and that he wished to use his remaining life to grow spiritually. A woman who had been persecuted said that she had experienced the worst in life and now does not care what happens next.

Some Tibetan refugees tried to break off the limitations of refugee life by finding newer and creative ways of discovering meaning in life. Some explored their artistic abilities to earn a living by painting and selling their works, especially *Thangkas,* the popular special Tibetan painting primarily that depicts Buddhist deities, the wheel of life, and other spiritual concepts. Others found new meaning in their life through volunteer work in the community and spiritual pursuits. All of these activities assisted refugees in shifting their self-perception from victim to survivor and living a more meaningful life.

Increased Community Bonding

Almost all interviewees in the study agreed that their individual and collective adversities had brought their family and community closer together and their mutual plight served as a unifying factor. Refugee life had a significant negative impact on family systems for almost all Tibetan refugees. Many were devastated by the loss of family members, which resulted in dysfunctional family dynamics that harmed individuals, particularly children. Some people lost contact with relatives who lived in Tibet whereas others stated that persecution led to the deaths of many of their friends and family members and many Tibetan children were orphaned after fleeing Tibet as children. These shared history and cumulative traumatic experiences had a profound effect on their psyches and brought the community of exiles closer together and prompted them to reconnect with their remaining family members as well as other members of the community who provided them with solace during the crisis. Their personal and collective trauma worked as a catalyst for a deeper and more meaningful engagement with their exiled family and community. The close connection with the community was important for their ability to survive and thrive in exile. Most of the participants reported that the support of their community in exile allowed them to survive and earn a living, offering a clear indication of the increased meaningful relationships with the community members following the struggle with the traumas of refugee life.

Conclusions and Implications

Narratives of Tibetan refugees revealed evidence of PTG, specifically of four major culture-specific dimensions of acceptance of traumatic events, development of a sense of compassion and responsibility, changes in self-perception from victim to survivor, and increased community bonding. Participants in qualitative research frequently reported the co-occurrence of distress and growth, which is consistent with the findings of the quantitative analysis and current literature.

Many studies on PTG have used a Western sample whereas research on other culturally diverse groups is scarce. Tibetan refugees had experienced PTG and their cultural world-views provided the required thrust and schemas. Protective schemas that exist in Tibetan Buddhist culture, especially the Dalai Lama, Buddhist resources, and community support act as a stimulus for coping and PTG. The Dalai Lama is seen as a fatherly figure who looked after refugees' necessities as well as a spiritual healer. His leadership and presence have aided them in surviving, coping, and thriving in exile. Tibetan Buddhism knowledge of the human mind and existence, rituals, and mind-training meditative techniques give them a variety of resources to help them cope and flourish. Lastly, their greatest source of coping and prosperity is the support of their community members in exile.

The use of a qualitative study to investigate PTG among Tibetan refugees demonstrated the necessity for emic views in order to widen our understanding and get culturally relevant insights into PTG and other trauma-related phenomena. Quantitative studies have indicated that people in different cultures recognize the possibility of PTG after trauma; however, there is a risk of falling victim to the fallacy that a certain construct exists in a given culture solely because the people responded in a certain way to items on an instrument. More research from an emic perspective is urgently needed, particularly to provide conceptual, theoretical, and cross-cultural insights into PTG. We need to learn more about how social narratives within a society influence people's perceptions, reactions, and healing processes during and after traumatic events and outcomes such as PTG.

References

Argyle, M., Furnham, A., & Graham, J. A. (1981). *Social situations*. Cambridge: Cambridge University Press.

Baker, A., & Shalhoub-Kevorkian, N. (1999). Effects of political and military traumas on children: The Palestinian case. *Clinical Psychology Review*, *19*(8), 935–950. doi:10.1016/S0272-7358(99)00004-5

Calhoun, L. G., Cann, A., & Tedeschi, R. G. (2010). The posttraumatic growth model: Sociocultural considerations. In T. Weiss, & R. Berger (Eds.), *Posttraumatic growth and culturally competent practice: Lessons learned from around the globe* (pp. 1–14). John Wiley & Sons Inc.

Castillo, R. (1997). *Culture and mental illness: A client-centered approach*. Pacific Grove, CA: Brooks/Cole.

Central Tibetan Administration (n.d.). Tibet in exile. Retrieved September 21, 2021, from https://tibet.net/about-cta/tibet-in-exile

Elsass, P., & Phuntsok, K. (2009). Tibetans' coping mechanisms following torture: An interview study of Tibetan torture survivors' use of coping mechanisms and how these were supported by Western counseling. *Traumatology*, *15*(1), 3–10. doi:10.1177/1534765608325120

Gelek, L. (2002). A general introduction to Tibetan culture and religion. *Chinese Sociology & Anthropology*, *34*(4), 15–31.

Hussain, D., & Bhushan, B. (2009). Development and validation of the refugee trauma experience inventory. *Psychological Trauma: Theory, Research, Practice, and Policy*, *1*(2), 107–117. doi:10.1037/a0016120

Hussain, D., & Bhushan, B. (2011a). Cultural factors promoting coping among Tibetan refugees: A qualitative investigation. *Mental Health, Religion & Culture*, *14*(6), 575–587. doi:10.1080/13674676.2010.497131

Hussain D., & Bhushan, B. (2011b). Posttraumatic stress and growth among Tibetan refugees: The mediating role of cognitive-emotional regulation strategies. *Journal of Clinical Psychology*, *67*(7), 720–735. doi:10.1002/jclp.20801

Hussain, D., & Bhushan, B. (2013). Posttraumatic growth experiences among Tibetan refugees: A qualitative investigation. *Qualitative Research in Psychology*, *10*(2), 204–216. doi:10.1080/14780887.2011.616623

Kashyap, S., & Hussain, D. (2018). Cross-cultural challenges to the construct "posttraumatic growth". *Journal of Loss and Trauma*, *23*(1), 51–69.

Kinsie, J. D. (1988). The psychiatric effects of massive trauma on Cambodian refugees. In J. P. Wilson, Z. Harel, & B. Kahana (Eds.), *Human adaptation to extreme stress* (pp. 305–319). New York, NY: Plenum Press.

Kinsie, J. D. (1993). Posttraumatic effects and their treatment among Southeast Asian refugees. In J. P. Wilson, & B. Raphael (Eds.), *International handbook of traumatic stress syndromes* (pp. 311–321). New York, NY: Plenum Press.

Mahmoudi, K. M. (1992). Refugee cross-cultural adjustment: Tibetans in India. *International Journal of Intercultural Relations*, *16*(1), 17–32. doi:10.1016/0147-1767 (92)90003-D

Mills, E. J., Singh, S., Holtz, T. H., Chase, R. M., Dolma, S., Santa-Barbara, J., & J Orbinski, J. J. (2005). Prevalence of mental disorders and torture among Tibetan refugees: A systematic review. *BMC International Health and Human Rights*, *5*(7). doi:10.1186/1472-698X-5-7

Pals, J. L., & McAdams, D. P. (2004). The transformed self: A narrative understanding of posttraumatic growth. *Psychological Inquiry*, *15*(1), 65–68.

Sachs, E., Rosenfeld, B., Lhewa, D., Rasmussen, A., & Keller, A. (2008). Entering exile: Trauma, mental health, and coping among Tibetan refugees arriving in Dharamsala, India. *Journal of Traumatic Stress*, *21*(2), 199–208. doi:10.1002/jts.20324

Servan-Schreiber, D., Le Lin, B., & Birmaher, B. (1998). Prevalence of posttraumatic stress disorder and major depressive disorder in Tibetan refugee children. *Journal of the American Academy of Child and Adolescent Psychiatry*, *37*(8), 874–879. doi:10.1097/00004583-199808000-00018

Shakespeare-Finch, J., & Copping, A. (2006). A grounded theory approach to understanding cultural differences in posttraumatic growth. *Journal of Loss and Trauma, 11*(5), 355–371.
Smith, S. G., & Cook, S. L. (2004). Are reports of posttraumatic growth positively biased? *Journal of Traumatic Stress, 17*(4), 353–358.
Sue, D. W., & Sue, S. (1990). *Counseling the culturally different.* New York, NY: Wiley.
Terheggen, M. A., Stroebe, M. S., & Kleber, R. J. (2001). Western conceptualizations and Eastern experience: A cross-cultural study of traumatic stress reactions among Tibetan refugees in India. *Journal of Traumatic Stress, 14*(2), 391–403. doi:10.1023/A:1011177204593
Wilson, J. P. (2007). The lens of culture: Theoretical and conceptual perspectives in the assessment of psychological trauma and PTSD. In J. P. Wilson & C. S. Tang (Eds.), *Cross-cultural assessment of psychological trauma and PTSD* (pp. 3–30). New York, NY: Springer Publisher.

11
POSTTRAUMATIC GROWTH AMONG FILIPINA/X/O AMERICANS

Kari Tabag

As the third largest Asian subgroup, Filipina/x/o Americans comprise 4.2 million, i.e., 18% of the Asian population in the United States (Budiman, 2021). Sixty percent of Filipina/x/o immigrants and 51% of native Filipina/x/o born to immigrants are women (Morelli et al., 2014; Stoney & Batalova, 2013; United States Census Bureau, 2017). As a result of Spanish, American, Chinese, and Japanese colonization, Filipina/x/o Americans have a unique relationship with the United States (David & Okazaki, 2006; Gabriel, 2017; Nadal, 2004; 2011). Filipinos were the first Asian subgroup to arrive in the United States in 1587 (Gomez, 1995) from their homeland, the Philippines, which is one of the few Asian countries where English is a second national language, and most of the educational systems adopted American curricula (Nadal, 2011). Nevertheless, Filipina/x/o Americans are underrepresented and misrepresented as Pacific Islanders (United States Census Bureau, 2016), and are often grouped with Asian Americans (Museus et al., 2013; Nadal, 2011; Takeda, 2016). The inconsistency in their classification is reflected in the United States Census Bureau (2016) classifying Filipina/x/o Americans as Asian American whereas the United States Department of Education categorizes them as Pacific Islanders (Horn & Maw, 1995). Filipinos and Filipina/x/o Americans have also been classified as "Hispanic" because of the Spanish colonization of the Philippines (Treviño, 1987), and are the only ethnic group to lobby for separation from the Asian American category (Hufana, 2021).

Furthermore, inconsistency in self-identification also exists due to the geographic location and history of the Philippines. The Philippine archipelago is located near Asia and the Pacific Islands and consists of 7,107 islands with 80 provinces divided into cities and municipalities maintaining their individual identity, ethnic languages, and cultural minority groups. Due to this history and regionalism, many Filipinos and Filipina/x/o Americans from the north self-identify as Asian, whereas those from the southeast islands self-identify as Pacific Islander, and may shift between self-identifying as "Asian," "Filipino/Pilipino," or "Pacific Islander" (Nadal, 2004; Sanchez & Gaw, 2007). Their unique experiences often led Filipina/x/o Americans to self-identify as "Brown Asians" as a means of differentiating their racialized experiences from East Asians (Nadal et al., 2022).

 DOI: 10.4324/9781032208688-13

Trauma among Filipina/x/o Americans

Collectively, crises have negatively affected the history of Filipinos, Filipino migrants and immigrants, and Filipina/x/o Americans. Such crises include multiple colonization (David, 2013a; David & Okazaki, 2006), natural disasters (Ladrido-Ignacio & Perlas, 1995), civil war (Gingrich, 2006), mistreatment of human rights (Ladrido-Ignacio & Perlas, 1995), child abuse and domestic violence (Carandang, 2002), and experiences with discrimination (Alvarez & Juang, 2010; Nadal et al., 2022; Sissoko & Nadal, 2021; Tabag, 2022). The aforementioned stressors led Filipinos and Filipina/x/o Americans to experience trauma differently compared to other Asian subgroups and generated psychological distress (Nadal et al., 2022).

Research examining traumatic experiences among Filipina/x/o Americans is scant. For example, one study focused on posttraumatic stress disorder (PTSD) among Filipinos in the Philippines (Gingrich, 2006) and found that Filipinos tend to dissociate when recalling their trauma. However, these findings may not be applicable to Filipina/x/o Americans. The few studies examining trauma among Filipina/x/o Americans, identified predicting factors including colonial mentality (David, 2008), internalized oppression (David, 2013b), racial microaggressions (Nadal et al., 2022), and gendered racial microaggressions (Tabag, 2022). However, little is known about the emotional effect of these factors on Filipina/x/o American's experiences with trauma, though some studies did demonstrate significantly higher correlations between posttraumatic stress experiences and poorer health in Filipina/x/o Americans compared to other Asian Americans (Kim et al., 2012; Klest et al., 2013).

Filipina/x/o Americans continue to experience discrimination as they are viewed as perpetual foreigners, historically associated with pandemics and epidemics, possibly exacerbating pre-existing mental health symptoms of anxiety and depression (Chen et al., 2020). For example, the socio-political upheaval surrounding the COVID-19 virus, unjustly labeled as the "Wuhan Virus," or "Chinese Virus", led to a rapid increase in racial acts of hatred towards Asians and Asian Americans, in the United States (Saw et al., 2021). Studies conducted during the COVID-19 pandemic examined the experiences of gendered racial microaggressions and psychological distress among Filipino American women (Tabag, 2022), perceived discrimination and psychological distress among Filipina/x/o women and men (Maglalang et al., 2021), and racial discrimination and depression and anxiety among Filipina/x/o Americans (Litam & Oh, 2022). The findings suggested that the anti-Asian sentiment that emerged during this time may have played a role in psychological distress, internalized oppression, and racial trauma.

The aforementioned colonization, economic and political instability, poverty, and internalized oppression generated negative effects on Filipina/x/o Americans (Austria, 2008; Gingrich, 2006). Internalized oppression is potentially invisible to and among Filipina/x/o Americans, across Filipino generations (David, 2008; 2013b; Millan & Alvarez, 2014). Internalized oppression potentially presents as psychological distress if untreated. Colonial debt, i.e., gratitude for being acclimated to one's culture, and covert colonial mentality, i.e., automatic preference for anything American and rejection of anything Filipina/x/o displayed in a covert manner are risk factors for psychological distress among Filipina/x/o Americans (David, 2010; 2013a; David & Okazaki, 2006; Ferrera, 2016). The psychological impacts of colonial mentality among Filipina/x/o Americans include depression (David, 2008), loss of cultural identity (David, 2013; Nadal, 2011), and loss of cultural values (David et al., 2017). Additionally, lack of role models (Nadal, 2004), low levels of Kapwa (connection; shared identity, and obligation to care for one another), *intergenerational family conflict* (Ferrera, 2017), hiya (shame), pakikisama (maintaining smooth interpersonal relations, and avoiding confrontation, Nadal, 2004) are risk factors for psychological distress among Filipina/x/o Americans.

Resiliency and Posttraumatic Growth among Filipina/x/o Americans

As a process of healing from the aforementioned trauma, posttraumatic growth (PTG) in Filipina/x/o Americans involves individual and communal aspects, specifically spirituality and religiosity, and social support.

Spirituality and Religiosity

Compared to other Asian subgroups and to populations in general, Filipino and Filipina/x/o Americans are interdependent with a strong Catholic religious and spiritual background involving rituals and spirit possession (Gingrich, 2006). Filipina/x/o's connection to Catholicism (Straiton et al., 2017) serves as a protective factor against psychological distress, and in overcoming adversity. Existing research suggests that Filipino American women have a higher level of resiliency than Filipino American men (Dial, 2007; Hufana & Morgan Consoli, 2020; Reyes et al., 2019). That resilience functions as a protective factor against PTSD particularly among Filipino American women (Reyes et al., 2019) can be attributed to their access to Filipino heritage and culture, which enables them to explore and develop their ethnic identity (Ferrera, 2017). Personal protective factors in Filipino American women also include a high socioeconomic status and high-income level (Ayres et al., 2013; Kiang & Takeuchi, 2009; Kuroki, 2015), optimism, the belief that good things will happen throughout one's lifetime (Reyes et al., 2019), a strong ethnic identity (Kiang & Takeuchi, 2009), and a connection to their religion (Straiton et al., 2017).

In pre-colonial Philippines, Babaylan who were Filipino shamans, i.e., healers specializing in communication with spirits of the dead and of nature, were predominantly women or individuals assigned a male gender at birth who adopted a feminine gender expression (known as *Bakla*). Various subtypes of Babaylan specialized in the arts of healing and herbalism, divination, and sorcery (Scott, 1992; Strobel, 2010). Whereas in Western culture, internal stimuli and hallucinations, i.e., schizoaffective disorder, schizophrenia, or dissociative disorder, are treated with medications, potentially leading to traumatic experiences, the Philippine culture views these symptoms as a gift, and the person is viewed as service to the community because their talents can be used and they are viewed as gifted, rather than diseased. Philippine culture associates enduring psychological struggle following adversity with positive growth including personal strength, appreciation for life, new possibilities in life, spiritual change, and relationships with others, all of which correspond with dimensions of PTG.

Social Support

Studies identified as significant to Filipina/x/o Americans' well-being, interpersonal factors such as strong levels of social support, especially from friends, family, and colleagues (Gee et al., 2006; Maramba, 2008; Nguyen, 2013; Singh et al., 2015), *Kapwa,* i.e., connection, shared identity, and obligation to care for one another (David et al., 2017), and *Bayanihan*, i.e., community and family cohesion (David & Nadal, 2013; Hufana & Morgan Consoli, 2020).

PTG has further evolved among later generations of Filipina/x/o Americans who strive to learn about their cultural backgrounds, ancestry, advocate for decolonization (Strobel, 1996), and formed their own *Kapwa* and *Bayanihan* in areas such as academia, the arts, feminist organizations, and Filipina/x/o owned entrepreneurship. Such efforts may potentially promote collaborative efforts towards PTG among different generations of Filipina/x/o Americans, including those with differing religions, races, and sexual orientations.

Interventions for the Promotion of PTG Filipina/x/o Americans

With the exception of mental health providers who identify as Filipina/x/o, many practitioners in the field are unfamiliar with the historical culture of the Philippines, including its customs, traditions, and view towards Western mental health. For example, Filipina/x/o Americans tend to report somatic symptoms, e.g., headache, dizziness, insomnia, to their primary care providers, without realizing that their symptoms could be somatizations of psychological distress (Nadal, 2011; Sabado-Liwag et al., 2022; Tompar-Tiu & Sustento-Seneriches, 1995).

Additionally, Filipina/x/o Americans' view disclosing one's family or personal issues such as experiences of racial discrimination, as *hiya*, i.e., shame, with the expectation that older generation Filipina/x/o family members seek out younger generation family members, e.g., grandchildren, for support and guidance. Thus, though they have the highest percentage of health insurance coverage of all Asian ethnic groups, Filipina/x/o Americans maintain one of the lowest rates of mental health care utilization (McNamara & Batalova, 2015). Psychosomatic symptoms and low mental health care utilization are possibly explained by *Sikolohiyang Pilipino*, i.e., the idea that rejects Western psychology as helpful to Filipinos and Filipina/x/o Americans because it reinforces colonization rather than respects indigenization. *Sikolohiyang Pilipino* combines Western psychological terminology and methods with Filipino language and culture in assessing Filipino experiences (Enriquez, 1975).

The Filipina/x/o American community requires culturally and linguistically skilled Filipina/x/o social workers and mental health practitioners who help improve access to mental health services and decrease crisis interventions (Ziguras et al., 2003). Specifically, services designed to enhance PTG should be compatible with the Filipina/x/o culture throughout the intervention process, including assessment, choosing an intervention modality, identifying a provider, and creating conditions conducive to PTG. Mental health providers should begin their service to clients with a thorough culture-informed assessment, including obtaining a full psychosocial and trauma history. This assessment needs to be conducted from a position of understanding the client's culture as a frame for assigning meaning to the situation, specifically the somatization of mental health problems and the abstention from using mental health services. It is imperative to determine if trauma was experienced as emotionally painful and unexpected, and to assess symptoms of psychological distress that a Filipina/x/o American client may be experiencing. This assessment can involve the Race-Based Traumatic Stress Symptom Scale (RBTSSS) (Carter, 2007; Carter & Muchow, 2017; Carter & Sant-Barket, 2015), which appraises psychological and emotional stress reactions to racism and racial discrimination by using open and closed-ended questions regarding experiences of racism within the past month that were sudden, emotionally painful, and out of an individual's control.

Mental health providers need to incorporate evidence-based interventions that promote PTG while respecting this cultural norm. As such, the inclusion of family members needs to be strongly considered in the provision of mental health treatment with Filipina/x/o Americans. Additionally, group therapy can help promotes self-awareness of the negative emotional effects of experiences of gendered racial microaggressions in combatting internalized oppression, preventing psychological distress, breaking down "otherness" by bridging together generations, and promoting mentorship and role modeling between/among Filipina/x/o Americans. Group therapy provides a sense of belonging, social support, promotes mutual aid, and self-advocacy, thereby reinforcing resiliency among Filipina/x/o Americans (Berger, 2009). Systemically, it is beneficial for mental health providers to work collaboratively with Filipina/x/o community-based organizations, and educational institutions to aid in the promotion of establishing peer support groups.

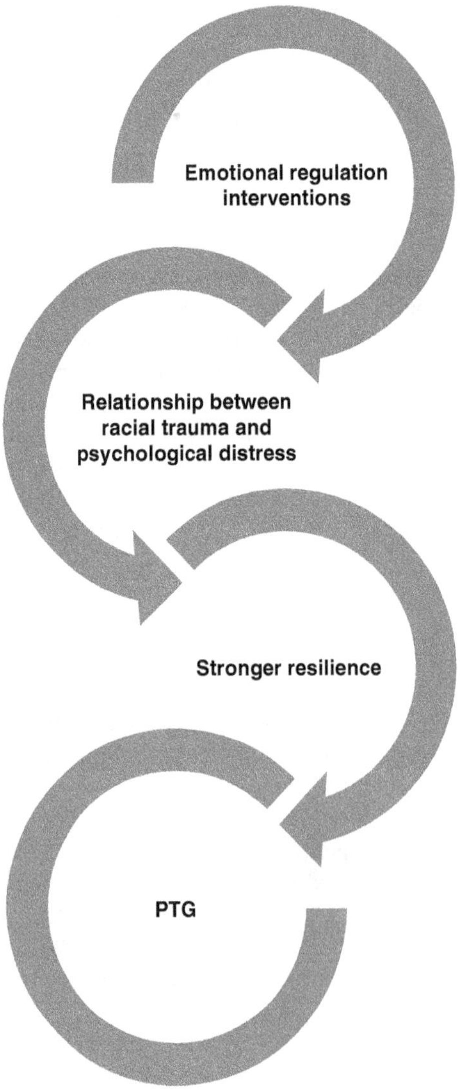

Figure 11.1 Psycho-educating Filipina/x/o Americans.

Knowledge about PTG among Filipina/x/o Americans and within the Filipino diaspora provides mental health practitioners with interventions conducive to the identification and promotion of PTG. The PTG model (Weiss & Berger, 2008) provides a way to understand the cognitive process potentially enabling growth. It is an intentional and proactive approach to identifying and understanding Filipina/x/o American clients' stressors and wellness, and to coping, i.e., surviving and managing negative mental health impacts (French et al., 2020; Tsong et al., 2021). Growth and distress occur concurrently, with cultural influences involving cognitive strategies, i.e., cognitively reestablishing beliefs, self-disclosure, and growth (Calhoun et al., 2010).

Psycho-educating Filipina/x/o Americans about the negative emotional impacts of racism and discrimination can contribute to their PTG (Figure 11.1). By being able to identify when a discriminatory act has occurred, Filipina/x/o Americans will be enabled to respond to such acts, preventing them from questioning if one occurred, and promoting awareness of negative emotions triggered by the discriminatory act, thereby empowering them, promoting PTG. Psycho-educating Filipina/x/o Americans in identifying when discriminatory acts have occurred strengthens the working alliance, protecting against a shift in the therapeutic relationship, and preventing early termination of services (Owen et al., 2018).

Including psycho-education and evidence-based interventions such as emotional regulation, e.g., identifying and reducing triggers, physical symptoms, and positive self-talk, in examining the relationship between racial trauma and psychological distress among Filipina/x/o Americans are helpful in strengthening their resilience, thereby promoting posttraumatic growth (Berger, 2015; Di Blasi et al., 2021).

References

Alvarez, A. N., & Juang, L. P. (2010). Filipino Americans and racism: A multiple mediation model of coping. *Journal of Counseling Psychology*, *57*(2), 167–178. 10.1037/a0019091

Austria, A. M. (2008). Spirituality and resilience of Filipinos. In C. A. Rayburn, & L. Comas-Diaz (Eds.), *Women's psychology. Woman soul: The inner life of women's spirituality* (pp. 119–126). Praeger Publishers.

Ayres, C., Mahat, G., & Atkins, R. (2013). Testing theoretical relationships: Factors influencing positive health practices (PHP) in Filipino college students. *Journal of American College Health*, *61*(2), 88.

Berger, R. (2009). Encounter of a racially mixed group with stressful situations. *Groupwork*, *19*(3), 57–76. 10.1921/gpwk.v19i3.684

Berger, R. (2015). *Stress, trauma, and posttraumatic growth: Social context, environment, and identities*. Routledge.

Budiman, A. (29 April 2021). *Filipinos in the U.S. Fact Sheet*. https://www.pewresearch.org/social-trends/fact-sheet/asian-americans-filipinos-in-the-u-s/

Calhoun, L. G., Cann, A., & Tedeschi, R. G. (2010). The posttraumatic growth model: Sociocultural considerations. In T. Weiss, & R. Berger (Eds.), *Posttraumatic growth and culturally competent practice: Lessons learned from around the globe* (pp. 1–14). John Wiley & Sons Inc.

Carandang, M. (2002). Children in pain: Studies on children who are abused, and are living in poverty, prison and prostitution. Quezon City, Philippines: Psychological Association of the Philippines.

Carter, R. T. (2007). Racism and psychological and emotional injury: Recognizing and assessing race-based traumatic stress. *The Counseling Psychologist*, *35*(1), 13–105. 10.1177/0011000006292033

Carter, R. T., & Muchow, C. (2017). Construct validity of the race-based traumatic stress symptom scale and tests of measurement equivalence. *Psychological Trauma*, *9*(6), 688–695. 10.1037/tra0000256

Carter, R. T., & Sant-Barket, S. M. (2015). Assessment of the impact of racial discrimination and racism: How to use the race-based traumatic stress symptom scale in practice. *Traumatology*, *21*(1), 32–39. 10.1037/trm0000018

Chen, J. A., Zhang, E., & Liu, C. H. (2020). Potential impact of COVID-19–related racial discrimination on the health of Asian Americans. *American Journal of Public Health*, *110*(11), 1624–1627. 10.2105%2FAJPH.2020.305858

David, E. (2010). Testing the validity of the colonial mentality implicit association test and the interactive effects of covert and overt colonial mentality on Filipino American mental health. *Asian American Journal of Psychology*, *1*(1), 31–45. 10.1037/a0018820

David, E. J. R. (2008). A colonial mentality model of depression for Filipino Americans. *Cultural Diversity and Ethnic Minority Psychology*, *14*(2), 118–127. 10.1037/1099-9809.14.2.118

David, E. J. R. (2013a). *Brown skin, white minds: Filipino/American postcolonial psychology*. Charlotte, NC: Information Age Publishing.

David, E. J. R. (2013b). *Internalized oppression: The psychology of marginalized groups*. Springer Publishing Company.

David, E. J. R., & Nadal, K. L. (2013). The colonial context of Filipino American immigrants' psychological experiences. *Cultural Diversity and Ethnic Minority Psychology*, *19*(3), 298–309. 10.1037/a0032903

David, E. J. R., & Okazaki, S. (2006). Colonial mentality: A review and recommendation for Filipino American psychology. *Cultural Diversity and Ethnic Minority Psychology*, *12*(1), 1–16. 10.1037/1099-9809.12.1.1

David, E. J. R., Sharma, D. K. B., & Petalio, J. (2017). Losing Kapwa: Colonial legacies and the Filipino American family. *Asian American Journal of Psychology*, *8*(1). 10.1037/aap0000068

Di Blasi, M., Albano, G., Bassi, G., Mancinelli, E., Giordano, C., Mazzeschi, C., Pazzagli, C., Salcuni, S., Lo Coco, G., Gelo, O. C. G., Lagetto, G., Freda, M. F., Esposito, G., Caci, B., Merenda, A., & Salerno, L. (2021). Factors related to women's psychological distress during the COVID-19 pandemic: Evidence from a two-wave longitudinal study. *International Journal of Environmental Research and Public Health*, *18*(21), 11656. 10.3390/ijerph182111656

Dial, M. N. (2007). Factors affecting the health of aging Filipino Americans [Ph.D.]. In *ProQuest Dissertations and Theses* (304836036). Loma Linda University.

Enriquez, V. G. (1975). Mga batayan ng Sikolohiyang Pilipino sa kultura at kasaysayan (The bases of Filipino psychology in culture and history). *General Education Journal*, *29*, 61–88.

Ferrera, M. J. (2016). The burden of colonial debt and indebtedness in second generation Filipino American families. *Journal of Sociology and Social Welfare*, *43*(3), 155–178. https://scholarworks.wmich.edu/jssw/vol43/iss3/10

Ferrera, M. J. (2017). The transformative impact of cultural portals on the ethnic identity development of second-generation Filipino-American emerging adults. *Journal of Ethnic & Cultural Diversity in Social Work*, *26*(3), 236–253. 10.1080/15313204.2016.1141739

French, B. H., Lewis, J. A., Mosley, D. V., Adames, H. Y., Chavez-Dueñas, N. Y., Chen, G. A., & Neville, H. A. (2020). Toward a psychological framework of radical healing in communities of color. *The Counseling Psychologist*, *48*(1), 14–46. 10.1177/0011000019843506

Gabriel, M. G. (2017). *The role of culture in the help-seeking behaviors of Filipino Americans* [Ph.D., Texas A & M University]. http://hdl.handle.net/1969.1/173132

Gee, G. C., Chen, J., Spencer, M. S., See, S., Kuester, O. A., Tran, D., & Takeuchi, D. (2006). Social support as a buffer for perceived unfair treatment among Filipino Americans: Differences between San Francisco and Honolulu. *American Journal of Public Health*, *96*(4), 677–684. 10.2105/AJPH.2004.060442

Gingrich, H. J. D. (2006). Trauma and dissociation in the Philippines. *Journal of Trauma Practice*, *4*(3–4), 245–269. 10.1300/J189v04n03_04

Gomez, B. E. G. (1995). Filipinos in Unamuno's California expedition of 1587. *Amerasia Journal*, *21*(3), 175–184. 10.17953/amer.21.3.q050756h25525n72

Horn, L., & Maw, C. (1995). *Minority undergraduate participation in postsecondary education. Statistical analysis report*. U.S. Dept. of Education, Office of Educational Research and Improvement.

Hufana, A. M. A. (2021). Exploring the lived experiences of second-generation Filipina American emerging adults: Navigating challenges and meaning-making of intersecting identities and cultural values [Ph.D., University of California, Santa Barbara]. In *ProQuest Dissertations and Theses* (2596628644). ProQuest Dissertations & Theses Global.

Hufana, A., & Morgan Consoli, M. L. (2020). "I push through and stick with it": Exploring resilience among Filipino American adults. *Asian American Journal of Psychology*, *11*(1), 3–13. 10.1037/aap0000171 10.1037/aap0000171

Kiang, L., & Takeuchi, D. T. (2009). Phenotypic bias and ethnic identity in Filipino Americans. *Social Science Quarterly*, *90*(2), 428–445. 10.1111/j.1540-6237.2009.00625.x

Kim, W., Kim, I., & Nochajski, T. H. (2012). Predictors of gambling behaviors in Filipino Americans living in Honolulu or San Francisco. *Journal of Gambling Studies*, *28*(2), 297–314. 10.1007/s10899-011-9248-y

Klest, B., Freyd, J. J., Hampson, S. E., & Dubanoski, J. P. (2013). Trauma, socioeconomic resources, and self-rated health in an ethnically diverse adult cohort. *Ethnicity & Health*, *18*(1), 97–113. 10.1080/13557858.2012.700916

Kuroki, Y. (2015). Risk factors for suicidal behaviors among Filipino Americans: A data mining approach. *American Journal of Orthopsychiatry*, *85*(1), 34–42. 10.1037/ort0000018

Ladrido-Ignacio, L., & Perlas, A. P. (1995). From victims to survivors: Psychosocial intervention in disaster management in the Philippines. *International Journal of Mental Health*, *24*(4), 3–51. 10.1080/00207411.1995.11449321

Litam, S. D. A., & Oh, S. (2022). Coping strategies as moderators of COVID-19 racial discrimination in Filipino Americans. *Asian American Journal of Psychology*, *13*(1), 18–29. 10.1037/aap0000253

Maglalang, D. D., Condor, B. J. L., Bañada, M. R., Nuestro, E., & Katigbak. (2021). *Perceived discrimination and psychological distress: A survey of Filipinx Americans in Massachusetts during the COVID-19 pandemic* [Preprint]. 10.21203/rs.3.rs-502283/v1

Maramba, D. C. (2008). Immigrant families and the college experience: Perspectives of Filipina Americans. *Journal of College Student Development*, *49*(4), 336–350. 10.1353/csd.0.0012

McNamara, K., & Batalova, J. (2015). *Filipino immigrants in the United States*. http://www.migrationpolicy.org/article/filipino-immigrants-united-states

Millan, J. B., & Alvarez, A. N. (2014). Asian Americans and internalized oppression: Do we deserve this? In E. J. R. David (Ed.), *Internalized oppression: The psychology of marginalized groups* (pp. 163–190). Springer.

Morelli, P. T., Trinidad, A., & Alboroto, R. (2014). Asian Americans: Filipinos. In P. T. Morelli, A. Trinidad, & R. Alboroto (Eds.), *Encyclopedia of social work*. NASW Press and Oxford University Press. 10.1093/acrefore/9780199975839.013.852

Museus, S. D., Maramba, D. C., & Teranishi, R. T. (2013). *The misrepresented minority: New insights on Asian Americans and Pacific Islanders, and the implications for higher education*. Stylus Publishing, LLC.

Nadal, K. L. (2004). Pilipino American identity development model. *Journal of Multicultural Counseling and Development*, *32*(1), 45–62. 10.1002/j.2161-1912.2004.tb00360.x

Nadal, K. L. (2011). *Filipino American psychology: A handbook of theory, research, and clinical practice*. John Wiley & Sons.

Nadal, K. L. Y., Corpus, G., & Hufana, A. (2022). The forgotten Asian Americans: Filipino Americans' experiences with racial microaggressions and trauma. *Asian American Journal of Psychology*, *13*(1), 51–61. 10.1037/aap0000261

Nguyen, V. J. (2013). *The daily impact of mood and social support on pain in Filipino-Americans (No. 3557821)*. [Ph.D.]. San Diego, CA: Alliant International University.

Owen, J., Tao, K. W., & Drinane, J. M. (2018). Microaggressions: Clinical impact and psychological harm. In G. C. Torino, D. P. Rivera, C. M. Capodilupo, K. L. Nadal, & D. W. Sue (Eds.), *Microaggression theory* (pp. 65–85). John Wiley & Sons, Inc. 10.1002/9781119466642.ch5

Reyes, A. T., Constantino, R. E., Cross, C. L., Tan, R. A., Bombard, J. N., & Acupan, A. R. (2019). Resilience and psychological trauma among Filipino American women. *Archives of Psychiatric Nursing*, *33*(6), 177–185. 10.1016/j.apnu.2019.08.008

Sabado-Liwag, M. D., Manalo-Pedro, E., Taggueg, R., Bacong, A. M., Adia, A., Demanarig, D., Sumibcay, J. R., Valderama-Wallace, C., Oronce, C. I. A., Bonus, R., & Ponce, N. A. (2022). Addressing the interlocking impact of colonialism and racism on Filipinx/a/o American health inequities: Article examines Filipinx/a/o American health inequities. *Health Affairs*, *41*(2), 289–295. 10.1377/hlthaff.2021.01418

Sanchez, F., & Gaw, A. (2007). Mental health care of Filipino Americans. *Psychiatric Services*, *58*(6), 810–815. 10.1176/ps.2007.58.6.810

Saw, A., Yellow Horse, A., & Jeung, R. (2021). *Stop AAPHI hate mental health report.* https://stopaapihate.org/wp-content/uploads/2021/05/Stop-AAPI-Hate-Mental-Health-Report-210527.pdf

Scott, W. H. (1992). *Looking for the prehispanic Filipino and other essays in Philippine history.* New Day Publishers.

Singh, S., Mcbride, K., & Kak, V. (2015). Role of social support in examining acculturative stress and psychological distress among Asian American immigrants and three sub-groups: Results from NLAAS. *Journal of Immigrant and Minority Health; New York*, *17*(6), 1597–1606. http://dx.doi.org.libproxy.adelphi.edu/10.1007/s10903-015-0213-1

Sissoko, D. R. G., & Nadal, K. L. (2021). Microaggressions toward racial minority immigrants in the United States. In P. Tummala-Narra (Ed.), *Trauma and racial minority immigrants* (pp. 85–102). American Psychological Association.

Stoney, S., & Batalova, J. (2013). *Filipino immigrants in the United States.* https://www.migrationpolicy.org/article/filipino-immigrants-united-states-0#10

Straiton, M. L., Ledesma, H. M. L., & Donnelly, T. T. (2017). A qualitative study of Filipina immigrants' stress, distress and coping: The impact of their multiple, transnational roles as women. *BMC Women's Health*, *17*(1). 10.1186/s12905-017-0429-4

Strobel, E. F. M. (1996). *Coming full circle: The process of decolonization among post-1965 Filipino-Americans.* University of San Francisco.

Strobel, L. M. (2010). *Babaylan: Filipinos and the call of the indigenous.* Center for Babaylan Studies.

Tabag, K. (2022). Experienced gendered racial microaggressions and psychological distress among Filipino American women [Ph.D., Adelphi University]. In *ProQuest Dissertations and Theses* (2677613880). Dissertations & Theses @ Adelphi University.

Takeda, O. (2016). A model minority? The misrepresentation and underrepresentation of Asian Pacific Americans in introductory American government textbooks. *Journal of Political Science Education*, *12*(4), 387–402. 10.1080/15512169.2016.1142449

Tompar-Tiu, A., & Sustento-Seneriches, J. (1995). *Depression and other mental health issues: The Filipino American experience.* Jossey-Bass.

Treviño, F. M. (1987). Standardized terminology for Hispanic populations. *American Journal of Public Health*, *77*(1), 69–72.

Tsong, Y., Tai, A. L., & Chopra, S. B. (2021). The emotional, cultural, and relational impact of growing up as parachute/satellite kids in Asian American transnational families. *Asian American Journal of Psychology*, *12*(2), 147–157. 10.1037/aap0000228

United States Census Bureau. (2016). *Asian/Pacific American heritage month: May 2016.* https://www.census.gov/newsroom/facts-for-features/2016/cb16-ff07.html

United States Census Bureau. (2017). *American community survey 1-year estimates.* https://factfinder.census.gov/faces/tableservices/jsf/pages/productview.xhtml?src=CF#

Weiss, T., & Berger, R. (2008). Posttraumatic growth and immigration: Theory, research, and practice implications. In S. Joseph, & P. A. Linley (Eds.), *Trauma, recovery, and growth: Positive psychological perspectives on posttraumatic stress* (pp. 93–104). Wiley.

Ziguras, S., Klimidis, S., Lewis, J., & Stuart, G. (2003). Ethnic matching of clients and clinicians and use of mental health services by ethnic minority clients. *Psychiatric Services*, *54*(4), 535–541. 10.1176/appi.ps.54.4.535

12
POSTTRAUMATIC GROWTH IN LGBTQ+ POPULATIONS

Claudia Zavala

The spectrum of sexual and gender identities is a manifestation of healthy, adaptive, and enriching human diversity (Wren et al., 2019). Within this spectrum, certain identities—namely heterosexual and cisgender—are seen as the norm and constitute the majority group, creating a power differential that allows them to treat the rest of identities unequally and pejoratively (Schaefer, 2019). This ascribes minority status to lesbian, gay, bisexual, transgender, queer, and other identities, i.e., LGBTQ+ (Galupo et al., 2015), who possess cultural and/or physical characteristics that are different from and not valued by the dominant group (Schaefer, 2019).

Estimates from North America, South America, and Europe show that around 6–8% of individuals openly identify as LGBTQ+ (Jones, 2021; Lam, 2016; Ministerio de Justicia y Derechos Humanos, 2020; Ortiz, 2018). However, Pachankis and Branstrom (2019) estimate that the actual number is much higher, with likely over 80% of LGBTQ+ individuals around the world concealing their identity due to fear of being stigmatized or discriminated against. Nonetheless, just taking the conservative estimate of 6% means that there are around 470,000,000 people in the world who identify as a sexual and/or gender minority (SGM).

Although this population is gaining social acceptance, homophobia and transphobia still continue to impart trauma on individual, interpersonal, and societal levels. Societal prejudice and discrimination pose an immense threat to the psychological well-being of SGMs as their minority identity leads to chronic exposure to additional stressors compared to the population at large, accounting for poorer health and well-being in these groups (Meyer, 2003). Alessi and Martin (2017) posit that these ubiquitous traumatic experiences that impact LGBTQ+ people's lives are associated with negative mental health outcomes, such as depression, anxiety, and Posttraumatic Stress Disorder (PTSD).

LGBTQ+ individuals face many types of minority stressors. Studies have shown that LGBTQ+ populations report adverse childhood experiences at a much greater rate than their heterosexual and cisgender peers because they are more likely to deviate from gender norms and be reprimanded for it (Bond et al., 2021; Schnarrs et al., 2019). As SGM youth grow and develop, they continue to encounter challenges related to potentially traumatic exposures such as managing their identity visibility, i.e., monitoring how they present their gender/sexuality to avoid discrimination (Cohen et al., 2016), coming out to significant others (Zavala & Waters, 2021), microaggressions (Vaccaro & Koob, 2019), and dealing

DOI: 10.4324/9781032208688-14

with family rejection and loss of support (Mills-Koonce et al., 2018). Additionally, LGBTQ+ individuals experience higher rates of victimization, intimate partner violence, physical violence, and sexual assault (Stenersen et al., 2019). Finally, because of the lack of workplace protections, housing instability, and stigma when accessing healthcare, LGBTQ+ individuals are chronically exposed to potential trauma through young, middle, and older adulthood (The Trevor Project, 2020).

The impact of these experiences may create a domino effect where SGMs begin to expect stigma, become hypervigilant, internalize negative societal attitudes, develop a negative identity, and begin concealing their identity to avoid stigma. Thus, negative psychological events emerge beyond concrete discriminatory events. Although these detrimental effects of minority stress on LGBTQ+ individuals have been well documented, a nascent approach has looked also at experiences of resilience, growth, and positive adjustment in this population following the struggle with the aforementioned stressors.

Posttraumatic Growth (PTG) in LGBTQ+ Populations

Research on PTG in LGBTQ+ persons to date clearly illustrates that this population can and does experience PTG after a host of minority stress events. Many LGBTQ+ individuals report manifestations of PTG including increased self-awareness, community connectedness, and strength building (Rhoads, 1995; Vaughan & Waehler, 2010; Vaughan et al., 2014). The presence of PTG in sexual and gender minorities following minority stress has been documented on individual, interpersonal, and societal levels.

Individual Level

Two quantitative studies of the experiences of gay men reported PTG (Kessinger, 2015; Yu et al., 2017). In a sample of Chinese gay men, alongside experiencing PTSD symptoms, participants reported the ability to make sense of adversity and thus build resilience, predicting PTG (Yu et al., 2017). Kessinger (2015) found that American gay men with an HIV diagnosis who were in monogamous relationships with a partner who also had an HIV diagnosis, experienced more PTG than participants in non-monogamous relationships, those who had an AIDS diagnosis, and those with HIV-negative partners. Higher PTG was related to lower levels of depression. Valls (2019) found in a qualitative study that participants cultivated growth through the process of integrating their HIV diagnosis into their identity, building a more caring relationship with themselves and others, and finding a community. These studies underscore the importance of support systems and community resilience in the process of making meaning of their HIV diagnosis and facilitating positive mental health outcomes.

Interpersonal Level

Studies have focused on identity disclosure (coming out) and homophobic bullying. *Identity disclosure* was found to lead to PTG in an American sample, with negative and positive social reactions positively influencing PTG, and internalized homophobia negatively influencing PTG (Solomon et al., 2015). In a Peruvian sample, Zavala and Waters (2021) found that posttraumatic stress symptoms predicted PTG through a curvilinear relationship, and that recalling strength-based parenting in childhood positively predicts PTG both directly and indirectly, by reducing stress symptoms. They also highlighted that bisexual individuals had significantly lower levels of PTG than other sexual minority identities. *Homophobic bullying* was found to be associated with PTG, particularly when participants perceived their sexual orientation as the reason for the bullying (Ratcliff et al., 2020).

Community and Societal Level

Two studies researched PTG and perceived institutional discrimination stigma in Latinx LGBTQ+ samples. Cárdenas et al. (2018) found that gay men and lesbian women in Chile who perceived their society as more hostile to sexual minority individuals experienced greater PTG if they used adaptive coping skills such as positive reappraisal and active coping to transform this trauma into growth. In a sample of Latina women in the US, García (2019) found that experiences of homophobic discrimination in society, having stronger religious beliefs, and being out all positively predicted PTG, while age, experiences of homophobic discrimination in the family, and the intersection of heterosexism and racial/ethnic discrimination negatively predicted PTG.

Hart and Shakespeare-Finch (2021), who conducted a qualitative study of experiences of pathologization of intersex bodies in healthcare settings, highlight two important processes in creating growth from trauma: accessing truth and connecting the pieces. *Accessing truth* entails gaining the language and conceptual framework to understand, accept, and validate their own identities and experiences. *Connecting the pieces* refers to bonding with others who have gone through similar experiences and creating a community of support to enable feelings of safety, normalization, and openness. These studies support the notion that some sort of stress levels are needed for PTG to occur (e.g., perceived stigma, heterosexism, discrimination in healthcare), but, at some point, too much stress is detrimental, particularly if this stress is coming from the familial sphere. Resources such as positive coping tools, family acceptance, social support, and community are vital in cultivating PTG in instances of societal stress.

Finally, Molina et al. (2019) examined how the community of LGBTQ+ people of color coped after the Pulse Nightclub shooting during *Noche Latina* in 2016. Although this study does not mention PTG per se, they report that the community faced the traumatic event by expanding and deepening their interpersonal relationships, becoming more open-minded and empathetic, and gaining awareness of their collective strengths. This coming together to create positive community transformation is one of many examples of collective PTG.

Culturally Responsive, Trauma-Informed Care as the Pathway to Growth

To promote favorable outcomes following trauma, it is vital that the practitioner keeps in mind how an LGBTQ+ client's culture facilitates and/or hinders their possibility to move through trauma into growth. Sue et al. (2019) define multicultural counseling and therapy as a process that centers the client's worldview, cultural values, and life experiences in the problem formulation, treatment, techniques, and goals. For example, for a lesbian Latina client, the cultural value of family centrality can promote PTG due to the unconditional family support even through difficult conversations, whereas the cultural importance given to Catholicism might deter PTG, if the client struggles with reconciling her religious and sexual orientation identities.

Simultaneously, incorporating a trauma-informed approach in counseling can help LGBTQ+ clients recognize instances of minority stress and name the systemic factors at play in their lives. With LGBTQ+ clients, a trauma-informed approach requires an understanding of how instances of heterosexist and/cissexist-related trauma can impact the person's development, cognitions, behavior, and emotions. For example, clients who constantly suffer invalidation of their gender or sexual identities might exhibit hypervigilance or have difficulty building trust with a therapist. To facilitate trust, therapists would benefit from creating a space where the client is free to share their identity, does not have to fight against heterosexist stigma, nor educate the therapist on general LGBTQ+ knowledge, and can be empowered to take the lead in their own narrative (SAMHSA, 2014).

The following case examples highlight two different counseling approaches to PTG in LGBTQ+. The first illustrates a counselor who demonstrates empathy and strives to understand the client's experience but lacks the awareness and knowledge to do so. The second showcases a culturally responsive, trauma-informed approach (Bishop et al., 2021; McNamara & Wilson, 2020; Schmitz et al., 2019).

Elena: A Case Example

Elena is a 28-year-old, second-generation Colombian-American lesbian woman living with her parents and two siblings in a large city in the Northeastern U.S. She works a stable job as a nurse and helps contribute to her family's finances while her siblings are still finishing school. Encouraged by her girlfriend, she sought therapy to discuss coming out to her extended family. While Elena's parents and siblings know about her sexuality and are learning to accept it, her parents do not want her to communicate this to other family members for fear of Elena being mistreated. Her parents' initial reaction to her coming out constituted a trauma for Elena, as she was kicked out of the home, was prohibited from contacting her siblings, and was verbally mistreated by her parents for a number of months. After some time, the family reconciled and Elena experiences some level of acceptance. Elena recognizes that she needs support and guidance since she wishes to come out to her whole family, but does not want to go against her parents' wishes or feel rejected again.

Counselor A

At intake, the counselor asks about Elena's age, socioeconomic status, and whether she has a boyfriend or is single. They question the importance Elena places on how her extended family views her, formulating it as an incomplete process of individuation. They wonder why Elena lives with her family given that she has the means to move out, and why she has not reached heteronormative milestones with her partner such as moving in together and/or getting engaged. When Elena discloses her sexual orientation and her fear of coming out, the counselor tries to show empathy by saying "we all know what it's like to have difficult conversations with others, you're not alone", unintentionally alienating Elena's experience of being minority stress. When Elena expresses anger at this statement, the counselor attributes this to a reactive personality rather than acknowledging that their statement inadvertently invalidated her previous traumatic experience of disclosing to her parents.

The counselor proposes to Elena that they work together on individuation and gaining independence from her family to help reduce the stress related to how they see her, without inquiring about the possibility of having family sessions, fearing further enmeshment. When Elena brings other areas of her life to the sessions, such as exploring changing her career path, the counselor overestimates how linked this is to her sexual orientation, wondering if she is trying to distract herself from the topic. To provide her with further resources, the counselor shares information about LGBTQ+ support groups in the area. Elena feels some support and acknowledges some gains from the therapy process, but feels retraumatized by the microinvalidations of the counselor, as well as the lack of understanding of her social identities.

Counselor B

At intake, the counselor asks Elena to describe all relevant aspects of her identity including gender, sexual orientation, race, ethnicity, age, ability status, relationship status, socioeconomic status, religion/spirituality, and any other aspect that is meaningful to her life experience. Whenever possible, the counselor uses intake forms with gender-affirming language and provides room for fill-in answers rather than checkboxes. As the counselor gathers information, they make sure to assess for individual and cultural strengths by using a strengths assessment tool, asking how Elena has successfully coped with the situation thus far, and what parts of her culture she used as sources of resilience for her. Understanding the nuances of being a lesbian Latina, the counselor realizes the importance of disclosure to the extended family due to the value of familismo (i.e., family centrality, loyalty, and closeness). The counselor identifies instances of minority stress such as the initial rejection by her parents, her parents referring to her girlfriend as a friend, or her aunts asking her when she will bring home a boyfriend. As Elena slowly opens up and remains hypervigilant of the counselor's behavior, the counselor expresses the understanding that this stems from previous traumatic experiences of being rejected/ invalidated; they respect her pace and openly acknowledge that it is reasonable that she might be afraid to share her inner world.

The counselor suggests bringing Elena's parents and siblings into some sessions to discuss how they might come to an agreement as a family regarding what is best for Elena in terms of disclosure to extended family, and how she can best be supported. Leaning on individual and cultural strengths such as creativity, integrity, and familismo, the counselor fosters collective meaning-making so the family can heal from Elena's initial coming out and move towards growth. Thus, in addition to reducing conflict in the family, reaching new levels of understanding and psychosocial functioning becomes a goal of counseling. Elena's family agrees to come to a few sessions, during which the counselor provides information on a psychoeducation group in their native Spanish language that supports LGBTQ+-membered families in the coming out.

Practitioners as Advocates for LGBTQ+-Related Social Change

As practitioners work with LGBTQ+ clients on an individual level, it is imperative that advocating for societal and systems-level equity increasingly takes a similar level of priority. Authors posit that, in addition to individual or interpersonal factors, systemic factors are also important in promoting PTG in the LGBTQ+ populations (Waters et al., 2021). Data from sexual minority women of color show that collective action can buffer the link between discriminatory experiences and distress by increasing a sense of agency and empowerment and by providing a wider lens through which experiences of oppression can be understood (DeBlaere et al., 2014). This illuminates further avenues for promoting PTG, such as encouraging involvement in activist groups and community gatherings, so that LGBTQ+ folks can transform systemic trauma into collective growth.

The same can be applied to different groups who are impacted by the same systems of oppression. For instance, transgender individuals who experience trauma due to barriers to accessing gender-affirming care might form an alliance with asexual individuals with traumatic experiences of pathologizing and medically unnecessary healthcare procedures. Although identities differ, both groups need the healthcare system to adopt a culturally appropriate, affirmative model of care. Such alliances can even be formed with those outside of the LGBTQ+ community; for instance, heterosexual women of color experience mistreatment by physicians due to the bias that people of color experience less pain (Hoffman et al., 2016). Systems-Informed Positive Psychology argues that the capacity for PTG in a system is influenced by how the different parts within the system interact with each other (Waters et al., 2021); thus, increasing possibilities for interaction and mutual support within different subgroups of the LGBTQ+ population and beyond can increase possibilities for PTG.

An additional avenue for clinicians to promote PTG is incorporating the roles of advocate, community worker, psycho-educator, and/or activist into their work, in accordance with social justice principles (Nadal, 2017). This can facilitate clinicians' ability to improve aspects of their clients' environment, and therefore alter it to be more conducive to growth. For example, a practitioner working with a gender minority client who is experiencing potentially traumatic events in school due to discrimination might reach out to the school and advocate for a more inclusive environment (e.g., helping change school policies around bullying and the use of bathrooms). A researcher might disseminate pertinent knowledge in a culturally accessible way to relevant communities, in addition to publishing a paper in a scholarly venue. Enriching the environment with such growth-promoting interventions or tools may be an effective way for cultivating PTG beyond the individual level, and thus promoting PTG for LGBTQ+ individuals in a holistic manner.

Future Research

The review of the literature presented above suggests that future research needs to seek to uncover systemic factors that may promote PTG given that the mental health of LGBTQ+ persons is influenced by all levels of the socio-ecological system (Rostosky & Riggle, 2017). One way to do this would be to conduct research on multiply-marginalized individuals, such as LGBTQ+ people of color, moving beyond an additive approach (e.g., studying the trauma of heterosexism and racism separately) to an intersectional approach (e.g., how heterosexism and racism show up in institutions to create barriers to diverse LGBTQ+ populations).

Another pathway would be to examine the moderating role of policies on the relationship between traumatic stress and PTG. For example, Tebbe et al. (2021) found that anti-trans legislation efforts strengthened the link between transgender discrimination and hopelessness. It seems fruitful for research to examine if healthcare, workplace, and school anti-discrimination laws can be conducive to PTG for LGBTQ+ individuals with experiences of trauma.

Further, most studies have focused on how individual, interpersonal, community/societal events lead to PTG in individuals. However, growth experiences can be found in systems as well such as parents grappling with their children's sexual/gender minority identity (Zavala & Waters, 2022), LGBTQ+ parents experiencing various forms of systemic stressors in their parenting journey (Prendergast & MacPhee, 2018), or LGBTQ+ communities suffering hate crimes (Molina et al., 2019). Future research should consider how PTG manifests in LGBTQ+-membered families and communities.

Finally, it is worth noting that certain subgroups within the LGBTQ+ community have not received enough attention in research. Most funding by the National Institutes of Health (NIH) for LGBTQ+ research is focused on sexual minority men and HIV (Bosse et al., 2020; Coulter et al., 2014). No studies have yet focused specifically on transgender/nonbinary or elder LGBTQ+ populations. This is concerning since those who challenge the gender binary experience greater levels of trauma (James et al., 2016), and older LGBTQ+ adults are often retraumatized in later life due to stigmatization by service providers and being forced to conceal their identity to receive care (Yang et al., 2018).

Conclusions

As we make our way toward social justice and equity, we must acknowledge that LGBTQ+ individuals, families, and communities continue to experience potentially traumatic events. Thus, it is vital that we acknowledge that PTG is not an automatic outcome of trauma; there are many facilitators at play, some of which can be modified and increased through interventions. Increasing individual coping skills, familial support and acceptance, and community resilience may ensure that we provide the highest level of care. However, while working to modify individual and community-level factors is necessary, it is insufficient. Clinicians can and should be engaged in system-level social justice work to ensure that future generations of LGBTQ+ people can be free of ubiquitous trauma exposure, with special attention to subgroups at the intersection of multiple systems of oppression. Beyond client empowerment, expanding our roles to include advocacy, activism, and social change is the ultimate road to positive transformational growth both for those we serve and for ourselves as professionals.

References

Alessi, E., & Martin, J. (2017). Intersection of trauma and identity. In K. L. Eckstrand, & J. Potter (Eds.), *Trauma, resilience, and health promotion in LGBT patients* (pp. 3–14). Springer International Publishing. 10.1007/978-3-319-54509-7_1

Bishop, J. et al. (2021). The real and ideal experiences of what culturally competent counselling or psychotherapy service provision means to lesbian, gay and bisexual people. *Counseling and Psychotherapy Research*, 1–10. 10.1002/capr.12469

Bond, M., Stone, A., Salcido, R., & Schnarrs, P. (2021). How often were you traumatized? Reconceptualizing adverse childhood experiences for sexual and gender minorities. *Journal of Affective Disorders*, *282*, 407–414. 10.1016/j.jad.2020.12.117

Bosse, J. D., Jackman, K. B., & Hughes, T. L. (2020). NINR funding dedicated to sexual and gender minority health: 1987–2018. *Nursing Outlook*, *68*(3), 293–300. 10.1016/j.outlook.2020.01.002

Cárdenas, M., Barrientos, J., Meyer, I., Gómez, F., Guzmán, M., & Bahamondes, J. (2018). Direct and indirect effects of perceived stigma on posttraumatic growth in gay men and lesbian women in Chile. *Journal of Traumatic Stress*, *31*(1), 5–13.

Cohen, J., Blasey, C., Barr Taylor, C., Weiss, B., & Newman, M. (2016). Anxiety and related disorders and concealment in sexual minority young adults. *Behavioral Therapy*, *47*(1), 91–101. 10.1016/j.beth.2015.09.006

Coulter, R. W. S., Kenst, K. S., Bowen, D. J., & Scout, P. (2014). Research funded by the national institutes of health on the health of lesbian, gay, bisexual, and transgender populations. *American Journal of Public Health*, *104*(2), e105–e112.

DeBlaere, C., Brewster, M., Bertsch, K., DeCarlo, A., Kegel, K., & Presseau, C. (2014). The protective power of collective action for sexual minority women of color: An investigation of multiple discrimination experiences and psychological distress. *Psychology of Women Quarterly*, *38*(1), 20–32. 10.1177/0361684313493252

Galupo, M., Mitchell, R., & Davis, K. (2015). Sexual minority self-identification: Multiple identities and complexity. *Psychology of Sexual Orientation and Gender Diversity*, 2(4), 355–364. 10.1037/sgd0000131

García, E. (2019). *Post-traumatic growth in sexual minority Latinas: An intersectional exploration of cumulative and systemic stress and trauma exposures*. [Master's thesis]. Purdue University.

Hart, B., & Shakespeare-Finch, J. (2021). Intersex lived experience: Trauma and posttraumatic growth in narratives. *Psychology & Sexuality*. 10.1080/19419899.2021.1938189

Hoffman, K. M., Trawalter, S., Axt, J. R., & Oliver, M. N. (2016). Racial bias in pain assessment and treatment recommendations, and false beliefs about biological differences between blacks and whites. *Proceedings of the National Academy of Sciences of the United States of America*, *113*(16), 4296–4301. 10.1073/pnas.1516047113

James, S. E., Herman, J. L., Rankin, S., Keisling, M., Mottet, L., & Anafi, M. (2016). *The report of the 2015 U.S. transgender survey* (December 2016 Report). Washington, DC: National Center for Transgender Equality.

Jones, J. (2021). *LGBT identification rises to 5.6% in latest U.S. estimate*. Retrieved from: https://news.gallup.com/poll/329708/lgbt-identification-rises-latest-estimate.aspx

Kessinger, A. (2015). *Posttraumatic growth as a moderator between relationship satisfaction and emotional wellbeing in a sample of gay men with HIV/AIDS*. Doctoral dissertation. Alliant International University. ProQuest Dissertations & Theses Global, 1658552073.

Lam, A. (2016). Counting the LGBT population: 6% of Europeans identify as LGBT. Retrieved from: https://daliaresearch.com/blog/counting-the-lgbt-population-6-of-europeans-identify-as-lgbt/

McNamara, G., & Wilson, C. (2020). Lesbian, gay and bisexual individuals experience of mental health services – A systematic review. *The Journal of Mental Health Training, Education, and Practice*, *15*(2), 59–70. 10.1108/JMHTEP-09-2019-0047

Meyer, I. H. (2003). Prejudice, social stress, and mental health in lesbian, gay, and bisexual populations: Conceptual issues and research evidence. *Psychological Bulletin*, *129*(5), 674–697. 10.1037/0033-2909.129.5.674

Mills-Koonce, W., Rehder, P., & McCurdy, A. (2018). The significance of parenting and parent-child relationships for sexual and gender minority adolescents. *Journal of Research on Adolescence*, *28*(3), 637–649. 10.1111/jora.12404

Ministerio de Justicia y Derechos Humanos. (2020). II Encuesta Nacional de Derechos Humanos: Población LGBT. Retrieved from: https://www.ipsos.com/sites/default/files/ct/news/documents/2020-06/presentacion_ii_encuesta_nacional_ddhh.pdf

Molina, O., Yegidis, B., & Jacinto, G. (2019). The Pulse nightclub mass shooting, and factors affecting community resilience following the terrorist attack. *Best Practices in Mental Health*, *15*(2), 2–15. Retrieved from: https://www.researchgate.net/publication/348249295_The_Pulse_Nightclub_Mass_Shooting_and_Factors_Affecting_Community_Resilience_Following_the_Terrorist_Attack

Nadal, K. (2017). "Let's get in formation": On becoming a psychologist–activist in the 21st century. *American Psychologist*, 72(9), 935–946. 10.1037/amp0000212

Ortiz, V. (2018). *En México, 6% de la población pertenece a la comunidad LGBT+*. Retrieved from: https://puedesdecirno.org/actualidad/en-mexico-6-de-la-poblacion-pertenece-a-la-comunidad-lgbt/

Pachankis, J., & Brãnstrom, R. (2019). How many sexual minorities are hidden? Projecting the size of the global closet with implications for policy and public health. *PLoS One*, *14*(6), 1–12. 10.1371/journal.pone.0218084

Prendergast, S., & MacPhee, D. (2018). Family resilience amid stigma and discrimination: A conceptual model for families headed by same-sex parents. *Family Relations*, *67*(1), 26–40. 10.1111/fare.12296

Ratcliff, J., Tombari, J. M., Miller, A. K., Brand, P. F., & Witnauer, J. E. (2020). Factors promoting posttraumatic growth in sexual minority adults following adolescent bullying experiences. *Journal of Interpersonal Violence*, 1–23. 10.1177/0886260520961867

Rhoads, R. A. (1995). Learning from the coming-out experiences of college males. *Journal of College Student Development*, *36*(1), 67–74.

Rostosky, S., & Riggle, D. (2017). Same-sex relationships and minority stress. *Current Opinion in Psychology*, *13*, 29–38.

Schaefer, R. (2019). *Racial and ethnic groups* (15th ed.). Hoboken, NJ: Pearson.

Schmitz, R. et al. (2019). LGBTQ1 Latino/a young people's interpretations of stigma and mental health: An intersectional minority stress perspective. *Society and Mental Health*, 1–17. 10.1177/2156869319847248

Schnarrs, P., Stone, A., Salcido, R., Baldwin, A., Georgiou, C., & Nemeroff, C. (2019). Differences in adverse childhood experiences (ACEs) and quality of physical and mental health between transgender and cisgender sexual minorities. *Journal of Psychiatric Research*, *119*(2019), 1–6. 10.1016/j.jpsychires.2019.09.001

Solomon, D., McAbee, J., Asberg, K., & McGee, A. (2015). Coming out and the potential for growth in sexual minorities: The role of social reactions and internalized homonegativity. *Journal of Homosexuality*, *62*(11), 1512–1538. 10.1080/00918369.2015.1073032

Stenersen, M., Ovrebo, E., Emery, H., Brown, E., New, C., Brasfield, C., & Turner, L. (2019). Interpersonal trauma, and PTSD symptomology among lesbian, gay, and bisexual individuals: A closer look at gender, minority stress, and help-seeking behaviors. *Journal of LGBT Issues in Counseling*, *13*(3), 216–231. 10.1080/15538605.2019.1627976

Substance Abuse and Mental Health Services Administration (SAMHSA). (2014). SAMHSA's Concept of *Trauma and Guidance for a Trauma-Informed* Approach. *SAMSHA*. Retrieved from: https://ncsacw.samhsa.gov/userfiles/files/SAMHSA_Trauma.pdf

Sue, D. W., Sue, D., Neville, H., & Smith, L. (2019). *Counseling the culturally diverse: Theory and Practice* (8th ed.). Hoboken, NJ: John Wiley & Sons.

Tebbe, E. A., Simone, M., Wilson, E., & Hunsicker, M. (2021). A dangerous visibility: Moderating effects of antitrans legislative efforts on trans and gender-diverse mental health. *Psychology of Sexual Orientation and Gender Diversity*. 10.1037/sgd0000481

The Trevor Project (2020). *National Survey on LGBTQ Youth Mental Health 2020*. Retrieved from: https://www.thetrevorproject.org/survey-2020/?section=Introduction

Vaccaro, A., & Koob, R. (2019). A critical and intersectional model of LGBTQ microaggressions: Toward a more comprehensive understanding. *Journal of Homosexuality*, *66*(10), 1317–1344. 10.1080/00918369.2018.1539583

Valls, L. (2019). *The lived experiences of posttraumatic growth in gay men after an HIV diagnosis: An interpretative phenomenological analysis*. Middlesex University, New School of Psychotherapy and Counselling. ProQuest 2411967690.

Vaughan, M. D., & Waehler, C. A. (2010). Coming out growth: Conceptualizing and measuring stress-related growth associated with coming out to others as a sexual minority. *Journal of Adult Development*, *17*(2), 94–109.

Vaughan, M. D., Miles, J., Parent, M. C., Lee, H. S., Tilghman, J. D., & Prokhorets, S. (2014). A content analysis of LGBT-themed positive psychology articles. *Psychology of Sexual Orientation and Gender Diversity*, *1*(4), 313–324. 10.1037/sgd0000060

Waters, L., Cameron, K., Nelson-Coffey, S. K., Crone, D. L., Kern, M. L., Lomas, T., Oades, L., Owens, R. L., Pawelski, J. O., Rashid, T., Warren, M. A., White, M. A., & Williams, P. (2021). Collective wellbeing and posttraumatic growth during COVID-19: How positive psychology can help families, schools, workplaces and marginalized communities. *The Journal of Positive Psychology*. 10.1080/17439760.2021.1940251

Wren, B., Launer, J., Reiss, M., Swanepoel, A., & Music, G. (2019). Can evolutionary thinking shed light on gender diversity? *British Journal of Psychological Advances*, *25*(6), 351–362. 10.1192/bja.2019.35

Yang, J., Chu, Y., & Salmon, M. A. (2018). Predicting perceived isolation among midlife and older LGBT adults: The role of welcoming aging service providers. *The Gerontologist*, *58*(5), 904–912. 10.1093/geront/gnx092

Yu, N., Chen, L., Ye, Z., Li, X., & Lin, D. (2017). Impacts of making sense of adversity on depression, posttraumatic stress disorder, and posttraumatic growth among a sample of mainly newly diagnosed HIV-positive Chinese young homosexual men: The mediating role of resilience. *AIDS Care*, *29*, 79–85. 10.1080/09540121.2016.121007

Zavala, C., & Waters, L. (2021). Coming out as LGBTQ +: The role strength-based parenting on posttraumatic stress and posttraumatic growth. *Journal of Happiness Studies*, *22*(3), 1359–1383. 10.1007/s10902-020-00276-y

Zavala, C., & Waters, L. (2022). "It's a family matter": A strengths-based intervention for parents of sexual minority individuals. *Journal of Gay & Lesbian Mental Health*. 10.1080/19359705.2022.2113948

PART 3

Developmental Aspects of PTG

13
POSTTRAUMATIC GROWTH IN CHILDREN AND YOUTH

Ryan P. Kilmer, Laura Marie Armstrong, and Janelle T. Billingsley

Posttraumatic growth (PTG), i.e., positive changes experienced as a result of the struggle with trauma (Tedeschi & Calhoun, 1995), has been the focus of considerable research attention (Helgeson et al., 2006; Liu et al., 2017; Prati & Pietrantoni, 2009; Xiaoli et al., 2019). The vast majority of this work has focused on adult populations. More recently, researchers have extended to children and youth explorations of PTG, which has now been documented in a range of child and youth populations (Armstrong et al., 2018; Kilmer et al., 2014; Meyerson et al., 2011), and researchers have sought to better understand the construct, its correlates, and the growth process in children and youth.

This chapter draws on this growing research base to outline the construct and provide a broad introduction to the study of PTG in children and youth, frame key developmental considerations, distinguish PTG from resilience, summarize current findings regarding factors associated with PTG in children and youth, highlight limitations of the extant literature base and needed future directions, and discuss relevant practice implications.

The Study of PTG in Children and Youth

Early studies of PTG in children and youth (e.g., Cryder et al., 2006) sought to address the question of whether the growth process was even possible in youngsters, and authors of initial writings in this area necessarily drew on parallel literature in their efforts to grapple with and hypothesize about the growth process in children and youth (Kilmer, 2006; Yaskowich, 2002).

Tedeschi and Calhoun (1995; 2004; also Calhoun & Tedeschi, 2006; Cann et al., 2010) conceptualized the PTG process in adults. They posited that trauma can shake an individual's basic assumptions and core beliefs (i.e., internal working models) about one's self, others, one's world, and expectations for their life (Cann et al., 2010). The disruption of one's beliefs and models of the world leads to efforts to cope, adapt to one's new reality, and understand its implications for their life. It is this struggle with the adversity and its aftermath that is thought to foster growth; the ongoing distress and the individual's efforts to understand and reconcile their posttrauma reality are believed to promote constructive cognitive processing of the trauma and the individual's life situation, a phenomenon that

DOI: 10.4324/9781032208688-16

has been labeled as productive or deliberate rumination (Calhoun & Tedeschi, 2006; Tedeschi et al., 2007). This constructive rumination process can help one make sense of their experience and integrate the trauma and its aftermath in a way that aligns with their prior working models or internal representations. This process is thought to yield schema change, which can consolidate new perspectives on the self, others, and one's life (Calhoun & Tedeschi, 2006). Available literature suggests that these changes, viewed as PTG, tend to be reported in multiple key domains: changed self-perception, such as a greater sense of one's personal strength, new perspectives regarding relationships, and a changed philosophy of life, such as an increased appreciation for life or spiritual growth (Calhoun & Tedeschi, 2006).

In light of this meaningful emphasis on the cognitive reprocessing of the trauma and its impact on one's life narrative in the PTG process, some scholars questioned whether children had the capacity to engage in the cognitive and affective processes thought necessary to foster growth. The evidence suggests that children and youth do experience growth as a result of the struggle with trauma and its aftermath (Armstrong et al., 2018; Kilmer et al., 2014). As the literature has grown, researchers have sought to better assess the construct (Kilmer et al., 2009), research factors that predict and contribute to PTG in youngsters (Andrades et al., 2018; Kilmer & Gil-Rivas, 2010; Taku et al., 2012), and describe the PTG process over time (Armstrong et al., 2018; Kilmer et al., 2014; Meyerson et al., 2011).

PTG has been reported in child and youth populations that have experienced a range of potentially traumatic events and adversities, including natural disasters (hurricanes, earthquakes) and wildfires (Andrades et al., 2018; Cryder et al., 2006; Felix et al., 2015; Kilmer & Gil-Rivas, 2010), parental loss (Salloum et al., 2019), cancer diagnosis (Barakat et al., 2006), and other potentially traumatic events (Milam et al., 2004; Taku et al., 2012). PTG in children and adolescents has been documented across cultures and contexts such as Spain (Andrades et al., 2018), Chile (Andrades et al., 2021), China (Xu et al., 2018), the Netherlands (Alisic et al., 2008), Norway (Hafstad et al., 2011), Israel (Laufer & Solomon, 2006; Levine et al., 2008), and Japan (Taku et al., 2012). Thus, evidence suggests that individuals who have not yet reached adulthood have the capacity to perceive and report positive change subsequent to potentially traumatic events.

Key Developmental Considerations

Key considerations regarding children's ability to experience PTG fall within at least three domains: emotional experience and regulation, cognitive capacity, and understanding of oneself and others.

Emotional Experience and Regulation

Children's ability to experience and regulate emotions is intimately linked to PTG because the experience of distress *and* an eventual increase in positive feelings about oneself and life, in general, are thought to be critical aspects of the PTG process (Calhoun & Tedeschi, 2006). Therefore, to experience PTG, children need to have the ability to experience positive and negative emotions about the trauma (Harter, 2006; Kilmer, 2006). While the capacity to experience emotions is present from birth, the ability to recognize and verbally describe both positive and negative emotions about the same event requires more advanced emotional skills, which typically emerge between 5 and 7 years old. By 5 years old, children are beginning to understand that multiple emotions can arise from one situation (Kestenbaum & Gelman, 1995; Zajdel et al., 2013); however, children at this age are better at explaining when multiple emotions might arise for *other* people rather than being able to articulate this possibility for oneself. Between ages 6 and 7, children are able to describe their own feelings of multiple, similarly valenced emotions in response to one situation (for example, feeling sad and angry when their mother tells them it is time to clean up their toys and get ready for bed), but they have trouble recognizing the possibility of feeling oppositely valenced emotions within the context of the same situation until about 7 years of age, e.g., feeling sad that the vacation is over and happy to be heading back to the comfort of their own home and friends (Heubeck et al., 2016; Wintre & Vallance, 1994).

The distress of the trauma can be so intense that it overwhelms the child's social-emotional and cognitive capacities. Some periods in the course of development such as toddlerhood are marked by frequent and sustained negative emotions (Potegal et al., 1996). However, the transition from toddlerhood to preschool age is critical for emotional development, as there is a developmental decline in anger that coincides with better-developed capacities for self-regulation (Cole et al., 2011; Roben et al., 2013). Because of individual differences in children's biological predisposition or temperament, some children, regardless of age, experience negative emotions more intensely and more often than others, are more emotionally reactive to environmental stimuli, and have a lower tolerance for frustration and distress (Rothbart & Bates, 2006). Thus, very young children and those with a greater temperamental proclivity toward negative emotionality may be less likely to experience PTG. While the limited cognitive and emotional capacities of toddlers likely preclude any possibility for PTG at that age, older children who experience more negative emotionality would likely require greater support and assistance from caregivers to manage their distress in ways that promote growth after trauma. Therefore, children's capacity for effective emotion regulation is a vital consideration in understanding experiences of PTG among youngsters.

While infants are born with rudimentary regulatory abilities for managing distress, preschool-age children can initiate and sustain regulatory behaviors in ways that are associated with less negative emotionality in the context of emotional situations (Cole et al., 2011). Furthermore, school-age children 6 years old and beyond can take the controllability of the situation into account as they select to employ regulatory behaviors that will be most effective in managing their emotions (Zimmer-Gembeck & Skinner, 2011). For example, school-age children report using problem-focused coping in controllable situations (e.g., peer difficulties, academic challenges) and emotion-focused coping in situations perceived as unfamiliar and less controllable e.g., accidents, medical emergencies (Altshuler & Ruble, 1989; Band & Weisz, 1988). Available evidence suggests that for PTG to emerge, children would need to engage flexibly in regulatory behaviors that manage acute and ongoing distress in the aftermath of the trauma. This requires a repertoire of regulatory behaviors from which to draw, as well as practice implementing emotion regulation skills during times of emotional distress that tax one's capacities.

The process of trying to make sense of, and struggling with, trauma consists of both cognitive and emotional elements that likely strain children's developmental competencies. Cognitive processing of the trauma to be constructive requires that children can regulate the distress that arises well enough and for long enough to reflect upon the trauma and its associated sequelae. Otherwise, processing the trauma could elicit distress too intensely, too quickly, and/or for such a prolonged amount of time that it contributes to emotional dysregulation, which in turn would be unlikely to yield positive effects. This type of cognitive processing of trauma that produces severe upset may have harmful consequences, as "unproductive" rumination is associated with negative outcomes for youth (Watkins, 2008; Watkins & Roberts, 2020). The apparent role of constructive rumination in PTG also means that children cannot rely on emotional suppression, avoidance, or distraction, as these would not allow the child to engage with the trauma in ways that promote growth. Rather, children would seem to need to harness specific emotion-focused coping and regulatory skills in order to struggle with the trauma in constructive ways. To experience PTG, children likely need the capacity to employ strategies that allow them to stay oriented toward and actively involved in processing the trauma, which is referred to as approach-oriented strategies in coping literature (Roth & Cohen, 1986), and as engagement strategies in emotion regulation literature (Sheppes, 2014).

Parents and other important adults can play a central role in this process of supporting the use of approach-oriented or emotional engagement strategies in ways that facilitate PTG among children and adolescents. This support can manifest through emotional expression, i.e., the purposeful sharing of emotions in relation to the trauma so that one can seek support, as well as make sense of the process and communicate feelings. Dialogues between children and more skilled peers or adults are thought to be critical to the co-construction of the trauma narrative, and the use of language, in particular, can provide an organizing framework that allows examining and potentially modifying thoughts and emotions associated with the trauma. These social dialogues can form the basis for children's more independent and sophisticated thinking (Vygotsky, 1964), which in turn may promote the child's constructive rumination in an effort to reconcile their post-trauma reality.

Constructive or deliberate rumination has been associated with higher levels of PTG among children (Kilmer & Gil-Rivas, 2010; Yoshida et al., 2016) and is a vital catalyst of PTG. Along with fostering constructive rumination, emotional expression may also increase the likelihood that children understand and accept their emotions and consider possible positive or growth-promoting aspects of their experience through the process of reappraisal. Several studies have shown that positive reappraisal is significantly related to greater PTG in childhood (Felix et al., 2015; Xiao et al., 2017). Given the developmental advances required for children to be able to view trauma in a positive light (i.e., reappraisal), children and youth likely rely on parent/adult conceptualizations of the post-trauma landscape to guide their new perspective on themselves, others, and the world (Janoff-Bulman, 2006). Kilmer and Gil-Rivas (2010) found that parental coping advice (including advice about positive reframing or reappraisal) was significantly associated with greater PTG among children. In sum, available evidence suggests that awareness, understanding, and acceptance of one's emotions, as well as the ability to express emotions in healthy ways and to reappraise or reinterpret the trauma, support the emergence of PTG among children and youth.

Cognitive Capacities

Certain cognitive capacities are necessary for PTG. For example, children and youth likely require the flexible deployment of attention (ability to engage and disengage from trauma and associated stimuli) as well as proficiency with abstract thought. The constructive processing of trauma depends on the maturation of the executive attention network (Rothbart et al., 2011), which allows effortful control of attention processes. For rumination to be constructive, children and youth need to be able to shift their attention intentionally and flexibly from thinking about the trauma to thinking about or focusing on other relevant aspects of daily life (e.g., school, friends) and vice versa. While the executive attention system develops rapidly during early childhood (Green et al., 2023; Ruff & Capozzoli, 2003), these executive processes continue developing over the course of childhood and are thought to increase and even accelerate between the ages 7 to 10, as other cognitive processes emerge and there are greater expectations and opportunities for self-control (Blair & Ursache, 2011; Simonds et al., 2007).

Maturity and the ability to think abstractly are also likely to support children's capacity for PTG (Kilmer, 2006). The ability to engage in abstract thought allows children to envision alternate realities or diverse paths forward, identify changes or benefits resulting from the trauma and its aftermath, better integrate the traumatic experience into their sense of self/identity, find meaning in the trauma, and develop a more complex understanding of themselves, others, and the world. The schema changes that occur within the PTG process for children might reflect the fact that events often do not unfold as expected even with the best of intentions, and that joys and sorrows (or gains and losses) can be simultaneously held in relation to the trauma.

Abstract thinking can also contribute to an increased potential for spiritual growth as it enables children and youth to conceptualize a spiritual life as a distinct part of the natural world (Fowler, 1981). More recent work on spirituality development suggests that children as young as 6 years old may have more sophisticated ideas about spirituality, prayer, and the soul than was previously thought (Richert & Harris, 2008; Vaden & Woolley, 2011; Woolley & Phelps, 2001). Grounded in bioecological theory, Boyatzis (2012) proposed that children's spirituality is shaped by the contexts within which they reside, such that dynamic interactions between children and key socializing agents, such as parents, religious groups, schools, and the cultural landscape contribute to children's spiritual or faith-based beliefs. Vaden and Woolley (2011) found that 4- to 6-year-old children were more likely to judge unfamiliar religious stories as true if they came from highly religious families in which there was involvement in religious educational activities. This suggests that the development of religious or spiritual understanding can expand children's beliefs about what might be possible. In relation to PTG, religious or spiritual development may support children's ability to imagine reasons for their traumatic experience from both natural and spiritual perspectives, as well as consider that many potential positive and negative paths might emerge in trauma's aftermath. In sum, the development of cognitive maturity and the transition from thought processes grounded in concrete experiences to a more flexible, unbounded, and abstract way of thinking may promote PTG among children.

Understanding of Oneself and Others

One's understanding of the self and others appears important in considering the potential for PTG among those who have not yet reached adulthood. This understanding begins in infancy and continues to develop over time (Rochat, 2015). Children's daily interactions within the family shape internal working models that are thought to provide the framework for understanding oneself and the world and, in turn, influence future interactions and well-being (Bowlby, 1969). When primary caregivers are sensitive and appropriately responsive to children's needs for closeness and autonomy over the first years of life, children are likely to view themselves as capable and lovable (Ainsworth et al., 1978). These caring and supportive interactions contribute to children's (healthy) assumptions that their world will be kind, safe, and predictable (Goldman, 2002). However, trauma may shatter this assumptive worldview, disrupting the child's sense of self and eroding their expectations for trust, safety, and consistency. Trauma can also interfere with the normative learning and exploration in which children typically engage to develop skillful social-emotional, cognitive, and behavioral functioning (Janoff-Bulman, 1992; Lieberman & Van Horn, 2004). Janoff-Bulman (1992) suggests that children's assumptive world is more pliable than that of adults, which can confer both greater risk and greater protection for children who have experienced trauma. Given that children's internal representations of the self and others evidence greater plasticity to environmental input, new experiences and outcomes may be incorporated into children's representational world with relative ease. Evidence suggests that children aged 9-10 may experience greater PTG than adolescents aged 14 years and older (Felix et al., 2015; Yoshida et al., 2016). Children may be more vulnerable to the trauma's potential disruption, as well as more receptive to protective forces that offer them needed support in its aftermath, such as caregivers who help children grapple with, understand, and construct meaning from the trauma so that it can be integrated into their new worldview in ways that promote growth.

In addition to basic assumptions about the self and others that emerge early on in life, children's and adolescents' views about their own abilities and expectations about their future may play an important role in experiencing growth after trauma. These perceptions, collectively referred to as the self-system (Sullivan, 1953) include "one's perceived competencies, optimism or positive future expectations, and appraisals, beliefs, and expectations regarding their ability to meet task demands, cope, and adjust in the face of stress" (Kilmer et al., 2020, p. 668). The resilience literature offers evidence that positive self-system factors are protective and growth-promoting for children and some self-system factors have shown meaningful associations with PTG and related processes in childhood. For example, Kilmer et al. (2020) found that among 6- to 10-year-olds who experienced Hurricane Katrina, those who reported greater coping competency also reported lower post-traumatic stress and those who reported more positive expectations about the future reported fewer depressive symptoms a year later. In their sample of bereaved 6- to 13-year-olds, Gabbay and colleagues (2022) found that children who self-reported higher levels of hope and more positive future expectations also reported higher levels of concurrent PTG. While the self-system is thought to be rooted in early experiences, it is continually shaped by the multiple contexts that children and adolescents are embedded within over time. The available evidence suggests that children as young as 6 years old hold views of their competence and efficacy, as well as beliefs about the future that matter for the emergence of growth in the aftermath of trauma.

Distinguishing PTG from Resilience in Children and Youth

A question has emerged in the literature regarding the degree to which PTG and resilience can be distinguished. While they are related constructs reflecting positively valenced responses post-adversity, writings in this area largely frame them as distinct, pointing to multiple differentiating characteristics (Clay et al., 2009; Cryder et al., 2006; Kilmer, 2006; Kilmer & Gil-Rivas, 2010; Kilmer et al., 2014). For example, resilience reflects a *dynamic developmental process* that manifests as effective coping and positive adaptation in the face of significant adversity (Cicchetti, 2003; Luthar et al., 2000; Masten, 2001), whereas PTG refers to *transformation* (e.g., Cryder et al., 2006; Tedeschi & Calhoun, 1995), i.e., individuals reporting PTG experience positive change as a result of the struggle with trauma and its aftermath that goes beyond sound adjustment.

Additionally, individuals reporting PTG may report less concurrent emotional well-being or positive adjustment than those evidencing resilience (Calhoun & Tedeschi, 2006; Cryder et al., 2006; Tedeschi et al., 2007). Consistent with conceptualizations of PTG that frame distress as necessary for catalyzing and, perhaps, maintaining growth, research suggests that PTG and distress (including posttraumatic stress symptoms; PTSS) regularly coexist (Kilmer et al., 2009; Laufer & Solomon, 2006; Levine et al., 2008; Shakespeare-Finch & Lurie-Beck, 2014). Therefore, models of PTG (and the results in the extant literature) are inconsistent with most conceptualizations of resilience in children and youth (Kilmer et al., 2014).

Factors Associated with PTG in Children and Youth

In the last two decades, researchers have sought to understand factors informing the development of PTG in children and youth as such insight could help promote growth (and, perhaps, resilience) in the face of trauma-based adversity. Studies examining PTG among children and youth have established relations between PTG and characteristics of the trauma, youth, and youths' social environment, particularly connecting the development of PTG in children and adolescents with the severity of trauma exposure, depressive and posttraumatic stress symptoms, cognitive processes, emotions, and perceptions of self, interpersonal dynamics and loss within the family, and broader social support.

Severity of Trauma Exposure

Studies examining the impact of trauma severity on youths' development of PTG have produced mixed results. For instance, Andrades and colleagues (2018) found a positive relationship between the severity of the trauma event and PTG among Chilean youth (aged 10-15 years) who survived the 2010 Chile earthquake. However, in a study examining Tibetan adolescents' development of PTG following the 2010 Yushu earthquake, Xie and colleagues (2020) found that youth reported less PTG following exposure to a greater number of disaster-related events. Similarly, Dawas and Thabet (2017) found that greater exposure to traumatic war-related events was negatively associated with PTG among adolescents in the Gaza Strip. Other studies suggest that experiencing few disaster-related events may promote youths' post-disaster growth (Laufer & Solomon, 2006; Tang et al., 2021). This variation may reflect meaningful differences between a time-limited natural disaster (and the subsequent secondary adversities) and a chronic ongoing conflict. Together, findings to date suggest that the optimal level or severity of exposure needed to promote growth may vary across populations and specific trauma circumstances.

Depressive and Posttraumatic Stress Symptoms

Results of studies examining associations between depressive symptoms and youths' development of PTG have also been mixed. While Chinese adolescents reporting higher depressive symptoms were more likely to report PTG following their exposure to a tornado (Xu et al., 2018), Tibetan youth reported higher PTG when they did not report depression following the Yushu earthquake (Xie et al., 2020). However, Bianchini and colleagues (2017) found that youth who experienced moderate levels of depression following the 2009 L'aquila earthquake also experienced greater PTG compared to youth who experienced higher or lower levels of depression. This finding aligns with other results that suggest the relationship between distress and growth may be curvilinear rather than linear (Kleim & Ehlers, 2009; Levine et al., 2008). The specific nature of these findings may also vary because of differences in culture, including individualistic versus collectivistic values as well as differing views and attributions regarding depression and related phenomena (Kilmer et al., 2014).

Studies examining the relationship between PTSS (post-traumatic stress symptoms) and youths' development of PTG indicate a positive relationship (Kilmer et al., 2009; Tang et al., 2021; Wilson et al., 2016). Tang and colleagues (2021) found that youth who reported greater avoidance facets of PTSS (e.g., avoidance of painful memories and negative thoughts) also reported greater PTG. While avoidance may seem incongruent with the cognitive engagement necessary for growth, this result may suggest the need to reduce distress to a manageable level to facilitate the PTG process. Consistent with theory and prior research supporting the salience of intrusive rumination, Wilson and colleagues (2016) found that youth who reported greater intrusive facets of PTSS reported higher PTG. These findings lend support to the suggestion that greater levels of post-traumatic stress may be needed to trigger the cognitive and emotional processes necessary for growth to occur among children and youth (Arpawong et al., 2013; Tedeschi & Calhoun, 2004).

Cognitive Processes, Emotions, and Perceptions of Self

Studies suggest that internal, cognitive coping processes are central to one's posttraumatic adjustment (Garland et al., 2015; Joseph et al., 2012; Tedeschi & Calhoun, 2004). Subsequently, researchers have focused on the roles that rumination and mindfulness may play in the development of PTG in children and youth (An et al., 2018; Andrades et al., 2018; Kilmer & Gil-Rivas, 2010; Xu et al., 2018; Yoshida et al., 2016; Zhang et al., 2018). Andrades and colleagues (2018) found that Chilean youth who reportedly engaged in deliberate rumination experienced PTG following their exposure to a 2010 earthquake. Studies with childhood cancer survivors (Tobin et al., 2018) and youth affected by the Great East Japan Earthquake (Yoshida et al., 2016) suggest that rumination prompted by religious or memorial service attendance and viewing trauma-related media coverage may facilitate youth PTG. Exposure to such stimuli may evoke traumatic memories or strong emotional reactions that elicit reflection and growth (Calhoun & Tedeschi, 1999; Yoshida et al., 2016).

Studies have also examined the associations between youths' emotions and self-perceptions and the development of PTG. Research has been mixed regarding the influence of children's coping competency beliefs. Cryder et al. (2006) found that children and youth who endorsed more positive views regarding their coping competency tended to report higher levels of PTG; however, in another sample (Kilmer & Gil-Rivas, 2010), these beliefs were not associated with PTG. Findings generally suggest that youth who report positively valenced emotions and perceptions of themselves are likely to report greater PTG (Salloum et al., 2019; Sleijpen et al., 2016; Tang et al., 2021; Wang et al., 2020; Wei et al., 2016). In their study of adolescents' PTG following the Wenchuan earthquake, Tang and colleagues (2021) found a positive relationship between adolescents' self-esteem and their development of PTG. Possibly, youth with higher self-esteem may feel more capable of handling stressful events (Dumont & Provost, 1999), and such assumed capability could serve as a precursor to growth (Tang et al., 2021). Similarly, studies demonstrated positive relationships between youths' self-reported PTG and their levels of hopefulness (Salloum et al., 2019; Wei et al., 2016) and optimism (Sleijpen et al., 2016). These findings support that hope and optimism are key resources associated with positive coping following trauma exposure (Fredrickson, 2001; Kilmer et al., 2014).

Family Dynamics and Loss

Studies examined the role of interpersonal familial dynamics in youths' development of PTG. Howard Sharp et al. (2017) found that greater parental support may have facilitated personal growth among children with cancer possibly because parental encouragement may help youth to positively reframe their stressful experiences (Kilmer & Gil-Rivas, 2010). Further, greater parental warmth (Koutná et al., 2017) and more positive family functioning (Wilson et al., 2016) were found to be associated with childhood cancer survivors reporting greater PTG. These findings support the importance of positive family relationships in promoting PTG (Tedeschi & Calhoun, 1995).

Regarding the impact of familial bereavement circumstances, McClatchey (2020) found that youth were more likely to experience PTG when the death of a parent was sudden rather than expected. Hirooka and colleagues (2017) found that parentally-bereaved youth reported greater PTG and grief reactions than youth who lost a grandparent, perhaps because youth likely feel a stronger connection to their parent and may also anticipate the death of an older grandparent. Preliminary data (Gabbay et al., 2022) suggest that child PTG is associated with multiple types of caregiver coping advice (e.g., positive reframing, active coping, emotional support, religious coping), underscoring the importance of parental and caregiver resources in supporting children and youth in the face of a loss.

Social Support

Research has considered the broader role that social support may have on youths' development of PTG (Sleijpen et al., 2016; Wang & Wu, 2020; Wei et al., 2016; Zhou et al., 2017). In a study of posttraumatic experiences in adolescent refugees and asylum seekers, Sleijpen and colleagues (2016) found that youth reporting greater social support from family, friends, and significant others also reported greater PTG, and Wang and Wu (2020) and Zhou et al. (2017) demonstrated a positive association between social support and Chinese youths' PTG following the Ya'an earthquake. The availability of social support may promote youths' PTG, as support sources may provide youth with a sense of security (Schaefer & Moos, 1992) and allow youth additional opportunities to discuss and reflect on their traumatic experiences (Sleijpen et al., 2016; Tedeschi & Calhoun, 2004).

Research Limitations and Future Directions

Although knowledge regarding PTG in children and youth has grown meaningfully in the last two decades, significant gaps remain and point to needed future directions for study. Ferris and O'Brien (2022) and Kilmer et al. (2014) asserted that the lack of longitudinal and prospective-longitudinal research limits understanding of PTG and its implications. Although some studies have employed short-term longitudinal designs (Kilmer & Gil-Rivas, 2010), much of the work in this area is cross-sectional, making it difficult to assess fully the process of PTG, draw conclusions about the time and support needed for PTG to emerge in non-adult populations, or examine how PTG's presentation may change over time. The effects associated with acute or ongoing adversities that occur subsequent to the event(s) or experience(s) that appeared to be the impetus for the growth process should also be examined. Greater convergence of developmental science and PTG research would shed light on the requisite emotional, cognitive, social, and self-system factors that would allow children to grapple with and create meaning from the trauma in ways that give rise to PTG in childhood and beyond.

Integrating explicitly developmental frameworks into PTG research is imperative, given the dynamic changes occurring for children and youth as they progress along their developmental and adjustment trajectories. Well-conceived longitudinal research is necessary to study if PTG influences the developmental and/or adjustment trajectories of children and youth. This has been identified as the "most substantive ongoing question in the area" (Kilmer et al., 2014, p. 509), as it is not yet clear if the experience of PTG relates to adjustment, well-being, or broader functioning over time. This crucial question could potentially inform intervention and programming. For instance, program leadership and staff in many settings (e.g., grief support) could learn if efforts to promote PTG contribute to an increased likelihood of positive posttrauma adaptation.

The lack of prospective research limits information about youngsters' pre-trauma functioning and prior adversity experiences as well as that of their caregiver(s) and families. Access to such data would enhance understanding of the PTG process and its impact on children and youth who have experienced trauma, and whether those who have experienced and navigated less severe, more normative life events and adversities successfully are better able to manage and potentially grow from trauma. Furthermore, such knowledge would help elucidate the role of caregivers in facilitating the PTG process. In light of the broader importance of the caregiving system for supporting children's coping and adaptation (Bernstein & Pfefferbaum, 2018; Kliewer et al., 1994), such work would also yield crucial information regarding PTG processes in the context of shared traumas or mass trauma events.

While some research suggests that continued distress or secondary adversities that emerge subsequent to the potentially traumatic event may influence posttraumatic responses, catalyze, and maintain the growth process (Hafstad et al., 2011), it is not fully clear what level of struggle and distress is necessary for PTG. While some work has supported a curvilinear, or "inverted U" association between PTSS and PTG (Levine et al., 2008; Shakespeare-Finch & Lurie-Beck, 2014), the relationship between distress that is subthreshold for PTSS and PTG remains undetermined.

The literature includes few examples of observation-based data or corroborating reports of youth PTG from parents, caregivers, other family members, classmates, or dating partners (Glad et al., 2019). Augmenting self-report data by child or youth participants with others' observations of behavioral changes can help enhance understanding of the construct and increase confidence in the validity of PTG self-reports (Glad et al., 2019; Helgeson, 2010).

To improve understanding of PTG and the growth process, future studies should employ methodologies grounded in ecological theory, or the bioecological model (Bronfenbrenner, 1977; Bronfenbrenner & Morris, 2006) and assess proximal and distal factors and conditions in youths' social contexts. While intra-individual factors (e.g., temperament or dispositional characteristics, cognitive processes such as rumination, self-system variables such as hope, efficacy beliefs, or future expectations) are believed to play a role in the growth process,

PTG research involving children and youth needs to go beyond a focus on the individual, with an increased focus on the caregiver-child dyad and the broader family system. Some researchers have recommended a family systems approach to examining PTG (Berger & Weiss, 2009), conceptualizing the family as the unit that grows, rather than simply the context for individual growth.

The salience of the caregiving and family contexts and their association with PTG has been established in the stress and coping literature (Kliewer et al., 1994; Masten & Coatsworth, 1998; National Child Traumatic Stress Network [NCTSN], 2010). PTG researchers have included caregiver factors and indicators of the caregiver-child relationship and family functioning in examinations of PTG (Felix et al., 2015; Hafstad et al., 2011; Kilmer & Gil-Rivas, 2010). Findings indicated the potential role of caregivers in helping children and youth understand what has taken place, providing emotional support and guidance in using adaptive coping approaches and specific coping strategies, such as positive reframing and assisting them in navigating the external world and their new normal (Felix et al., 2015; Gabbay et al., 2022; Kilmer & Gil-Rivas, 2010; Wolchik et al., 2009).

In sum, to improve the understanding of PTG in children and youth and its potential impact, research will be enhanced by assessing a broader network of variables with potential associations with PTG, employing designs that include multiple respondents (caregivers and their children), recruiting larger and more diverse samples (including increased sociodemographic diversity within and across cultures), collecting data over multiple time points and for a longer duration of time (Kilmer et al., 2014), and considering cultural and spiritual aspects.

Implications for Practice

Multiple authors have identified facilitating PTG as a "legitimate aim" in serving those who have faced notable trauma (Calhoun & Tedeschi, 1999; Kilmer & Gil-Rivas, 2008; Linley & Joseph, 2004; Tedeschi & Calhoun, 2009). Kilmer and colleagues (2014) describe the clinical implications of PTG research involving children and youth and highlight their application in the context of a center that provides comprehensive grief support. Supporting and guiding parents or caregivers can be critical in working with children and youth subsequent to trauma to help caregivers meet their children's needs and support them (Kilmer et al., 2014). Therefore, practitioners should ensure that caregivers receive support and psychoeducation regarding children and youths' posttrauma reactions and adjustment, building caregivers' capacity and efficacy expectations to support their children emotionally and help them cope (Gil-Rivas et al., 2004; Kilmer & Gil-Rivas, 2008). They can also help caregivers in tolerating and validating their children's distress and other posttrauma responses, and caregivers can coach coping responses and help children regulate their emotional and behavioral reactions as well as interpret what has taken place and its meaning going forward (Gil-Rivas et al., 2004; Kilmer, 2006; Kilmer & Gil-Rivas, 2008; 2010).

Practitioners can also give children and youth critical support subsequent to trauma by providing a safe space, listening actively, helping children regulate their emotions in an accepting setting, guiding their coping efforts, and modeling adaptive strategies (Calhoun & Tedeschi, 2006; Kilmer, 2006; Kilmer & Gil-Rivas, 2008; Tedeschi & Kilmer, 2005). Practitioners can also take steps that may facilitate PTG, including listening for youths' statements about possible benefits that may align with PTG or changed beliefs about their worlds, prompting for elaboration about perceived changes or benefits or, if appropriate, guiding positive reframes of the youth's situation (Kilmer & Gil-Rivas, 2008; Tedeschi & Kilmer, 2005; Tedeschi & Calhoun, 2009). Such attempts to recognize or reinforce a perceived positive change must be done judiciously (Tedeschi & Kilmer, 2005).

Practitioners can also try to promote the development or enhancement of socio-emotional resources, cognitive processes, and interpersonal supports that are associated with PTG in children and youth. PTG research supports a focus on active coping, positive reappraisal or positive reframing coping advice, deliberate rumination, social support and connection, and self-system resources such as positive future expectations, hope, and optimism (Armstrong et al., 2018; Ferris & O'Brien, 2022; Kilmer et al., 2014; Meyerson et al., 2011) as many of these domains are linked positively with positive adjustment outcomes, symptom reduction and child and youth adjustment subsequent to adversity.

Practitioners' efforts to strengthen children's socioemotional competencies may have potential benefits. Specifically, existing research supports the potential positive influence of building children and youths' self-system resources that reflect their self-views, self-perceptions, and self-representations, such as enhancing their positive beliefs about their coping competency or efficacy, their expectations for their future, and their sense of hope or optimism (Kilmer et al., 2014; 2020; Wei et al., 2016; Wyman et al., 1993). These resources are broadly associated with PTG and can serve a meaningful protective or promotive function for children and youth (Kilmer, 2006; Luthar et al., 2000; Masten, 2001).

Practitioners can facilitate children and youths' use of constructive deliberate productive rumination (Calhoun & Tedeschi, 2006), to help children and youth reflect on and share verbally or through art or play their experience(s) of and reactions to trauma and loss. Such practices can reduce avoidance, help youth recognize how they may have coped or adapted effectively, and provide scaffolding for ongoing dialogue to make sense of their traumatic experience(s) and understand what the event(s) and their subsequent new reality may mean for them and their future life (Kilmer et al., 2014). During such activities, practitioners can attend to child or youth reports of perceived positive change and follow up sensitively, recognizing and reinforcing such notions as appropriate (Kilmer & Gil-Rivas, 2008; Kilmer et al., 2014), supporting children and youth in discussing these possible benefits and integrating them into their life narrative (Tedeschi & Kilmer, 2005).

Practitioners can also consider ways to connect children, youth, and families with those with similar experiences. Although research documenting the effectiveness of support-based approaches is limited in settings serving those who have experienced trauma or loss, peer support models are widely employed in the context of grief support (Gabbay et al., 2022). Peer-based, mutual support can help children and their caregivers feel less alone and isolated, learn new ways of dealing with their feelings and understanding their experiences.

Concluding Thoughts

Every day the news includes stories of large-scale trauma – from natural disasters (earthquakes, hurricanes, tsunamis, wildfires) to train derailments, mass shootings, terrorism, or war. Sometimes lost in these stories are the impacts of these experiences on the survivors and the ongoing challenges they may face, as well as the experiences of children and youth who face trauma that does not occur as part of a large-scale event. Important resources and networks exist (e.g., the National Child Traumatic Stress Network; nctsn.org), and our knowledge continues to grow regarding trauma's effects on children and youth, factors that influence their adaptation, and their potential posttrauma outcomes. Pursuing research on PTG in children and youth, particularly via designs that address the aforementioned limitations and are grounded in developmental frameworks, can have the heuristic benefit of increasing knowledge and enhancing understanding in the area and yield findings with implications for practitioners and their interventions.

References

Ainsworth, M. D. S., Blehar, M. C., Waters, E., & Wall, S. (1978). *Patterns of attachment: A psychological study of the strange situation.* Lawrence Erlbaum.

Alisic, E., van der Schoot, T. A. W., van Ginkel, J. R., & Kleber, R. J. (2008). Looking beyond posttraumatic stress disorder in children: Posttraumatic stress reactions, posttraumatic growth, and quality of life in a general population sample. *Journal of Clinical Psychiatry, 69*(9), 1455–1461. 10.4088/jcp.v69n0913

Altshuler, J. L., & Ruble, D. N. (1989). Developmental changes in children's awareness of strategies for coping with uncontrollable stress. *Child Development, 60*(6), 1337–1349. 10.2307/1130925

An, Y., Yuan, G., Zhang, N., Xu, W., Liu, Z., & Zhou. (2018). Longitudinal cross-lagged relationships between mindfulness, posttraumatic stress symptoms, and posttraumatic growth in adolescents following the Yancheng tornado in China. *Psychiatry Research, 266*, 334–340. 10.1016/j.psychres.2018.03.034

Andrades, M., García, F. E., Calonge, I., & Martínez-Arias, R. (2018). Posttraumatic growth in children and adolescents exposed to the 2010 earthquake in Chile and its relationship with rumination and posttraumatic stress symptoms. *Journal of Happiness Studies, 19*(5), 1505–1517. 10.1007/s10902-017-9885-7

Andrades, M., García, F., & Kilmer, R. P. (2021). Posttraumatic stress symptoms and posttraumatic growth in children and adolescents 12 months and 24 months after the earthquake and tsunamis in Chile in 2010: A longitudinal study. *International Journal of Psychology, 56*, 48–55. 10.1002/ijop.12718

Arpawong, T. E., Oland, A., Milam, J. E., Ruccione, K., & Meeske, K. A. (2013). Post-traumatic growth among an ethnically diverse sample of adolescent and young adult cancer survivors. *Psycho-Oncology, 22*, 2235–2244.

Armstrong, L. M., Basquin, C., & Tedeschi, R. (2018). Posttraumatic growth and resilience. In J. D. Osofsky, & B. M. Groves (Eds.), *Violence and trauma in the lives of children: Prevention and intervention* (pp. 51–72). Praeger/ABC-CLIO.

Band, E. B., & Weisz, J. R. (1988). How to feel better when it feels bad: Children's perspectives on coping with everyday stress. *Developmental Psychology, 24*(2), 247–253. 10.1037/0012-1649.24.2.247

Barakat, L. P., Alderfer, M. A., & Kazak, A. E. (2006). Posttraumatic growth in adolescent survivors of cancer and their mothers and fathers. *Journal of Pediatric Psychology, 31*, 413–419. 10.1093/jpepsy/jsj058

Berger, R., & Weiss, T. (2009). The Posttraumatic Growth model: An expansion to the family system. *Traumatology, 15*(1), 63–74. 10.1177/1534765608323499

Bernstein, M., & Pfefferbaum, B. (2018). Posttraumatic growth as a response to natural disasters in children and adolescents. *Current Psychiatry Reports, 20*(5), 1–10. 10.1007/s11920-018-0900-4

Bianchini, V., Giusti, L., Salza, A., Cofini, V., Cifone, M., Casacchia, M., Fabiani, L, & Roncone, R. (2017). Moderate depression promotes posttraumatic growth (PTG): A young population survey 2 years after the 2009 L'Aquila earthquake. *Clinical Practice and Epidemiology in Mental Health, 13*(1), 10–19. 10.2174/1745017901713010010

Blair, C., & Ursache, A. (2011). A bidirectional model of executive functions and self-regulation. In K. D. Vohs, & R. F. Baumeister (Eds.), *Handbook of self-regulation: Research, theory, and applications* (pp. 300–320). Guilford Press.

Bronfenbrenner, U. (1977). Toward an experimental ecology of human development. *American Psychologist, 32*, 513–531.

Bronfenbrenner, U., & Morris, P. A. (2006). The bioecological model of human development. In R. M. Lerner, & W. R. Damon (Eds.), *Handbook of child psychology: Theoretical models of human development* (6th ed., Vol. 1, pp. 793–828). Hoboken, NJ: Wiley.

Bowlby, J. (1969). *Attachment and loss: Vol. 1. Attachment.* New York, NY: Basic Books.

Boyatzis, C. J. (2012). Spiritual development during childhood and adolescence. In L. J. Miller (Ed.), *The Oxford handbook of psychology and spirituality* (pp. 151–164). New York, NY: Oxford University Press.

Calhoun, L. G., & Tedeschi, R. G. (1999). *Facilitating posttraumatic growth: A clinician's guide.* Routledge.

Calhoun, L. G., & Tedeschi, R. G. (2006). The foundations of posttraumatic growth: An expanded framework. In L. G. Calhoun, & R. G. Tedeschi (Eds.), *Handbook of posttraumatic growth: Research and practice* (pp. 1–23). Mahwah, NJ: Erlbaum.

Cann, A., Calhoun, L. G., Tedeschi, R. G., Kilmer, R. P., Gil-Rivas, V., Vishnevsky, T., & Danhauer, S. C. (2010). The Core Beliefs Inventory: A brief measure of disruption in the assumptive world. *Anxiety, Stress, and Coping: An International Journal, 23*, 19–34. 10.1080/10615800802573013

Cicchetti, D. (2003). Foreword. In S. Luthar (Ed.), *Resilience and vulnerability: Adaptation in the context of childhood adversities* (pp. xix–xxvii). New York, NY: Cambridge University Press.

Clay, R., Knibbs, J., & Joseph, S. (2009). Measurement of posttraumatic growth in young people: A review. *Child Clinical Psychology and Psychiatry, 14*(3), 411–422. 10.1177/1359104509104049

Cole, P. M., Tan, P. Z., Hall, S. E., Zhang, Y., Crnic, K. A., Blair, C. B., & Li, R. (2011). Developmental changes in anger expression and attention focus: Learning to wait. *Developmental Psychology, 47*(4), 1078–1089. 10.1037/a0023813

Cryder, C. H., Kilmer, R. P., Tedeschi, R. G., & Calhoun, L. G. (2006). An exploratory study of posttraumatic growth in children following a natural disaster. *American Journal of Orthopsychiatry, 76*, 65–69. 10.1037/0002-9432.76.1.65

Dawas, M. K., & Thabet, A. A. (2017). The relationship between traumatic experience posttraumatic stress disorder resilience and posttraumatic growth among adolescents in Gaza Strip. *JOJ Nurse Health Care, 5*(1), 10–17. 10.19080/JOJNHC.2017.05.555652

Dumont, M., & Provost, M. A. (1999). Resilience in adolescents: Protective role of social support, coping strategies, self-esteem, and social activities on experience of stress and depression. *Journal of Youth and Adolescence, 28*(3), 343–363. 10.1023/A:1021637011732

Felix, E., Afifi, T., Kia-Keating, M., Brown, L., Afifi, W., & Reyes, G. (2015). Family functioning and posttraumatic growth among parents and youth following wildfire disasters. *American Journal of Orthopsychiatry, 85*(2), 191–200. 10.1037/ort0000054

Ferris, C., & O'Brien, K. (2022). The ins and outs of posttraumatic growth in children and adolescents: A systematic review of factors that matter. *Journal of Traumatic Stress, 35*, 1305–1317. 10.1002/jts.22845

Fowler, J. (1981). *Stages of faith: The psychology of human development and the quest for meaning.* New York, NY: Harper Collins.

Fredrickson, B. L. (2001). The role of positive emotions in positive psychology: The broaden-and-build theory of positive emotions. *American Psychologist, 56*(3), 218–226. 10.1037//0003-066x.56.3.218

Gabbay, P., Snyder, L. M., & Kilmer, R. P. (June 2022). *Examining posttraumatic growth in children's peer support grief groups: A pilot study.* Paper presentation at the 25th National Alliance Symposium on Children's Grief, Orlando, FL.

Garland, E. L., Farb, N. A., Goldin, P., & Fredrickson., B. L. (2015). Mindfulness broadens awareness and builds eudaimonic meaning: A process model of mindful positive emotion regulation. *Psychological Inquiry, 26*(4), 293–314. 10.1080/1047840X.2015.1064294

Gil-Rivas, V., Holman, E. A., & Silver, R. C. (2004). Adolescent vulnerability following the September 11th terrorist attacks: A study of parents and their children. *Applied Developmental Science, 8*(3), 130–142. 10.1207/s1532480xads0803_3

Glad, K. A., Kilmer, R. P., Dyb, G., & Hafstad, G. S. (2019). Caregiver-reported positive changes in young survivors of a terrorist attack. *Journal of Child and Family Studies, 28*(3), 704–719. 10.1007/s10826-018-1298-7

Green, L. M., Genaro, B. G., Ratcliff, K. A., Cole, P. M., & Ram, N. (2023). Investigating the developmental timing of self-regulation in early childhood. *International Journal of Behavioral Development, 47*(2), 101–110. 10.1177/01650254221111788

Goldman, L. (2002). The assumptive world of children. In J. Kauffman (Ed.), *Loss of the assumptive world: A theory of traumatic loss* (pp. 193–202). Routledge.
Hafstad, G. S., Kilmer, R. P., & Gil-Rivas, V. (2011). Posttraumatic growth among Norwegian children and adolescents exposed to the 2004 tsunami. *Psychological Trauma: Theory, Research, Practice, and Policy*, *3*(2), 130–138. 10.1037/a0023236
Harter, S. (2006). Self-processes and developmental psychopathology. In D. Cicchetti, & D. J. Cohen (Eds.), *Developmental psychopathology: Theory and method* (Vol. 1, 2nd ed., pp. 370–418). John Wiley & Sons.
Helgeson, V. S. (2010). Corroboration of growth following breast cancer: Ten years later. *Journal of Social and Clinical Psychology*, *29*(5), 546–574. 10.1521/jscp.2010.29.5.546
Helgeson, V., Reynolds, K. A., & Tomich, P. L. (2006). A meta-analytic review of benefit finding and growth. *Journal of Consulting and Clinical Psychology*, *74*, 797–806. 10.1037/0022-006x.74.5.797
Heubeck, B. G., Butcher, P. R., Thorneywork, K., & Wood, J. (2016). Loving and angry? Happy and sad? Understanding and reporting of mixed emotions in mother–child relationships by 6-to 12-year-olds. *British Journal of Developmental Psychology*, *34*(2), 245–260. 10.1111/bjdp.12128
Hirooka, K., Fukahori, H., Ozawa, M., & Akita, Y. (2017). Differences in posttraumatic growth and grief reactions among adolescents by relationship with the deceased. *Journal of Advanced Nursing*, *73*(4), 955–965. 10.1111/jan.13196
Howard Sharp, K. M., Willard, V. W., Barnes, S., Tillery, R., Long, A., & Phipps, S. (2017). Emotion socialization in the context of childhood cancer: perceptions of parental support promotes posttraumatic growth. *Journal of Pediatric Psychology*, *42*(1), 95–103. 10.1093/jpepsy/jsw062
Janoff-Bulman, R. (1992). *Shattered assumptions*. New York: The Free Press.
Janoff-Bulman, R. (2006). Schema-change perspectives on posttraumatic growth. In L. G. Calhoun, & R. G. Tedeschi (Eds.), *The handbook of posttraumatic growth: Research and practice* (pp. 81–99). Lawrence Erlbaum.
Joseph, S., Murphy, D., & Regal, S. (2012). An affective–cognitive processing model of posttraumatic growth. *Clinical Psychology & Psychotherapy*, *19*(4), 316–325. 10.1002/cpp.1798
Kestenbaum, R., & Gelman, S. A. (1995). Preschool children's identification and understanding of mixed emotions. *Cognitive Development*, *10*(3), 443–458. 10.1016/0885-2014(95)90006-3
Kilmer, R. P. (2006). Resilience and posttraumatic growth in children. In L. G. Calhoun, & R. G. Tedeschi (Eds.), *Handbook of posttraumatic growth: Research and practice* (pp. 264–288). Mahwah, NJ: Lawrence Erlbaum Associates.
Kilmer, R. P., & Gil-Rivas, V. (2008). Posttraumatic growth in youth following disasters. *The Prevention Researcher*, *15*(3), 18–20.
Kilmer, R. P., & Gil-Rivas, V. (2010). Exploring posttraumatic growth in children impacted by Hurricane Katrina: Correlates of the phenomenon and developmental considerations. *Child Development*, *81*, 1211–1227. 10.1111/j.1467-8624.2010.01463.x
Kilmer, R. P., Gil-Rivas, V., Griese, B., Hardy, S. J., Hafstad, G. S., & Alisic, E. (2014). Posttraumatic growth in children and youth: Clinical implications of an emerging research literature. *American Journal of Orthopsychiatry*, *84*, 506–518. 10.1037/ort0000016
Kilmer, R. P., Gil-Rivas, V., & Roof, K. A. (2020). Associations between children's self-system functioning and depressive and posttraumatic stress symptoms following disaster. *American Journal of Orthopsychiatry*, *90*(6), 667–676. 10.1037/ort0000487
Kilmer, R. P., Gil-Rivas, V., Tedeschi, R. G., Cann, A., Calhoun, L. G., Buchanan, T., & Taku, K. (2009). Use of the revised Posttraumatic Growth Inventory for Children (PTGI-C-R). *Journal of Traumatic Stress*, *22*, 248–253. 10.1002/jts.20410
Kleim B., & Ehlers A. (2009). Evidence for a curvilinear relationship between posttraumatic growth and posttrauma depression and PTSD in assault survivors. *Journal of Traumatic Stress*, *22*(1), 45–52. 10.1002/jts.20378
Kliewer, W., Sandler, I. N., & Wolchik, S. A. (1994). Family socialization of threat appraisal and coping: Coaching, modeling, and family context. In F. Nestmann, & K. Hurrelmann (Eds.), *Social networks and social support in childhood and adolescence* (pp. 271–291). Waler de Gruyter.
Koutná, V., Jelínek, M., Blatný, M., & Kepák, T. (2017). Predictors of posttraumatic stress and posttraumatic growth in childhood cancer survivors. *Cancers (Basel)*, *9*(3), 26. 10.3390/cancers9030026

Laufer, A., & Solomon, Z. (2006). Posttraumatic symptoms and posttraumatic growth among Israeli youth exposed to terror incidents. *Journal of Social and Clinical Psychology*, *25*(4), 429–447. 10.1521/jscp.2006.25.4.429

Levine, S. Z., Laufer, A., Hamama-Raz, Y., Stein, E., & Solomon, Z. (2008). Posttraumatic growth in adolescence: Examining its components and relationship with PTSD. *Journal of Traumatic Stress*, *21*(5), 492–496. 10.1002/jts.20361

Lieberman, A. F., & Van Horn, P. (2004). Assessment and treatment of young children exposed to traumatic events. In J. D. Osofsky (Ed.), *Young children and trauma: Intervention and treatment* (pp. 111–138). Guilford Press.

Linley, P. A., & Joseph, S. (2004). Positive change following trauma and adversity: A review. *Journal of Traumatic Stress*, *17*(1), 11–21. 10.1023/B:JOTS.0000014671.27856.7e

Liu, A. N., Wang, L. L., Li, H. P., Gong, J., & Liu, X. H. (2017). Correlation between posttraumatic growth and posttraumatic stress disorder symptoms based on Pearson correlation coefficient: A meta-analysis. *Journal of Nervous Mental Disease*, *205*(5), 380–389. 10.1097/NMD.0000000000000605

Luthar, S. S., Cicchetti, D., & Becker, B. (2000). The construct of resilience: A critical evaluation and guidelines for future work. *Child Development*, *71*, 543–562. 10.1111/1467-8624.00164

Masten, A. S. (2001). Ordinary magic: Resilience processes in development. *American Psychologist*, *56*, 227–238. 10.1037//0003-066X.56.3.227

Masten, A. S., & Coatsworth, J. D. (1998). The development of competence in favorable and unfavorable environments. *American Psychologist*, *53*(2), 205–220. 10.1037//0003-066x.53.2.205

Meyerson, D. A., Grant, K. E., Smith Carter, J., & Kilmer, R. P. (2011). Posttraumatic growth among children and adolescents: A systematic review. *Clinical Psychology Review*, *31*, 949–964. 10.1016/j.cpr.2011.06.003

McClatchey, I. S. (2020). Trauma-informed care and posttraumatic growth among bereaved youth: A pilot study. *Omega - Journal of Death and Dying*, *82*(2), 196–213. 10.1177/0030222818804629

Milam, J. E., Ritt-Olson, A., & Unger, J. (2004). Posttraumatic growth among adolescents. *Journal of Adolescent Research*, *19*, 192–204. 10.1177/0743558403258273

National Child Traumatic Stress Network. (2010). *Age-related reactions to a traumatic event*. Retrieved from http://www.nctsn.org/nctsn_assets/pdfs/age_related_reactions.pdf

Potegal, M., Kosorok, M. R., & Davidson, R. J. (1996). The time course of angry behavior in the temper tantrums of young children. *Annals of the New York Academy of Sciences*, *794*, 31–45. 10.1111/j.1749-6632.1996.tb32507.x

Prati, G., & Pietrantoni, L. (2009). Optimism, social support, and coping strategies as factors contributing to posttraumatic growth: A meta-analysis. *Journal of Loss and Trauma*, *14*, 364–388. 10.1080/15325020902724271

Richert, R. A., & Harris, P. L. (2008). Dualism revisited: Body vs. mind vs. soul. *Journal of Cognition and Culture*, *8*(1–2), 99–115. 10.1163/156770908x289224

Roben, C. K. P., Cole, P. M., & Armstrong, L. M. (2013). Longitudinal relations among language skills, anger expression, and regulatory strategies in early childhood. *Child Development*, *84*(3), 891–905. 10.1111/cdev.12027

Rochat, P. (2015). Layers of awareness in development. *Developmental Review*, *38*, 122–145. 10.1016/j.dr.2015.07.009

Roth, S., & Cohen, L. J. (1986). Approach avoidance and coping with stress. *American Psychologist*, *41*(7), 813–819. 10.1037/0003-066X.41.7.813

Rothbart, M. K., & Bates, J. E. (2006). Temperament. In N. Eisenberg, W. Damon, & R. M. Lerner (Eds.), *Handbook of child psychology: Social, emotional, and personality development* (Vol. 3, 6th ed., pp. 99–166). John Wiley & Sons.

Rothbart, M. K., Sheese, B. E., Rueda, M. R., & Posner, M. I. (2011). Developing mechanisms of self-regulation in early life. *Emotion Review*, *3*(2), 207–213. 10.1177/1754073910387943

Ruff, H. A., & Capozzoli, M. C. (2003). Development of attention and distractibility in the first 4 years of life. *Developmental Psychology*, *39*(5), 877–890. 10.1037/0012-1649.39.5.877

Salloum, A., Bjoerke, A., & Johnco, C. (2019). The associations of complicated grief, depression, posttraumatic growth, and hope among bereaved youth. *Omega: Journal of Death and Dying*, *79*(2), 157–173. 10.1177/0030222817719805

Schaefer, J. A., & Moos, R. H. (1992). Life crises and personal growth. In B. Carpenter (Ed.), *Personal coping: Theory, research and application* (pp. 149–170). Westport, CT: Praeger.

Shakespeare-Finch, J., & Lurie-Beck, J. (2014). A meta-analytic clarification of the relationship between posttraumatic growth and symptoms of posttraumatic distress disorder. *Journal of Anxiety Disorders*, *28*(2), 223–229. 10.1016/j.janxdis.2013.10.005
Sheppes, G. (2014). Emotion regulation choice: Theory and findings. In J. J. Gross (Ed.), *Handbook of emotion regulation* (2nd ed., pp. 126–136). Guilford Publications.
Simonds, J., Kieras, J. E., Rueda, M. R., & Rothbart, M. K. (2007). Effortful control, executive attention, and emotional regulation in 7–10-year-old children. *Cognitive Development*, *22*(4), 474–488. 10.1016/j.cogdev.2007.08.009
Sleijpen, M., Haagen, J., Mooren, T., & Kleber, R. J. (2016). Growing from experience: An exploratory study of posttraumatic growth in adolescent refugees. *European Journal of Psychotraumatology*, *7*. 10.3402/ejpt.v7.28698
Sullivan, H. S. (1953). *The interpersonal theory of psychiatry*. New York, NY: Norton.
Taku, K., Kilmer, R. P., Cann, A., Tedeschi, R. G., & Calhoun, L. G. (2012). Exploring posttraumatic growth in Japanese youth. *Psychological Trauma: Theory, Research, Practice, and Policy*, *4*(4), 411–419. 10.1037/a0024363
Tang, W., Wang, Y., Lu, L., Lu, Y., & Xu, J. (2021). Post-traumatic growth among 5195 adolescents at 8.5 years after exposure to the Wenchuan earthquake: Roles of post-traumatic stress disorder and self-esteem. *Journal of Health Psychology*, *26*(3), 2450–2459. 10.1177/1359105320913947
Tedeschi, R. G., & Calhoun, L. G. (1995). *Trauma and transformation: Growing in the aftermath of suffering*. Thousand Oaks, CA: Sage.
Tedeschi, R. G., & Calhoun, L. G. (2004). Posttraumatic growth: Conceptual foundations and empirical evidence. *Psychological Inquiry*, *15*, 1–18. 10.1207/s15327965pli1501_01
Tedeschi, R. G., & Calhoun, L. G. (2009). The clinician as expert companion. In C. L. Park, S. Lechner, A. Stanton, & M. Antoni (Eds.), *Medical illness and positive life change: Can crisis lead to personal transformation* (pp. 215–235). Washington, DC: American Psychological Association.
Tedeschi, R. G., Calhoun, L. G., & Cann, A. (2007). Evaluating resource gain: Understanding and *misunderstanding* posttraumatic growth. *Applied Psychology: An International Review*, *56*, 396–406. 10.1111/j.1464-0597.2007.00299.x
Tedeschi, R. G., & Kilmer, R. P. (2005). Assessing strengths, resilience, and growth to guide clinical interventions. *Professional Psychology: Research and Practice*, *36*(3), 230–237. 36(3), 230–237. 10.1037/0735-7028.36.3.230
Tobin, J., Allem, J. P., Slaughter, R., Unger, J. B., Hamilton, A. S., & Milam, J. E. (2018). Posttraumatic growth among childhood cancer survivors: Associations with ethnicity, acculturation, and religious service attendance. *Journal of Psychosocial Oncology*, *36*(2), 175–188. 10.1080/07347332.2017.1365799
Vaden, V. C., & Woolley, J. D. (2011). Does God make it real? Children's belief in religious stories from the Judeo-Christian tradition. *Child Development*, *82*(4), 1120–1135. 10.1111/j.1467-8624.2011.01589.x
Vygotsky, L. S. (1964). *Thought and Language*. MIT Press.
Wang, W. C., & Wu, X. C. (2020). Mediating roles of gratitude, social support and posttraumatic growth in the relation between empathy and prosocial behavior among adolescents after the Ya'an earthquake. *Acta Psychologica Sinica*, *52*, 307–316. 10.3389/fpsyg.2018.02131
Watkins, E. R. (2008). Constructive and unconstructive repetitive thought. *Psychological Bulletin*, *134*(2), 163–206. 10.1037/0033-2909.134.2.163
Watkins, E. R., & Roberts, H. (2020). Reflecting on rumination: Consequences, causes, mechanisms and treatment of rumination. *Behaviour Research and Therapy*, *127*. 10.1016/j.brat.2020.103573
Wei, W., Li, X., Tu, X., Zhao, J., & Zhao, G. (2016). Perceived social support, hopefulness, and emotional regulations as mediators of the relationship between enacted stigma and post-traumatic growth among children affected by parental HIV/AIDS in rural China. *AIDS Care*, *28*, 99–105. 10.1080/09540121.2016.1146217
Wilson, J. Z., Marin, D., Maxwell, K., Cumming, J., Berger, R., Saini, S., Ferguson, W., & Chibnall, J. T. (2016). Association of posttraumatic growth and illness-related burden with psychosocial factors of patient, family, and provider in pediatric cancer survivors. *Journal of Traumatic Stress*, *29*(5), 448–456. 10.1002/jts.22123

Wintre, M. G., & Vallance, D. D. (1994). A developmental sequence in the comprehension of emotions: Intensity, multiple emotions, and valence. *Developmental Psychology*, *30*(4), 509–514. 10.1037/0012-1649.30.4.509

Wolchik, S. A., Coxe, S., Tein, J. Y., Sandler, I. N., & Ayers, T. S. (2009). Six-year longitudinal predictors of posttraumatic growth in parentally bereaved adolescents and young adults. *Omega: Journal of Death and Dying*, *58*(2), 107–128. 10.2190/OM.58.2.b

Woolley, J. D., & Phelps, K. E. (2001). The development of children's beliefs about prayer. *Journal of Cognition and Culture*, *1*(2), 139–166. 10.1163/156853701316931380

Wyman, P. A., Cowen, E. L., Work, W. C., & Kerley, J. H. (1993). The role of children's future expectations in self-system functioning and adjustment to life stress: A prospective study of urban at-risk children. *Development and Psychopathology*, *5*(4), 649–661. 10.1017/S0954579400006210

Xiao, Z., Xinchun, W., & Rui, Z. (2017). Understanding the relationship between social support and posttraumatic stress disorder/posttraumatic growth among adolescents after Ya'an earthquake: The role of emotion regulation. *Psychological Trauma: Theory, Research, Practice & Policy*, *9*(2), 214–221. 10.1037/tra0000213

Xiaoli, W., Kaminga, A. C., Wenjie, D., Jing, D., Zhipeng, W., Xiongfeng, P. & Aizhong, L. (2019). The prevalence of moderate-to-high posttraumatic growth: A systematic review and meta-analysis. *Journal of Affective Disorders*, *243*, 408–415. 10.1016/j.jad.2018.09.023

Xie, Y., Wu, J., & Shen, G. (2020). Posttraumatic growth in Tibetan adolescent survivors 6 years after the 2010 Yushu earthquake: Depression and PTSD as predictors. *Child Psychiatry & Human Development*, *51*(1), 94–103. 10.1007/s10578-019-00913-5

Xu, W., Ding, X., Goh, P. H., & An, Y. (2018). Dispositional mindfulness moderates the relationship between depression and posttraumatic growth in Chinese adolescents following a tornado. *Personality and Individual Differences*, *127*, 15–21. 10.1016/j.paid.2018.01.032

Yaskowich, K. M. (2002). *Posttraumatic growth in children and adolescents with cancer*. Unpublished doctoral dissertation. Calgary, Alberta: University of Calgary.

Yoshida, H., Kobayashi, N., Honda, N., Matsuoka, H., Yamaguchi, T., Homma, H., & Tomita, H. (2016). Post-traumatic growth of children affected by the Great East Japan Earthquake and their attitudes to memorial services and media coverage. *Psychiatry and Clinical Neurosciences*, *70*(5), 193–201. 10.1111/pcn.12379

Zajdel, R. T., Bloom, J. M., Fireman, G., & Larsen, J. T. (2013). Children's understanding and experience of mixed emotions: The roles of age, gender, and empathy. *The Journal of Genetic Psychology*, *174*(5–6), 582–603. 10.1080/00221325.2012.732125

Zhang, Y., Xu, W., & Yuan, G. (2018). The relationship between posttraumatic cognitive change, posttraumatic stress disorder, and posttraumatic growth among Chinese adolescents after the Yancheng tornado: The mediating effect of rumination. *Frontiers in Psychology*, *9*, 474–481. 10.3389/fpsyg.2018.00474

Zhou, X., Wu, X., & Zhen, R. (2017). Understanding the relationship between social support and posttraumatic stress disorder/posttraumatic growth among adolescents after Ya'an earthquake: The role of emotion regulation. *Psychological Trauma: Theory, Research, Practice and Policy*, *9*(2), 214–221. 10.1037/tra0000213

Zimmer-Gembeck, M. J., & Skinner, E. A. (2011). The development of coping across childhood and adolescence: An integrative review and critique of research. *International Journal of Behavioral Development*, *35*(1), 1–17. 10.1177/0165025410384923

14

POSTTRAUMATIC GROWTH IN GROWN ORPHANED CHILD SURVIVORS OF GENOCIDE IN GUATEMALA

Shirley A. Heying and David C. Witherington

In December 1996, representatives of the Guatemalan government and the leftist guerilla movement signed formal peace accords that ended the country's 36-year internal armed conflict and genocide (Schirmer, 1998). The nearly four decades of violence resulted in 200,000 murders and disappearances, 626 massacres, 440 razed villages, over one million displaced persons, and roughly 45,000 widowed women—although some estimates are as high as 80,000 (CEH, 1999; Heying, 2022). A United Nations-supported truth report revealed that 83 percent of victims were non-combative Maya Indigenous civilians and that the government perpetrated 93 percent of the documented abuses, clearly committing acts of genocide that intensified during the period between 1980 to 1983 (CEH, 1999; Oglesby & Ross, 2009). Among those who survived the brutality were an estimated 150,000 to 200,000 orphaned children (CITGUA, 1989; WOLA, 1989). Informed by his work with Holocaust child survivors, Durst (2003) notes, "Wherever there is war, children are the most injured and the most silent; therefore, they easily become the most forgotten victims" (p. 499). This chapter aims to validate and memorialize both the trauma Guatemalan orphaned child survivors endured and their posttraumatic growth (PTG).

Child Survivors of Genocide

It is difficult to determine how many children have survived genocides, in particular, in the 20th and 21st centuries. It is equally challenging to establish how many of those children were orphaned during those horrendous experiences. However, statistics from several genocides that took place since 1900 give some insight into the magnitude and frequency of orphaned child survivorship. For example, in the early 1900s, an estimated 65,000 Herero were murdered by German colonizers and their military forces (Chalk & Jonassohn, 1990). Children were among the many who were murdered and tens of thousands more lost their parents to the brutal attacks. Similarly, the genocide of Armenians by the Ottoman Empire in the early 1900s left over one million dead and, consequently, an unfathomable number of children orphaned (Jones, 2016). Less than twenty years later, the Nazi regime carried out the Holocaust executing over eight million people, mostly Jews (six million) with as

DOI: 10.4324/9781032208688-17

many as 1.5 million of them children (Jones, 2016; US Holocaust Memorial Museum, 2020). Nine to ten thousand Jewish children who survived were safely transported to Great Britain via the *Kindertransport* (children's transport) rescue effort by public and private organizations between 1938 and 1940 (Heberer, 2011). Many thousands of children were also saved because they were successfully hidden by non-Jewish families in Nazi-occupied territories during World War II (US Holocaust Memorial Museum, 2020). Thus, likely tens of thousands of orphaned Jewish children survived the Holocaust and faced a future of uncertainty.

Despite the powerful phrase "Never Again!" that arose after the Holocaust, a multitude of genocides occurred in the last half of the 20th century. For example, in the Cambodian genocide, nearly two million people, constituting roughly one-quarter of the entire national population at the time, were executed, (Chalk & Jonassohn, 1990). Children were among the victims, as well as among the millions of survivors. Likewise, numerous southern Sudanese children were orphaned during Sudan's second civil war where an estimated two million people were killed (Parkhurst Moss, 2008). Over 20,000 Sudanese boys were among the child survivors forced to flee their homes in the late-1980s. Without adult support, they made a long, arduous walk for three months across dangerous desert terrain with no provisions to refugee camps in Ethiopia. In 1991, the group was forced, once again, to set out on foot after the fall of the Ethiopian government made conditions untenable. The boys walked back to Sudan and then onward to a Kakuma refugee camp in Kenya. By the time they reached the camp, only half of the original 20,000 boys had survived and most had no idea what had happened to their remaining family members (Hazard, 2017; U.S. Office of Refugee Resettlement, 2014).

In the last half of the 20th century, genocides were also perpetrated in places such as Guatemala, Argentina, Bosnia and Herzegovina, Rwanda, Burundi, and Syria. Despite efforts in the international community to hold perpetrators of past genocides accountable, genocides show no signs of diminishing in the 21st century (Ibreck & de Waal, 2022; Jones, 2016; Mohajan, 2018). The frequency and magnitude of current and likely future genocides mean that thousands, if not millions, more children will become survivors and many will lose one or both parents, leaving them orphaned. Losing primary caregivers forces orphaned child survivors to face their traumatic experiences and the ensuing consequences of their orphan status without their primary centers of socialization and enculturation. Their experiences are further compounded by not having the evaluative abilities and coping skills of adults (De Young et al., 2011; Saarni et al., 2006). Given their particular experiences as children, child survivors clearly constitute a distinct group of survivors that warrants attention in research and praxis.

Child Survivors as a Distinct Group of Survivors

Children are particularly vulnerable to the brutality of war, armed conflict, and genocide. Young children do not have the physical strength necessary to withstand grave bodily harm and precarious living conditions; yet overwhelming evidence from genocides around the world shows that children were deliberate targets of perpetrators despite their known vulnerability (Heying, 2022). Child survivors have been often overlooked in early research because scholars and practitioners commonly assumed that children were too young to remember what happened, lacked the cognitive skills necessary to understand the gravity of what was occurring, or had experiences indistinct from those of adults (Heberer, 2011;

Robinson et al., 1994). However, their experiences, particularly their relationship with trauma, are worthy of further exploration.

Trauma is a relational phenomenon that inheres in the relation of persons to events rather than in the events themselves (i.e., no event, situation, or circumstance is inherently traumatizing). For example, those subjected to genocide do not invariably experience trauma, despite genocide's prototypical status as an event *that* traumatizes. It is by virtue of how individuals *evaluate* an event like genocide, specifically whether they appraise it as posing a serious and overwhelming threat to their physical or psychological well-being, that such events come to constitute a trauma for those individuals (Cicchetti & Toth, 1997; Frijda, 1986; Lazarus, 1991; Pynoos et al., 1995). Consequently, what does or does not traumatizes depends on the evaluations individuals make and the coping skills they have at their disposal for addressing the challenges that they appraise as such. Both the evaluative abilities and coping skills of children differ qualitatively from those of adults and undergo reorganization as the child moves from prelinguistic foundations in infancy to the immature conceptual foundations of preschoolers and to the increasingly adult-like abilities of school-age children (De Young et al., 2011; Lieberman & Knorr, 2007; Pynoos et al., 1995; Saarni et al., 2006). Hence, what constitutes a traumatic experience must be developmentally contextualized.

At no point in development are children immune from trauma (Shahinfar & Fox, 1997). Given their limited coping skills, both infants and young children may be at particular risk for experiences of trauma since events they appraise as threatening can easily signal to them overwhelming danger (Lieberman & Knorr, 2007). Preschoolers' misattributions of causality and misconceptions of personal responsibility can render an event traumatic that, for a school-aged child or adult, would be considered perfectly innocuous. Furthermore, infants and young children's reliance on caregivers for protection and for making emotional sense of the world can buffer them from experiencing events as traumatic and render them more susceptible to being overwhelmed by events appraised as threatening, depending on the availability and communicative skills of trusted caregivers in their lives (De Young et al., 2011; Pynoos et al., 1995).

Appraisals of events are predicated on sets of generalized assumptions about self and world that develop gradually and consolidate during early childhood, i.e., assumptions constructed through individual life experiences and developmental histories of interacting with others and the world. Such assumptions lie at the heart of Janoff-Bulman's (1992) relational framework for conceptualizing the psychology of trauma, a framework that has figured prominently in both trauma and PTG literature (e.g., Calhoun & Tedeschi, 1998; Calhoun et al., 2010; Cicchetti & Toth, 1997). Janoff-Bulman posits that events become traumatic to the degree that they challenge and ultimately shatter individuals' deep-seated, most fundamental assumptions about the world and people as good and trustworthy, as well as about themselves as worthy of comfort and security. Such an undermining of fundamental assumptions precipitates a psychological crisis constitutive of trauma.

Whereas adults' assumptive frameworks tend to be stable, well-consolidated, and more resistant to shattering, those of children, especially in infancy and early childhood, are still undergoing construction. This renders children's assumptive frameworks more fragile and easily violated but also more open to reformulation and new levels of stability. As Janoff-Bulman (1992) argues, the "plasticity of the child's inner world provides the possibilities for both greater psychological protection from trauma as well as for greater psychological devastation" (p. 84). Children orphaned during the genocide are particularly susceptible as their trauma experiences are not limited to just a single event. Rather, they often experience a series of distressing events that occur throughout childhood and even into adulthood because of their orphan status and often result in sequential traumatization that contributes to their distinct survivorship.

Sequential Traumatization in Orphaned Child Survivors of Genocide

Conducting one of the earliest and most influential studies with orphaned Holocaust child survivors, German-Dutch child psychologist Hans Keilson (1979) used the term "sequential traumatization" to encapsulate the full scope of child survivors' experiences with a succession of cumulative trauma prior to, during, and following the Holocaust. His work inspired a new era of research, prompting an array of publications specifically centered on Holocaust child survivors and the long-term effects of their sequential traumatization (Durst, 2003).

Psychiatrist Robert Krell (1985), a Holocaust child survivor himself, worked with Holocaust child survivors in the early 1980s. Understanding their experiences first-hand, he conducted a comparative analysis of adult and child survivor eyewitness accounts. Krell found that child survivors expressed little pride or dignity in survivorhood and had few to no pre-war memories of establishing their early footing in life. Furthermore, child survivors were scattered in the post-war period rather than living in survivor communities because they sought to be "normal" (p. 399). In contrast, adult survivors expressed a sense of pride and emphasized their personal initiative in survival, as well as preserving a legacy of pre-war memories, sharing their experiences with other adult survivors, and banding together. Krell's research was instrumental in highlighting how child survivors of genocide experience sequential traumatization and feel its long-term effects throughout childhood and into adulthood.

Studies with child survivors of the Holocaust that continued through subsequent decades offer additional insights into the long-term sequential traumatization that orphaned child survivors face over their lifetimes. In addition to losing parents and most semblance of typical childhood during the Holocaust, they also continued to experience loss and psychological distress long after the war ended (Durst, 2003). At the same time, they have shown remarkable coping skills and resilience even decades later.

Studies with Holocaust child survivors have spurred subsequent research focused specifically on child survivor experiences with trauma related to more recent wars, armed conflicts, and genocides. However, much of this research, while imperative and offering vital insights, has been limited in scope, focusing on child survivors' psychological distress and trauma while they are still in childhood (e.g., Dyregrov et al., 2002; Kravić et al., 2013; Thabet & Vostanis, 2000). Some studies have centered on the trauma experienced by adolescent refugee child survivors who lived outside of their home countries at the time of assessment (Geltman et al., 2005; Papageorgiou et al., 2000; Sack et al., 1997). Other studies have assessed child survivors' sequential traumatization experiences by focusing on their experiences with poverty, sexual and physical abuse, and taking on adult responsibilities in their child-headed households while still children (Ng et al., 2015; Reddy, 2003; Whetten et al., 2011). While most studies have focused on trauma associated with the short-term or immediate aftermath of war, armed conflict, and genocide, fewer have conducted extended longitudinal analyses with child survivors at either adolescence or early adulthood, a field that needs to be expanded (Betancourt et al., 2015; Munyandamutsa et al., 2012). More recent longitudinal research with orphaned child survivors in Guatemala, conducted by the first author of this chapter, is helping with that expansion.

Grown Orphaned Child Survivors in Guatemala

Despite the considerable number of orphaned child survivors during the genocide, research on this segment of Guatemala's survivor population, who are now in middle adulthood, remains limited. Heying (2022) and colleagues (Heying et al., 2016) studied 20 mostly Maya Indigenous orphaned child survivors in Guatemala who are now adults in their 30s and 40s. These individuals were orphaned when one or both unarmed, non-combative parents disappeared (kidnapped and murdered) or were murdered by the Guatemalan state during the heightened years of genocide, a period they refer to as "the violence." They were raised for the majority of their childhoods at a permanent residential home founded in the majority Maya highlands town of Santa Teresa by a group of mainly Guatemalan Catholic sisters dedicated to social justice. The residential home consisted of eight small homes that replicated typical family homes in the region. Each home was staffed with several caregivers, called "*tías*" (or aunts), who spoke various Mayan languages to help child survivors maintain their primary languages while they also learned Spanish. Many *tías* had been widowed during the genocide and were invited to bring their own children to live at the residential home as well. The average caregiver-to-child ratio was one-to-five for older children and one-to-three for the youngest children.

In addition to providing basic care, the Catholic sisters enrolled school-aged child survivors in the local schools where they could better socialize with peers from the town. Child survivors also attended vocational skills training and received academic tutoring and reinforcement at the residential home. The Catholic sisters helped the children preserve cultural and religious traditions, customs, and practices, offering them some consistency in their enculturation, identity, and spirituality. Family members were encouraged to visit as often as possible, and the transfer of legal custody of children back to their birth family members could be restored at any time as long as those family members could demonstrate that they had the means to care for the children and would commit to continuing their education. At the height of operations in the mid-1990s, 120 children from newborns to 18-year-olds were enrolled in the residential home.

Heying, who served as a volunteer at the residential home for two years in the mid-1990s, returned to Santa Teresa years later to evaluate how child survivors in their adulthood perceived and experienced the long-term effects of the armed conflict and the genocide. She found that they perceived and expressed having experienced sequential traumatization, which continues to affect them today. As orphaned child survivors, they have had to contend with the lingering trauma of losing one or both of their parents and experiencing brutal violence as well as the traumatic distress of transitioning from living with surviving family members to living in a permanent residential home quite different and distant from their natal homes and communities. While child survivors mostly acknowledged and appreciated that the permanent residential home provided them with a safe, stable, and structured environment and access to resources that their impoverished surviving family members could not offer, the transition to living there was extremely distressing and traumatizing for nearly all of them.

Child survivors reported experiencing trauma, once again, when they transitioned to early adulthood as the permanent residential home did not have the funding to financially support them once they became adults. However, some who did not graduate from high school by the time they turned 18 (several had never attended school before being enrolled in the residential home at older ages) were able to maintain financial support until they completed their high school education by the age of 19 or 20. Regardless, all faced transitioning to adulthood on their own and without an economic, familial, or emotional safety net because of their orphan status. The transition was distressing for most, adding to their sequential traumatization.

Both the qualitative and quantitative research findings of Heying's (2022) research confirm that their experiences with trauma cannot be confined simply to single events occurring during the genocide such as losing parents, witnessing atrocities, and suffering brutality. Rather, they have experienced a sequence of cumulative trauma that includes distress caused by marked life transitions made especially difficult by their orphan status. The distress of these life transitions is unique to orphaned child survivors, as demonstrated by Heying (2022) comparing them with non-orphaned survivors and same-age peers from the same community.

While these orphaned child survivors are fully aware of the enduring distress, hardships, and repercussions they faced in childhood and adulthood because of their orphan status, they also report positive, well-adjusted behaviors and resilience, which are further reflected in their experiences with and reporting of PTG. Using the Spanish version of the Posttraumatic Growth Inventory (Weiss & Berger, 2006), participants were asked to respond relative to their experiences with sequential traumatization, general psychological distress, and how they felt that day. Findings revealed that orphaned child survivors perceived themselves as having grown psychologically from their experiences at a significantly higher rate than their peers (Heying et al., 2016), illuminating how the particular experiences of orphaned child survivors differed from those of other children born and raised in the highlands during the armed conflict and genocide. The instrument was especially useful in elucidating child survivors' and peers' life-long experiences with childhood trauma and distress because it revealed information not otherwise explicitly captured via trauma-focused ethnographic questions, and the results corroborated child survivors' perceptions of their abilities to positively confront sequential traumatization. These results are insightful and warrant further exploration of factors that may have helped foster child survivors' PTG.

Heying (2022) identified four factors that likely influenced child survivors' PTG, including quality of care and low caregiver-to-child ratios, self-disclosure and emotional expressiveness, perceived stability, and improved access to economic resources.

Quality of Care and Low Caregiver-to-Child Ratios

The rations offered by the residential home enabled an intensive, loving, nurturing, family-like relationship between child survivors and their caregivers (Heying et al., 2016). Such childcare is vital for positive child development (Betancourt & Khan, 2008; McCall, 2011; Whetten et al., 2009). Furthermore, close ties with caregivers have been shown to help diminish psychological distress resulting from armed conflict, genocide, and other disasters (Bragin, 2007; Calhoun et al., 2010; Ungar et al., 2007).

Specifically, social support seems to play a primary complex role in facilitating PTG. Across contexts of traumatization, nuanced results characterize the relationship between PTG and social support in children and adolescents (Kilmer et al., 2014; Meyerson et al., 2011). Some research suggests that greater caregiver and family support positively correlates with greater PTG (e.g., Kimhi et al., 2009; Wolchik et al., 2009) whereas other research suggests that no significant correlation exists (e.g., Cryder et al., 2006; Kilmer & Gil-Rivas, 2010), or that teacher and peer but not parental support is key to the facilitative effect (e.g., Yu et al., 2010). What is clear from these findings, and those of Heying (2022) as well, is that the facilitative nature of social support is both person and context-specific, with factors like socioeconomic status and rural versus urban settings playing critical roles in individual differences (Kilmer et al., 2014; Meyerson et al., 2011; Shah & Mishra, 2021). In fact, the commonsense idea that emotionally warm caregiver support is a natural breeding ground for PTG itself requires qualification, given empirical findings demonstrating no correlation between the two (e.g., Kilmer & Gil-Rivas, 2010). Kilmer et al. (2014) have argued that "warm, supportive caregiving" may actually minimize the shattering of world assumptions deemed critical to the promotion of PTG (Calhoun et al., 2010; Janoff-Bulman, 1992), thereby limiting the conditions for fueling such growth per se. Additional support has emerged from recent work by Panjikidze et al. (2020) showing that informational support, practical assistance, and problem-solving skill-building were far more valuable in promoting PTG, especially in the long term, than emotional support. For adolescents, peer groups and the support they offer, rather than the family context, are often more conducive to such aims (Panjikidze et al., 2020; Shah & Mishra, 2021).

Self-Disclosure and Emotional Expressiveness

Sharing experiences and building peer attachments, which were fostered in child survivors by the residential home (Heying et al., 2016), have been shown to strengthen child survivors' critical emotional and social support systems (Johnson et al., 2009; Mota & Matos, 2013). Having the opportunity to share personal stories and emotions through self-disclosure can help child survivors develop coping skills and create strong connections with others, facilitating PTG (Calhoun et al., 2010; Tedeschi & Calhoun, 2004). Studies with child survivors of war have shown similar positive correlations between strong peer attachments and increased wellbeing (Dyregrov et al., 2000; Schaal & Elbert, 2006).

Child survivors' self-disclosure and emotional expressiveness reflect rumination, which plays a critical role in Tedeschi and Calhoun's (1995; 2004) model of PTG, and work with adults has borne out its importance (e.g., Calhoun et al., 2010; Kilmer et al., 2014; Linley & Joseph, 2004). Findings regarding relationships between the amount of rumination and PTG in adolescents are somewhat mixed. This may be explained by the various types of rumination, some of which are constructive whereas others are counterproductive (Watkins, 2008). Research on rumination that revolves around intrusive thoughts, which arrive unbidden and compulsively capture one's attention, yielded mixed findings; however, research specifically targeting rumination characterized by deliberate activities of reflection and rooted in problem-solving strategies, found positive relations between rumination and PTG in adolescent populations (Kilmer et al., 2014; Meyerson et al., 2011; Zhou et al., 2015). Rumination can motivate, inform, and be informed by the inclination toward self-disclosing conversations among peers that is so prominent during the period of adolescence, enhancing peer support networks, especially among individuals who have shared in a country's collective trauma (Panjikidze et al., 2020).

Perceived Stability

Living in the residential home may have afforded a sense of stability. Studies confirm that restoring and maintaining formal education and other vocational training offers children a feeling of security, hope, and predictability even during times of war, violence, and armed conflict (Betancourt & Khan, 2008). Literature on PTG further demonstrates that routine involvement in cultural practices, formal education, vocational training, and similar activities can help children develop skills that foster their sense of self-reliance and self-confidence and bolster their hope for the future, which are important for PTG (Calhoun et al., 2010; Tedeschi & Calhoun, 1996).

Positive future expectations of children and youth following exposure to major distress or trauma can influence PTG via children's and youth's perception of and response to stress or trauma (Cryder et al., 2006; Kilmer et al., 2014). They also factor into the degree of effort children and youth put into making sense of what occurred (Vloet et al., 2017). Several studies have shown that positive future expectations and beliefs about one's own competency correlate positively with PTG (Kilmer, 2006; Wyman et al., 1993).

Improved Access to Economic Resources

Coming to live in the residential home meant that child survivors instantly had improved access to economic resources, including sufficient food, clothing, and school supplies. They could go to school and get medical care not readily available to their surviving family members or communities. Having consistent access to various resources may have furthered child survivors' sense of stability and well-being, helping foster their PTG (Heying et al., 2016). However, further examination of the relationship between increased economic resources and PTG is needed and should involve various orphaned child survivor groups in residential settings around the world.

Future Research

While the PTG experienced by grown orphaned child survivors in Guatemala in the face of adversity is remarkable given their experiences with sequential traumatization and the long-reaching effects of the armed conflict and genocide on their lives, their concurrent experiences of trauma and PTG are not uncommon among other child survivors who experience trauma related to war, armed conflicts, and genocide. Therefore, the relationship between trauma and PTG among such child survivors both necessitates and is deserving of expanded future research. Conducting studies across a wide range of contexts, such as with orphaned children and adolescents who have survived the war, armed conflicts, and genocides is imperative for both research and praxis.

Research has shown that individuals who experience distress and trauma in childhood, particularly in relation to war, armed conflict, and genocide, are more likely to face psychological repercussions for years to come and well into adulthood if they do not have a favorable recovery context in childhood (e.g., Andersson, 2011; Kellermann, 2001, Llabre et al., 2015). As demonstrated in Heying's (2022) research with grown Guatemalan child survivors, children and youth provided with a favorable context can fare reasonably well and even grow from their trauma experiences. However, advanced research involving longitudinal analyses of childhood trauma is needed to more fully understand the lifelong repercussions that child survivors confront and the varied trajectories of their PTG processes. Furthermore, longitudinal analyses of the correlation of sequential traumatization with PTG can contribute to a more extensive and better-informed understanding of how child survivors cope with childhood trauma and what impact it has on their well-being as they progress through their various developmental stages (Masten et al., 2015).

Looking toward the future, researchers suggest that studies also expand analyses of how various factors influence PTG, particularly in child survivors of war, armed conflict, and genocide (Kilmer et al., 2014). For example, psychosocial factors (e.g., age, ethnicity, education levels, optimism) have been shown to correlate with PTG in children and adolescents. However, the direction of correlation (positive or negative) has been inconsistent across studies. Furthermore, because most studies of children's reactions to war and genocide have focused on PTG assessments of children in middle childhood and adolescence, less is known about the levels of PTG in younger populations. Expanded research with younger children, as well as with adolescents, is necessary to flesh out how age correlates with PTG, in which contexts, and to what degree. Further research can help illuminate such varying correlations and help determine what other factors may be influencing correlations as well. Likewise, cultural differences can impact how PTG is experienced and how various cultural practices and products correlate with it. Examining how cultural norms and practices influence PTG is paramount for understanding such growth in diverse cultural contexts (Calhoun et al., 2010).

Distinct types of trauma are also important to consider in future research. Working with Iraqi students living in Turkey who experienced severe war-related trauma, Kiliç et al. (2016) found that different trauma types can lead to differing levels of PTG and that the differences may be further influenced by gender. They also concluded that while trauma type correlates with PTG, the severity of trauma does not. Thus, the relationship between war-related trauma and PTG is not uniform. Kira et al. (2013) found similar dynamics of PTG across different trauma types in their research with Palestinians. They concluded that PTG was not associated with all types of trauma and was even seriously impeded by some trauma such as collective identity trauma (e.g., discrimination and poverty). They suggest that future research considers the trauma profiles of individuals and groups when examining PTG and interventions.

Based on Heying's (2022) research in Guatemala, we further contend that future research, especially with orphaned child survivors of war, armed conflict, and genocide, be expanded to include a wider sampling of orphaned survivors, including those raised in institutionalized care and in noninstitutionalized setting (e.g., with extended family, foster care, adoption). Involving multiple institutionalized care facilities, forms of care, regions of the country, as well as various time periods (e.g., during vs. after the armed conflict) is also imperative. Additionally, we suggest using mixed qualitative and quantitative research methods to facilitate a broader examination of survivor experiences and promote a more systematic analysis of the combinations of care that can help facilitate PTG and resiliency for orphaned children in addition to the aftermath of war, armed conflict, and genocide, throughout their life trajectories. Recognizing and incorporating a diverse range of participants and contexts into trauma and PTG analyses and assessing various factors influencing both can cast a wider light on child survivors' life experiences, leading to a more holistic understanding and much improved practices that can ameliorate their suffering and foster their growth, resilience, and well-being throughout their life spans.

References

Andersson, P. (2011). Post-traumatic stress symptoms linked to hidden Holocaust trauma among adult Finnish evacuees separated from their parents as children in World War II, 1939–1945: A case-control study. *International Psychogeriatrics*, *23*(4), 654–661. doi:10.1017/S1041610210001791

Betancourt, T. S., & Khan, K. T. (2008). The mental health of children affected by armed conflict: Protective processes and pathways to resilience. *International Review of Psychiatry*, *20*(3), 317–328.

Betancourt, T. S., Gilman, S. E., Brennan, R. T., Zahn, I., & VanderWeele, T. J. (2015). Identifying priorities for mental health interventions in war-affected youth: A longitudinal study. *Pediatrics*, *136*(2), e344–e350.

Bragin, M. (2007). The psychological effects of war on children: A psychosocial approach. In E. K. Carl (Ed.), *Trauma psychology: Issues in violence, disaster, health, and illness* (Vol. 195–229). Westport, CT: Praeger.

Calhoun, L. G., Cann, A., & Tedeschi, R. G. (2010). The posttraumatic growth model: Sociocultural considerations. In T. Weiss & R. Berger (Eds.), *Posttraumatic growth and culturally competent practice: Lessons learned from around the globe* (pp. 1–14). Hoboken, NJ: Wiley.

Calhoun, L. G., & Tedeschi, R. G. (1998). Posttraumatic growth: Future directions. In R. G. Tedeschi, C. L. Park, & L. G. Calhoun (Eds.), *Posttraumatic growth: Positive changes in the aftermath of crisis* (pp. 215–238). Mahwah, NJ: Erlbaum.

Chalk, F., & Jonassohn, K. (1990). *The history and sociology of genocide*. New Haven, CT: Yale University Press.

Cicchetti, D., & Toth, S. L. (Eds.). (1997). *Developmental perspectives on trauma: Theory, research and intervention*. Rochester, NY: University of Rochester Press.

Ciencia y Tecnología para Guatemala (CITGUA). (1989). *Situación de la mujer en Guatemala IV*. México City, México: CITGUA.

CEH (Comisión para el Esclarecimiento Histórico. (1999). *Guatemala: Memoria del silencio*. Guatemala City, Guatemala: Comisión para el Esclarecimiento Histórico.

Cryder, C. H., Kilmer, R. P., Tedeschi, R. G., & Calhoun, L. G. (2006). An exploratory study of posttraumatic growth in children following a natural disaster. *American Journal of Orthopsychiatry*, *76*(1), 65–69. doi:10.1037/0002-9432.76.1.65

De Young, A. C., Kenardy, J. A., & Cobham, V. E. (2011). Trauma in early childhood: A neglected population. *Clinical Child Family Psychological Review*, *14*(3), 231–250. doi:10.1007/s10567-011-0094-3

Durst, N. (2003). Child survivors of the Holocaust: Age-specific traumatization and the consequences for therapy. *American Journal of Psychotherapy*, *57*(4), 499–518.

Dyregrov, A., Gjestad, R., & Raundalen, M. (2002). Children exposed to warfare: A longitudinal study. *Journal of Traumatic Stress*, *15*(1), 59–68.

Dyregrov, A., Gupta, L., Gjestad, R., & Mukanoheli, E. (2000). Trauma exposure and psychological reactions to genocide among Rwandan children. *Journal of Traumatic Stress*, *13*(1), 3–21. doi: 10.1023/A:1007759112499

Frijda, N. (1986). *The emotions*. Cambridge, England: Cambridge University Press.

Geltman, P. L., Grant-Knight, W., Mehta, S. D., Lloyd-Travaglini, C., Lustig, S., Landgraf, J. M., & Wise, P. H. (2005). The 'Lost Boys of Sudan': Functional and behavioral health of unaccompanied refugee minors resettled in the United States. *Archives of Pediatrics & Adolescent Medicine*, *159*(6), 585–591.

Hazard, C. (2017). John Dau, one of the lost boys of Sudan: A story about courage, suffering and redemption. Richmond.com. Retrieved May 4, 2009, from https://www.richmond.com/news/local/john-dau-one-of-the-lost-boys-of-sudan-a/article65e72860-dfb5-58dd-9661-5acf63d3fad8.html

Heberer, P. (2011). *Children during the Holocaust*. Lanham: AltaMira Press.

Heying, S. A. (2022). *Child survivors of genocide: Trauma, resilience, and identity in Guatemala*. Lanham, MD: Lexington Books.

Heying, S. A., Witherington, D. C., Smith, J. E., & Gibbons, J. L. (2016). Post-traumatic distress and growth among Guatemalan war orphans in adulthood. *International Perspectives in Psychology: Research, Practice, Consultation*, *5*(1), 18–33. doi:10.1037/ipp0000047

Ibreck, R., & de Waal, A. (2022). Introduction: Situating Ethiopia in genocide debates. *Journal of Genocide Research*, *24*(1), 83–96.

Janoff-Bulman, R. (1992). *Shattered assumptions: Towards a new psychology of trauma*. New York, NY: Free Press.

Johnson, H., Thompson, A., & Downs, M. (2009). Non-western interpreters' experiences of trauma: The protective role of culture following exposure to oppression. *Ethnicity & Health*, *14*(4), 407–418. doi:10.1080/13557850802621449

Jones, A. (2016). *Genocide: A comprehensive introduction* (3rd edition). New York: Routledge.

Keilson, H. (1979). *Sequentielle traumatisierung bei kindern: Deskriptiv-klinische und quantifizierend-statistische follow-up untersuchung zum schicksal der jüdischen kriegswaisen in den Niederlanden.* Stuttgart: Enke.

Kellermann, N. P. F. (2001). The long-term psychological effects and treatment of Holocaust trauma. *Journal of Loss &Trauma*, *6*(3), 197–218. doi:10.1080/108114401753201660

Kılıç, C., Magruder, K. M., & Koryürek, M. M. (2016). Does trauma type relate to posttraumatic growth after war? A pilot study of young Iraqi war survivors living in Turkey. *Transcultural Psychiatry*, *53*(1), 110–123. doi:10.1177/1363461515612963

Kilmer, R. P. (2006). Resilience and posttraumatic growth in children. In L. G. Calhoun & R. G. Tedeschi (Eds.), *Handbook of posttraumatic growth: Research and practice* (pp. 264–288). Mahwah, NJ: Erlbaum.

Kilmer, R. P., & Gil-Rivas, V. (2010). Exploring posttraumatic growth in children impacted by Hurricane Katrina: Correlates of the phenomenon and developmental considerations. *Child Development*, *81*(4), 1211–1227. doi:10.1111/j.1467-8624.2010.01463.x

Kilmer, R. P., Gil-Rivas, V., Griese, B., Hardy, S. J., & Hafstad, G. S. (2014). Posttraumatic growth in children and youth: Clinical implications of an emerging research literature. *American Journal of Orthopsychiatry*, *84*(5), 506–518. doi:10.1037/ort0000016

Kimhi, S., Eshel, Y., Zysberg, L., & Hantman, S. (2009). Getting a life: Gender differences in postwar recovery. *Sex Roles*, *61*, 554–565. doi:10.1007/s11199-009-9660-2

Kira, I. A., Aboumediene, S., Ashby, J. S., Odenat, L., Mohanesh, J., & Alamia, H. (2013). The dynamics of posttraumatic growth across different trauma types in a Palestinian sample. *Journal of Loss and Trauma*, *18*(2), 120–139. doi:10.1080/15325024.2012.679129

Kravić, N., Pajević, I., & Hasanović, M. (2013). Surviving genocide in Srebrenica during the early childhood and adolescent personality. *Croatian Medical Journal*, *54*(1), 55–64.

Krell, R. (1985). Therapeutic value of documenting child survivors. *Journal of the American Academy of Child Psychiatry*, *24*(4), 397–400.

Lazarus, R. S. (1991). *Emotion and adaptation.* New York: Oxford University Press.

Lieberman, A. F., & Knorr, K. (2007). The impact of trauma: A developmental framework for infancy and early childhood. *Psychiatric Annals*, *36*(4), 209–215.

Linley, P. A., & Joseph, S. (2004). Positive change following trauma and adversity: A review. *Journal of Traumatic Stress*, *17*(1), 11–21. doi:10.1023/B:JOTS.0000014671.27856.7e

Llabre, M. M., Hadi, F., La Greca, A. M., & Lai, B. S. (2015). Psychological distress in young adults exposed to war-related trauma in childhood. *Journal of Clinical Child & Adolescent Psychology*, *44*(1), 169–180. doi:10.1080/15374416.2013.828295

Masten, A. S., Narayan, A. J., Silverman, W. K., & Osofsky, J. D. (2015). Children in war and disaster. In M. H. Bornstein & T. Leventhal (Eds.), *Handbook of child psychology and developmental science* (volume 4, pp. 704–745). Hoboken, NJ: John Wiley & Sons.

McCall, R. B. (2011). Research, practice, and policy perspectives on issues of children without permanent parental care. *Monographs of the Society for Research in Child Development*, *76*(4), 223–272. doi:10.1111/j.1540-5834.2011.00634.x

Meyerson, D. A., Grant, K. E., Carter, J. S., & Kilmer, R. P. (2011). Posttraumatic growth among children and adolescents: A systematic review. *Clinical Psychology Review*, *31*(6), 949–964. doi:10.1016/j.cpr.2011.06.003

Mohajan, H. K. (2018). The Rohingya Muslims in Myanmar are victim of genocide!. *ABC Journal of Advanced Research*, *7* (2), 95–108.

Mota, C. P., & Matos, P. M. (2013). Peer attachment, coping, and self-esteem in institutionalized adolescents: The mediating role of social skills. *European Journal of Psychology of Education*, *28*(1), 87–100. doi:10.1007/s10212-012-0103-z

Munyandamutsa, N., Nkubamugisha, P. M., Gex-Fabry, M., & Eytan, A. (2012). Mental and physical health in Rwanda 14 years after the genocide. *Social Psychiatry and Psychiatric Epidemiology*, *47*(11), 1753–1761.

Ng, L. C., Ahishakiye, N., Miller, D. E., & Meyerowitz, B. E. (2015). Narrative characteristics of genocide testimonies predict post-traumatic stress disorder symptoms years later. *Psychological Trauma: Theory, Research, Practice, and Policy*, *7*(3), 303–311. doi:10.1037/tra0000024

Oglesby, E., & Ross, A. (2009). Guatemala's genocide determination and the spatial politics of justice. *Space and Polity*, *13*(1), 21–39.
Panjikidze, M., Beelmann, A., Martskvishvili, K., & Chitashvili, M. (2020). Posttraumatic growth, personality factors, and social support among war-experienced young Georgians. *Psychological Reports*, *123*(3), 687–709. doi:10.1177/0033294118823177
Papageorgiou, V., Frangou-Garunovic, A., Iordanidou, R., Yule, W., Smith, P., & Vostanis, P. (2000). War trauma and psychopathology in Bosnian refugee children. *European Child and Adolescent Psychiatry*, *9*(2), 84–90. doi:10.1007/s007870050002
Parkhurst Moss, B. (2008). *Dark exodus: The lost girls of Sudan*. Dallas, TX: The P3 Press.
Pynoos, R. S., Steinberg, A. M., & Wraith, R. (1995). A developmental model of childhood traumatic stress. In D. Cicchetti & D. J. Cohen (Eds.), *Manual of developmental psychopathology* (pp. 72–95). New York, NY: Wiley.
Reddy, S. N. (2003). The agonising plight of orphans of war: A national survey. *Indian Journal of Social Work*, *64*(3), 307–332.
Robinson, S., M. Rapaport-Bar-Sever, M., & Rapaport, J. (1994). The present state of people who survived the Holocaust as children. *Acta Psychiatrica Scandinavica*, *89*(4), 242–245.
Saarni, C., Campos, J. J., Camras, L. A., & Witherington, D. (2006). Emotional development: Action, communication, and understanding. In W. Damon & R. M. Lerner (Series Eds.) & N. Eisenberg (Vol. Ed.), *Handbook of child psychology: Vol. 3. Social, emotional and personality development* (6th ed., pp. 226–299). New York: Wiley.
Sack, W. H., Seeley, J. R., & Clarke, G. N. (1997). Does PTSD transcend cultural barriers? A study from the Khmer adolescent refugee project. *Journal of the American Academy of Child and Adolescent Psychiatry*, *36*(1), 49–54.
Schaal, S., & Elbert, T. (2006). Ten years after the genocide: Trauma confrontation and post-traumatic stress in Rwandan adolescents. *Journal of Traumatic Stress*, *19*(1), 95–105. doi:10.1002/jts.20104
Schirmer, J. (1998). *The Guatemalan military project: A violence called democracy*. Philadelphia, PA: University of Pennsylvania Press.
Shah, H., & Mishra, A. K. (2021). Trauma and children: Exploring posttraumatic growth among school children impacted by armed conflict in Kashmir. *American Journal of Orthopsychiatry*, *91*(1), 132–148. doi:10.1037/ort0000523
Shahinfar, A., & Fox, N. A. (1997). The effects of trauma on children: Conceptual and methodological issues. In D. Cicchetti, & S. L. Toth, (Eds.), *Developmental perspectives on trauma: Theory, research and intervention* (pp. 115–139). Rochester, NY: University of Rochester Press.
Tedeschi, R. G., & Calhoun, L. G. (1995). *Trauma and transformation: Growing in the aftermath of suffering*. Thousand Oaks, CA: Sage.
Tedeschi, R. G., & Calhoun, L. G. (1996). The Post-traumatic Growth Inventory: Measuring the positive legacy of trauma. *Journal of Traumatic Stress*, *9*(3), 455–472. doi:10.1007/BF02103658
Tedeschi, R. G., & Calhoun, L. G. (2004). Posttraumatic growth: Conceptual foundations and empirical evidence. *Psychological Inquiry*, *15*(1), 1–18. doi:10.1207/s15327965pli1501_01
Thabet, A. A., & Vostanis. P. (2000). Post traumatic stress disorder reactions in children of war: A longitudinal study. *Child Abuse & Neglect*, *24*(2), 291–298.
Ungar, M., Brown, M., Liebenberg, L., Othman, R., Kwong, W. M., Armstrong, M., & Gilgun, J. (2007). Unique pathways to resilience across cultures. *Adolescence*, *42*(166), 287–310.
US Holocaust Memorial Museum. (2020). Introduction to the Holocaust. Ushmm.org. Retrieved March 21, 2022, from https://encyclopedia.ushmm.org/content/en/article/introduction-to-the-holocaust\
US Office of Refugee Resettlement. (2014). The lost boys of Sudan. *Annual ORR Reports to Congress*. Retrieved April 6, 2022, from https://www.acf.hhs.gov/orr/resource/annual-orr-reports-to-congress-2005-iii-the-lost-boys-of-sudan
Vloet, T. D., Vloet, A., Bürger, A., & Romanos, M. (2017). Post-traumatic growth in children and adolescents. *Journal of Trauma Stress Disorders & Treatment*, *6*(4), 1–7. doi:10.4172/2324-8947.1000182
WOLA (Washington Office on Latin America. (1989). *The administration of injustice: Military accountability in Guatemala*. Washington, DC: WOLA.

Watkins, E. R. (2008). Constructive and unconstructive repetitive thought. *Psychological Bulletin, 134*(2), 163–206. doi:10.1037/0033-2909.134.2.163

Weiss, T., & Berger, R. (2006). Reliability and validity of a Spanish version of the post-traumatic growth inventory. *Research on Social Work Practice, 16*(2), 191–199. doi:10.1177/1049731505281374

Whetten, K., Ostermann, J., Whetten, R., O'donnell, K., Thielman, N., & Positive Outcomes for Orphans (POFO) Research Team. (2011). More than the loss of a parent: Potentially traumatic events among orphaned and abandoned children. *Journal of Traumatic Stress, 24*(2), 174–182.

Whetten, K., Ostermann, J., Whetten, R. A., Pence, B. W., O'donnell, K., Messer, L. C., & Thielman, N. M. (2009). A comparison of the wellbeing of orphans and abandoned children ages 6–12 in institutional and community-based care settings in 5 less wealthy nations. *PLoS One, 4*(12), e8169. doi:10.1371/journal.pone.0008169

Wolchik, S. A., Coxe, S., Tein, J. Y., Sandler, I. W., & Ayers, T. S. (2009). Six-year longitudinal predictors of posttraumatic growth in parentally bereaved adolescents and young adults. *Omega: Journal of Death and Dying, 58*(2), 107–128. doi:10.2190/om.58.2.b

Wyman, P. A., Cowen, E. L., Work, W. C., & Kerley, J. H. (1993). The role of children's future expectations in self-system functioning and adjustment to life stress: A prospective study of urban at-risk children. *Development and Psychopathology, 5*(4), 649–661. doi:10.1017/S0954579400006210

Yu, X., Lau, J. T. F., Zhang, J., Mak, W. W. S., Choi, K. C., Lui, W. W. S., Zhang, J., & Chan, E. Y. (2010). Posttraumatic growth and reduced suicidal ideation among adolescents at month 1 after the Sichuan earthquake. *Journal of Affective Disorders, 123*(1–3), 327–331. doi:10.1016/j.jad.2009.09.019

Zhou, X., Wu, X., Fu, F., & An, Y. (2015). Core belief challenge and rumination as predictors of PTSD and PTG among adolescent survivors of the Wenchuan earthquake. *Psychological Trauma: Theory, Research, Practice, and Policy, 7*(4), 391–397. doi:10.1037/tra0000031

15
PTG IN EMERGING ADULTS

Steven D. Schmidt

According to Erikson (1968), critical developmental milestones that many adolescents and young adults are expected to reach include identity development, commencement of postsecondary education and/or career, and establishing interpersonal relationships including marriage and family. Emerging adulthood was proposed by Arnett (2000) as a stage of development, roughly between the ages of 18–25, conceptually and operationally separate from both adolescence and adulthood. Arnett (2007) further describes this stage of development as characterized by identity formation, instability, establishing autonomy, transition, and new possibilities. In essence, this stage of development theoretically bridges adolescence and adulthood providing a transition from the dependent nature of adolescence to the independence of adulthood and is a time for people to imagine what their adult life could be like (e.g., a rewarding career, happy marriage, and family). The experience of trauma during or prior to emerging adulthood, however, can disrupt the path to achieving one or more of these developmental goals.

In pursuing the goals of education/career and marriage/family, it is common, though not universal, for children to leave the home of their parents before the age of 20 (Arnett, 2014), a change that fosters a greater level of independent decision-making; however, these changes can also leave emerging adults with a sense of confusion regarding who they are and questioning their actual status as adults (Yi et al., 2017). As such, emerging adulthood is also marked by a sense of uncertainty regarding what the future holds due to anticipated pending milestones (e.g., the commencement of a career, marriage, or starting a family). However, despite the uncertainty of the future or, perhaps *because* of this uncertainty, there is ample opportunity for growth during the emerging adult years following a traumatic event. Santacroce et al. (2010) refer to uncertainty as a central feature of experiencing childhood trauma, and this uncertainty manifests via rumination over the potential for long-term effects, quality of life, and control over the trauma.

Although some scholars (e.g., Wood et al., 2017) have argued that emerging adulthood is only applicable to a limited subset of the population for whom access to critical resources is available, it may be that emerging adulthood is experienced differently by people based on the resources that are available to them, and not all emerging adults are privileged enough to have the freedom to explore options that will set their path into adulthood

 DOI: 10.4324/9781032208688-18

(Arnett, 2014). However, a discussion on the validity of emerging adulthood as a distinct stage of development is beyond the scope of this chapter, and thus, the focus will be on the Arnett (2000) definition and the task of identity formation.

In using Arnett's (2000) definition of emerging adulthood, much of the research on posttraumatic growth (PTG) that has included this population has also included adolescents and young children and/or older adults making it difficult to truly identify how and to what degree PTG is typically realized by this age cohort. Thus, in the review of the literature presented here, studies were excluded if the sample was not limited to 18 to 25; exceptions were made for studies that included samples as young as 12 and as old as 30 providing that the majority of the sample was between 18 and 25. This literature on PTG and emerging adults has reported on the nature of PTG in this cohort and on resources that have been found to be related to reports of growth among emerging adults including identity development, cognitive processing of trauma, event centrality, coping skills, and social support.

The Nature of PTG in Emerging Adulthood

Considering the developmental stage of emerging adulthood, it should be expected with a great deal of certainty that most will attain some personal growth during this life stage. An argument can be made that growth in the domain of new possibilities within the model of PTG is likely to be achieved by most emerging adults. As they fully transition to adulthood and become more independent, many have a focus on "what can be" including work and love opportunities. However, for emerging adults who have experienced a traumatic event, this may not be the case.

Devine et al. (2010) documented reports by emerging adults about their experiences with a serious childhood illness. The majority of the responses were negative (e.g., physical/health problems, medical requirements), and the negative aspects were reported at a much higher rate than positive ones; however, this may reflect the easier recall of negative characteristics due to adverse and unpleasant connotations associated with serious illnesses. When asked specifically about the positive aspects of having a serious childhood illness, between a quarter and a third of participants mentioned a shift in perspective, personal strength, appreciation for life, and/or increased support/closeness from family and friends. These last three aspects are very much in line with the domains of PTG (absent from this list are the domains of new possibilities and spiritual change). Regarding traumatic events that span over time, such as serious childhood illnesses, Yi et al. (2017) posited that the time that is consumed by the trauma fosters a new perspective of time and life, which can lead to growth in one's appreciation for life. Parry and Chesler (2005) noted that after dealing with a serious illness such as cancer, survivors became more empathetic and compassionate due to their own feelings of being different, which led to a fuller appreciation for life.

In another study, Gottlieb et al. (2007) collected from college students data about changes experienced in the past couple of years, though not specifically about events that were perceived as traumatic, and found positive endorsements for the domains of personal strength and new possibilities. Although personal strength was endorsed by samples in both studies by Gottlieb et al. (2007) and Devine et al. (2010), the other domains in which growth was identified differed indicating that growth realized during emerging adulthood may differ between those who have experienced a traumatic event and those who have not. The former experienced more changes in personal strength, appreciation for life, and relations with others, whereas the latter experienced the aforementioned new possibilities often associated with the transition from dependent child to independent adult.

Moreover, Gottlieb et al. (2007) reported in addition to the domain of new possibilities being highly endorsed, that contrary to Devine et al. (2010), growth (positive) items were more often endorsed than decline (negative) items. This can be explained, in part, by the type of experiences reported because the events in the Gottlieb et al. (2007) study were significant but not necessarily traumatic. Thus, it is likely that experiencing new possibilities is a typical achievement during emerging adulthood, but for those who have had to deal with a traumatic event that has affected their development, new possibilities may be interfered with as they process and adjust to their trauma experience.

In support of these findings, Schmidt et al. (2019) found no difference in personal strength and relationships with others between a group of trauma survivors and a comparison group, but they did report two significant differences between these groups in reports of PTG. First, the comparison group, which reported on their transition to college, reported more growth in the domain of new possibilities, which supports the idea that major non-traumatic events may not impede the pursuit of new possibilities typical during emerging adulthood. In essence, this is not surprising considering that college is a time for exploring new opportunities, and certain traumas (e.g., serious/chronic illnesses) may limit the number and type of opportunities that can be explored. Second, it was also found that the group of trauma survivors reported a higher level of appreciation for life (Schmidt et al., 2019). When dealing with a trauma, particularly if the trauma is life-threatening or life-altering, worldviews are challenged, and perspectives change leading to the potential for a greater appreciation for life.

Identity Development

Although many factors go into one's identity, college/career and marriage/family are among the more salient characteristics that are considered by many to be developmental milestones for emerging adults, and interruptions during this stage of development can be disruptive to the achievement of these goals (Kim et al., 2018; McDonnell et al., 2018; Tavernier et al., 2019; Yi et al., 2017). Through the process of exploring options for work and love, emerging adults learn more about who they are and what is important to them (Yi et al., 2017). Because establishing one's identity and worldview is a critical milestone that is typically achieved during emerging adulthood, researchers have investigated how experiencing a traumatic event can interfere with identity development. For example, Bellizzi et al. (2012) reported that a third of adolescent and young adult cancer survivors experienced negative effects on their career plans as a result of their cancer.

Emerging adults typically explore employment interests and romantic relationships, both of which are critical to identity development (Erikson, 1968; Yi et al., 2017). Experiencing a traumatic event is a potential interruption that can have a salient impact on this exploration and establishment of a career and family. Lingering or late effects of a traumatic experience have the potential to interfere with these pursuits, which can impede identity development during emerging adulthood (Yi et al., 2017). However, this developmental period is also marked by instability, and cognitions and meaning-making abilities are quite malleable, possibly resulting in the realization of new possibilities (Arnett, 2014;

Cook et al., 2021; Parry & Chesler, 2005). The powerful nature of living through a traumatic experience may provide emerging adults with new considerations when pursuing career interests or serious romantic relationships. For example, these young adults may consider a career that is linked to the type of trauma experienced (which may not have previously been on their radar) or focus on deep and meaningful, rather than shallow and casual, relationships. To this end, emerging adults who have experienced a trauma may select a career or choose a mate that differs from their ideals prior to their exposure to a traumatic event, but whether these changes are perceived as growth has not been empirically examined.

How and to what degree a traumatic experience affects a person (including the potential for PTG) depends, in part, on the resources available to them and their ability to use them. Young children and adolescents who experience trauma are likely to also experience delays in pursuing and achieving their goals related to career and family, and the resources available to help them respond to and manage the traumatic event and its impact, such as cognitive development, event centrality, coping, and perceived and actual use of social support, are likely to differ from individuals who are more settled in their adulthood (Schmidt et al., 2019).

Cognitive Processing of Trauma

Several of the aforementioned resources tend to covary with age and developmental stage. Devine et al. (2010) found that age at diagnosis of a serious or chronic childhood illness was not associated with PTG, whereas Tremolada et al. (2016a) reported younger age at diagnosis to be a predictor of PTG. This difference can be partly explained by the fact that some of these studies collected data specifically from cancer survivors, which can be more serious and life-threatening than many other chronic illnesses. Another possible reason for this contradiction regarding the influence on PTG is that for traumas experienced at younger ages, there is more time to process the impact, and older individuals in this age group are also more likely to have the cognitive skills needed to realize PTG. However, trauma at the older end of this spectrum of ages may be more impactful as there is less time for adjustments before the typical transition to independence which is a marker of adulthood.

Other researchers (McDonnell et al., 2018; Tremolada et al., 2016a; Tremolada et al., 2018) have shown that within samples of adolescent and young adult cancer survivors, older age at data collection was a predictor of PTG. This may be due to more developed cognitive processing skills. The cognitive processing of a traumatic event can impact one's identity, however, the research is mixed. In one study on post-breakup distress, Norona et al. (2018) reported that emotional suppression predicted lower levels of growth, and higher cognitive processing was related to more growth. Tavernier et al. (2019) and Tremolada et al. (2018) note that, compared with those younger than them, emerging adults possess more developed coping skills and higher cognitive and emotional development, which likely coincide with deeper processing of personal experiences.

In their study on female college students in Dominica following exposure to tropical storm Erika, Tavernier et al. (2019) suggest that "rumination may be part of the cognitive process through which individuals emerge with a sense of renewed psychological well-being in the face of trauma" (p. 91) and reported significant positive associations between rumination and PTG in their sample of emerging adults. In another study investigating college students' reports on various traumas, Shigemoto et al. (2017) found that several types of rumination predicted PTG for men but not women with the exception of deliberate rumination, which was significant for both genders. Although not broken down by gender, Lancaster et al. (2015) also found deliberate rumination, but not intrusive rumination, to be a predictor of PTG. Similarly, meaning-making was associated with growth in a sample of college students whose mothers had been diagnosed with a mental illness (Abraham & Stein, 2015). These findings suggest that interventions aimed at the cognitive processing of a traumatic event could be one path to facilitating PTG in emerging adults.

Event Centrality

Event centrality, i.e., the significance that an event has for one's understanding of themself and the world, has been reported to be positively correlated with PTG (Lancaster et al., 2015; Wamser-Nanney et al., 2018). For instance, Cook et al. (2021) studied 196 adolescent and emerging adult cancer survivors and 131 healthy comparisons and found that those diagnosed with cancer reported more event centrality than those who reported on non-cancer traumatic events (the correlation between event centrality and PTG in the cancer group was .37); this was also true for cancer survivors who reported an event other than their cancer diagnosis as being the most traumatic. Thus, it appears that the cancer experience (and perhaps other serious health conditions) can become a significant part of an emerging adult's identity (Yi et al., 2017).

When an event is perceived as traumatic, it can be particularly detrimental to one's self-concept and Cook et al. (2021) comment that the centrality of an event can be critical in identity development. Lancaster et al. (2015) further identified a relationship between core beliefs and event centrality, suggesting that, traumatic events may be significantly impactful when one's worldviews have been seriously disrupted, which has been related to PTG. Moreover, it appears that the type of trauma does not moderate the relations between event centrality and PTG, making event centrality, similar to cognitive processing, a potential target for approaches to foster PTG in trauma survivors (Wamser-Nanney et al., 2018).

Coping Skills

Schmidt et al. (2019) found that emerging adult survivors of trauma reported more use of self-distraction, denial, disengagement, acceptance, and turning to religion as coping strategies than a comparison group of emerging adults who reported regarding their transition to college. This comparison group reported greater use of active coping, use of instrumental support, positive reframing, planning, humor, and self-blame. These findings suggest that emerging adults who had experienced a traumatic event are less likely to engage in approach/active-oriented coping strategies. Possibly, the emotional distress associated with a traumatic event may interfere with emerging adults' ability to engage in more active approach-oriented styles of coping.

For those in the Schmidt et al. (2019) study who reported exposure to trauma, the strongest predictors of PTG were active coping ($r = .35$), use of emotional support ($r = .38$), use of instrumental support ($r = .41$), positive reframing ($r = .39$), planning ($r = .36$), and turning to religion ($r = .37$). However, with the exceptions of use of emotional support and turning to religion, those in the trauma group, were also less likely than the comparison group to use these coping strategies. Although religious coping has often been found to be correlated with PTG, Although religious coping has been found to be correlated with PTG, this relationship may be confounded because spiritual growth is part of the operationalization of PTG.

In addition to these coping strategies, resilience has been defined as "... a class of phenomena characterized by *good outcomes in spite of serious threats to adaptation or development* [emphasis added]" (Masten, 2001, p. 228). Resilience may be a trait that fosters the use of approach/active-oriented coping abilities in response to a stressor (Wamser-Nanney et al., 2018). Studies have reported moderate to strong correlations ranging from .39 to .79 (Ergün et al., 2018; Li et al., 2018; Wamser-Nanney et al., 2018) between resilience and PTG in samples of emerging adults. These studies support the notion of resilience as a resource that enables people to cope with and overcome stressful adversity (Li et al., 2018).

One study that tested an intervention aimed at promoting resilience in a sample of adolescents and emerging adults with cancer found a small effect for adolescents 12 to 17 and a larger effect for emerging adults 18 to 25 suggesting that there may be a developmental component involved in the coping abilities that benefits emerging adults (Lau et al., 2020). Arnett (2014) posits that emerging adults' cognitive abilities related to self-knowledge and self-understanding may make it possible for them to transform their lives, because when compared with adolescents, emerging adults have a greater ability to appreciate their capacity to change aspects of their lives.

Social Support

Researchers have assessed the perceived quality and use of instrumental and emotional support within samples of emerging adults (Milam & Schmidt, 2018; Parry & Chesler, 2005); Schmidt et al., 2019). For example, Parry and Chesler (2005), in their qualitative study on the psychosocial adjustment of emerging adults to childhood cancer, conducted interviews with 50 participants who reported that relationships with close family members and friends were important in their psychosocial adjustment, whereas participants who reported a lack of social support tended to identify it as a contributing factor to their poor psychosocial adjustment. In another study of 232 college students whose parents had divorced, Milam and Schmidt (2018) found that perceived support from family and friends as well as the use of instrumental and emotional support were positively, though weakly, associated with reports of PTG (correlations coefficients = .28, .15, .22, respectively). However, when entered into a regression model, perceived support, but not the use of instrumental or emotional support, remained a significant contributor to the variance in PTG. Thus, it can be argued that perceived support may be more important in the context of PTG than the actual use of support.

Researchers have also compared aspects of social support between those who have experienced trauma with those who have not (Schmidt et al., 2019; Tremolada et al., 2016b). Schmidt et al. (2019) investigated PTG in 329 emerging adult trauma survivors and found that received emotional/instrumental support ($r = .24$), use of emotional support ($r = .38$), and use of instrumental support ($r = .41$) were all significant predictors of PTG. However, when comparing these data with a group of emerging adults who reported on their experiences of transition to college, there was no significant difference between the groups in overall perceived support or use of emotional support, whereas the use of instrumental support was reported more by the comparison group. Moreover, a study comparing emerging adult cancer survivors with a control group found less support from family and partners for the cancer survivors (Tremolada et al., 2016b), while another study on emerging adult cancer survivors found support from family, but not from other sources, to be predictive of reports of PTG (Tremolada et al., 2016a).

Thus, it is plausible that as individuals move through the transition period from adolescence to adulthood, changes in relationships with family, friends, and partners may moderate the support available to them and the influence this support can have on experiencing PTG. It appears that the use and perception of support can provide unique contributions to the development of PTG, but Milam and Schmidt (2018) suggest that the perception of support may be more important in the context of dealing with a traumatic event. More research is needed to understand the different influences of perceived and actual social support on adjustment.

Conclusion

PTG is commonly reported by emerging adults who have experienced a traumatic event. However, traumatic events have the potential to interfere with the developmental tasks of identity formation, embarking on a career, pursuing a college degree, and getting married or starting a family. Individuals may have to put off college, change career plans, or delay marriage and starting a family. All these factors – trauma, career/college, and spouse/family – are critical components in a person's identity. Challenges to these developmental tasks caused by traumatic events can force individuals to reexamine their worldviews and core beliefs. These challenges can foster rumination and meaning-making processes to reconceptualize what is important and valued. In one mixed-methods study, when asked to report positive outcomes from being diagnosed and living with a chronic or serious childhood illness, emerging adults responded with comments related to shifts in perspectives and worldviews 36 percent of the time, and this category of responses was the most common among all positive comments (Devine et al., 2010). These changes in worldviews and core beliefs can then be realized as growth, which can be achieved during this life stage because of the malleability of cognitive processes and the instability of transitioning from a dependent adolescent to an independent adult.

Scores of PTG collected from emerging adults do not appear to differ from those reported by older adults. The review of the limited available studies with emerging adults shows that personal strength was most frequently reported to be the highest (Devine et al., 2010; Li et al., 2018; Tremolada et al., 2016a) or second highest (Schmidt et al., 2019) level of growth. Scores for appreciation for life were also endorsed at or near the top of PTG domains (Devine et al., 2010; Li et al., 2018; Schmidt et al., 2019; Tremolada et al., 2016a). In two studies that investigated various traumas, new possibilities scored high for individuals who reported events that were not necessarily traumatic. Schmidt et al. (2019) found that trauma survivors' scores were lower on the domain of new possibilities than the scores from a comparison group who reported on their transition to college, and Gottlieb et al. (2007), who asked participants to report on changes experienced in recent years, reported that new possibilities were endorsed higher than all other domains of PTG. Arnett (2014) comments "there is something about reaching adulthood that opens up new possibilities for transformation for people who have had more than their share of adversity during their early years" (pp. 307–308). However, this opening up of new possibilities may be more applicable to individuals who have not had to deal with a great deal of adversity.

After all, this transition stage is a time when most are considering what lies ahead and what could be, but for those who have lived through a traumatic event, this may not be the case.

Finally, there is a large gap in the literature regarding samples and populations. Many studies on emerging adults have been conducted with college students, and the majority of participants in these studies are Caucasian females. Research needs to be conducted with more diverse and marginalized populations to answer critical research questions. Are the domains of PTG differently valued by different populations? Do the paths to achieving PTG differ among populations and cultures? To better understand the in-between developmental stage of emerging adulthood and how trauma affects these young individuals across populations and cultures, researchers need to focus specifically on the 18–25 cohort as defined by Arnett (2000) and include more diverse populations.

References

Abraham, K. M., & Stein, C. H. (2015). Stress-related personal growth among emerging adults whose mothers have been diagnosed with mental illness. *Psychiatric Rehabilitation Journal, 38*(3), 227–233. 10.1037/prj0000128

Arnett, J. J. (2000). Emerging adulthood: A theory of development from the late teens through the twenties. *American Psychologist, 55*(5), 469–480. 10.1037/0003-066X.55.5.469

Arnett, J. J. (2007). Emerging adulthood: What is it, and what is it good for? *Child Development Perspectives, 1*(2), 68–73. https://doi-org.ezproxy.lib.uconn.edu/10.1111/j.1750-8606.2007.00016.x

Arnett, J. J. (2014). *Emerging adulthood: The winding road from the late teens through the twenties.* Oxford University Press.

Bellizzi, K. M., Smith, A., Schmidt, S., Keegan, T. H. M., Zebrack, B., Lynch, C. F., Deapen, D., Shnorhavorian, M., Tompkins, B. J., & Simon, M. (2012). Positive and negative psychosocial impact of being diagnosed with cancer as an adolescent or young adult. *Cancer, 118*(20), 5155–5162. https://doi-org.ezproxy.lib.uconn.edu/10.1002/cncr.27512

Cook, J. L., Russell, K., Long, A., & Phipps, S. (2021). Centrality of the childhood cancer experience and its relation to post-traumatic stress and growth. *Psycho-Oncology, 30*(4), 564–570. 10.1002/pon.5603

Devine, K. A., Reed-Knight, B., Loiselle, K. A., Fenton, N., & Blount, R. L. (2010). Posttraumatic growth in young adults who experienced serious childhood illness: A mixed-methods approach. *Journal of Clinical Psychology in Medical Settings, 17*(4), 340–348. 10.1007/s10880-010-9210-7

Ergün, G., Gümüş, F., & Dikeç, G. (2018). Examining the relationship between traumatic growth and psychological resilience in young adult children of parents with and without a mental disorder. *Journal of Clinical Nursing, 27*(19–20), 3729–3738. 10.1111/jocn.14533

Erikson, E. H. (1968). *Identity: Youth and crisis.* Norton & Co.

Gottlieb, B. H., Still, E., & Newby-Clark, I. R. (2007). Types and precipitants of growth and decline in emerging adulthood. *Journal of Adolescent Research, 22*(2), 132–155. 10.1177/0743558406298201

Kim, B., Patterson, P., & White, K. (2018). Developmental considerations of young people with cancer transitioning to adulthood. *European Journal of Cancer Care, 27*(6), 1–7.

Lancaster, S. L., Klein, K. R., Nadia, C., Szabo, L., & Mogerman, B. (2015). An integrated model of posttraumatic stress and growth. *Journal of Trauma & Dissociation, 16*(4), 399–418. 10.1080/15299732.2015.1009225

Lau, N., Bradford, M. C., Steineck, A., Scott, S., Bona, K., Yi-Frazier, J. P., McCauley, E., & Rosenberg, A. R. (2020). Examining key sociodemographic characteristics of adolescents and young adults with cancer: A post hoc analysis of the promoting resilience in stress management randomized clinical trial. *Palliative Medicine, 34*(3), 336–348. 10.1177/0269216319886215

Li, Y., Xing, A., Chen, X., Lou, F., & Cao, F. (2018). Posttraumatic growth and parental bonding in young adults of parents with physical disabilities: Testing mediation model of resilience. *Psychology, Health & Medicine, 23*(6), 661–667. 10.1080/13548506.2017.1417608

Masten, A. S. (2001). Ordinary magic: Resilience processes in development. *American Psychologist*, *56*(3), 227–238. 10.1037/0003-066X.56.3.227

McDonnell, G. A., Pope, A. W., Schuler, T. A., & Ford, J. S. (2018). The relationship between cancer-related worry and posttraumatic growth in adolescent and young adult cancer survivors. *Psycho-Oncology*, *27*(9), 2155–2164. 10.1002/pon.4785

Milam, S. R. B., & Schmidt, C. K. (2018). A mixed methods investigation of posttraumatic growth in young adults following parental divorce. *The Family Journal*, *26*(2), 156–165. 10.1177/1066480718781518

Norona, J. C., Scharf, M., Welsh, D. P., & Shulman, S. (2018). Predicting post-breakup distress and growth in emerging adulthood: The roles of relationship satisfaction and emotion regulation. *Journal of Adolescence*, *63*, 191–193. 10.1016/j.adolescence.2018.01.001

Parry, C., & Chesler, M. A. (2005). Thematic evidence of psychosocial thriving in childhood cancer survivors. *Qualitative Health Research*, *15*(8), 1055–1073. 10.1177/1049732305277860

Santacroce, S. J., Asmus, K., Kadan-Lottick, N., & Grey, M. (2010). Feasibility and preliminary outcomes from a pilot study of coping skills training for adolescent-young adult survivors of childhood cancer and their parents. *Journal of Pediatric Oncology Nursing*, *27*(1), 10–20. 10.1177/1043454209340325

Schmidt, S. D., Blank, T. O., Bellizzi, K. M., & Park, C. L. (2019). Posttraumatic growth reported by emerging adults: A multigroup analysis of the roles of attachment, support, and coping. *Current Psychology: A Journal for Diverse Perspectives on Diverse Psychological Issues*, *38*(5), 1225–1234. 10.1007/s12144-017-9670-0

Shigemoto, Y., Low, B., Borowa, D., & Robitschek, C. (2017). Function of personal growth initiative on posttraumatic growth, posttraumatic stress, and depression over and above adaptive and maladaptive rumination. *Journal of Clinical Psychology*, *73*(9), 1126–1145. 10.1002/jclp.22423

Tavernier, R., Fernandez, L., Peters, R. K., Adrien, T. V., Conte, L., & Sinfield, E. (2019). Sleep problems and religious coping as possible mediators of the association between tropical storm exposure and psychological functioning among emerging adults in Dominica. *Traumatology*, *25*(2), 82–95. 10.1037/trm0000187

Tremolada, M., Bonichini, S., Basso, G., & Pillon, M. (2016a). Post-traumatic stress symptoms and post-traumatic growth in 223 childhood cancer survivors: Predictive risk factors. *Frontiers in Psychology*, *7*, Article 287. 10.3389/fpsyg.2016.00287

Tremolada, M., Bonichini, S., Basso, G., & Pillon, M. (2016b). Perceived social support and health-related quality of life in AYA cancer survivors and controls. *Psycho-Oncology*, *25*(12), 1408–1417. 10.1002/pon.4072

Tremolada, M., Bonichini, S., Basso, G., & Pillon, M. (2018). Adolescent and young adult cancer survivors narrate their stories: Predictive model of their personal growth and their follow-up acceptance. *European Journal of Oncology Nursing*, *36*, 119–128. 10.1016/j.ejon.2018.09.001

Wamser-Nanney, R., Howell, K. H., Schwartz, L. E., & Hasselle, A. J. (2018). The moderating role of trauma type on the relationship between event centrality of the traumatic experience and mental health outcomes. *Psychological Trauma: Theory, Research, Practice, and Policy*, *10*(5), 499–507. 10.1037/tra0000344

Wood, D., Crapnell, T., Lau, L., Bennett, A., Lotstein, D., Ferris, M., & Kuo, A. (2017). Emerging adulthood as a critical stage in the life course. In N. Halfon, R. M. Lerner, E. M. Faustman, & C. B. Forrest (Eds.), *Handbook of life course health development* (pp. 123–143). Springer.

Yi, J., Tian, T., & Kim, J. (2017). Emerging adults who have flourished through a physical health challenge. In L. M. Padilla-Walker, & L. J. Nelson (Eds.), *Flourishing in emerging adulthood: Positive development during the third decade of life* (pp. 559–579). Oxford University Press.

16
POST-TRAUMATIC GROWTH AMONG OLDER ADULTS

Emre Senol-Durak and Mithat Durak

Post-traumatic growth (PTG) is a universally accepted concept that expresses the increase in the individual's functionality level after traumatic or extremely challenging experiences (Weiss & Berger, 2010). Calhoun and Tedeschi (2010) describe it as making significant changes in people's lives, philosophy, thinking about themselves, and interactions with others after a traumatic event. Traumatic experiences change individuals' assumptive worlds since these events have seismic value (Calhoun & Tedeschi, 1998). The original PTG domains of appreciation of life, personal strength, social connections, new possibilities, and spirituality were later expanded to include considerations of cultural variations (Tedeschi et al., 2017). Cross-cultural research shows that expanded PTG fields are ubiquitous (Taku et al., 2021). Positive transformations are seen among individuals and their families (Berger & Weiss, 2009). In therapeutic settings, emphasizing PTG improves patients' well-being (Calhoun & Tedeschi, 1998), suggesting that clinicians should focus on an individual's strengths rather than on their symptoms (Berger & Weiss, 2009).

Although positive shifts following a traumatic event persist throughout one's life, the bulk of studies on PTG since its inception has been on adults (Berger & Weiss, 2009; Grad & Zeligman, 2017; Senol-Durak & Ayvasik, 2010; Taku et al., 2021; Zeligman et al., 2018). While it has been noted that older people may face difficulty as a result of any change (Merecz et al., 2012), studies on the occurrence of PTG in older adults support Calhoun and Tedeschi's (1998) idea that PTG can be observed at any developmental stage, regardless of age. Nevertheless, PTG in the older population has received little attention in studies (Kadri et al., 2022), even though the global population of older people is on the rise (Wilson & Saklofske, 2018). It is anticipated that by the year 2050, the proportion of older people will make up 35% of the population in Europe, 28% of the population in Northern America, 25% of the population in Latin America and the Caribbean, 24% of the population in Asia, 23% of Oceania, and 9% of the population in Africa (United Nations, 2017). As the global population ages, it will be crucial to implement a process of radical social transformation that brings about positive changes in areas such as family structures and intergenerational relationships.

Most explorations of positive life experiences in older people focused on resiliency (Gaffey et al., 2016; MacLeod et al., 2016; Resnick, 2014). Resilience in later life is associated with

DOI: 10.4324/9781032208688-19

longevity (MacLeod et al., 2016) and successful aging, defined as maintaining high levels of physical, psychological, and social functioning and the absence of severe illness (Taylor & Carr, 2021). Resilient older individuals can understand and make meaning of their lives and integrate their identity and high-level interpersonal abilities (Nuccio & Stripling, 2021). Studies on resilience in older people suggest that studying PTG at this age in a therapeutic context may be useful (Stein et al., 2020; Tedeschi & Blevins, 2017).

In addition to the term resiliency, positive reappraisal has also been cited by those over 65 who have succeeded in making changes in the face of adversity (Nowlan et al., 2015). Aging is associated with a strengthening of positive appraisal (Shiota & Levenson, 2009), i.e., the act of extracting good personally significant meaning from an unpleasant situation (Nowlan et al., 2015) by focusing on emotions (Liang et al., 2017). Higher levels of positive affect, positive social ties, and self-acceptance were all independently linked to the meaning-based coping technique of positive reappraisal in a sample of older adults concerning their health problems at a residential care facility (Schanowitz & Nicassio, 2006). Similarly, a higher positive appraisal was associated with higher positive affect and lower unpleasant emotions in a sample of community-dwelling older adults (Liang et al., 2017). Increased problem-focused and positive reappraisal coping, as well as higher levels of perceived control and life involvement, accounted for the higher levels of emotional well-being associated with wisdom in a sample of retired older adults (Etezadi & Pushkar, 2013).

The literature suggests that self-compassion and a positive appraisal are increasingly helpful in helping older adults cope with life challenges such as physical health problems (Allen et al., 2012). A compassionate viewpoint toward oneself and one's experiences is essential to self-compassion, defined as developing and sustaining such a perspective (Seligowski et al., 2015). Higher self-compassion moderated the relationship between poor physical health and higher psychological well-being (Allen et al., 2012). In a sample of traumatized older adults, self-compassion through positive reframing helped people lessen their tendency to overidentify with negative feelings (Munroe et al., 2022).

Traumatic Experiences and PTG among Older Adults

Inevitably, the world's population will continue to get older year after year (Durak & Senol-Durak, 2018b). As a result, the number of seniors suffering from mental health concerns is rising, and 15 million older people are expected to be diagnosed with a mental illness by 2030 (Jeste et al., 1999) while availability to receive psychological help is poor (Bartels, 2003). Preventive and evidence-based strategies are needed to address older adults' problems (Bartels, 2003) and it is necessary to integrate positive reframing into those strategies (Munroe et al., 2022).

Research has demonstrated a rise in the incidence of distressing events among older adults (Pless Kaiser et al., 2019; VanBockel, 2020; van Zelst et al., 2003). A comprehensive epidemiological study (N = 9463) of older adults living in the United States reveals that the lifetime prevalence of post-traumatic stress disorder (PTSD) ranges from 4.5% to 5.5% (Pietrzak et al., 2012). Pless Kaiser et al. (2019) found that many older people (50–90%) say they have had at least one traumatic event in their adult lives. Specifically, only a few studies have been conducted on older women experiencing trauma (Thorp et al., 2011). Older adults have higher PTSD scores than younger adults, particularly those who have lost a loved one, had a loved one becomes sick or injured, or were exposed to the 9/11 terrorist attacks (Pietrzak et al., 2012). Childhood tragedies like being deported or witnessing the

Holocaust profoundly impact the lives of many older individuals (Durak & Senol-Durak, 2019; Greenblatt-Kimron, 2021; van Zelst et al., 2003). The intensity of PTSD symptoms was shown to be greater in older people (N = 1995) who had been physically assaulted when they were adults or had been violently abused as children (Ogle et al., 2014).

While studies have focused extensively on the negative psychological outcomes of traumatic experiences in old age (Cook & Niederehe, 2007; Cook & Simiola, 2017; Durak & Senol-Durak, 2019; Pietrzak et al., 2012), similar to other age groups, older adults might also experience a positive transformation, i.e., PTG in the aftermath of traumatic experiences or big life events. These changes can include gaining a new appreciation for life, becoming more spiritual, more connected to others, and evaluating new alternatives in life. PTG levels in older persons have been found to range from moderate to high (Kadri et al., 2022); however, compared to younger people, older adults are predicted to have less PTG (Boyle et al., 2017) possibly because they have more life experiences (Bellizzi & Blank, 2006). In contrast to common assumptions, research has found that older persons are more prone to exhibit happy feelings (Carstensen et al., 2011). Moreover, activating positive transitions helps older people improve their quality of life (Wilson & Saklofske, 2018), as encountering diverse life events may strengthen their coping abilities (Henson et al., 2021). Studies of PTG in older adults are less common than in other age groups, presenting a challenge to understanding the nature and expression of PTG in older people. This challenge is further increased by the exceedingly diverse reactions of older people to life's challenges (Kadri et al., 2022). Of the few studies that exist, a systematic evaluation of 16 studies showed a moderate to high level of PTG among older adults (Kadri et al., 2022). Greenblatt-Kimron (2021) posited that meaning-making is critical for PTG in older adults and ideas, knowledge, and wisdom gained with age boost the capacity to adjust to new conditions.

Because ideas about death are also associated with advancing years, community-dwelling older people (N = 339) were surveyed regarding their views of mortality and subjective judgment of age (Palgi, 2016). Surprisingly, neither closure to death nor subjective age assessment was found to be significantly related. However, those factors were a moderator between post-traumatic stress (PTS) and PTG. Findings indicated that the desire to live and the sensation of youth were predictors of PTG in older adults such that older people who felt younger than their objective age and reported feeling not close to dying scored considerably higher on PTG and lower on PTS measurements.

The amount of time since the traumatic incident influences PTG in older adults. Several studies on older people have shown that traumatic events many years ago positively impacted individuals (Greenblatt-Kimron, 2021; Greenblatt Kimron et al., 2019; Palgi, 2016; Stein et al., 2020). It is possible that previous experiences might have contributed to a beneficial positive transformation in older adults. Further, traits like high crystallized intellect and a strong capacity for long-term memory demonstrate that memories from the past can also help people learn and grow.

Several studies have shown contradictory results. For example, research on community-dwelling adults revealed negative relationships between PTS and PTG (Palgi, 2016), whereas a study of Holocaust survivors revealed positive relationships between these variables (Greenblatt-Kimron, 2021). Furthermore, PTG and PTSD symptoms were found to be more prevalent in Holocaust survivors (Greenblatt Kimron et al., 2019) than in matched control group and veterans who survived the war after 18 and 45 years, respectively (Stein et al., 2020). As a result, it seems as if this kind of traumatic experience has a role in mediating the relationship between PTS and PTG in older individuals.

Domains of PTG among Older Adults

The domains of PTG include appreciation in life, relationships with others, personal strength, new possibilities, and spirituality (Tedeschi & Calhoun, 2004). Differential reactions can be seen in these domains because of how the aftershocks happen (Calhoun & Tedeschi, 1998); for instance, one individual may feel more robust than the other, but his/her relationship may not get closer after an event. Several studies on older adults examined the existence of these domains and the possible causes for each.

Appreciation of Life

Realizing the greatness and value of one's life is at the heart of the concept of "life appreciation." Older adult breast cancer patients (Błaszczyński & Turek, 2013; Brix et al., 2013), cancer patients (Hoogland, 2016), Holocaust survivors (Greenblatt Kimron et al., 2019), and decorated veterans (Stein et al., 2020) reported elevated scores of appreciation of life. This domain scored the highest among PTG domains studied in older adults with cancer in the study by Hoogland (2016) who also reported an adverse association between time since diagnosis and enjoyment of life, whereas being married and older and problem-focused coping were connected positively with an appreciation of life among cancer patients.

Relationship with Others

Relationships with others refer to feeling more connected socially and realizing the significance of social ties. Higher scores in relationships with others were seen in older persons who experienced grief (Oksuzler & Dirik, 2019), cancer (Brix et al., 2013; Hoogland, 2016), and those with military decoration (Stein et al., 2020) compared to healthy older adults or those without such experiences. Patients with stronger problem-focused coping reported more positive improvements in their interactions with others (Hoogland, 2016). Oksuzler and Dirik (2019) found that social support from friends and significant others was linked to the relationships with others domain of PTG in older people who had recently lost a loved one.

Personal Strength

A stronger reliance on oneself in the face of the challenges presented by life is one definition of the concept of personal strength. Decorated veterans (Stein et al., 2020), older adults who have experienced bereavement (Oksuzler & Dirik, 2019), and cancer patients (Hoogland, 2016) rated higher on personal strength than healthy older adults or those without bereavement experiences. Women and older adults living longer in nursing institutions reported having higher personal strength after losing a loved one (Oksuzler & Dirik, 2019). Higher levels of self-reported personal strength were also associated positively with religious and problem-focused coping (Hoogland, 2016). Demographic aspects might also lead to differences in the sense of strength. For instance, in his study of cancer patients, Hoogland (2016) found a negative association between age and personal strength and those who shared their home with a child or grandkids reported lower levels of personal strength than those who shared their home with a spouse or were living alone.

New Possibilities

Developing new life priorities is linked to establishing new life objectives that one wishes to achieve in one's lifetime. However, the lower levels of voluntary change seen among older adults may explain why this area is less likely to be highlighted in this population. Only one study with cancer patients demonstrated higher scores in this domain (Hoogland, 2016). Factors related to the new possibilities dimension of cancer patients were being married, living with a spouse, and greater problem-focused coping.

Spirituality

Spirituality includes greater religious faith and an understanding of the value of spirituality and existential matters. Bereaved seniors rated higher than non-bereaved ones on spirituality (Oksuzler & Dirik, 2019). Hoogland (2016) reported higher religiosity and spirituality among older adult cancer patients, an adverse association between the period since diagnosis and spirituality and a positive association between spirituality and emotion-focused and meaning-focused coping but not with problem-focused coping.

PTG across Types of Traumas and Significant Life Events

A few studies compared PTG in older adults following the struggle with different kinds of trauma. A study examining several traumatic experiences, such as violent personal attacks, bereavement, illness, and medical intervention, revealed that older adults experiencing less stressful events had higher PTG scores (Lopez et al., 2015). No significant difference was found between widowed and non-widowed participants regarding PTG. A comprehensive examination of the types of trauma experienced by older people found that Holocaust survivors had lower PTG scores than those experiencing war-related or historical trauma (Kadri et al., 2022); however, results reported in the literature are controversial. For instance, a study comparing older women suffering sexual trauma reported higher scores of PTG than non-sexual war trauma in World War II (Kuwert et al., 2014).

PTG has been explored in relation to numerous key life experiences in older adults, especially health issues, surviving the Holocaust, and bereavement (Figure 16.1).

Health Issues

A study of older adult cancer patients conducted more than a year post-diagnosis showed that higher PTG was significantly associated with lower depression and higher hope (Heidarzadeh et al., 2016). Those positive transformations were mostly observed in the dimensions of appreciation of life (Brix et al., 2013; Heidarzadeh et al., 2016) and relations with others (Brix et al., 2013). Treatment-related variables, including larger tumor size, having a mastectomy (rather than lumpectomy), and having endocrine treatment, were also related to a higher incidence of PTG. Higher PTG was found in cancer patients who used more problem-, emotional-, and meaning-focused coping (Hoogland, 2016). Even after accounting for the effects of emotion-focused and meaning-focused coping, the associations between PTG and problem-focused coping remained statistically significant. Other studies comparing older and younger cancer patients found that older patients who perceived cancer negatively reported higher PTG scores, no significant association existed between

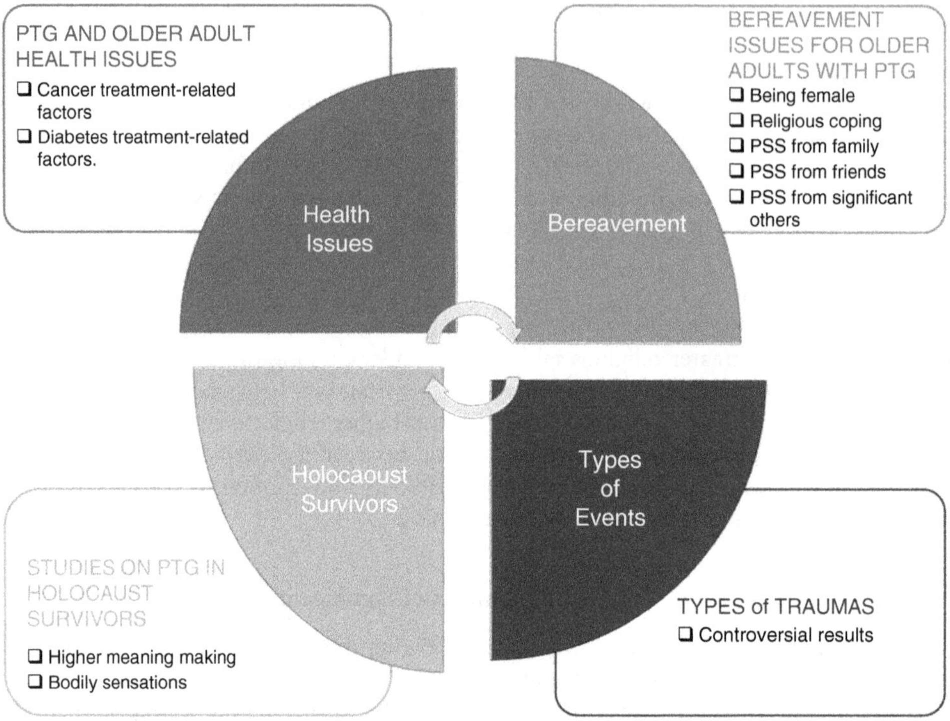

Figure 16.1 Life issues and PTG in older adults.

approach-oriented coping and PTG and the effect of altruistic behaviors (e.g., being mentors of younger patients, sharing wisdom with younger generations) on the PTG was questioned (Boyle et al., 2017).

One study addressed the effect of diabetes on older people and found that PTG was strongly associated with having more children, better diet adherence, and being an outpatient as well as greater levels of perceived social support from family members and cognitive avoidance (Senol-Durak & Durak, 2018b).

Recently, the impact of COVID-19 on PTG responses in people over the age of 55 has been studied in Barcelona (Celdran et al., 2021), and about a quarter of the participants (N=1009) said that they had greater PTG due to the Spanish lockdown, during which they learned more about PTG dimensions. Older people infected by COVID-19 who had suffered the loss of a close relative because of the pandemic reported more PTG than other participants. Increased PTG was shown to be substantially associated with younger age, having meaningful daily interactions with others, and changing their view about loneliness (either more fabulous or lower). The PTG scores of males were lower than those of women.

Holocaust Survivors

Meaning-making appears to be an important predictor of PTG (Grad & Zeligman, 2017). In a study of 159 senior Holocaust survivors (Greenblatt-Kimron, 2021), positive worldviews about life, a high degree of personal worth, and higher levels of PTSD were significantly associated with PTG. Further, this study found that meaning in life and post-traumatic stress mediated the relationship between world assumptions and PTG, such that those who reevaluated their preconceived notions about the world reported enhanced post-traumatic feelings as well as a newfound sense of purpose, both of which were associated with a higher PTG score. These studies show the importance of having strong beliefs about the meaning of life and the world.

The developers of the PTG model highlighted that PTG and PTSD might be experienced simultaneously (Tedeschi & Calhoun, 1995). Higher PTG and PTSD were seen among Holocaust survivors when compared with non-Holocaust survivors and older adults (N = 159 and N = 87 respectively; Greenblatt Kimron et al., 2019). Older adults with greater PTG had increased heart rate variability, whereas older adults with higher PTSD had lower heart rates. PTG mediated the relationship between PTSD and heart rate variability and older adults with superior subjective health ratings reported greater PTG. The results may be explained by how individuals think and how their bodies respond.

Bereavement

Older people commonly face the death of a loved one during their senior years. However, the role of bereavement in PTG has received little attention in the literature. In research on bereaved older females living in nursing facilities, having stronger religious coping and more social support from family, friends, and significant others were related to higher PTG (Oksuzler & Dirik, 2019). The findings showed that widows fared better than widowers when it came to PTG and religious coping strategies. Interestingly, self-esteem was not substantially related to PTG in older people who had lost a loved one. The researchers underlined the fact that they collected data only from older adults who were living in nursing homes, which limited the findings' generalizability to a larger population. Staff was primarily responsible for meeting the unique requirements of the facility's older adult residents.

Social Resources and Psychological Aspects Associated with PTG in Older Adults

The influence of social resources on PTG in older people has significant therapeutic implications. Many studies have concluded that social resources and PTG are intertwined (Berger & Weiss, 2009). Older people who exhibit a greater interest in social interactions (Grad & Zeligman, 2017), those who got more support from family members (Senol-Durak & Durak, 2018b), friends, and significant others (Oksuzler & Dirik, 2019) were more likely to report PTG. More recently, while investigating COVID-19-related experiences, it has been revealed that changes in social ties during a lockdown may trigger a sense of growth (Celdran et al., 2021) showing how adaptable people are in nature. Furthermore, social support includes, in addition to the family, an extended environment. For example, support from religious communities is highlighted among older adults who have experienced the loss of a spouse (Lopez et al., 2015).

Several psychological aspects have been identified in the literature as related to PTG. They include coping, cognitive processing, hopefulness, self-compassion, and personality traits. As Calhoun and Tedeschi (1998) pointed out, coping helps individuals manage their post-traumatic resources as well as their anxiety-related feelings. Research on coping in relation to PTG has shown that bereaved older people exhibited higher levels of religious coping (Oksuzler & Dirik, 2019) whereas cancer survivors showed higher levels of problem-focused, emotion-focused, and meaning-focused coping (Hoogland. 2016). Many studies have focused on the importance of cognitive processing in PTG (Berger & Weiss, 2009; Senol-Durak & Ayvasik, 2010; Tedeschi et al., 2017); however, only one study looked at cognitive processing and PTG in older people and showed an association between greater cognitive avoidance among older people with diabetes and higher PTG (Senol-Durak & Durak, 2018b). Some of this may be attributable to the fact that diabetes consequences (such as eyesight loss and renal failure) are more difficult for older people to understand mentally. PTG has also been linked to higher hopefulness in cancer survivors (Heidarzadeh et al., 2016), higher meaning-making in Holocaust survivors (Greenblatt-Kimron, 2021), and better affective well-being in cancer patients (Boyle et al., 2017). A positive association was reported in a group of traumatized older adults between self-compassion and PTG, both of which were also associated with higher active coping, instrumental support, and positive reframing (Munroe et al., 2022)., Only one study examined how personality and PTG are linked by examining the effect of self-esteem on PTG and failed to find a correlation between bereaved older people's self-esteem and PTG (Oksuzler & Dirik, 2019).

Practice Implications

PTG research with older people indicates the feasibility of beneficial transformations. Learning throughout life struggles is vital for older people (Kadri et al., 2022) who encounter daily personal health concerns and social challenges. In dealing with losses experienced in old age, boosting older adults for PTG is a significant finding that suggests that professionals who work with people who have been through traumatic events can use psychological and social resources to help them cope. Figure 16.2 presents an overview of practice implications for enabling and enhancing PTG in older adults.

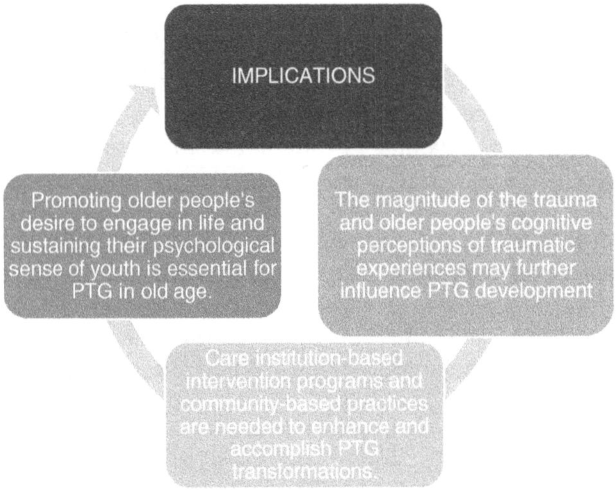

Figure 16.2 Overview of Implications.

Considering the high number of older adults around the world and the psychological difficulties they experience, both institution-based and community-based intervention programs are needed to enhance and accomplish good transformations. The aforementioned empirical findings can potentially obtain a systematized momentum using therapy approaches that monitor older adults who report a traumatic life event, bring to the agenda positive consequences that occurred after the event, and construct positive transformations in individuals.

Clinicians need to consider the various variables that influence PTG in older people. This review shows that the intellect and long-term memory of older individuals become more securely established as they age, and "notebooks" containing early life experiences are automatically opened and shared with younger generations potentially helping older adults to recuperate from earlier memories. The period following the traumatic incident and how the event is viewed are essential. From the standpoint of lifespan development, it is possible to assess how traumatic events in past stages of life, paired with present stressful circumstances, impact PTG. As a result, similar PTG levels may be predicted following various lifetime traumas. However, this may not be the case for all childhood traumas.

For older adults who have recently experienced chronic illness and loss, providing professional assistance to preserve internal resources (hope, self-perception, and coping) and external resources (social and rapidly growing technology and health care systems) and to improve the quality of life (emotional state, a sense of purpose, sustaining connections and activities) is critical (Senol-Durak & Durak, 2018a). Specifically, strengthening social support networks and reconfiguring social relationships in a more positive manner may help older adults acquire PTG. Promoting older people's desire to engage in life and sustaining their psychological sense of youth is essential for PTG. Professionals may investigate designing strategies to enhance PTG in older people.

As several studies have shown that there is a greater demand than ever for PTG interventions that address the special requirements of older people confronting various life issues, these actions will undoubtedly assist older adults in remaining safe in an aging society.

Future Directions

Studies to date have focused on the impact of recent single trauma. Given that life is filled with stress, it is more probable that older adults would have several painful experiences (Durak & Senol-Durak, 2018b; Nuccio & Stripling, 2021). Specifically, looking at bereavement through the lens of PTG requires more research, including on community-dwelling older people. Several trauma types connected to PTSD among older people, such as physical violence, natural disasters, and terrorist acts, have not been highlighted regarding PTG (Durak & Senol-Durak, 2019; Ogle et al., 2014; Pietrzak et al., 2012). Thus, future PTG studies should examine the impact of various types of traumas and the challenges in one's life as well as the nature of PTG in older people with a variety of traumatic experiences.

No research compares the PTG of older adults depending on their location of residence. It is generally believed that community-dwelling older people and older adults staying in institutions are different. The only research that compared older people depending on whom they lived with was Hoogland's study (2016). More research is needed to compare PTG outcomes based on living location. This will help enhance both institution-based treatments and community-based interventions to enable aging adults to continue to live independently (Durak & Senol-Durak, 2018a).

Because the role of spousal support and active engagement to solve problems are considered important for new possibilities in life dimension, additional research should investigate new opportunities in older adults struggling with traumatic exposure.

Further studies examining a broad range of psychological variables will aid in elucidating their effects on PTG in older people as well as the positive mechanisms underlying the relative flexibility of PTG and older individuals' ability to improve in late life. Also, exploring cultural differences in the PTG of older adults is crucial (Weiss & Berger, 2010). Therefore, it is advised to compare cross-cultural research to find culture-related characteristics in positive transformations. Finally, older people are being considered in relatively few clinical trials regarding PTG compared to other age groups and future research should augment such studies

References

Allen, A. B., Goldwasser, E. R., & Leary, M. R. (2012). Self-compassion and well-being among older adults. *Self and Identity*, *11*(4), 428–453. 10.1080/15298868.2011.595082

Bartels, S. J. (2003). Improving system of care for older adults with mental illness in the United States. Findings and recommendations for the President's New Freedom Commission on Mental Health. *American Journal of Geriatric Psychiatry*, *11*(5), 486–497. 10.1097/00019442-200309000-00003

Bellizzi, K. M., & Blank, T. O. (2006). Predicting posttraumatic growth in breast cancer survivors. *Health Psychology*, *25*(1), 47–56. 10.1037/0278-6133.25.1.47

Berger, R., & Weiss, T. (2009). The posttraumatic growth model: An expansion to the family system. *Traumatology*, *15*(1), 63–74. 10.1177/1534765608323499

Błaszczyński, P., & Turek, R. (2013). Lepsze życie po traumie: Stowarzyszenie stomijne jako środowisko rozwoju potraumatycznego pacjentów ze stomią jelitową. *Psychiatria i Psychologia Kliniczna*, *3*(13), 164–173.

Boyle, C. C., Stanton, A. L., Ganz, P. A., & Bower, J. E. (2017). Posttraumatic growth in breast cancer survivors: Does age matter? *Psycho-Oncology*, *26*(6), 800–807. 10.1002/pon.4091

Brix, S. A., Bidstrup, P. E., Christensen, J., Rottmann, N., Olsen, A., Tjonneland, A., Johansen, C., & Dalton, S. O. (2013). Post-traumatic growth among elderly women with breast cancer compared to breast cancer-free women. *Acta Oncologica*, *52*(2), 345–354. 10.3109/0284186X.2012.744878

Calhoun, L. G., & Tedeschi, R. G. (1998). Posttraumatic growth: Future directions. In L. G. Calhoun, Tedeschi, R. G., (Ed.), *Posttraumatic Growth: Positive Changes in the Aftermath of Crisis* (1 ed., pp. 215–238). Routledge. 10.4324/9781410603401

Calhoun, L. G., & Tedeschi, R. G. (2010). Beyond recovery from trauma: Implications for clinical practice and research. *Journal of Social Issues*, *54*(2), 357–371. 10.1111/j.1540-4560.1998.tb01223.x

Carstensen, L. L., Turan, B., Scheibe, S., Ram, N., Ersner-Hershfield, H., Samanez-Larkin, G. R., Brooks, K. P., & Nesselroade, J. R. (2011). Emotional experience improves with age: Evidence based on over 10 years of experience sampling. *Psychology and Aging*, *26*(1), 21–33. 10.1037/a0021285

Celdran, M., Serrat, R., & Villar, F. (2021). Post-traumatic growth among older people after the forced lockdown for the COVID-19 pandemic. *Spanish Journal of Psychology*, *24*, e43, Article e43. 10.1017/SJP.2021.40

Cook, J. M., & Niederehe, G. (2007). Trauma in older adults. In M. J. Friedman, T. M. Keane, & P. A. Resick (Eds.), *Handbook of PTSD: Science and Practice* (pp. 252–276). Guilford Press.

Cook, J. M., & Simiola, V. (2017). Trauma and PTSD in older adults: Prevalence, course, concomitants and clinical considerations. *Current Opinion in Psychology*, *14*, 1–4. 10.1016/j.copsyc.2016.08.003

Durak, M., & Senol-Durak, E. (2018a). The characteristics and life preferences of Turkish older adults. *Journal of Aging and Long-Term Care*, *1*(3), 115–129. 10.5505/jaltc.2018.54154

Durak, M., & Senol-Durak, E. (2018b). İleri yaştaki danışanlarla psikoterapi [psychotherapy with older adults]. In I. Tufan & M. Durak (Eds.), *Gerontoloji: Sağlık ve Bakım [Gerontology: Health, Care]* (1 ed., pp. 577–625). Nobel Academic Publishing.

Durak, M., & Senol-Durak, E. (2019). Re-experiencing trajectories of posttraumatic stress disorder among older adults exposed to an exile. *Journal of Aging and Long-Term Care*, *2*(2), 51–58. 10.5505/jaltc.2019.09719

Etezadi, S., & Pushkar, D. (2013). Why are wise people happier? An explanatory model of wisdom and emotional well-being in older adults. *Journal of Happiness Studies*, *14*(3), 929–950. 10.1007/s10902-012-9362-2

Gaffey, A. E., Bergeman, C. S., Clark, L. A., & Wirth, M. M. (2016). Aging and the HPA axis: Stress and resilience in older adults. *Neuroscience and Biobehavioral Reviews*, *68*, 928–945. 10.1016/j.neubiorev.2016.05.036

Grad, R. I., & Zeligman, M. (2017). Predictors of post-traumatic growth: The role of social interest and meaning in life. *Journal of Individual Psychology*, *73*(3), 190–207. 10.1353/jip.2017.0016

Greenblatt-Kimron, L. (2021). World assumptions and post-traumatic growth among older adults: The case of Holocaust survivors. *Stress and Health*, *37*(2), 353–363. 10.1002/smi.3000

Greenblatt Kimron, L., Marai, I., Lorber, A., & Cohen, M. (2019). The long-term effects of early-life trauma on psychological, physical and physiological health among the elderly: The study of Holocaust survivors. *Aging and Mental Health*, *23*(10), 1340–1349. 10.1080/13607863.2018.1523880

Heidarzadeh, M., Dadkhah, B., & Gholchin, M. (2016). Post-traumatic growth, hope, and depression in elderly cancer patients. *International Journal of Medical Research & Health Sciences*, *5*(9), 455–461. WOS:000395762300068

Henson, C., Truchot, D., & Canevello, A. (2021). What promotes post traumatic growth? A systematic review. *European Journal of Trauma & Dissociation*, *5*(4), 100195. 10.1016/j.ejtd.2020.100195

Hoogland, A. I. (2016). *Posttraumatic growth among older adults with late-life cancer diagnoses* University of Kentucky]. http://uknowledge.uky.edu/gerontol_etds/10

Jeste, D. V., Alexopoulos, G. S., Bartels, S. J., Cummings, J. L., Gallo, J. J., Gottlieb, G. L., Halpain, M. C., Palmer, B. W., Patterson, T. L., Reynolds, C. F., 3rd, & Lebowitz, B. D. (1999). Consensus statement on the upcoming crisis in geriatric mental health: Research agenda for the next 2 decades. *Archives of General Psychiatry*, *56*(9), 848–853. 10.1001/archpsyc.56.9.848

Kadri, A., Gracey, F., & Leddy, A. (2022). What factors are associated with posttraumatic growth in older adults? A systematic review. *Clinical Gerontologist*, 1–18. 10.1080/07317115.2022.2034200

Kuwert, P., Glaesmer, H., Eichhorn, S., Grundke, E., Pietrzak, R. H., Freyberger, H. J., & Klauer, T. (2014). Long-term effects of conflict-related sexual violence compared with non-sexual war trauma in female World War II survivors: a matched pairs study. *Archives of Sexual Behavior*, *43*(6), 1059–1064. 10.1007/s10508-014-0272-8

Liang, Y., Huo, M., Kennison, R., & Zhou, R. (2017). The role of cognitive control in older adult cognitive reappraisal: Detached and positive reappraisal. *Frontiers in Behavioral Neuroscience*, *11*. 10.3389/fnbeh.2017.00027

Lopez, J., Camilli, C., & Noriega, C. (2015). Posttraumatic growth in widowed and non-widowed older adults: Religiosity and sense of coherence. *Journal of Religion and Health*, *54*(5), 1612–1628. 10.1007/s10943-014-9876-5

MacLeod, S., Musich, S., Hawkins, K., Alsgaard, K., & Wicker, E. R. (2016). The impact of resilience among older adults. *Geriatric Nursing*, *37*(4), 266–272. 10.1016/j.gerinurse.2016.02.014

Merecz, D., Waszkowska, M., & Wezyk, A. (2012). Psychological consequences of trauma in MVA perpetrators: Relationship between post-traumatic growth, PTSD symptoms and individual characteristics. *Transportation Research Part F: Traffic Psychology and Behaviour*, *15*(5), 565–574. 10.1016/j.trf.2012.05.008

Munroe, M., Al-Refae, M., Chan, H. W., & Ferrari, M. (2022). Using self-compassion to grow in the face of trauma: The role of positive reframing and problem-focused coping strategies. *Psychological Trauma: Theory, Research, Practice, and Policy*, *14*(S1), S157–S164. 10.1037/tra0001164

Nowlan, J. S., Wuthrich, V. M., & Rapee, R. M. (2015). Positive reappraisal in older adults: a systematic literature review. *Aging & Mental Health*, *19*(6), 475–484. 10.1080/13607863.2014.954528

Nuccio, A. G., & Stripling, A. M. (2021). Resilience and post-traumatic growth following late life polyvictimization: A scoping review. *Aggression and Violent Behavior*, *57*, 101481. 10.1016/j.avb.2020.101481

Ogle, C. M., Rubin, D. C., & Siegler, I. C. (2014). Cumulative exposure to traumatic events in older adults. *Aging and Mental Health*, *18*(3), 316–325. 10.1080/13607863.2013.832730

Oksuzler, B., & Dirik, G. (2019). Investigation of post-traumatic growth and related factors in elderly adults experience of spousal bereavement. *Turkish Journal of Geriatrics*, *22*(2), 181–190. 10.31086/tjgeri.2019.91

Palgi, Y. (2016). Subjective age and perceived distance-to-death moderate the association between posttraumatic stress symptoms and posttraumatic growth among older adults. *Aging & Mental Health*, *20*(9), 948–954.

Pietrzak, R. H., Goldstein, R. B., Southwick, S. M., & Grant, B. F. (2012). Psychiatric comorbidity of full and partial posttraumatic stress disorder among older adults in the United States: results from wave 2 of the National Epidemiologic Survey on Alcohol and Related Conditions. *American Journal of Geriatric Psychiatry*, *20*(5), 380–390. 10.1097/JGP.0b013e31820d92e7

Pless Kaiser, A., Cook, J. M., Glick, D. M., & Moye, J. (2019). Posttraumatic stress disorder in older adults: A conceptual review. *Clinical Gerontologist*, *42*(4), 359–376. 10.1080/07317115.2018.1539801

Resnick, B. (2014). Resilience in older adults. *Topics in Geriatric Rehabilitation*, *30*(3), 155–163. 10.1097/tgr.0000000000000024

Schanowitz, J. Y., & Nicassio, P. M. (2006). Predictors of positive psychosocial functioning of older adults in residential care facilities. *Journal of Behavioral Medicine*, *29*(2), 191–201. 10.1007/s10865-005-9034-3

Seligowski, A. V., Miron, L. R., & Orcutt, H. K. (2015). Relations among self-compassion, PTSD symptoms, and psychological health in a trauma-exposed sample. *Mindfulness*, *6*(5), 1033–1041. 10.1007/s12671-014-0351-x

Senol-Durak, E., & Ayvasik, H. B. (2010). Factors associated with posttraumatic growth among myocardial infarction patients: Perceived social support, perception of the event and coping. *Journal of Clinical Psychology in Medical Settings*, *17*(2), 150–158. 10.1007/s10880-010-9192-5

Senol-Durak, E., & Durak, M. (2018a). İleri yaş yetişkinlerde psikopatoloji [psychopathology among older adults]. In I. Tufan & M. Durak (Eds.), *Gerontoloji: Sağlık ve Bakım [Gerontology: Health, Care]* (1 ed., pp. 577–625). Nobel Academic Publishing.

Senol-Durak, E., & Durak, M. (2018b). Posttraumatic growth among Turkish older adults with diabetes. *Journal of Aging and Long-Term Care*, *1*(2), 55–63. 10.5505/jaltc.2018.36844

Shiota, M. N., & Levenson, R. W. (2009). Effects of aging on experimentally instructed detached reappraisal, positive reappraisal, and emotional behavior suppression. *Psychology and Aging*, *24*(4), 890–900. 10.1037/a0017896

Stein, J. Y., Bachem, R., Lahav, Y., & Solomon, Z. (2020). The aging of heroes: Posttraumatic stress, resilience and growth among aging decorated veterans. *Journal of Positive Psychology*, *16*(3), 390–397. 10.1080/17439760.2020.1725606

Taku, K., Tedeschi, R. G., Shakespeare-Finch, J., Krosch, D., David, G., Kehl, D., Grunwald, S., Romeo, A., Di Tella, M., Kamibeppu, K., Soejima, T., Hiraki, K., Volgin, R., Dhakal, S., Zięba, M., Ramos, C., Nunes, R., Leal, I., Gouveia, P., …Calhoun, L. G. (2021). Posttraumatic growth (PTG) and posttraumatic depreciation (PTD) across ten countries: Global validation of the PTG-PTD theoretical model. *Personality and Individual Differences*, *169*, 110222. 10.1016/j.paid.2020.110222

Taylor, M. G., & Carr, D. (2021). Psychological resilience and health among older adults: A comparison of personal resources. *Journals of Gerontology - Series B Psychological Sciences and Social Sciences*, *76*(6), 1241–1250. 10.1093/geronb/gbaa116

Tedeschi, R. G., & Blevins, C. L. (2017). Posttraumatic growth: A pathway to resilience. In U. Kumar (Ed.), *The Routledge International Handbook of Psychosocial Resilience* (pp. 324–333). Routledge/Taylor & Francis Group.

Tedeschi, R. G., & Calhoun, L. (1995). *Trauma & Transformation: Growing in the Aftermath of Suffering*. SAGE Publications, Inc. 10.4135/9781483326931

Tedeschi, R. G., & Calhoun, L. G. (2004). Target article: "Posttraumatic growth: Conceptual foundations and empirical evidence". *Psychological Inquiry*, *15*(1), 1–18. 10.1207/s15327965pli1501_01

Tedeschi, R. G., Cann, A., Taku, K., Senol-Durak, E., & Calhoun, L. G. (2017). The posttraumatic growth inventory: A revision integrating existential and spiritual change. *Journal of Traumatic Stress*, *30*(1), 11–18. 10.1002/jts.22155

Thorp, S. R., Sones, H. M., & Cook, J. M. (2011). Posttraumatic stress disorder among older adults. In K. H. Sorocco & S. Lauderdale (Eds.), *Cognitive Behavior Therapy With Older Adults: Innovations Across Care Settings* (pp. 189–217). Springer Publishing Company.

United Nations. (2017). *World Population Ageing 2017 - Highlights (ST/ESA/SER.A/397)*. Department of Economic and Social Affairs-Population Division. https://www.un.org/en/development/desa/population/publications/pdf/ageing/WPA2017_Highlights.pdf

van Zelst, W. H., de Beurs, E., Beekman, A. T., Deeg, D. J., & van Dyck, R. (2003). Prevalence and risk factors of posttraumatic stress disorder in older adults. *Psychotherapy and Psychosomatics*, *72*(6), 333–342. 10.1159/000073030

VanBockel, F. (2020). *A qualitative study of posttraumatic growth among older adults* (Publication Number 28151243) Northcentral University]. California. https://www.proquest.com/dissertations-theses/qualitative-study-post-traumatic-growth-older/docview/2465716219/se-2?accountid=15310

Weiss, T., & Berger, R. (2010). *Posttraumatic Growth Around the Globe: Research Findings and Practice Implications*. Wiley.

Wilson, C. A., & Saklofske, D. H. (2018). The relationship between trait emotional intelligence, resiliency, and mental health in older adults: The mediating role of savouring. *Aging and Mental Health*, *22*(5), 646–654. 10.1080/13607863.2017.1292207

Zeligman, M., Varney, M., Grad, R. I., & Huffstead, M. (2018). Posttraumatic growth in individuals with chronic illness: The role of social support and meaning making. *Journal of Counseling & Development*, *96*(1), 53–63. 10.1002/jcad.12177

PART 4

PTG in Relational Systems

PART 4A

PTG in Couples

17
PTG IN COUPLES STRUGGLING WITH INFERTILITY

Marilyn S. Paul

Case Vignette

Anna and Jair were referred to a couples' therapist for counseling following a required psychological screening for egg donation at a local fertility clinic. The clinic's referring practitioner noted the couple to have endured a pregnancy loss after natural conception, numerous failed in-vitro fertilization cycles, one miscarriage following an in-vitro cycle, and most recently, the diagnosis of poor egg quality. The practitioner further noted that while the couple presented as "sorting out donor options," e.g. using Anna's sister as a known direct donor versus using a donor agency or an anonymous donor, there was more hesitation and ambivalence than is commonly seen in potential egg donor recipients, and thus the referral was made for couple counseling to facilitate clarity. At the initial appointment, the couple's therapist identified a plethora of loss issues yet to be addressed, and it was therefore recommended that the couple engage in 4–6 sessions to achieve a full history, clarity on the presenting problem, and determine a path for infertility resolution. The couple agreed with this determination and began weekly couple counseling sessions.

The initial 4–6 session contract with the couple served the purpose of completing psychosocial histories on each and gaining a sense of how the married couple functioned as a unit. Anna, age 38, a first-generation Italian immigrant, spent her early years going back and forth between Italy and the US, largely as a function of her father's work, both in New York and in Milan, and had never developed a solid peer support network. Anna clearly harbored resentment toward her parents and her younger sister for what she considered "a lost childhood." She experienced her sister as frail and emotionally needy and claimed that through childhood she was required to demonstrate strength and perseverance, even when she was emotionally struggling. Jair, age 40, a first-generation Cuban immigrant, was brought to New York at age 14 by his parents along with two college-age siblings. Jair's history revealed trauma of separation from and loss of his grandparents in Cuba who had raised him, and of trauma associated with the challenges of trying to fit in and even survive in a new and often hostile city environment, with little parental support.

In early sessions, Anna and Jair became easily triggered by one another and were both highly reactive. There seemed to be familial, cultural, and survival mechanisms in place,

DOI: 10.4324/9781032208688-22

that for Anna manifested in heightened emotionality in voice, tone, and body language, which she revealed as "typical for Italians, and especially for her family", and for Jair manifested in distancing followed by hostility, anger and volatility. These were learned behaviors from his adolescence that, at the time, protected him from feelings of inadequacy, shame, and fear of abandonment. As the episodes of reactivity continued, the couple agreed to maintain ongoing counseling sessions for the purpose of improving communication in addition to achieving a resolution of infertility and a path to parenthood.

Anna and Jair had a history together, and a foundation on which to build their relationship, if they chose to use it. They had known each other for a long time, having met in college while completing bachelor's degrees in business, and were friends for many years before they became a couple. The skill of reaching into the reactive enactments that unfolded organically during their weekly sessions drew from the structural family therapy model (Nichols, 2021), and allowed for observation of and reflection on deep cultural differences between the two, as well as their residual traumas. These enactments illustrated repetitive dysfunctional cycles of behavior, which were seen and labeled as vulnerability cycles, a mutual activation process whereby within the couple interaction, individual vulnerabilities are triggered and corresponding survival positions are taken that end up being at odds with each other (Scheinkman & Fishbane, 2004). The use of sustained empathy and holding (Cooper & Granucci- Lesser, 2015; Nichols, 2021) allowed for a pause to draw each member of the couple's attention to their own and their partner's vulnerability, understand the history and meaning of the survival position, as well as its negative effect in the current context. Most importantly, it was noted how each partner's vulnerability was associated with the trauma and loss related to infertility as well as the layers of trauma and loss that came before it. The use of the session process, including transference, countertransference, and interpretations helped the couple develop mutual empathy.

While their traumatic infertility experience was layered on earlier, unprocessed trauma and loss, life continued to present Anna and Jair with challenges. There were job losses for Jair, health crises for each, and Anna's elderly parents endured health complications due to chronic and degenerative illnesses. However, as the couple dealt with each stressor event, their reactivity began to diminish through further developing their mutual empathy and sustaining healthy discourse. For example, when there was a flood in the couple's home and Anna reacted to it with a high level of emotionality and accusation toward Jair, Jair was able to reflect back to Anna the recognition she was upset and anxious, and an offer to work with her to find a plumber. Similarly, when Jair reacted with hostility and road rage toward another driver, while Anna reflected recognition of his anger at the other driver, she did not engage in it. This newly found ability to tune in to the other's feelings was noted and labeled by the practitioner as a strength of the couple. As time went on, the couple rejected egg donation as a family-building option, realizing that they were uncomfortable with the imbalance of genetic ties to the child that would result. They continued attempting to conceive naturally and through in-vitro fertilization (IVF) using Anna's eggs, but endured several failed IVF cycles, and another pregnancy loss. Through all these experiences, the couple observed their ability to address and manage each crisis as a function of their improved communication, mutual empathy, and stronger bond, which was empowering and built strength and resilience.

The treatment approach used in this case was a multi-theoretical one that drew on object relations couples' therapy, structural, strategic, Bowenian family therapy, and narrative therapy. From the very first session, it was clear that there needed to be a safe holding environment to support and contain the enactments as they occurred and to create a space for observing and analyzing the dysfunctional patterns that were framed in deep historical roots as they unfolded. The use of transference, countertransference, and interpretation allowed Anna and Jair to build their skills of self-awareness and develop deeper mutual empathy. Bowenian strategies drew on the use of "I" statements to convey feelings and minimize defensive responses in the other, and narrative strategies externalized the infertility, defined the losses, and sought out and highlighted individual and couple strengths. Credit was always assigned to the couple for their progress and growth.

As time went on, and the couple continued longing to be parents, they concluded that adoption was the best remaining option. Grieving and mourning their individual loss experience, and achieving mutual empathy facilitated a realistic and thorough adoption exploration e.g. private, agency, domestic or international. During the process of their adoption home study and while building an adoption portfolio, the couple endured yet another health crisis for Jair. At this time, Anna had passed age 40 and Jair had passed age 42, and the couple began to explore the possibility of a child-free option, based on their health challenges, ages, and life context. The painful reality they faced was that any possibility of parenting in the way they had envisioned had faded. Time was invested in grieving and mourning pregnancy and parenthood. That the two were able to engage in the grieving and mourning process and use their observing egos (Goldstein, 1995) to see themselves and their infertility within a deeper context of their lives, demonstrated growth and maturity.

PTG: A Process and an Outcome

Calhoun and Tedeschi (2001) defined posttraumatic growth (PTG) as the individual's process of positive psychological change, which results in improvement from pre-traumatic functioning following the struggle with highly challenging life circumstances. The PTG model identifies six components: pre-trauma characteristics, a traumatic or highly stressful event, challenges, rumination, social context, and posttraumatic growth. PTG outcome is then categorized into any of five areas; new possibilities, relationship to others, personal strength, appreciation of life, and spiritual change (Tedeschi & Calhoun, 1996). Berger and Weiss (2008) applied the PTG model to couples and families noting parallel process and outcome categories.

Anna and Jair's commitment and engagement in the couple therapy process may well be the most important variable in the growth that occurred for them thus far, as the one correlate that has been consistently identified as important in PTG research is the availability of and satisfaction with social support (Paul et al., 2009), and the most important factor in the success of therapy has long been identified as the worker-client relationship (O'Neill, 2002). Anna and Jair came to couples' therapy eager for the support, which they willingly engaged in, and through the process learned skills and strategies for better supporting each other and for seeking and utilizing support from family and community. The therapy room acted as a microcosm of the couple's real world, where interpersonal communication skills were tried, practiced, and ultimately transferred to daily living. Inherent in this process were traumatic ruptures (Deutch, 2014) where either partner or the therapist failed to communicate with empathy. Noting and working through the ruptures was a necessary ingredient for building trust and healing from a lifelong pile-up of stress and trauma.

Through the challenges of Anna and Jair's infertility and a context rooted in couple counseling allowing for rumination and building of social support, the couple found new possibilities for generativity and meaning-making. They deepened their interpersonal relationship as well as relationships with extended family, including Anna's parents, sister and brother-in-law, Jair's mother, brother and sister-in-law, and especially Jair's nieces and nephews. This development may be viewed as reflecting the domain of relating to others of PTG. They also found a deeper appreciation for life manifested through travel and engaging together in new activities and hobbies. Individually, Jair grew in spirituality, becoming more active and involved with the Catholic Church, and taking on a leadership role, which manifest the PTG domain of religiosity and spirituality as well as recognizing personal strengths. He also invested in self-care, exercising regularly, and eating healthy. For Anna there has been less observed individual PTG thus far, which may be in large part associated with the burden she feels, based on her culture and her gender, to prioritize caring for her elderly and ailing parents, and the role conflict it often creates, e.g. work and marriage. Thus, Anna and Jair's movement toward a satisfying child-free life manifests their growth post the challenges of infertility both individually and as a couple.

References

Berger, R., & Weiss, T. (2008). The posttraumatic growth model: An expansion to the family system. *Traumatology*, *15*(1), 63–74.doi:10.1177/1534765608323499

Calhoun L. G., & Tedeschi, R. G. (2001). Posttraumatic growth: The positive lessons of loss. In R. A. Neimeyer (Ed.), *Meaning reconstruction and the experience of loss* (pp. 157–172). Washington, DC: American Psychological Association.

Carter, D., Misri, S., & Tomfohr, L. (2007). Psychological aspects of early pregnancy loss. *Clinical Obstetrics & Gynecology*, *50*(1), 154–165. DOI: 10.1097/GRF.0b013e31802f1d28

Cooper, M. G., & Granucci- Lesser, J. (2015). *Clinical social work practice: An integrated approach* (5th ed.). Needham Heights, MA: Allyn and Bacon.

Deutch, R. A. (Ed.) (2014). *Traumatic ruptures: Abandonment and betrayal in the analytic relationship*. New York: Routledge.

Goldstein, E. (1995). *Ego psychology and social work practice* (2nd ed.). New York: The Free Press.

Nichols, M. (2021). *Family therapy: Concepts and methods* (12th ed.). Boston: Pearson Education.

O'Neill, J. V. (2002). Therapy technique may not matter much. *NASW News*, March.

Paul, M. S., Berger, R., Berlow, N., Rovner-Ferguson, H., Figlerski, L., Gardner, S., & Malave, A. F. (2009). Posttraumatic growth and social support in individuals with infertility. *Human Reproduction*, *25*(1), 133–141. doi:10.1093/humrep/dep367

Peoples, D., & Rovner-Ferguson, H. (2000). *Experiencing infertility*, New York: WW Norton & Company.

Scheinkman, M. and Fishbane, M. D. (2004). The vulnerability cycle: Working with impasses in couple therapy. *Family Process*, 43(3), 279–299.

Shapiro, V. B., Shapiro, J. R., & Paret, I. H. (2001). *Complex adoption and assisted reproductive technology: A developmental approach to clinical practice*. New York: The Guilford Press.

Tedeschi, R. G., & Calhoun, L. G. (1996). The posttraumatic growth inventory: Measuring the positive legacy of trauma. *Journal of Traumatic Stress*, 9(3), 455–471.

PART 4B

PTG in Families

18

PTG IN PARENTS OF YOUNG ADULTS DIAGNOSED WITH AUTISM SPECTRUM DISORDER

Victoria Grinman

Autism Spectrum Disorder (ASD) is a neuro-developmental disorder characterized by deficits in social communication and social reciprocity, nonverbal communicative behaviors, and skills needed to initiate, maintain and understand relationships, as well as stereotyped and repetitive patterns of behaviors (e.g., head banging, flipping objects, or use of idiosyncratic phrases) or interests (e.g., strong attachment to or preoccupation with unusual objects) (APA, 2013). ASD is distinct from other developmental and chronic childhood conditions due to its multifactorial origin, attributed to a combination of genetic, metabolic, biochemical, and neurological factors, as well as the fact that it represents an umbrella for various separate disorders and syndromes (Faras et al., 2010). ASD is not easily categorized as a genetic disorder (as is Down syndrome), or as a biological/anatomical disorder (as in brain malformations), and it is not a definite metabolic/nutritional disorder (like childhood diabetes). Because ASD does not show up in a static and predictable way, the experience of parenting children with ASD is uniquely difficult to adjust to (Huws et al., 2001; O'Brien, 2007).

While it is difficult to "see" ASD on brain scans, behaviors associated with this diagnosis are usually overt, visible, often misunderstood, and socially "unacceptable." It is often assumed that they are the result of *bad parenting* (Neely-Barnes et al., 2011), a stigma that often results in the exclusion, stereotyping, and rejection of these children, complicating the parenthood experience and potentially contributing to parents' and families' challenges, especially when children integrate into the larger social context (Kinnear et al., 2016).

ASD is considered the second most common serious developmental disability next to mental retardation or intellectual disability (Newschaffer et al., 2007). As per the CDC, the number of children diagnosed with ASD in the United States has increased consistently, regardless of racial, ethnic, and socioeconomic affiliation. From one in every 68 children in 2014, the number increased to one in every 59 in 2018 (CDC, 2018), and one in every 44 eight-year-old old children in 2021 (Maenner et al., 2021). This exponential increase brought in a new need of looking "wholistically" at the parenthood experiences in the ASD family community, to capture the duality of trauma, with stresses and benefits transformative aspects of such experience, as well as a retrospective cumulative look at one's self-reported experience after their child with ASD is grown (Grinman 2020).

DOI: 10.4324/9781032208688-24

Parents of children with ASD encounter numerous specific stressors related to their child's needs and issues due to ASD, issues shared by parents of children with various types of chronic conditions or disabilities, and general parenthood stressors. Similar to a Russian doll or the layers-of-an-onion phenomena, the layers of stressors are piling up producing a parenthood experience laced with multilayered compounding stress experience (Grinman, 2020). These stresses can cause physical and mental health conditions in parents (Avison et al., 2007; Paulson et al., 2006; Saxbe et al., 2016; Smith-Nielsen et al., 2016; Taylor, 2009), which increases the underlying stressors even more.

Stressors Associated with Parenting a Child with ASD

Existing knowledge supports that parents of children with ASD experience multilayered stress (Bluth et al., 2013; Derguy et al., 2016; Derguy et al., 2018). Grinman (2020) offers that those layers of stress are compounding, with related challenges mutually potentiating and/or generating within and between the layers. Past research portrayed the experience of these parents as a linear set of stresses (Hill, 1958; Miodrag & Hodapp, 2010), the outcomes dichotomously as either adaptation ***or*** a crisis (Hill, 1958; McCubbin, & Patterson, 1983), and focused mostly on individual parents' (Perry, 2004) or couple's outcomes (Bluth et al., 2013). Grinman (2020) proposed a more comprehensive ecological approach, highlighting the multilayered nature of the stress experience presented in Figure 18.1.

Figure 18.1 shows that challenges experienced by parents of children with ASD incorporate the challenges experienced by parents in general (especially during the transition to parenthood) (Crnic et al., 2005; Crouter & Booth, 2003; Glass et al., 2016)), challenges

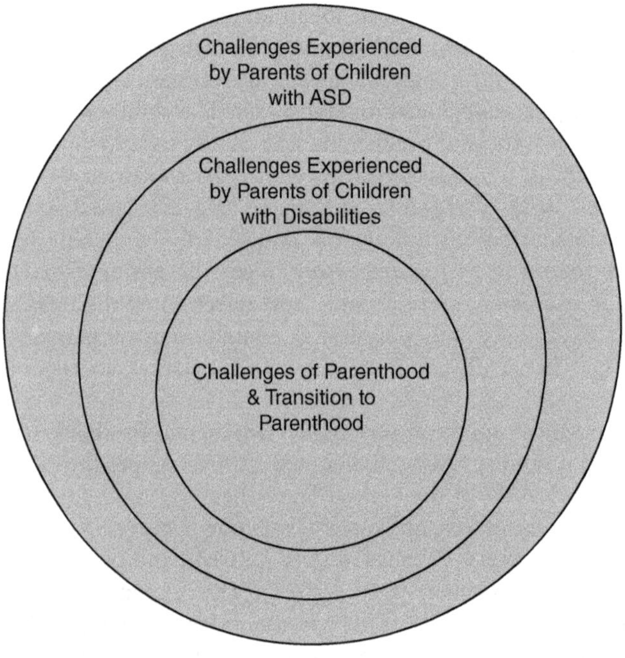

Figure 18.1 Challenges Experienced by Parents of Children with ASD.

experienced by parents of children with chronic illnesses or disabilities (Compas et al., 2012; Juster et al., 2010; Yamaoka et al., 2015) and challenges unique to parents rearing children with an ASD diagnosis (Bonis, 2016; Ooi et al., 2016) and that each layer adds to the weight of the whole structure.

The multitude of negative effects brought on by the universal challenges (represented in Layer 1) includes stressors prior to birth, and difficulties with the birth (Nomaguchi & Milkie, 2003; Ross & Van Willigen, 1996; Simon & Nath 2004; Umberson & Gove, 1989). These impacts may comprise worsened physical well-being and mental conditions such as depression and postpartum disorder (Evenson & Simon, 2005), increased health risk (Wickrama et al., 2001), and negative effects on marital, social and parent-child relationships (Huston, & Holmes, 2004; Knoester & Eggebeen, 2006).

Negative experiences related to children's chronic illnesses and/or disabilities (represented in layer 2) may include isolation from other parents, children, and their own families, especially when children exhibit intellectual, neurological, mental, and behavioral problems (Einfeld et al., 2006; Feldman et al., 2004; Lecavalier et al., 2006; Muscara et al., 2015; Nachshen et al., 2005), as well as added stresses because of the chronic caregiving role and the need for reorganization of the family (Epifanio et al., 2013).

Parents of children with ASD have higher stress levels than any other group of parents (Bonis, 2016; Ooi et al., 2016; Pisula, 2002), with the reported additional parental stresses being related specifically to the ASD diagnosis (Grinman, 2020). These include a lengthy diagnostic process lacking clarity, lack of parental education (Kozlowski et al., 2011) and post-ASD diagnosis challenges including ongoing symptoms (Davis & Carter, 2008; Zwaigenbaum et al., 2005), loss of "normality" (Ruiz-Robledillo et al., 2014), mourning the "ambiguous loss" of a child they will never have (Boss, 2007; O'Brien, 2007), societal stigma and judgments (Kinnear et al., 2016), low level of societal (Breevaart & Bakker, 2012) and of family support (Coulthard & Fitzgerald, 1999; Keenan et al., 2010), and lack of effective interventions for their families (Catalano et al., 2018).

A compounding quality of the multilayered stress that accumulates over time is not a new concept in trauma literature, and it was described in other populations, e.g., asylum seekers (Sinnerbrink et al., 1997) and victims of sexual or domestic abuse (Edmund & Bland, 2011). Parenting a child with ASD is also characterized by stress proliferation (Benson, 2006; Ward, 2014), allostatic stress overload (Barker et al., 2011; Fava et al., 2019; McEwen, 2017) and circularity principle (Lazarus & Folkman, 1986).

Stress Proliferation heightens one's stress level, causing dysfunction in physical, and mental health, and relationships (Benson & Karlof, 2009; LeBlanc et al., 2015). In the aforementioned model, stress proliferation is responsible for the same type of stressor present in each layer of parental experience becoming the compounding "add-on" (Grinman, 2020). For parents of children with ASD, challenges with accessing needed resources and support exist at each layer of their parental experience. In the first layer, these challenges may be caused by financial strain during the transition to parenthood. In the second layer, the challenges are heightened by additional causes (home-based services, lack of professional support, and communication between providers). In the third layer, there is even greater stress related to accessing resources and support because the symptoms of ASD are unpredictable, pervasive (and never "go away"), and stigmatized by the general population. This potentiates the stress of accessing resources and support that was already strained in the first place.

Allostatic stress refers to the cumulative effects over time of daily stress that may lead to disease in the body (Fava et al., 2019), which occurs when an individual's coping mechanisms are overwhelmed by the long-term exposure to varying or heightened neural and systemic physiological responses, known as "toxic stress." The allostatic stress (over)load explains the biological effect of pile-up of stresses experienced by parents as measurable chronic stress, which can eventually lead to posttraumatic stress syndrome (PTSS) that develops over time (Casey et al., 2012).

Circular Causality (Kelledy & Lyons, 2019; Lazarus & Folkman, 1986) explains how some effects of the original stressors become stressors themselves because of the non-linear relationships among stressors. The construct of circular causality posits that while all effects result from multiple causes, they in turn influence the causal pathways. This is best illustrated by the metaphor of a "hamster wheel," or circular interactions of mutual influence, creating an interactional rather than cause-and-effect pattern (Kelledy & Lyons, 2019). In parents of children with ASD, frustrations related to communications with family and professionals impact parents' satisfaction with their role as a parent, which in turn may impact their marital relationships causing more frustrations around parental roles (Grinman, 2020).

PTG in Parents of Children with ASD

Despite the challenges, parents of children with ASD may also experience joy, appreciation of life and personal strengths, see new opportunities, become better at relating to others, and be more spiritual than they were before their child's ASD diagnosis. These changes are domains of PTG, which is both a process and an outcome of finding benefits and growth from the struggle following a traumatic event (Calhoun & Tedeschi, 2006a).

PTG as aprocess

The first stage in the PTG process is a seismic traumatic event that is felt as a "before-and-after" experience. While this is exactly how parents describe the start of their journey of parenting a child with ASD, their specific traumatic events vary. For some parents, it is the diagnosis itself and the lengthy process leading to it, the meaning parents attributed to it (e.g., that their child may never be independent, be accepted, or integrated into society), the lack of clarity of what was wrong, as well as ASD related behavior and the associated societal stigma. For others, the manner of diagnosis delivery was traumatic, as they experienced a lack of professionals' empathy for the (assumed) glooming future of their child, a lack of validation of their parental intuition and concerns prior to and during the diagnostic process, lack of empowerment related to their role in their children's development, as well as lack of information about available support (Grinman, 2020).

Parents' experience of multiple traumatic/seismic "the-hardest-time," events at different times of their parenthood journey may lead to "budding," cascading, and evolving of PTG. Each "seismic event" triggers its own "independent" PTG process. This can be seen as parents continuously go through the process described in the PTG model, and their automatic ruminations are changing to reflective and more productive ones; this process is never over, especially because of the ever-evolving, "cascading," PTG process. Figure 18.2 presents the process of PTG in parents of children with ASD.

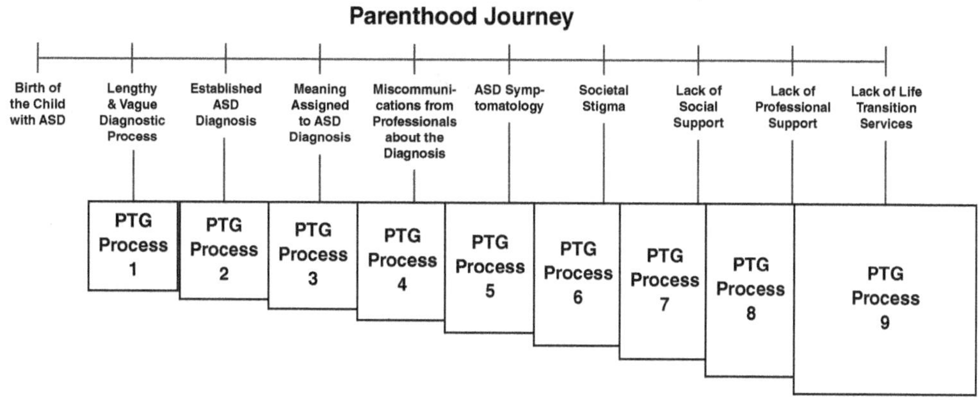

Figure 18.2 Evolving/ "Budding" / "Cascading" PTG in Parents of Children with ASD.

PTG as an Outcome

The PTG Model includes five main domains of growth: (1) seeing new possibilities, (2) relating to others, (3) personal strength, (4) spiritual change, and (5) appreciation of life, although the authors allowed changes beyond this common core specific to the struggle with particular stressors (Tedeschi & Calhoun, 1996). Parents of children diagnosed with ASD reported finding benefits from their parenthood experience, improved well-being (Bayat, 2007), and PTG (Myers et al., 2009; Samios et al., 2009; Strecker et al., 2014). Specifically, studies describe changes in parents' beliefs and self-reflection, gaining greater patience, appreciation, and a new philosophy of life (Zhang et al., 2015), as well as enriched relationships and a sense of support when they became advocates and helped others through their parenthood journeys (Fleischmann, 2004). In the aforementioned narrative analysis of reports from 16 parents of children with ASD that reached young adulthood, Grinman (2020) found that all the parents reported at least one domain of PTG, and more than half reported two or more domains. This PTG is expressed in a "budding" manner, i.e., finding unique ways of coping and functioning as the "ASD family unit" (Grinman, 2020) in service of helping their child with ASD. Parents become "expert companions" for their children, just as clinicians are trained to be for people they support (Calhoun & Tedeschi, 2006b).

Parents of children with ASD manifest various domains of PTG. For example, they may develop a new philosophy and change priorities to focus on understanding their child's well-being and happiness rather than on social status, career, and how things "should be" (Ekas et al., 2010; Manning et al., 2011; Safe et al., 2012). Some undertake new paths in life and get involved in new careers and leadership including servicing the ASD community and becoming its advocates (Boshoff et al., 2018; Ewles et al., 2014), expressing creative ideas for improving the lives of families in the ASD world, and sharing their wisdom of addressing the challenges presented by the child's ASD diagnosis with parents who are just starting their parenthood journeys (Grinman, 2020). Parents change their relationships with their children by joining them in their world, rather than pushing-and-pulling to get the child into the parent's world and support the children in a unique, collaborative way, expressing increased compassion and relatedness to their children in service of the latter's needs, sometimes failing to recognize their own resulting in isolation from society, spouses, children, and family members (Grinman, 2020). Some parents also report improved relationships with extended family members and especially with parents with similar struggles. They change their perception of self, feeling that they gained the freedom to be themselves, uncover strengths they did not know they possessed, and gain wisdom (Grinman, 2020). Parents of children with ASD may experience a deepened sense of spirituality and faith, a belief that their child is an expression of God's will and that they themselves were chosen to experience this journey (Ekas et al., 2009).

PTG can be shaped by proximate and distal sociocultural factors (Calhoun & Tedeschi, 2004). One *proximate factor* is the perceived presence of social support from peers, other parents of children with ASD, family, friends, and professionals that have been identified as facilitators of PTG in this population (Schroevers et al., 2010; Zhang et al., 2015). However, more than half of the participants in Grinman's (2020) study reported having experienced PTG despite the lack of social support and dissatisfaction with professional support throughout their parenting journeys. *Distal sociocultural influences*, including societal, ethnic, religious, and cultural themes, vary for different parents and help them manage emotional distress or/and cause redirection of ruminations into deliberate reflective constructive ones, resulting in revisions in parents' narratives and schemas (Grinman, 2020; Zuckerman et al., 2014). For example, a mother of Peruvian cultural background who lives in Japan reported that societal cultural themes of both her foreign and native cultures affected her well-being and peace of mind in both negative and positive ways. An Orthodox Jewish mother experienced ethnic religious cultural influences in the form of acceptance of her child as God's will.

Part of the PTG of parents of children diagnosed with ASD is developing new ways of coping and managing stress while taking on a multitude of roles. The "ASD family unit" includes the dynamic nature of the roles that parents take on as well as the decisions they have to make, the new collaborative parenting style they use, and the roles that siblings of children diagnosed with ASD take on as collaborators in caretaking (Grinman, 2020).

Parents experience an accumulation of parenting roles of a caretaker, a playmate, a mentor, and a guide and expert companion as their children with ASD grow older. For many parents of children diagnosed with ASD, these roles become integrated into an expanding parenting role. Decisions that parents have to make include treatment approaches, medical care, and appropriate school settings, and are more dynamic and complex than they could have ever imagined at every stage of their child's development (Grinman, 2020).

In addition to a pile-up of roles, parents develop a unique way of coping that contributes to growth and benefit finding in the parenthood experience. Since ASD is not a state that "goes away," parents cannot rely solely on problem-focused coping mechanisms to help them solve problems and need to find new and innovative ways to respond to the many challenges that they face (Grinman, 2020). In addition to biology-focused coping (Wilson, 2010), problem-focused coping, and emotion-focused coping, parents of children diagnosed with ASD universally exhibit a "collaborative," parenting style characterized by full immersion and joining in their child's life (Grinman, 2020). This style is based on parents' empathic and understanding stance, and willingness to isolate from others in service of their child, while providing a voice and being an advocate for their child, unconditionally, without expecting reciprocity from their children with ASD. A coping strategy employed by parents of children with ASD was becoming an expert, the chief operating officer, in their child's care (Grinman, 2020). During the post-ASD diagnosis period, parents (rather than the professionals) take on the responsibility for making decisions related to their child's diet and use of medication oftentimes relying on methods, research, and guidance beyond the scope of prescription or information provided by professionals, which offer comfort, value, and peace of mind for parents coping, as they know their child better than anyone (Grinman, 2020).

Recommendations for Professionals Serving Parents of Children with ASD

Several directions and principles for professionals working with parents of young adults with ASD can be offered to support the facilitation of PTG. To this end, professionals need to be educated in effective communication skills and knowledge about ASD and parents' experiences, especially about the scope of ASD and available avenues for families to explore as they navigate the ASD realm from the point of diagnosis.

Professionals, such as doctors or therapists, have a significant influence on decisions regarding the care of children with Autism Spectrum Disorder (ASD) and their families. However, communicating with these professionals can be challenging because they may not always understand or appreciate the difficulties and challenges that parents face when raising a child with ASD, which can result in a lack of empathy or understanding of these professionals.

Communication skills training, specifically for breaking bad news (Vandekieft, 2001), facilitating prompt and effective treatment planning and follow-ups with parents, as well as promoting effective communication strategies pre, during, and post-diagnosis should be prioritized. Practitioners should focus on being empathic listeners, communicate compassion, trust parents' intuition, and explore parents' concerns and instincts about their child.

Parents need to have better involvement in making decisions regarding available ASD treatment and services and being adequately informed about available policies and resources. Practitioners who are equipped with education and understanding of the information can involve parents at a greater scale and present to them clear information about early ASD symptomatology, the diagnostic process, prognosis, treatment options, and goals associated with their child's care and family support. Within this scope of information, there should be an understanding of potential positive outcomes of parents' struggle with their very negative experiences, resilience, and PTG (Calhoun & Tedeschi, 2006a; Luthar, 2006).

Finally, professionals working with this population group would benefit from training aimed at recognizing the signs of traumatic stress as well as growth, which includes identifying what is going well for the parent, the child, and the family, and recognizing any positive outcomes of traumatic experiences of these parents, including manifestations of all PTG domains. This could be supported by becoming familiar with the PTG model, specific manifestations of PTG in this population, and ways for listening for it and helping facilitate it. This can be done by utilizing cognitive, narrative, and existentially based interventions (Calhoun & Tedeschi, 2006a), which may inform the provision of effective support of parents' self-agency, hope, guidance, encouragement, and empowerment to families, as well as help create a new meaning of the traumatic experience. This ability to facilitate and foster PTG can give a way for professionals to become expert companions who work in tandem with the parents, focusing on benefits finding and growth in people who struggle with traumatic experiences in addition to traditional trauma-sensitive practice techniques of exposure and desensitization (Calhoun & Tedeschi, 2006a). Rather than a new way of therapy, it offers a lens that can be used with any intervention, especially cognitive, existential, and narrative treatments.

To empower parents, professionals can further provide psychoeducation to normalize parents' experiences, especially breaking down assumptions of what "should be" expected, thus decreasing their stress and empowering them about all the possible (positive and negative) outcomes. To support parents' desire to focus on their child's strengths (rather than only on limitations), interventions should also highlight the promotion of children's social skills and connection with others, and bridging the children's internal world with the world around them, by using models such as the Developmental, Individual-difference and Relationship-based "DIR Floortime" Model (Casenhiser et al., 2015; Greenspan & Wieder, 2007), and Relationship Development Intervention (RDI) (Gutstein, 2002; 2009).

Since parents often express a lack of available effective interventions (Grinman, 2020) it is suggested that professionals utilize also alternative or controversial interventions such as complementary medicine, mindfulness practice, self-regulation biological interventions, and psychoeducation focused on self-regulation (Kurtz, 2008), which can potentially achieve a double benefit by parents' getting a handle on their own self-regulation, and being able to guide their children to self-regulate (Beer et al., 2013; Ferraioli & Harris, 2013; Singh et al., 2014).

Finally, family unit-based practices that are supported by parents, like the Son-Rise Program (Kaufman & Kaufman, 1995) should be considered, rather than the current dominance of problem-focused or individual-focused interventions that emphasize the child's pathology (Dillenburger & Keenan, 2009). These family-oriented interventions may improve the family's functioning while improving the child's behaviors because as professionals support parents, they indirectly support the child.

Conclusion

Many insights and inspirations come from the look at PTG as it relates to parents of children diagnosed with ASD. While most of the available literature focuses on the stress associated with this parenthood experience, the medical and mental health fields would benefit from more exploration of PTG and its benefits as well as effective approaches to helping facilitate this growth for parents of newly diagnosed children and their families.

References

American Psychiatric Association (2013). What is Autism Spectrum Disorder? Retrieved from http://www.psychiatry.org/patients-families/autism/what-is-autismspectrum-disorder

Avison, W. R., Ali, J., & Walters, D. (2007). Family structure, stress, and psychological distress: A demonstration of the impact of differential exposure. *Journal of Health and Social Behavior*, *48*(3), 301–317. DOI: 10.1177/002214650704800307

Baker, D. L., & Drapela, L. A. (2010). Mostly the mother: Concentration of adverse employment effects on mothers of children with autism. *The Social Science Journal*, *47*(3), 578–592. DOI: 10.1016/j.soscij.2010.01.013

Barker, E. T., Hartley, S. L., Seltzer, M. M., Floyd, F. J., Greenberg, J. S., & Orsmond, G. I. (2011). Trajectories of emotional well-being in mothers of adolescents and adults with autism. *Developmental Psychology*, *47*(2), 551–561. DOI: 10.1037/a0021268

Bayat, M. (2007). Evidence of resilience in families of children with Autism. *Journal of Intellectual Disability Research*, *51*(Pt 9), 702–714. DOI: 10.1111/j.1365-2788.2007.00960.x

Beer, M., Ward, L., & Moar, K. (2013). The relationship between mindful parenting and distress in parents of children with an autism spectrum disorder. *Mindfulness*, *4*(2), 102–112. DOI: 10.1007/s12671-012-0192-4

Benson, P. L. (2006). *All kids are our kids: What communities must do to raise caring and responsible children and adolescents*. Jossey-Bass.
Benson, P. R., & Karlof, K. L. (2009). Anger, stress proliferation, and depressed mood among parents of children with ASD: A longitudinal replication. *Journal of Autism and Developmental Disorders, 39*(2), 350–362. DOI: 10.1007/s10803-008-0632-0
Bluth, K., Roberson, P. N., Billen, R. M., & Sams, J. M. (2013). A stress model for couples parenting children with autism spectrum disorders and the introduction of a mindfulness intervention. *Journal of Family Theory & Review, 5*(3), 194–213. DOI: 10.1111/jftr.12015
Bonis, S. (2016). Stress and parents of children with autism: A review of literature. *Issues in Mental Health Nursing, 37*(3), 153–163. DOI: 10.3109/01612840.2015.1116030
Boss, P. (2007). Ambiguous loss theory: Challenges for scholars and practitioners. *Family Relations, Special Issue: Ambiguous Loss, 56*(2), 105–110. DOI: 10.1111/j.1741-3729.2007.00444.x
Boshoff, K., Gibbs, D., Phillips, R. L., Wiles, L., & Porter, L. (2018). Parents' voices: "Our process of advocating for our child with autism." A meta-synthesis of parents' perspectives. *Child: Care, Health and Development, 44*(1), 147–160. DOI: 10.1111/cch.12504
Breevaart, K., & Bakker, A. B. (2012). The influence of job and parental strain on typically and atypically developing children: a vicious circle? *Community, Work & Family, 15*, 173–188. DOI: 10.1080/13668803.2011.609657
Calhoun, L. G., & Tedeschi, R. G. (2004). The foundations of posttraumatic growth: New considerations. *Psychological Inquiry, 15*(1), 93–102. DOI: 10.1207/s15327965pli1501_03
Calhoun, L. G., & Tedeschi, R. G. (2006a). *Handbook of posttraumatic growth: Research and practice*. Lawrence Erlbaum Associates.
Calhoun, L. G., & Tedeschi, R. G. (2006b). Expert companions: Posttraumatic growth in clinical practice. In L. G. Calhoun & R. G. Tedeschi (Eds.), *Handbook of posttraumatic growth: Research & practice* (pp. 291–310). Lawrence Erlbaum Associates Publishers.
Casenhiser, D. M., Binns, A., McGill, F., Morderer, O., & Shanker, S. G. (2015). Measuring and supporting language function for children with autism: evidence from a randomized control trial of a social-interaction-based therapy. *Journal of Autism and Developmental Disorders, 45*(3), 846–857. DOI: 10.1007/s10803-014-2242-3
Casey, L. B., Zanksas, S., Meindl, J. N., Parra, G. R., Cogdal, P., & Powell, K. (2012). Parental symptoms of posttraumatic stress following a child's diagnosis of Autism Spectrum Disorder: A pilot study. *Research in Autism Spectrum Disorders, 6*(3), 1186–1193.
Catalano, D., Holloway, L., & Mpofu, E. (2018). Mental health interventions for parent carers of children with Autistic Spectrum Disorder: Practice guidelines from a critical interpretive synthesis (CIS) systematic review. *International Journal for Environmental Research and Public Health, 15*(2), 341–364. DOI: 10.3390/ijerph15020341
Center for Disease Control and Prevention (CDC) (2018). Data on Autism: Five facts to know. Retrieved from https://www.cdc.gov/features/new-autism-data/index.html
Compas, B. E., et al. (2012). Coping with chronic illness in childhood and adolescence. *Annual Review of Clinical Psychology, 8*, 455–480. DOI: 10.1146/annurev-clinpsy-032511-143108
Coulthard, P., & Fitzgerald, M. 1999. In God we trust? Organised religion and personal beliefs as resources and coping strategies, and their implications for health in parents with a child on the autistic spectrum. *Mental Health, Religion & Culture*, 2(1), 19–33. DOI: 10.1080/136746799084 06329
Crnic, K. A., Gaze, C., & Hoffman, C. (2005). Cumulative parenting stress across the preschool period: Relations to maternal parenting and child behavior at age 5. *Infant and Child Development, 14*(2), 117–132. DOI: 10.1002/icd.384
Crouter, A. C., & Booth, A. (Eds.). (2003). *Children's influence on family dynamics: The neglected side of family relationships*. Routledge.
Davis, N. O., & Carter, A. S. (2008). Parenting stress in mothers and fathers of toddlers with autism spectrum disorders: Associations with child characteristics. *Journal of Autism and Developmental Disorders, 38*(7), 1278–1291. DOI: 10.1007/s10803-007-0512-z
Derguy, C., M'Bailara, K., Michel, G., Roux, S., & Bouvard, M. (2016). The need for an ecological approach to parental stress in Autism Spectrum Disorders: The combined role of individual and environmental factors. *Journal of Autism and Developmental Disorders, 46* (6), 1895–1905. DOI: 10.1007/s10803-016-2719-3

Derguy, C., Roux, S., Portex, M., & M'bailara, K. (2018). An ecological exploration of individual, family, and environmental contributions to parental quality of life in autism. *Psychiatry Research*, *268*, 87–93. DOI: 10.1016/j.psychres.2018.07.006

Dillenburger, K., & Keenan, M. (2009). None of the As in ABA stand for autism: Dispelling the myths. *Journal of Intellectual & Developmental Disability*, *34*(2), 193–195. DOI: 10.1080/13668250902845244

Edmund, D. S., & Bland, P. J. (2011). *Real tools: Responding to multi-abuse trauma. A tool kit to help advocates and community partners better serve people with multiple issues*. Alaska Network on Domestic Violence & Sexual Assault.

Ekas, N. V., Lickenbrock, D. M., & Whitman, T. L. (2010). Optimism, social support, and well-being in mothers of children with Autism Spectrum Disorder. *Journal of Autism and Developmental Disorders*, *40*(10), 1274–1284. DOI: 10.1007/s10803-010-0986-y

Ekas, N. V., Whitman, T. L., & Shivers, C. (2009). Religiosity, spirituality, and socioemotional functioning in mothers of children with autism spectrum disorder. *Journal of autism and developmental disorders*, *39*(5), 706–719. DOI: 10.1007/s10803-008-0673-4

Epifanio, M. S., Genna, V., Vitello, M. G., Roccella, M., & La Grutta, S. (2013). Parenting stress and impact of illness in parents of children with coeliac disease. *Pediatric Reports*, *5*(4), e19. DOI: 10.4081/pr.2013.e19

Einfeld, S. L., Piccinin, A. M., Mackinnon, A., Hofer, S. M., Taffe, J., Gray, K. M., Bontempo, D. E., Hoffman, L. R., Parmenter, T., & Tonge, B. J. (2006). Psychopathology in young people with intellectual disability. *JAMA*, *296*(16), 1981–1989. DOI: 10.1001/jama.296.16.1981

Evenson, R. J., & Simon, R. W. (2005). Clarifying the relationship between parenthood and depression. *Journal of Health and Social Behavior*, *46*(4), 341–358. DOI: 10.1177/002214650504600403

Ewles, G., Clifford, T., & Minnes, P. (2014). Predictors of advocacy in parents of children with autism spectrum disorders. *Journal on Developmental Disabilities*, *20*(1), 73–82.

Faras, H., Al Ateeqi, N., & Tidmarsh, L. (2010). Autism spectrum disorders. *Annals of Saudi Medicine*, *30*(4), 295–300. DOI: 10.4103/0256-4947.65261

Fava, G. A., McEwen, B. S., Guidi, J., Gostoli, S., Offidani, E., & Sonino, N. (2019). Clinical characterization of allostatic overload. Psychoneuroendocrinology, *108*, 94–101. DOI: 10.1016/j.psyneuen.2019.05.028

Feldman, R., Sussman, A. L., & Zigler, E. (2004). Parental leave and work adaptation at the transition to parenthood: Individual, marital, and social correlates. *Journal of Applied Developmental Psychology*, *25*(4), 459–479.

Ferraioli, S. J., & Harris, S. L. (2013). Comparative effects of mindfulness and Skills-based parent training programs for parents of children with autism: Feasibility and preliminary outcome data. *Mindfulness*, *4*(2), 89–101. DOI: 10.1007/s12671-012-0099-0

Fleischmann, A. (2004). Narrative published on the Internet by parents of children with autism: What do they reveal and why is it important? *Focus on Autism and Other Developmental Disabilities*, *19*(1), 35–43. DOI: 10.1177/10883576040190010501

Glass, J., Simon, R. W., & Andersson, M. A. (2016). Parenthood and happiness: Effects of work-family reconciliation policies in 22 OECD countries. *American Journal of Sociology*, *122*(3), 886–929. DOI: 10.1086/688892

Greenspan, S. I., & Wieder, S. (2007). The developmental individual-difference, relationship-based (DIR/Floortime) model approach to Autism Spectrum Disorders. In E. Hollander, & E. Anagnostou (Eds.), *Clinical manual for the treatment of autism* (pp. 179–209). American Psychiatric Publishing.

Grinman, V. (2020). *A retrospective exploration of the experience, interpretation and perception of growth in parents of young adults diagnosed with Autism Spectrum Disorder*. Adelphi University. https://adelphi.idm.oclc.org/login?url= https://www.proquest.com/dissertations-theses/retrospective-exploration-experience/docview/2480659167/se-2

Gutstein, S. E. (2002). *Relationship development intervention with young children: Social and emotional development activities for Asperger syndrome, Autism, PDD and NLD* (Kindle Edition). Jessica Kingsley Publishers.

Gutstein, S. E. (2009). Empowering families through Relationship Development Intervention: An important part of the biopsychosocial management of Autism Spectrum Disorders. *Annals of Clinical Psychiatry*, *21*(3), 174–182.

Hill, R. (1958). Generic features of families under stress. *Social Casework*, *39*, 139–150.
Huston, T. L., & Holmes, E. K. (2004). Becoming parents. In A. Vangelisti (Ed.), *Handbook of family communication* (pp. 105–133). Lawrence Erlbaum Associates.
Huws, J. C., Jones, R. S., & Ingledew, D. K. (2001). Parents of children with autism using an email group: A grounded theory study. *Journal of Health Psychology*, *6*(5), 569–584.
Juster, R.-P., McEwen, B. S., & Lupien, S. J. (2010). Allostatic load biomarkers of chronic stress and impact on health and cognition. *Neuroscience and Biobehavioral Reviews*, *35*(1), 2–16. DOI: 10.1016/j.neubiorev.2009.10.002
Kaufman, B. N., & Kaufman, R. (1995). *Son-Rise: The miracle continues*. H.J. Kramer.
Keenan, M., Dillenburger, K., Doherty, A., Byrne, T., & Gallagher, S. (2010). The experiences of parents during diagnosis and forward planning for children with autism spectrum disorder. *Journal of Applied Research in Intellectual Disabilities*, *23*(4), 390–397. DOI: 10.1080/13668803.2011.609657
Kelledy, L., & Lyons, B. (2019). Circular causality in a family systems theory In J. L. Lebow, A. L. Chambers, & D. C. Breunlin, (Eds). *Encyclopedia of Couple and Family Therapy* (pp. 431–434). Springer. DOI: 10.1007/978-3-319-49425-8_248
Kinnear, S. H., Link, B. G., Ballan, M. S., & Fischbach, R. L. (2016). Understanding the experience of stigma for parents of children with Autism Spectrum Disorder and the role stigma plays in families' lives. *Journal of Autism and Developmental Disorders*, *46*(3), 942–953. DOI: 10.1007/s10803-015-2637-9
Kurtz, L. A. (2008). *Understanding controversial therapies for children with autism, attention deficit disorder, and other learning disabilities: A guide to complementary and alternative therapies*. Singing Dragon Books.
Kozlowski, A. M., Matson, J. L., Horovitz, M., Worley, J. A., & Neal, D. (2011). Parents' first concerns of their child's development in toddlers of Autism Spectrum Disorder. *Developmental Neurorehabilitation*,*14*(2), 72–78. DOI: 10.3109/17518423.2010.539193
Knoester, C., & Eggebeen, D. J. (2006). The effects of the transition to parenthood and subsequent children on men's well-being and social participation. *Journal of Family Issues*, *27*, 1532–1560. DOI: 10.1177/0192513X06290802
Lazarus, R. S., & Folkman, S. (1986). Cognitive theories of stress and the issue of circularity. In M. H. Appley & R. Trumbull (Eds.), *Dynamics of stress* (pp. 63–80). The Plenum Series on Stress and Coping. Springer.
LeBlanc, A. G., Katzmarzyk, P. T., Barreira, T. V., Broyles, S. T., Chaput, J. P., Church, T. S., Fogelholm, M., Harrington, D. M., Hu, G., Kuriyan, R., Kurpad, A., Lambert, E. V., Maher, C., Maia, J., Matsudo, V., Olds, T., Onywera, V., Sarmiento, O. L., Standage, M., Tudor-Locke, C., Zhao, P., Tremblay, M. S., & ISCOLE Research Group. (2015). Correlates of total sedentary time and screen time in 9–11 year-old children around the world: the international study of childhood obesity, lifestyle and the environment. *PloS One*, *10*(6), e0129622. DOI: 10.1371/journal.pone.0129622
Lecavalier, L., Leone, S., & Wiltz, J. (2006). The impact of behaviour problems on caregiver stress in young people with Autism Spectrum Disorders. *Journal of Intellectual Disability Research: JIDR*, 50. 172–183. DOI: 10.1111/j.1365-2788.2005.00732.x
Luthar, S. S. (2006). Resilience in development: A synthesis of research across five decades. In D. Cicchetti, & D. J. Cohen (Eds.), *Developmental Psychopathology, Vol. 3: Risk, Disorder, and Adaptation* (pp. 739–795) (2nd ed.). Wiley.
Maenner, M. J., Graves, S. J., Peacock, G., Honein, M. A., Boyle, C. A., & Dietz, P. M. (2021). Comparison of 2 case definitions for ascertaining the prevalence of Autism Spectrum Disorder among 8-year-old children. *American Journal of Epidemiology*, *190*(10), 2198–2207. DOI: 10.1093/aje/kwab106
Manning, M. M., Wainwright, L., & Bennett, J. (2011). The double ABCX model of adaptation in racially diverse families with a school-age child with autism. *Journal of Autism and Developmental Disorders*, *41*(3), 320–331. DOI: 10.1007/s10803-010-1056-1
McCubbin, H. I., & Patterson, J. M. (1983). The family stress process: The double ABCX model of adjustment and adaptation. *Marriage and Family Review*, *6*(1-2), 7–37.
McEwen, B. S. (2017). Stress: Homeostasis, rheostasis, reactive scope, allostasis and allostatic load. In S. Fiedler (Ed.), *Reference Module in Neuroscience and Biobehavioral Psychology*. NY: The Rockefeller University. DOI: 10.1016/B978-0-12-809324-5.02867-4

Miodrag, N., & Hodapp, R. M. (2010). Chronic stress and health among parents of children with intellectual and developmental disabilities. *Current Opinions in Psychiatry*, *23*(5), 407–411. DOI: 10.1097/YCO.0b013e32833a8796. PMID: 20592593.

Muscara, F., Mccarthy, M. C., Woolf, C., Hearps, S. J., Burke, K., Anderson, V. A., (2015). Early psychological reactions in parents of children with a life threatening illness within a pediatric hospital setting. *European Psychiatry*, *30*(5), 555–561. DOI: 10.1016/j.eurpsy.2014.12.008

Myers, B. J., Mackintosh, V. H., & Goin-Kohel, R. P. (2009). "My greatest joy and my greatest heart ache:" Parents' own words on how having a child in the autism spectrum has affected their lives and their families' lives. *Research in Autism Spectrum Disorders*, *3*(3), 670–684. DOI: 10.1016/j.rasd.2009.01.004

Nachshen, J. S., Garcin, N., & Minnes, P. (2005). Problem behavior in children with intellectual disabilities: Parenting stress, empowerment and school services. *Mental Health Aspects of Developmental Disabilities*, *8*(4), 105–114.

Neely-Barnes, S. L., Hall, H. R., Roberts, R. J., & Graff, J. C. (2011). Parenting a child with an autism spectrum disorder: Public perceptions and parental Conceptualizations. *Journal of Family Social Work*, *14*(3), 208–225. DOI: 10.1080/10522158.2011.571539

Newschaffer, C. J., Croen, L. A., Daniels, J., Giarelli, E., Grether, J. K., Levy, S. E., & Reynolds, A. M. (2007). The epidemiology of Autism Spectrum Disorders. *Annual Review of Public Health*, *28*, 235–258. DOI: 10.1146/annurev.publhealth.28.021406.144007

Nomaguchi, K. M., & Milkie, M. A. (2003). Costs and rewards of children: The effects of becoming a parent on adults' lives. *Journal of Marriage and Family*, *65*(2), 356–374.

O'Brien, M. (2007). Ambiguous loss in families of children with Autism Spectrum Disorders. *Family Relations*, *56*(2), 135–146. DOI: 10.1111/j.1741-3729.2007.00447.x

Ooi, K. L., Ong, Y. S., Jacob, S. A., & Khan, T. M. (2016). A meta-synthesis on parenting a child with autism. *Neuropsychiatric Disease and Treatment*, *12*, 745–762. DOI: 10.2147/NDT.S100634

Paulson, J. F., Dauber, S., & Leiferman, J. A. (2006). Individual and combined effects of postpartum depression in mothers and fathers on parenting behavior. *Pediatrics*, *118*(2), 659–668. DOI: 10.1542/peds.2005-2948

Perry, A. (2004). A model of stress in families of children with developmental disabilities: Clinical and research applications. *Journal on Developmental Disabilities*, *11*(1), 1–16.

Pisula, E. (2002). Parents of children with autism: recent research findings. *Psychiatria Polska*, *36*(1), 95–108.

Ross, C. E., & Van Willigen, M. (1996). Gender, parenthood, and anger. *Journal of Marriage and the Family*, *58*(3), 572–584. DOI: 10.2307/353718

Ruiz-Robledillo, N., De Andrés-García, S., Pérez-Blasco, J., González-Bono, E., & Moya-Albiol, L. (2014). Highly resilient coping entails better perceived health, high social support and low morning cortisol levels in parents of children with Autism Spectrum Disorder. *Research in Developmental Disabilities*, *35*(3), 686–695. DOI: 10.1016/j.ridd.2013.12.007

Safe, A., Joosten, A., & Molineux, M. (2012). The experiences of mothers of children with Autism: Managing multiple roles. *Journal of Intellectual & Developmental Disability*, *37*(4), 294–302. DOI: 10.3109/13668250.2012.736614

Samios, C., Pakenham, K. I., & Sofronoff, K. (2009). The nature of benefit finding in parents of a child with Asperger syndrome. *Research in Autism Spectrum Disorders*, *3*(2), 358–374. DOI: 10.1 016/j.rasd.2008.08.003

Saxbe, D. E., Schetter, C. D., Guardino, C. M., Ramey, S. L., Shalowitz, M. U., Thorp, J., & Vance, M. (2016). Sleep quality predicts persistence of parental postpartum depressive symptoms and transmission of depressive symptoms from mothers to fathers. *Annals of Behavioral Medicine*, *50*(6), 862–875. DOI: 10.1007/s12160-016-9815-7

Schroevers, M. J., Helgeson, V. S., Sanderman, R., & Ranchor, A. V. (2010). Type of social support matters for prediction of posttraumatic growth among cancer survivors. *PsychoOncology*, *19*(1), 46–53. DOI: 10.1002/pon.1501

Simon, R. W., & Nath, L. E. (2004). Gender and emotion in the United States: Domen and women differ in self-reports of feelings and expressive behavior? *American Journal of Sociology*, *109*(5), 1137–1176. DOI: 10.1086/382111

Singh, N. N., Lancioni, G. E., & Winton, A. S. (2014). Mindfulness-based positive behavior support (MBPBS) for mothers of adolescents with autism spectrum disorder: Effects of adolescents' behavior and parental stress. *Mindfulness*, *5*, 646–657. DOI: 10.1007/s12671-014-0321-3

Sinnerbrink, I., Silove, D., Field, A., Steel, Z., & Manicavasagar, V. (1997). Compounding of premigration trauma and postmigration stress in asylum seekers. *The Journal of psychology*, *131*(5), 463–470. DOI: 10.1080/00223989709603533

Smith-Nielsen, J., Tharner, A., Steele, H., Cordes, K., Mehlhase, H., &Vaever, M. S. (2016). Postpartum depression and infant-mother attachment security at one year: The impact of co-morbid maternal personality disorders. *Infant Behavior and Development*, *44*, 148–158. DOI: 10.1016/j.infbeh.2016.06.002

Strecker, S., Hazelwood, Z. J., & Shakespeare-Finch, J. E. (2014) Post-diagnosis personal growth in an Australian population of parents raising children with developmental disability. *Journal of Intellectual and Developmental Disability*, *39*(1), 1–9. DOI: 10.3109/13668250.2013.835035

Taylor, J. L. (2009). Midlife impacts of adolescent parenthood. *Journal of Family Issues*, *30*(4), 484–510. DOI: 10.1177/0192513X08329601

Tedeschi, R. G., & Calhoun, L. G. (1996). The posttraumatic growth inventory: Measuring the positive legacy of trauma. *Journal of Traumatic Stress*, *9*(3), 455–471. DOI: 10.1007/BF02103658

Umberson, D., & Gove, W. R. (1989). Parenthood and psychological well-being theory, measurement, and stage in the family life course. *Journal of Family Issues*, *10*(4), 440–462. DOI: 10.1177/019251389010004002

VandeKieft, G. (2001). Breaking bad news. *American Family Physician*, *64*(12), 1975–1979.

Ward, E. (2014). *Parental accounts of sharing an autism spectrum diagnosis with their Child: a thematic analysis* (Doctoral dissertation, University of Nottingham).

Wickrama, K. A. S., Lorenz, F. O., Wallace, L. E., Peiris, L., Conger, R. D., & Elder, G. H. (2001). Family influence on physical health during the middle years: The case of onset of hypertension. *Journal of Marriage and Family*, *63*(2), 527–539. DOI: 10.1111/j.1741-3737.2001.00527.x

Wilson, D. R. (2010). Stress management for adult survivors of childhood sexual abuse: A holistic inquiry. *Western Journal of Nursing Research*, *32*(1), 103–127. DOI: 10.1177/0193945909343703

Yamaoka, Y., Tamiya, N., Moriyama, Y., Garrido, F. A. S., Sumazaki, R., & Noguchi, H. (2015). Mental health of parents as caregivers of children with disabilities: Based on Japanese nationwide survey. *PloS One*, *10*(12), e0145200. DOI: 10.1371/journal.pone.0145200

Zhang, W., Yan, T. T., Barriball, K. L., While, A. E., & Liu H. X. (2015). Post-traumatic growth in mothers of children with autism: A phenomenological study. *Autism*, *19*(1), 29–37. DOI: 10.1177/1362361313509732

Zuckerman, K. E., Sinche, B., Mejia, A., Cobian, M., Becker, T., & Nicolaidis, C. (2014). Latino parents' perspectives of barriers to autism diagnosis. *Academic Pediatrics*, *14*(3), 301–308. DOI: 10.1016/j.acap.2013.12.004

Zwaigenbaum, L., Bryson, S., Rogers, T., Roberts, W., Brian, J., & Szatmari, P. (2005). Behavioral manifestations of autism in the first year of life. *International Journal of Developmental Neuroscience*, *23*(2-3), 143–152. DOI: 10.1016/j.ijdevneu.2004.05.001

19

POSTTRAUMATIC GROWTH IN ADULTHOOD FOLLOWING CHILD, EARLY, AND FORCED MARRIAGES

Ayten Zara and Zeynep Akbudak

Child, early, and forced marriage (CEFM) is a formal marriage or informal union of living with a partner as if married, of a girl or boy before the age of 18 (Unicef, 2021a). CEFM is a human rights crisis that violates the Declaration on the Elimination of Violence Against Women, which defines violence against women as "any act of gender-based violence that results in or is likely to result in, physical, sexual or psychological harm or suffering to women, including threats of such acts, coercion or arbitrary deprivation of liberty, whether occurring in public or private life" (UNHR, 1993).

Although rates have been dropping thanks to civil society efforts, CEFM is still very frequent, especially in poor, traditional, gender-segregated countries. Approximately 90% of child marriages take place in Africa, Asia, and the Middle East. There are more than 700 million child marriages worldwide and at least 12 million girls are married off before they reach the age of 18. In the least developed countries, 40% of girls are married before age 18, and 12% are married before age 15. South Asia is home to almost half (42%) of all child brides worldwide and India accounts for one-third of the global total (UNICEF, 2020). Niger is considered to have the highest prevalence rate of CEFM, and Turkey has the highest rate in Europe. It has also been estimated that 115 million boys are married before the age of 18, out of whom 23 million were married before they turned 15 (UNICEF, 2021b). However, boys who get married early do not face the same risks of sexual violence and increased social pressure as girls do (Veenema et al., 2015).

The practice of CEFM is particularly widespread in conflict-affected situations such as the Gaziantep provinces of Turkey, among the 4.5 million Syrians who have fled the war that has been going on since 2011 to take refuge in Turkey and struggle to survive by selling their children. The number of men who marry underage Syrian girls as second wives in Turkey is growing substantially as post-disaster marriages are seen as generating income and protecting orphaned girls from rape.

Girls in CEFM struggle with responsibilities for building a family, taking care of a home, raising children at an early age, separation from parents and peers, conflicts with their spouses and their families, low social support, and economic difficulties.

 DOI: 10.4324/9781032208688-25

Factors Associated with CEFM

Multiple factors are associated with early marriage; specifically, traditional attitudes and cultural beliefs and educational, economic, and domestic violence levels of the family.

Traditional Attitudes and Cultural Beliefs

Early marriages are a continuous and ongoing problem, which is culturally produced and sustained in many societies based on culturally constructed gender roles. Roles assigned to women in the patriarchal system are one of the mechanisms that put early marriage into motion. Beliefs and traditions, which legitimize and ensure unequal treatment of women and girls, support the early marriage of girls (Burn & Evenhuis, 2014).

In Islamic culture, marriage is sacred, valuable, the only way to obtain identity, and is strongly recommended on religious, moral, social, and psychological grounds. Consequently, many Islamic countries do not view child marriage as a crime. Traditional families see female children as an asset entrusted to them for a certain period of time whereas they consider the girl's "real home" to be the home of her husband and deem it necessary for her to be married at an early age in order to adapt to this home. It is also believed that girls can be protected from sexual harassment and violence if they are brought under the shield of a man as soon as possible (Iustitiani & Ajisuksmo, 2018; Nurmala et al., 2020).

Traditional practices that encourage early marriage and are supported by norms of ethnic and religious groups with common and similar cultural values include bride price, berdel (a bride or bridegroom is exchanged with a bride or bridegroom of another family), cradle notch (betrothing a baby boy to a baby girl by their fathers), and blood price marriage. Knowledge of ancestry, better understanding between children of relatives, traditions, and customs are reasons cited for these marriages, which are concentrated in the rural and poor regions of Middle East countries (Güneş et al., 2016; Malatyalı, 2014; Yount et al., 2016).

Such beliefs perpetuate early marriage and sexual violence against children. For example, in sub-Saharan Africa, there is a widespread myth that having sex with a virgin woman, girl, or child of their own cures HIV and many other diseases in men. In addition to encouraging early marriages, this belief also increases the rape of young girls.

Early marriages usually take place in the form of religious rituals with no formalities, legally binding rights, or a marriage ceremony. The relations are shaped by tradition, and custom solutions are used to resolve issues, especially those related to matters of honor. When traditional customs cannot resolve child marriage-related issues, social pressure, isolation, blood feud, and even death are used (Iustitiani & Ajisuksmo, 2018; Soylu & Ayaz, 2013). Because the traditional social structure is authority-based, marital relationships are often based on the sense of "we" and fatalism, causing violence to be seen as a form of rightful "discipline" both in the family and in public life.

Educational, Economic, and Domestic Violence Levels of the Family

CEFM is impacted by the economic and educational level of the family and by domestic violence, all of which can push girls into early marriage (Montazeri et al., 2016). Girls who are married at a young age have typically never received any education and most of their mothers are illiterate and did not receive any education either (Kasim et al., 2015). These families usually lack knowledge about the effects that early marriage can have on children. They try to protect the girls from assault, offenses, or teasing that occurs against unmarried girls by marrying them off soon after they hit puberty (Soylu & Ayaz, 2013).

In poor countries, gender-based discrimination prevails such that girls are often denied equal access to common resources when a family is poor. While families treat male children as future assets and the economic base of the family, they view female children as a burden. Due to this discrimination in spending on children's education, female children are given the least or no priority at all. Thus, poor families resort to child marriage to avoid possible troubles that may become female children. Early marriages are often seen as an economic salvation for the family and may be perceived as a hidden form of selling girls by poorer families for money, gold, a house, or land. Because the price is determined by the age of the child and decreases with age, families tend to sell the girls while they are young.

Effects of Child, Early, and Forced Marriage

CEFM hinders children's education, limits their social, psychological, physical, and cultural development, and restricts their freedom. Marrying girls off before they have completed their development is a form of human rights violation and is the most common form of sexual abuse, which may generate severe trauma and grief with present and future devastating effects that may change one's personality (Tenkorang, 2019; Wodon et al., 2017).

Marriage at a young age has always meant life imprisonment for girls. It destroys their childhood, innocence, and dreams, and pushes onto them huge responsibilities related to early pregnancy, childrearing, and house chores. High rates of physical and sexual violence, unintended pregnancy, abortion, preterm labor, delivery of low-birth-weight babies, and fetal and maternal mortality can be seen in CEFM (Eray et al., 2019; Gage, 2013).

Girls who get married at a young age are two times more likely to be exposed to physical violence, and three times more likely to be exposed to sexual violence compared to women in other age groups. Married children become vulnerable to exploitation, all kinds of violence, abuse, and poverty at home. For example, 14.6% of girls who were married at an early age in Turkey were exposed to spousal physical violence and abuse, and 27.1% were exposed to emotional violence and abuse. Possible reasons for spousal violence in these marriages include lack of education, the child's economic level, age difference, power imbalance between spouses, social isolation, and lack of women's autonomy. Pregnancy of girls who have not yet completed their physical development increases risks for permanent physical and psychological damage, mother-child mortality, exposure to HIV infections, and postnatal depression (Güneş et al., 2016; Kidman, 2016; Soylu & Ayaz, 2013).

The aforementioned experiences may potentially cause posttraumatic stress and accompanying depression (Fisher et al., 2011; Kidman, 2016; Malatyalı, 2014), acute stress disorder, major depressive disorder, and anxiety disorder. Moreover, it has been reported that 15.8%–29.2% of girls in CEFM developed suicidal ideation, and 5.3%–20.8% of them attempted suicide (Soylu & Ayaz, 2013). The lifetime suicide attempt rate was 1.5–10.1%, and the annual incidence of suicidal ideation was 6.0% (Bridge et al., 2006). However, symptoms of posttraumatic stress disorder and postpartum depression are often ignored in early marriages.

The first author witnessed the effects of CEFM firsthand. Her mother was the smartest and hardest-working child in her village. Her dream was to be a teacher, but she was forced into marriage when she was 14. Her daughter grew up witnessing her mother's never-ending mourning and grief. She has nightmares of a "blackened corpse," which her daughter understood later to refer to her lost childhood and a life she always dreamed of yet never experienced.

Posttraumatic Growth in CEFM

Growth is a long road and knowing they are not alone on this journey, survivors can feel more comfortable. Psychological growth requires working through the pain and the distress of the trauma. This process involves cognitive restructuring where cognitive schemas are challenged, reshaped, and changed since the traumatic reality demolished the basic assumptions about the world. The development of PTG is influenced by event-related factors (e.g., the type, intensity, and duration of the trauma), environmental factors (e.g., social network), and personal factors (e.g., coping and personality) (Tedeschi & Calhoun, 1996).

Lessons learned from years of working with survivors of early and forced marriages have shown that as children of early and forced marriages grow and develop, the trauma grows with them. The effect of the traumatic experiences related to CEFM is agonizing and hurtful and the pain caused by such traumatic experiences cannot die out and remains a somber shadow that accompanies them their whole life. However, some survivors of CEFM grow from this experience as the following real-life examples illustrate.

Hatice Nur Uzgenç is the founder of "Strong Woman" Association which empowers and supports young women of CEFM who openly shares on social media being a survivor of child marriage. Hatice had no one to trust and support her, working hard to take care of herself and her two daughters after escaping from an abusive marriage. When she managed to save enough money, she established an association to help women who are going through similar experiences. Similarly, Dilek Demir, the sole female neighborhood head in Diyarbakır Turkey, who during her term of office saved more than forty girls from CEFM, self-identifies as a survivor of CEFM. She was forced by her father to marry at the age of 14. When she resisted she and her mother were brutally abused by her father finally accepting to avoid further abuse. At the age of 15, she had a baby. Because she was also a child, she could not recognize her baby's health problem, which was suffering a seizure and eventually mental disabilities. After suffering repeated violence during her marriage and struggling in her abusive marriage for 15 years, she succeeded to escape from it. With support from her children, she established a new life for her family. She won the elections to become a neighborhood representative and is helping girls who seek her help to avoid being forced to marry and continue their education. To date, she has saved 40 girls from marriage by convincing their families (Kamer, 2021).

PTG in CEFM is a multidimensional process that unfolds gradually over a period of time because, like traumatic events generally, it requires massive schematic changes. The growth in survivors of CEFM relates to putting back the self's pieces together as a coherent unit. The most important step is for individuals to evaluate themselves as survivors rather than victims. Survivors may learn to connect better with their sense of self, which can give a sense of victory, control over their perspectives towards life, increase self-efficacy, and fosters self-confidence (Wood, 2009). Gaining awareness of what they went through serves to provide a better understanding of the self and gain the ability for questioning the value of life, understand priorities that are important in life, and know how to deal with challenges (Jackson, 2017; Tedeschi & Calhoun, 1998; Zeligman et al., 2019).

PTG and resilience do not necessarily entail denial of the psychopathological effects of trauma; rather, they help reveal paths leading to the light at the end of the tunnel after trauma. Helgeson et al. (2006) stated, "growth outcomes may reflect a variety of processes, some of which have to do with actual changes in one's life, some of which have to do with coping, and others of which have to do with cognitive manipulations on the order of self-enhancement biases meant to alleviate distress." (p. 812).

Especially striking is the demonstration of growth in survivors' career preferences such as using strategies that deal with traumatic events to guide drawing a career path (Prescod & Zeligman, 2018). Sheridan and Carr (2020) found that survivors can be drawn to helping others who have lived through similar experiences. It is likely that helping others deal with similar issues, helps the survivor-helper as well. Thus, it is not surprising that a major motive of survivors is interlinked with their own sense of healing. For example, survivors who voluntarily worked at sexual assault crisis centers hope to soothe their wounds and create positive meaning for their trauma by providing help to others and creating a change in society's attitude towards sexual abuse (Gueta et al., 2020). Two main factors that shape the ability of survivors to progress well from a negative trajectory toward PTG are coping and problem-solving behavior and social support.

Coping and Problem-Solving Behavior

PTG in CEFM is an ongoing oscillating rather than a straight linear process. Survivors of CEFM can experience both PTS and PTG simultaneously. The ability for active coping and problem-solving behavior enables individuals to deal with the pain of the loss, tolerate a wide range of emotions, and cope with the demands of marriage is especially important (Archambeault, 2010; Walker-Williams, 2012). A critical turning point is when survivors accept, name, and talk about the abuse they experienced and eliminate negative attitudes toward the self, allowing positive progress to start (Hill, 2017; Sheridan & Carr, 2020). Emotional coping through the expression of anger, sadness, shame, and guilt towards the abuser might dissipate the survivors' feelings of guilt and sense of victimization (Vilenica et al., 2013). As Tedeschi and Calhoun (2004) stated: "The degree to which individuals engage in self-disclosure about their emotions and about their perspective on their crisis, and how others respond to that self-disclosure, may also play a role in growth" (p. 7). By actively thinking about the abuse survivors can create for themselves new meanings, which provides a fresh perspective and a sense of motivation (Lev-Wiesel, 2008).

Religious coping may help survivors give meaning and re-construct their demolished trauma-related life narrative and grief (Kirkner & Ullman, 2019). Believing that things happen for a reason and that events develop due to a fate beyond their control can reduce the feelings of responsibility, guilt, and anger of survivors. When acknowledging the distressing reality of loss within a social exchange and companionship, affection, and humor might provide a sense of well-being as well as a source of reliance that helps soothe the debilitating effect of abuse and loss. Religious coping can also help survivors achieve a sense of control over a difficult situation, provide intimacy with the members of the religious community, and assist in making major life transformations (Pargament, 2000).

Survivors who are more actively processing the stressor tend to process and incorporate the traumatic reality more efficiently. This may help them come to terms with the conflict and the irreversible changes that the loss and trauma brought to their lives. Using active coping with violence, loss, grief, and burden as a guide for drawing a career path predicts growth in survivors. For example, helping others who have lived through a similar experience or working towards preventing CEFM promotes a pathway for growth (Yilmaz & Zara, 2016) because the beneficial effect of personal and social resources is partially mediated by coping responses; i.e., coping strategies promote PTG as they arise from active efforts to deal with the problem or the consequent emotions.

Social Support

Perceived social and emotional support helps survivors acknowledge the pain of the loss and tolerate a wide range of emotions such as delayed reactions, quiet reflections, intense crying, expression of guilt, anger, and emptiness. They also maintain survivors individuals' integrity and ability to function in the presence of stress (Hartley et al., 2016; Nanfuka et al., 2020).

Tedeschi and Calhoun (2004) posit that "Supportive others can aid in posttraumatic growth by providing a way to craft narratives about the changes that have occurred, and by offering perspectives that can be integrated into schema change" (p. 8). Social relations, especially those involving emotional support from significant others, are vital for survivors of CEFM. Growth takes place when survivors can establish meaningful relations with their environments and organize them within their autonomy. Having emotional support from significant others helps survivors feel loved and allows them to cope better with the effects of abuse and the demands of marriage. The social support in the relationships provides them with time to develop new opportunities, facilitates growth, and allows them to discover themselves in areas they could not express before (Nelson et al., 2019; Zeligman et al., 2019).

Conclusions

Given the prevalence, characteristics, and potential PTG, community and mental health centers should create comprehensive and competent programs for offering survivors of CEFM psychological, social, and legal support and engage in prevention. Detecting abuse, providing support, and preventing revictimization is vital to secure the health of individuals and the community. Promoting strategies focusing on girls' education and targeting social inequalities are potentially effective strategies for preventing child marriage. Empowering girls, improving their access to education, providing economic support for their families, and strengthening legal policies are some of the most important measures to prevent CFEM. Efforts should aim to change the gender-biased attitudes of parents and society and prevent discrimination against girls. Civil communities and governments should challenge traditional customs and religious beliefs that surround early marriage and educate health and community workers about its dangers. The police, judges, and persecutors, should be trained and directed to enforce the law against early marriage.

One example of community-focused work is Active in rural areas of Turkey, Africa, and Asia. Aiming to prevent CEFM, the organization enables thousands of girls to enjoy the childhood they deserve by raising awareness among families, community members, and youth of the negative consequences of early marriage and empowering girls to negotiate with their parents. Further, a strong support system is developed to keep girls in school, provide scholarships where necessary, and encourage teachers to support girls. Meetups are organized with leading professional women in communities to be role models and a source of inspiration for the younger girls. In addition, psychological support is provided to children and adult survivors of CEFM.

References

Archambeault, M. (2010). *How women of color conceptualize and cope with their history of childhood sexual abuse: A preliminary investigation* (Unpublished master's thesis). Pepperdine University. Theses and Dissertations. 96. https://digitalcommons.pepperdine.edu/etd/96

Burn, J. M., & Evenhuis, M. (2014). *'Just Married, Just a Child': Child Marriage in the Indo-Pacific Region.* Plan International Australia.

Bridge, J. A., Goldstein, T. R. & Brent, D. A. (2006). Adolescent suicide and suicidal behavior. *Journal of Child Psychology and Psychiatry, 47*(3-4), 372–394. 10.1111/j.1469-7610.2006.01615.x

Eray, Ş., Uçar, H. N., & Murat, D. (2019). Early marriage and related mental illnesses. *Van Medical Journal, 26*(4), 445–451. 10.5505/vtd.2019.50146

Fisher, J., Cabral de Mello, M., Izutsu, T., Vijayakumar, L., Belfer, M., & Omigbodun, O. (2011). Nature, prevalence and determinants of common mental health problems and their management in primary health care. *International Journal of Social Psychiatry, 57*(1_suppl), 9–12. 10.1177/0020764010397628

Gage, A. J. (2013). Association of child marriage with suicidal thoughts and attempts among adolescent girls in Ethiopia. *Journal of Adolescent Health, 52*(5), 654–656. 10.1016/j.jadohealth.2012.12.007

Gueta, K., Cohen-Leibovich, Y., & Ronel, N. (2020). "Even crap can be fertilizer": The experience of volunteering at sexual assault crisis centers for women survivors of sexual assault. *Feminism & Psychology, 31* (1). 10.1177/0959353520955141

Güneş, M., Selcuk, H., Demir, S., Ibiloglu, A., Bulut, M., Kaya, M., Yilmaz, A., Atli, A., & Sir, A. (2016). Marital harmony and childhood psychological trauma in child marriage. *Journal of Mood Disorders,* 6(2), 63–70. 10.5455/jmood.20160425l0034

Hartley, S., Johnco, C., Hofmeyr, M., & Berry, A. (2016). The nature of posttraumatic growth in adult survivors of child sexual abuse. *Journal of Child Sexual Abuse, 25*(2), 201–220. 10.1080/10538712.2015.1119773

Helgeson, V. S., Reynolds, K. A., & Tomich, P. L. (2006). A meta-analytic review of benefit finding and growth. *Journal of Consulting and Clinical Psychology, 74*(5), 797–816. 10.1037/0022-006x.74.5.797

Hill, L. L. (2017). *Post traumatic growth among African American women survivors of childhood sexual abuse: the roles of spirituality, locus of control, and self-concept* (Unpublished master's thesis). The University of North Carolina at Charlotte (2002342600).

Iustitiani, N. S., & Ajisuksmo, C. R. (2018). Supporting factors and consequences of child marriage. *ANIMA Indonesian Psychological Journal, 33*(2), 100–111. 10.24123/aipj.v33i2.1581

Jackson, C. J. M. (2017). *Women's lived experience of recovery from childhood sexual abuse, and their perception of the role of mental health services* (Unpublished Doctoral dissertation 10767620). Cardiff University.

Kamer, H. (2021, December 1). *Diyarbakır'ın Merkezdeki Tek kadın muhtarı dilek demir: 'Kimsenin çocuk Gelin Olmasına Izin Vermeyeceğim'.* BBC News Türkçe. Retrieved December 2, 2021, from https://www.bbc.com/turkce/haberler-turkiye-59484627

Kasim, B., Cem, U., Mustafa, K., Süleyman, S., İsmail, B., Ubeydullah, D., Yaşar, T., & Süleyman, G. (2015). Evaluation of the early age married girls applying to our department. *Open Journal of Pediatrics, 05*(04), 334–338. 10.4236/ojped.2015.54050

Kidman, R. (2016). Child marriage and intimate partner violence: A comparative study of 34 countries. *International Journal of Epidemiology,* 46(2), 662–675. 10.1093/ije/dyw225

Kirkner, A., & Ullman, S. E. (2019). Sexual assault survivors' post-traumatic growth: Individual and community-level differences. *Violence against Women, 26*(15–16), 1987–2003. 10.1177/1077801219888019

Lev-Wiesel, R. (2008). Child sexual abuse: A critical review of intervention and treatment modalities. *Children and Youth Services Review, 30*(6), 665–673. 10.1016/j.childyouth.2008.01.008

Malatyalı, M. K. (2014). Türkiye'de Çocuk Gelin Sorunu. *Nesne Psikoloji Dergisi.* 2(3), 27–38. DOI: 10.7816/nesne-02-03-03

Montazeri, S., Gharacheh, M., Mohammadi, N., Alaghband Rad, J., & Eftekhar Ardabili, H. (2016). Determinants of early marriage from married girl's perspectives in Iranıan setting: A qualitative study. *Journal of Environmental and Public Health, 2016,* 1–8. 10.1155/2016/8615929

Nanfuka, E., Turyomurugyendo, F., Ochen, E., & Gibbs, G. (2020). Leaving a violent child Marriage: Experiences of adult survivors in Uganda. *Social Sciences*, *9*(10), 172–190. 10.3390/socsci9100172

Nelson, K. M., Hagedorn, W. B., & Lambie, G. W. (2019). Influence of attachment style on sexual abuse survivors' posttraumatic growth. *Journal of Counseling & Development*, *97*(3), 227–237. 10.1002/jcad.12263

Nurmala, I., Astutik, F. N., & Devi, Y. P. (2020). Surrounding the reason for women to continue the tradition of child marriage. *Utopía y Praxis Latinoamericana*, *25*(2), 24–32. 10.5281/zenodo.3808599

Pargament, K. I. (2000). Interventions based in religious congregations. In A. E. Kazdin (Ed.), *Encyclopedia of psychology* (Vol. 4, 359–360). American Psychological Association.

Prescod, D. J., & Zeligman, M. (2018). Career adaptability of trauma survivors: The moderating role of posttraumatic growth. *The Career Development Quarterly*, *66*(2), 107–120. 10.1002/cdq.12126

Sheridan, G., & Carr, A. (2020). Survivors' lived experiences of posttraumatic growth after institutional childhood abuse: An interpretative phenomenological analysis. *Child Abuse & Neglect*, *103*, 104430. 10.1016/j.chiabu.2020.104430

Soylu, N., & Ayaz, M. (2013). Adli değerlendirme için yönlendirilen küçük yaşta evlendirilmiş kız çocuklarının sosyodemografik özellikleri ve ruhsal değerlendirmesi. *Anadolu Psikiyatri Dergisi*, *14*(2), 136–144.

Tedeschi, R. G., & Calhoun, L. G. (1996). The posttraumatic growth inventory: Measuring the positive legacy of trauma. *Journal of Traumatic Stress*, *9*(3), 455–471. 10.1002/jts.2490090305

Tedeschi, C. L., & Calhoun, L. (1998). Posttraumatic growth: Conceptual issues. *Posttraumatic Growth*, 9–30. 10.4324/9781410603401-5

Tedeschi, R. G., & Calhoun, L. G. (2004). Posttraumatic Growth: Conceptual foundations and empirical evidence. *Psychological Inquiry*, *15*(1), 1–18. 10.1207/s15327965pli1501_01

Tenkorang, E. Y. (2019). Explaining the links between child marriage and intimate partner violence: Evidence from Ghana. *Child Abuse & Neglect*, *89*, 48–57. 10.1016/j.chiabu.2019.01.004

UNICEF. (2020, March 11). Child marriage around the world. Retrieved November 19, 2021, from https://www.unicef.org/stories/child-marriage-around-world

UNICEF. (2021a, March 7). *Child marriage*. Retrieved September 27, 2021, from https://www.unicef.org/protection/child-marriage

UNICEF DATA. (2021b, August 16). *Child marriage*. Retrieved September 27, 2021, from https://data.unicef.org/topic/child-protection/child-marriage/

United Nations Human Rights Office of the High Commissioner (UNHR, 1993). *Declaration on the elimination of violence against women*. Retrieved September 27, 2021, from https://www.ohchr.org/en/professionalinterest/pages/violenceagainstwomen.aspx.32. 10.5281/zenodo.3808599

Veenema, T. G., Thornton, C. P., & Corley, A. (2015). The public health crisis of child sexual abuse in low and middle income countries: An integrative review of the literature. *International Journal of Nursing Studies*, *52*(4), 864–881. 10.1016/j.ijnurstu.2014.10.017

Vilenica, S., Shakespeare-Finch, J., & Obst, P. (2013). Exploring the process of meaning making in healing and growth after childhood sexual assault: A case study approach. *Counselling Psychology Quarterly*, *26*(1), 39–54. 10.1080/09515070.2012.728074

Walker-Williams, H. J. (2012). *Coping behaviour, posttraumatic growth and psychological well-being in women who experienced childhood sexual abuse* (Unpublished dissertation) North-West University.

Wodon, Q., Male, C., Onagoruwa, A., Savadogo, A., & Yedan, A. (2017). Child marriage, early child-bearing, low educational attainment for girls, and their impacts in Uganda: The cost of not investing in girls. World Bank, Washington, DC. https://openknowledge.worldbank.org/handle/10986/29039

Wood, K. E. (2009). *Women's narratives of healing from the effects of child sexual abuse* (Dissertation thesis1314614018). Saskatoon: University of Saskatchewan.

Yılmaz, M. & Zara, A. (2016). Traumatic loss and posttraumatic growth: The effect of traumatic loss related factors on posttraumatic growth. *Anadolu Psikiyatri Dergisi*, *17*(1), 5–11. 10.5455/apd.188311

Yount, K. M., Crandall, A. A., Cheong, Y. F., Osypuk, T. L., Bates, L. M., Naved, R. T., & Schuler, S. R. (2016). Child marriage and intimate partner violence in rural Bangladesh: A longitudinal multilevel analysis. *Demography*, *53*(6), 1821–1852. 10.1007/s13524-016-0520-8

Zeligman, M., Grossman, L., & Tanzosh, A. (2019). Posttraumatic growth in trauma survivors: Meaning making and locus of control. *Journal of Counselor Practice*, *10*(2), 1–21. 10.22229/ptg1022019

20

POSTTRAUMATIC GROWTH IN SURVIVORS OF DOMESTIC ABUSE IN SCOTLAND

Julien le Jeune d'Allegeershecque, Breda Cullen, and Clare McFeely

Domestic Abuse (DA) is a worldwide social issue, which affects one in three women (WHO, 2021). DA, also referred to as intimate partner violence (IPV) or intimate terrorism, is defined as "behaviour by an intimate partner or ex-partner that causes physical, sexual or psychological harm, including physical aggression, sexual coercion, psychological abuse and controlling behaviours" (WHO, 2021, *Introduction,* para. 1). DA, therefore, meets the DSM-5 criteria for a traumatic event, as it involves "exposure to actual or threatened death, serious injury, or sexual violence" (APA, 2013, p. *271*), and has been linked to a range of negative psychological and physical outcomes, including Post Traumatic Stress Disorder (PTSD), depression, and physical injuries.

DA may involve exposure to multiple instances of physical, sexual, and psychological abuse over a period of time. The burden of DA is overwhelmingly borne by women, with 30% of women worldwide reporting they have experienced an event of physical or sexual violence by an intimate partner during their lifetime (WHO, 2021). It has been reported that 85% of all violent crimes experienced by women in the United States are cases of DA, compared to only 3% of violent crimes experienced by men (Rennison, 2003). Thus, while men can be victims of DA, it is a social problem, which disproportionately affects women.

While posttraumatic Growth (PTG) has been identified in survivors of DA, there is little research in this area (Anderson et al., 2012). PTG refers to the potential of individuals who have lived through a traumatic event to move beyond a pre-trauma level of functioning (Splevins et al., 2010). Within a PTG framework, a traumatic experience represents a potential catalyst for positive psychological and interpersonal growth (Grubaugh & Resick, 2007). As DA is a pervasive problem, which affects over a million women a year in the UK alone (ONS, 2018), research into how best to promote growth in survivors of DA is vital.

There is little information on the reliability and acceptability of tools used to study PTG in populations of survivors of DA, or on other practical feasibility factors, such as recruitment and support provision. In this chapter, we present a collaborative approach to identifying potential barriers and increasing acceptability, accessibility, and participation in research on PTG in survivors of DA, and emphasize the importance of safeguarding participants.

 DOI: 10.4324/9781032208688-26

Posttraumatic Growth in Survivors of Domestic Abuse: Literature Review

The majority of research into the psychological outcomes of survivors of DA describes the negative impact of living with DA (Grubaugh & Resick, 2007). In the first study to examine quantitatively PTG in survivors of IPV specifically, Cobb and colleagues (2006) studied the correlates of PTG in survivors of IPV in a sample of 60 women utilizing DA shelter services in the United States. Using the Post-Traumatic Growth Inventory (PTGI; Tedeschi & Calhoun, 1996), they found that 67% of the participants reported at least a moderate degree of change, showing that growth was experienced in this sample. The severity of abuse did not appear to be correlated with levels of growth, possibly due to the majority of participants reporting high amounts of abuse as measured by the Index of Spouse Abuse (Hudson & McIntosh, 1981). Grubaugh and Resick (2007) examined PTG in a sample of 100 treatment-seeking female assault victims in the United States. They measured PTG using the PTGI, as well as symptom severity of PTSD and depression. In their sample, 77% of participants reported experiencing at least a moderate degree of positive change. Their results show that there does not appear to be a direct relationship between PTG and posttraumatic distress, meaning that one can, but does not always occur in the presence of the other. In other words, the results of the study support the idea of a "double-track" for PTG and distress and contradict the simplistic understanding that following exposure to a traumatic event, an individual will experience *either* distress *or* growth. However, Grubaugh and Resick did not state how many of the women were victims of violence in the context of DA. Furthermore, the use of the PTGI is problematic since the authors state that this is the first time it was used with this specific population, and that it was not checked for acceptability.

The results of Cobb and colleagues' (2006) and Grubaugh and Resick's (2007) studies are reflected in the findings of a later study by Valdez and Lilly (2015). The study, which was based on a sample of 23 women survivors of IPV from Northern Illinois in the USA, focused on the way in which an individual sees the world and their place within it, and how challenges to these assumptions can influence PTG. The study also measured PTG more generally through the use of the PTGI. In this sample, the mean score on the PTGI was 62.74 (SD = 29.47), equating to a "moderate degree of change." However, the high standard deviation observed highlights the need for further research with larger samples to confirm the results of this study. Furthermore, while the authors of this study discuss ways in which they overcame barriers to participation, such as providing childcare and transportation, there is no mention of the support measures implemented to ensure the safeguarding of the women taking part in the study. Nor is it discussed whether the measures used were piloted for acceptability within the target population.

Qualitative studies have also been undertaken to examine PTG in survivors of DA. A study by Senter and Caldwell (2002), which involved a sample of nine women who had previously been in abusive relationships, found that women who have survived DA reported stronger interpersonal relationships and increased control over their lives, amongst other signs which are seen as demonstrating growth. Again, the methodology of the study does not include any mention of safeguarding measures that ensure the well-being of participants. Anderson, Renner, and Danis (2012) studied recovery and resilience in a sample of 37 women formerly in abusive relationships. Semi-structured interviews focused on the contexts in which participants found solutions, which helped them recover and grow following their experience of DA. These interviews were then analyzed using a grounded theory approach. Although not asked specifically about growth, some women in this study shared experiences of personal growth in the aftermath of an abusive relationship and identified conditions, which enabled them to "recover ***and grow***" (Anderson et al., 2012, p. 1288, *emphasis added*). Spirituality and social support were found to be central to many women's recovery.

The importance of religion and spirituality as factors, which can potentially promote PTG is also reflected in Bloom's (2021) findings. This qualitative study examined PTG in a sample of 30 Latina immigrants who had been exposed to DA and were recruited from a center that provides IPV support services. The results of the study showed that after experiencing IPV, participants reported changes in their faith, including a "deepening" of their relationship with God and experiencing growth through regular prayer practice. Once again, the study does not discuss the safeguarding of participants in the study design or implementation.

Research has also been undertaken on factors and opportunities, which facilitate PTG in survivors of DA (Burnette, 2018; Brosi et al., 2020; D'Amore et al., 2018; Mushonga et al., 2020). These studies were all qualitative in nature and utilized semi-structured interviews. The factors highlighted in these studies include cultural values, which promote non-violence (Burnette, 2018) and motherhood (Mushonga et al., 2020). In these studies, these factors were found to promote resilience in survivors of DA, therefore fostering an environment in which PTG was more likely to take place.

The studies discussed above illustrate gaps in the study of PTG in the context of DA. First, there are few studies to date. Furthermore, in the three quantitative studies on PTG and DA, the PTGI was not checked for acceptability, which is especially important considering the vulnerability of the population being studied. Obtaining information as to the acceptability of the measures used in these studies would allow for the relevance of the items included in the measures to be confirmed, as well as to identify aspects of PTG that may not be included in the measure. Further, the studies summarized above also give little information as to the ethical issues which are involved in this field, and the steps taken by the authors to ensure safeguarding of the participants. However, the evidence-base which has resulted from these studies is promising.

A Pilot Study of PTG in DA Survivors in Scotland

This section discusses a pilot study of PTG in DA violence survivors in Scotland, which attempted to address challenges in the research to date.

Overview of the Study

We describe a mixed-methods design used to explore PTG in female survivors of DA living in the West of Scotland in order to provide information and guidelines for future research on this topic in this specific population. The study design and methodology were developed based on the guidelines presented in the WHO's Ethical and Safety Recommendations for Intervention Research on Violence against Women (2016).

The study involved two phases: a planning phase and a data-collection phase. Both phases were delivered in partnership with a community-based local Non-Governmental Organisation (NGO) which specializes in supporting survivors of DA. Two local services operating in the west of Scotland were involved in running the study.

During the planning phase, two members of staff from each of the local services were recruited to be interviewed. The aim of this phase of the project was to identify potential challenges, which may arise in involving survivors of DA in research focusing on PTG. One of the key topics considered during this phase was the safeguarding of survivors of DA during data collection. These staff members had professional experience in working with and providing support to survivors of DA and were therefore well-positioned to provide useful and actionable recommendations. Through the interviews, staff members provided feedback regarding the study materials and other logistic aspects planned to be implemented as part of the data collection. The interviews were transcribed and analyzed in order to highlight insight and suggestions, which required a change ahead of the second phase of the project.

Once the changes and other recommendations had been implemented, the data-collection phase was carried out. Potential participants were recruited from the organizational partner's service users. Staff members were asked to identify and contact service users who they thought were eligible and may be interested in participating in the study. Once recruited, participants were asked to complete a data-collection "pack", which included a socio-demographic questionnaire, a question whether the participant could identify an "anchor point" (i.e., could they remember a point from before they experienced abuse to which they could compare their current self), the Psychological-Wellbeing – Post-Traumatic Changes Questionnaire (PWB-PTCQ; Joseph et al., 2012), an open-ended questionnaire on PTG, and acceptability questionnaires. A summary of the main contributions of the study to the evidence-base on researching PTG in survivors DA is provided below. This study will then be used to illustrate and explain the recommendations we make in the section aiming to provide guidance to researchers who wish to study PTG in survivors of DA.

Contributions of the Study to the Evidence-Base

The study provided an important contribution to understanding effective processes for collaborating with third-sector organizations or non-governmental organizations to design feasible, acceptable, and accessible research with survivors of domestic abuse. The study demonstrated a feasible research design, which investigates PTG in female survivors of DA as well as confirmed the acceptability and internal reliability of the PWB-PTCQ for use with women survivors of DA. Furthermore, the study provided some insight as to aspects of the materials used and of the study design, which could be modified in future research, such as including a narrative interview-based approach to support the quantitative data.

The study showed that it is possible to work in partnership with specialist NGOs to conduct research on PTG in the context of DA. Establishing an effective working partnership with an NGO partner facilitated recruitment and strengthened the study design, as well as ensuring the ethical principles of nonmaleficence, beneficence, and confidentiality.

Recommendations for Effective and Acceptable Research on PTG in DA Survivors

The aforementioned study offers recommendations for conducting research about PTG in the context of DA. One of the principal recommendations, which can be made in light of the results of the study is that, when possible, researchers conducting studies on PTG in survivors of DA should try to work in collaboration with NGOs operating in the field of DA as such collaboration offers multiple benefits discussed below.

Access to Participants and to Experts

Creating a partnership with a specialized organization facilitates access to survivors of DA as well as provides access to staff members who can share their professional expertise.

Effective Dissemination of Findings

The link between organizations and researchers provides avenues for the dissemination of research findings beyond traditional academic pathways. For example, findings can be shared within the organization via newsletters or simply communication between staff members, who can then share the findings with other relevant stakeholders working in the field of DA. This approach allows for a direct link to be created between the researchers, the organizational partner, and by extension the organization's service users. As a result, collaboration with a third-sector organization provides participants with a clear pathway to accessing the results of the study they were involved in. Evidence suggests that women survivors of abuse often find participating in research on abuse to be a beneficial experience (Becker-Blease & Freyd, 2006; Newman et al., 1999). Furthermore, it has been reported that women survivors of DA often want to help other survivors of DA once they have exited their abusive relationship as a way of finding greater purpose within their life (Anderson et al., 2012). Ensuring that survivors can access the results of the studies they are involved in is therefore important, as it can further encourage PTG. It is thus strongly recommended that future researchers should try and work in partnership with specialized NGOs, as this facilitates both the design and delivery of ethical research and the communication of relevant study results to stakeholders in the field of DA, with the survivors themselves being a key sub-set of this group. This collaboration could also lead to faster and more effective implementation of recommendations resulting from academic research in third-sector practices (Hardwick et al., 2015).

Safeguarding

Working in partnership with an NGO allowed for safeguarding measures to be built into the study design. Accessing the organizational partner's service users meant that there was no need to screen potential participants for exposure to DA, as being a service user implied that the participant was a survivor. The use of screening tools to measure exposure to DA can be a distressing experience, as it forces participants to relive the abuse they were subjected to. The inclusion of a preliminary phase in which staff members with professional expertise screened the tools and planned methodology allowed for potential problems to be resolved before the service users interacted with the study materials, and the study in general. Indeed, the feedback from the staff members during the preparation phase accurately anticipated the service users' experience during the feasibility study. For example, the staff members believed that all of the participants would be able to identify an "anchor point" as part of the second phase of the study, and indeed, all 13 participants were able to identify an anchor point.

Working with Women's Aid ensured that staff members had the necessary training and professional experience to provide support to participants before, during, and after the study, which is in line with recommended practice when researching sensitive issues

(Bergen, 1993; Liamputtong, 2007). Ensuring that adequate support was made available to survivors was an important aspect of safeguarding participants, and contributed to the creation of an environment that could potentially encourage PTG. Collaboration with the partner organization's staff members in the planning phase ensured that the context in which survivors would take part in the study was as safe as possible. Furthermore, using feedback from the survivors to improve the design and methods used in future research in the field was potentially empowering for survivors.

The collaboration with the service organization also created challenges, specifically overcoming sampling bias resulting from the role of staff members from the partner organization in identifying potential participants and ensuring accessibility. It is understandable why staff members were reluctant to involve certain service users in the study, as they were considered too vulnerable to cope with the potential distress. As the partner organization has a duty of care toward its service users, it took this cautious approach. However, from an ethical point of view, these service users have just as much a right to take part in research as service users who are less vulnerable. To ensure accessibility, future studies focusing on PTG in survivors of DA should include choices, which are made available to all service users, so that they are able to decide for themselves whether they are able to take part in research. Ensuring that a range of options are available increases the accessibility of the study.

A second major recommendation that emerged from discussions with staff members was that the root of all decisions should be the survivor. Ensuring that participants were in control in terms of *how* they took part in the study was also designed to potentially promote empowerment in the group of survivors who participated in the research. The participants were provided choices in terms of the following:

Location

Participants could decide if they wished to complete the study at home, in the offices of the organizational partner, or in another location of their choice.

Support

Participants could decide if a staff member would be present in the room while they completed the data-collection pack, if a staff member would be available nearby should support be necessary but not present in the room, or if no support was requested.

Method of Participation

Participants could decide between completing a paper copy of the data-collection pack or completing it online.

It is important to note that participants were made aware of pathways to access support even in cases where they did not identify any specific support requirements. Loss of control is a key part of the experience of domestic abuse; thus providing these choices to participants could potentially promote empowerment in the context of the study.

The inclusion of choices in the study design was important because it increased the accessibility of the study and could potentially promote the empowerment of survivors of DA and also. Indeed, across all 13 participants, each option within each category was chosen at least once. Employing a similar approach in future studies would allow for issues relating to the study materials and the study design to be modified to minimize the potential for distress once survivors become actively involved in the study and have the potential to empower participants and promote PTG.

As the study was organized in collaboration with a third-sector organization, and participants were recruited among the service users of the partner organization, it is important to consider the potential for implied coercion. Indeed, as participants were individuals who were using, or had previously used, the services provided by the partner organization, it is possible that potential participants may feel that participation in the study is obligatory, and that continuation of the support they receive from the organization may be contingent on participation. In order to address this, it was made clear in the participant information sheet that participation was fully voluntary and that participants were free to exit the study at any stage. However, future studies may benefit from being even clearer on this topic and making it explicit that not taking part in the study will have absolutely no impact on the service they are receiving from the partner organization.

A third recommendation is using a narrative approach to study PTG because it allows survivors to talk about their experiences with more freedom, as they are not restricted by pre-set expectations of what PTG-related outcomes are. While the research showed that the PWB-PTCQ was relevant to the sample population and reflective of their experiences, it also showed that it did not fully encompass aspects of PTG as reflected in comments made by the participants. One participant stated that "while the statements were valid, [the questionnaire] may not completely reflect the extent of post-traumatic growth experienced by the person later in life." Another participant commented that "bunching up [their] feelings of life into a 5-number scale was inaccurate to say the least, […] after dealing with abuse the turmoil of feelings cannot be confined to a number scale." Future studies could therefore employ a mixed-methods approach, in which the results from the PWB-PTCQ are supplemented by qualitative data recorded using a narrative approach. In recent years, researchers have effectively used narrative and ethnographic approaches to examine factors that mediate PTG in survivors of DA (Burnette, 2018; D'Amore et al., 2018; Mushonga et al., 2020).

The use of a narrative approach also allows for a greater acknowledgment of the role of contextual factors in shaping PTG in survivors of DA, including culture (Bent-Goodley, 2007), sexuality (Counselman-Carpenter & Redcay, 2018; Donovan & Hester, 2014), and gender (Perryman & Appleton, 2016). While the concept of PTG is cross-cultural in nature, the aspects of PTG, which are presented in measures such as the PWB-PTCQ represent a Westernized conception of PTG and may not be applicable cross-culturally. Therefore, it seems plausible that the way in which survivors of DA experience growth and the factors which may promote it may also vary across cultures. A cross-cultural approach to studying PTG in survivors of DA would be beneficial to the field. It is also important for future studies to look at the experiences of survivors of DA in relationships with diverse sexualities. Evidence suggests that the experience of heterosexual relationships is not representative of same-sex relationships, in both the experience of abuse and access to support (Donovan & Hester, 2014). This highlights further the importance of recognizing diversity and acknowledging the role it can play in mediating the experiences of PTG. Building our understanding of the influence of these mediating factors could provide a foundation on which to examine the role intersectionality plays in shaping PTG following exposure to DA.

Acknowledgments

We would like to thank the staff members and service users from East Ayrshire Women's Aid and South Ayrshire Women's Aid for their help in planning this project and for participating in this research.

References

American Psychiatric Association (2013). *Diagnostic and statistical manual of mental disorders: DSM-5* (5th ed). Arlington, VA.

Anderson, K. M., Renner, L. M., & Danis, F. S. (2012). Recovery: Resilience and growth in the aftermath of domestic violence. *Violence against Women*, *18*(11), 1279–1299. 10.1177/1077801212470543

Becker-Blease, K. A., & Freyd, J. J. (2006). Research participants telling the truth about their lives: The ethics of asking and not asking about abuse. *American Psychologist*, *61*(3), 218–226. 10.1037/0003-066X.61.3.218

Bent-Goodley, T. B. (2007). Health disparities and violence against women: Why and how cultural and societal influences matter. *Trauma, Violence & Abuse*, *8*(2), 90–104. 10.1177/1524838007301160

Bergen, R. K. (1993). Interviewing survivors of marital rape: Doing feminist research on sensitive topics. In R. M. Lee, & C. M. Renzetti, (Eds.), *Researching sensitive topics* (pp. 197–211). SAGE Publications Ltd.

Bloom, A., (2021). Faith in the future: Posttraumatic growth through evangelical Christianity for immigrant survivors of intimate partner violence. *Medical Anthropology*, *40*(7), 626–638. 10.1080/01459740.2020.1860961

Brosi, M., Rolling, E., Gaffney, C., & Kitch, B. (2020). Beyond resilience: Glimpses into women's posttraumatic growth after experiencing intimate partner violence. *The American Journal of Family Therapy*, *48*(1), 1–15. 10.1080/01926187.2019.1691084

Burnette, C. E., (2018). Family and cultural protective factors as the bedrock of resilience and growth for Indigenous women who have experienced violence. *Journal of Family Social Work*, *21*(1), 45–62. 10.1080/10522158.2017.1402532

Cobb, A. R., Tedeschi, R. G., Calhoun, L. G., & Cann, A. (2006). Correlates of posttraumatic growth in survivors of intimate partner violence. *Journal of Traumatic Stress* *19*(6), 895–903. 10.1002/jts.20171

Counselman-Carpenter, E., & Redcay, A. (2018). Mining for posttraumatic growth (PTG) in sexual minority women who survive intimate partner violence: A conceptual perspective. *Behavioural Sciences*, *8*(9), 77. 10.3390/bs8090077

D'Amore, C., Martin, S. L., Wood, K., & Brooks, C. (2018). Themes of healing and posttraumatic growth in women survivors' narratives of intimate partner violence. *Journal of Interpersonal Violence*, *36*(5-6), NP2697–NP2724. 10.1177/0886260518767909

Donovan, C., & Hester, M. (2014). *Domestic violence and sexuality: What's love got to do with it?* Policy Press.

Grubaugh, A. L., & Resick, P. A. (2007). Posttraumatic growth in treatment-seeking female assault victims. *Psychiatric Quarterly*, *78*(2), 145–155. 10.1007/s11126-006-9034-7

Hardwick, R., Anderson, R., & Cooper, C. (2015). How do third sector organisations use research and other knowledge? A systematic scoping review. *Implementation Science*, *10* (1), 1–12. 10.1186/s13012-015-0265-6

Hudson, W. W., & McIntosh, S. R. (1981). The assessment of spouse abuse: Two quantifiable dimensions. *Journal of Marriage and Family*, *43*(4), 873–885. 10.2307/351344

Joseph, S., Maltby, J., Wood, A. M., Stockton, H., Hunt, N., & Regel, S., 2012. The Psychological Well-Being-Post-Traumatic Changes Questionnaire (PWB-PTCQ): Reliability and validity. *Psychological Trauma: Theory, Research, Practice and Policy*, *4*(4), 420–428. 10.1037/a0024740

Liamputtong, P. (2007). *Researching the vulnerable*. SAGE.

Mushonga, D. R., Rasheem, S., & Anderson, D. (2020). And still I rise: Resilience factors contributing to posttraumatic growth in African American women. *Journal of Black Psychology*, *47*(2-3), 151–176. 10.1177/0095798420979805

Newman, E., Walker, E. A., & Gefland, A. (1999). Assessing the ethical costs and benefits of trauma-focused research. *General Hospital Psychiatry*, *21*(3), 187–196. 10.1016/S0163-8343(99)00011-0

Office for National Statistics (ONS, 2018). *Domestic abuse in England and Wales: Year ending March 2018*. London: UK. [Available at: https://www.ons.gov.uk/peoplepopulationandcommunity/crimeandjustice/bulletins/domesticabuseinenglandandwales/yearendingmarch2018] (accessed 17.03.21).

Perryman, S. M. & Appleton, J. (2016). Male victims of domestic abuse: Implications for health visiting practice. *Journal of Research in Nursing*, *21*(5-6), 386–414. 10.1177/1744987116653785

Rennison, C. M. (2003). *Intimate partner violence*, 1993-2001. Department of Justice Bureau of Justice Statistics.

Senter, K. E., & Caldwell, K. (2002). Spirituality and the maintenance of change: A phenomenological study of women who leave abusive relationships. *Contemporary Family Therapy*, *24*(4), 543–564. 10.1023/A:1021269028756

Splevins, K., Cohen, K., Bowley, J., & Joseph, S., (2010). Theories of post-traumatic growth: Cross-cultural perspectives. *Journal of Loss and Trauma*, *15*(3), 259–277. 10.1080/15325020903382111

Tedeschi, R. G., & Calhoun, L. G. (1996). The Post-Traumatic Growth Inventory: Measuring the positive legacy of trauma. *Journal of Traumatic Stress*, *9*(3), 455–471. 10.1007/BF02103658

Valdez, C. E., & Lilly, M. M. (2015). Posttraumatic growth in survivors of intimate partner violence: An assumptive world process. *Journal of Interpersonal Violence*, *30*(2), 215–231. 10.1177/0886260514533154

World Health Organisation (2016). *Ethical and safety recommendations for intervention research on violence against women*. World Health Organisation.

World Health Organisation (2021). *Violence against women*. Geneva: WHO. [Available at: http://www.who.int/news-room/fact-sheets/detail/violence-against-women] (accessed 02.11.21).

21

PERINATAL BEREAVEMENT AND POSTTRAUMATIC GROWTH

Research Findings and Clinical Implications

Olga O. Thomadaki

Of all major life stressors, the death of a child has been identified as the most grievous of losses (Braun & Berg, 1994; Klass, 1986–87; Sanders, 1980). Literature suggests that non-normative ("off-time"), violent or unnatural deaths, and sudden, unexpected losses are more likely to precipitate longer and more intense grief reactions (Currier et al., 2006; Stroebe & Schut, 2005). These losses combine the characteristics of both grief and trauma reactions (Neria & Litz, 2003; Rubin et al., 2003), causing people to embark on a process of searching to find meaning and trying to rebuild a shattered life. This chapter presents definitions and statistics on perinatal bereavement, reviews available research findings on PTG and perinatal bereavement, and discusses the clinical implications of PTG for therapists working with perinatally bereaved parents.

Definitions, Prevalence, and Impact of Perinatal Death

Definitions of what is considered a stillbirth and a neonatal death differ; however, both stillbirths and neonatal deaths constitute *perinatal deaths*. According to the World Health Organization (WHO), perinatal mortality refers to the number of stillbirths i.e., a baby born with no signs of life at or after 28 weeks' gestation and deaths in the first week of life. However, in the UK, babies are considered stillborn when they are born dead after 24 weeks of gestation, while before this mark they are labeled as *miscarriages*. Death within the first four weeks of life is defined as a *neonatal death*, while in later weeks it is labeled as *infant death*. The lack of agreement over the definition of these losses is possibly indicative of the limited attention they have received.

In 2009, there were 2.6 million stillbirths globally with more than 8200 of them occurring on any single day. Among the 133 million babies born alive each year, 2.8 million die in the first week of life with 265.000 stillbirths (3.5 per 1000 births) happening in high-income countries (Flenady et al., 2016). When compared with the leading global causes of death in all age categories, all-cause stillbirths rank fifth among the global health burdens- before diarrhea, HIV/AIDS, tuberculosis, traffic accidents, and any form of cancer (Frøen et al., 2011).

In spite of its prevalence, stillbirth has received limited public attention. Comparing how often the media have covered AIDS-related deaths to perinatal deaths, it becomes apparent

DOI: 10.4324/9781032208688-27

that it may not be the numbers that draw public attention to certain problems. Reducing the number of stillbirths was never included in the Millennium Development Goals of the United Nations, unlike the reduction of infant deaths. In April 2011, the widely respected medical journal The Lancet launched a series of articles on stillbirth (www.thelancet.com/series/stillbirth) and returned to the topic in 2016 (de Bernis et al., 2016) in a series titled "ending preventable deaths," in which the editor-in-chief, Richard Horton (2013; the Lancet, 2011, 00:25), commented that "stillbirth has been a neglected, marginalized, and stigmatized issue" and that is "bizarre and wrong".

Despite the common occurrence of perinatal loss, current society and the media promote the message that good maternal health, proper prenatal care, and modern medical science ensure perfect babies. A perinatal death is often an isolating, marginalizing experience for parents and there exists a social discrepancy in the degree to which grief after the death of a stillborn or a newborn child is legitimate, as opposed to the death of an older child (Cacciatore & Bushfield, 2008). This may intensify, complicate or even prolong grief (Doka, 1989). Doka (1989) introduced the term *disenfranchised grief*, which refers to grief that "persons experience when they incur a loss that is not or cannot be openly acknowledged, publicly mourned, or socially supported" (p. 4), a definition that captures the experience of the vast majority of perinatally bereaved parents. In the case of a perinatal loss, especially of firstborns, the parents usually are not perceived by society as "real" parents, and the death, as well as their relationship with the baby, are disenfranchised, as society fails or is unwilling to acknowledge this as the death of a real person (Corr, 1998–9; Doka, 1989).

That society fails to recognize those parent's parental identity is related to the difficulty to recognize the "person" identity of unborn children, resulting in the discouragement of open grieving for this type of loss (Cacciatore & Bushfield, 2008; Keefe-Cooperman, 2004; Layne, 2003; Uren & Wastell, 2002). The social status of a fetus is central to public and scientific debates on abortion, genetic research, in-vitro fertilization, and the legal status of an unborn child, when issues of abortion or protection from drug and alcohol-abusive mothers are raised (Heriot, 1996; Layne, 2003; Morgan, 2002). The definitions of life and death depend on social and cultural criteria (Kovit, 1978); however, the social debates of who is a person that deserves to be mourned and who is not, are not always relevant to the needs of a traumatized parent who has lost a newborn or an unborn wanted child unexpectedly.

PTG and Perinatal Parental Bereavement

While research has sporadically reported positive outcomes or growth after parental bereavement (Braun & Berg, 1994; Davis et al., 2000; Lehman et al., 1987; Lehman et al., 1993; Miles & Crandall, 1983; Moulton Milo, 1997; Riley et al., 2007; Wheeler, 2001), knowledge about this type of bereavement is relatively limited. In early 2021, a search in the PsychInfo database for the keyword *Posttraumatic Growth* yielded 2.320 journal articles and book chapters, whereas for *Bereavement and PTG* the number was lowered to 137 (including a model presentation of PTG and Grief by Calhoun et al. in 2010 and a systematic literature review by Michael & Cooper in 2013). The search for *Parental Bereavement and PTG* yielded 14 entries (Albuqueque et al., 2018; Bogensperger & Lueger- Schuster, 2014; Calhoun et al., 2000; Calhoun & Tedeschi, 1989–90; Davis et al., 2007; Engelkemeyer & Marwit, 2008; Gerrish et al., 2010; Martinčeková & Klatt, 2017; Moore et al., 2015; Pan et al., 2016; Polatinsky & Esprey, 2000; Waugh et al., 2018; Xiu et al., 2018; Znoj & Keller, 2002).

Literature exploring positive changes and PTG of bereaved parents after a perinatal loss, although very limited, comes from across the globe. The vast majority of studies on perinatally bereaved parents reported parallel processes of ongoing mourning, yearning, and pain, but also positive changes and growth. For example, an Australian survey of 109 perinatally bereaved mothers, two months to 17 years after their loss, reported an ongoing emotional bond with the deceased child irrespective of the time elapsed since the loss, and a predominance and perseverance of acute emotional experiences of yearning and despair (Uren & Wastell, 2002). The authors concluded that common conceptualizations of bereavement recovery are simplistic and misplaced and that the term bereavement adaptation or resolution might be more appropriate. In agreement with Janoff-Bulman's (1992) assumptive world model, perinatal loss appeared to shatter the mothers' sense of invulnerability and elicited typical responses to loss when an attachment has been achieved and lost, experiencing yearning and despair; however, they also reported a perception of favorable changes in mothers' self-identity as they were able to see themselves as stronger or wiser, a finding that supports the development of PTG in perinatally bereaved parents.

Büchi and colleagues (2007) in Switzerland, assessed grief, depression, anxiety, and PTG of 54 bereaved parents, two to six years after an early stillbirth (24–26 weeks of gestation). The results revealed that 80% of the parents were still experiencing grief for their dead baby, with mothers having higher scores on this measure. Despite the grief reactions, 78% of the mothers and 44% of the fathers had high scores on the subscale of *appreciation of life* (changed priorities) of the PTGI measure of PTG (Tedeschi & Calhoun, 1996). Furthermore, there were significant gender-based differences both on grief intensity and PTG with the majority of mothers (63–67%) compared to 30–40% of the fathers scoring high in all other four subscales of the PTGI (*relating to others*, *personal strength*, *spiritual change*, *new possibilities*). In agreement with Calhoun and colleagues (2000) who concluded that high-intensity grief and trauma reactions are not inhibiting nor excluding the possibility of PTG, Büchi and colleagues (2007) reported that parents' suffering was largely determined by the severity of their grief but minimally influenced by their personal growth following the death of their baby.

Thomadaki (2012, 2017) in the UK used Interpretative Phenomenological Analysis (Smith et al., 2009) to explore how mothers experience personal growth after a perinatal loss. She conducted eight semi-structured interviews with women who had lost their firstborn baby perinatally, 18 months to eight years following the loss. The analysis revealed four super-ordinate themes including the traumatic qualities of this type of bereavement, the multiple losses involved, coping mechanisms that participants activated to work through their loss, and positive changes following the experience. Positive changes were growth as an affirmation of the baby's importance and as an outcome of the awareness of personal vulnerability. Participants reported transformations in self-perception (self-worth and self-efficacy), attitude (appreciation of life and changed priorities), and relationships (empathy and companionship).

Krosch and Shakespeare-Finch (2017) conducted an online survey in Australia with 328 women in perinatal loss support groups, including women who had suffered both miscarriages and stillbirths, with four years mean time since their loss. The study found that women reported moderate levels of both PTG and posttraumatic stress (PTSD) symptoms. Perinatal grief scores significantly predicted both PTSD and PTG, while core belief disruptions played a significant role in post-trauma outcomes confirming Calhoun et al.'s (2010) claim that for growth to be experienced, the individual needs to be deeply affected by the loss and their struggle to rebuild their world may give rise to growth.

In 2018, Cacciatore and colleagues in the United States, used a subset of earlier data (Cacciatore et al., 2018), to analyze the answers of 39 parents about choosing to do volunteer work after their babies' perinatal death, and the parents' scores on the PTGI. They found that those who had started volunteering after their perinatal loss had significantly higher scores on PTGI than those who did not, indicating that volunteering could be a behavioral expression of growth.

In spite of its aforementioned sparsity, empirical evidence in the last two decades across the globe is consistently showing that PTG in perinatally bereaved parents is possible and high-intensity grief reactions can be a positive predictor of it. Parents who suffer the most, experience their loss as seismic, and engage in deliberate rumination, actively trying to reconstruct meaning in their lives, are the ones who might experience PTG, and the most important mediator for that has been found to be the quality of social support (Ozer et al., 2003; Polatinsky & Esprey, 2000; Prati & Pietrantoni, 2009; Taku et al., 2009). Consequently, psychotherapists can play a catalytic role in supporting parents to work through feelings of shame, guilt, and despair, construct meaning, and integrate the traumatic event into their life narrative.

PTG in Psychotherapy

Traditional schools of psychotherapy do not explicitly address growth as a part or goal of psychological interventions. Since World War II, psychology has been dominated and absorbed by the medical model of treating illnesses and damage (Seligman & Csikszentmihalyi, 2000). Clients are commonly referred to as suffering from distressing symptoms, negative emotions, or impaired functionality affecting their interpersonal, social, and professional lives. Thus, the focus of their treatment is on alleviating symptoms, to allow the person to return to a "normal" pre-crisis level of functioning.

Theorists of the humanistic-existential schools of thought, like Rogers (1951), Frankl (1969), and Yalom (1980), have addressed growth implicitly through closely related phenomena and terminologies, such as becoming self-actualized, finding meaning, or being transformed through adversity and trauma. Rollo May (1981) discussed the transformative power of trauma "... giving up the delusion of false hopes [...] Then and only then can this person begin to rebuild himself" (p. 236). Since most individuals seek psychotherapy after or while they are going through some sort of crisis or trauma, which they perceive as exceeding their coping capacity, it is reasonable to consider growth as an integral part of psychotherapy.

With the emergence of the Positive Psychology paradigm, the last two decades, have witnessed developments in psychodynamic (Zoellner & Maercker, 2006) and cognitive behavioral therapies (CBT) with recent therapy manuals addressing growth as a treatment goal for depression (Karwoski et al., 2006), posttraumatic stress disorder (Schubert et al., 2019; Zoellner et al., 2011), and grief (Bartl et al., 2018; Wagner et al., 2007).

Joseph and Linley (2006; Joseph, 2004; Linley & Joseph, 2004), Calhoun and Tedeschi (1998; 1999; Tedeschi & Calhoun, 2004b; Tedeschi et al., 2015) have offered advice for a clinical application of their theories as traditional grief counseling has been criticized repeatedly, both theoretically and empirically, for being possibly ineffective (Allumbaugh & Hoyt, 1999; Jordan & Neimeyer, 2003). When working with traumatically bereaved individuals, therapists ought to realize that trauma does not necessarily lead to psychopathology and damaged lives and to be aware of the possibility of growth after struggling with a traumatic event. Both of these realizations do not question the psychological distress resulting from trauma, nor do they suggest that all trauma survivors should or can experience growth because dismissing the distress of trauma survivors and forcing them to experience growth can have detrimental effects on their psychological well-being (Calhoun & Tedeschi, 1999; Joseph & Linley, 2006; Tennen & Affleck, 1999).

The organismic valuing theory of growth (Joseph & Linley, 2005, 2008) and the person-centered model (Rogers, 1951) postulate that traumatized individuals actualize their innate tendency for growth and reach personal growth when provided the appropriate environment that facilitates rather than impedes this process. Psychotherapists are supposed to provide their clients with such a social environment, realize that growth is a very gradual and slow process, and respect each client's personal needs of time. Additionally, Joseph (2004) underlines the need for therapists to understand that, regardless of their personal desire to facilitate change, they should not take the responsibility for trauma resolution away from their clients' hands. Accordingly, Calhoun and Tedeschi (1999) underline that therapists can provide a therapeutic context conducive to PTG, but PTG can only be achieved by the clients themselves.

Parental bereavement is a very long journey (Gerrish et al., 2010), requiring therapists to accompany parents on this long path to resolution whereas short-term therapy may not be appropriate for bereaved parents. As this is not always possible because of setting restrictions (e.g., managed public care), clinicians might at least try to spread out the number of sessions allowed in their setting to accommodate the needs of bereaved parents.

PTG in Psychotherapy for Perinatally Bereaved Parents

Following a perinatal loss, the initial stage of establishing a relationship between the bereaved parents and the therapist is crucial. Tedeschi and Calhoun (2004b) provided a general framework for interventions and emphasized major differences between bereaved parents and other client groups. Although bereaved parents may appear in therapy to be in great psychological distress, in most cases, they were psychologically healthy individuals before their loss. Consequently, the clinician should be able to trust them to find their own way to grieve and survive, rather than proceed to various psychopathology-centered psychological interventions. However, treatment approaches focusing on trauma might well be an integral part of psychotherapy for bereaved parents. Especially important are the therapeutic stance, safeguarding social support, working with cultural and religious influences, and, adopting a growth perspective.

The Therapeutic Stance

A therapist working with perinatally bereaved parents needs to fundamentally accept and respect the deceased fetus or newborn as a person and their clients as bereaved parents with the right to mourn. Therapists need to be aware of the special characteristics and the traumatic qualities of this loss where the non-birthing parent in both types of neonatal death witnesses the unexpected death of their child, which is the traumatic exposure that is the starting point of parental bereavement. Mothers who experienced a stillbirth meet all criteria for trauma exposure as they unexpectedly learn that their assumed healthy baby is dead and their lives are in increased danger during the delivery of a dead baby (RCOG, 2010), while they witness an event that involves death; mothers experiencing a neonatal death witness the unexpected death of their newborn baby although their own life is not in danger.

Mothers who lost their baby to stillbirth can be considered a highly traumatized group because, in addition to the conditions of their potentially traumatic loss, they may be exposed to additional iatrogenic trauma due to ineffective and insensitive hospital practices (Cacciatore et al., 2009; Thomadaki, 2012; Trulsson & Rädestad, 2004). Because hospital practices vary greatly, therapists need to explore, acknowledge and consider them.

The central clinical stance for practitioners serving bereaved parents is that of an *expert companion*, who downplays professional clinical expertise (Tedeschi & Calhoun, 2004b; Tedeschi et al., 2015). This stance may promote safety and trust in individuals, who have often felt avoided, isolated, misunderstood, and in great despair related to the unnatural loss of their children. In accordance with the suggested therapeutic stance and assuming that bereaved parents are psychologically healthy individuals, rather than being directive, the therapist should be open to the parents' expectations and suggestions of what is helpful to them in therapy. Providing very structured sessions following any specific psychotherapeutic approach might not be the type of therapy that a bereaved parent needs or finds helpful.

As a companion, the therapist can offer parents what their social environment has often denied them by staying with them as they talk about their children's lives and deaths. The therapist must seek to learn the special meanings and qualities that the life and death of their clients' children hold for the parents and the circumstances surrounding the death to allow parents to feel safer when the clinician wants to know about their children and respects their memory. Parents should be encouraged to help the therapists know their children by inviting the sharing of pictures, videos, and stories (Tedeschi & Calhoun, 2004b). This might be especially important for parents of stillborn babies who typically cannot share pictures of their dead fetus with their social networks nor display them in their living room. In the perinatal loss, keepsakes can serve as evidence of the existence of their babies and enhance grief rituals, thus embracing whatever parents want to share from their baby (lock of hair, hand or footprint, pictures). Inviting such sharing is an essential gesture of acceptance and respect by the therapist whereas the lack of keepsakes can be harmful for parents, as their existence can have prophylactic effects on their psychological well-being (Rädestad et al., 1996). The therapist who comments on the looks of the baby in the pictures might offer parents a chance to feel pride in their baby, potentially helping them rebuild their sense of self-worth.

Many therapists are unaware of the medical procedures involved in perinatal death and allowing parents to explain their personal journey may assist the therapist in understanding the particular experience of each client. An expert companion allows parents the space to talk about their loss, acknowledge its importance, does not rush them to move on and have other babies, as their social contexts often do, and does not end the conversation with an uncomfortable silence, or avoids them altogether. Because perinatally bereaved parents often experience a great incongruence between the intensity of their grief and the limited societal acknowledgment and validation of that grief, the presence of an expert companion provides the needed validation, allowing parents a space to comprehend their loss and work through its traumatic aspects. Parental deliberate rumination is essential for grief and trauma resolution, and the therapeutic context can offer a facilitating environment for this process (Calhoun, Tedeschi et al., 2000).

As an expert companion, the therapist should focus on being a fully present listener, since it is essential for the parent to feel free to talk about all the details of their loss.

Although most clinicians feel compelled to intervene and reduce the emotional distress, or to solve a problem, Tedeschi and Calhoun (2004b) suggest that passivity adopted by therapists is a building block towards growth. They further suggest that "... therapists will be most effective when they listen in a way that allows them to be changed by their clients' experience rather than being intent on promoting certain changes in the client" (Calhoun & Tedeschi, 2007, p. 168). This kind of respect for the bereaved parent is powerful. When clinicians acknowledge their limitations, and provide their full attention, they acknowledge at the same time how profound this loss is and how much it takes to endure it, thus providing recognition of parents' struggle. When therapists are willing to learn and be changed, they value the parental experience and allow the legacy of the dead baby to touch them as well.

Safeguarding Social Support

Tedeschi and Calhoun (2004b) prompted therapists to initially explore and identify the primary groups of reference and support that parents have and later proceed in exploring any behavioral or attitudinal changes in those groups that parents experience. A clinician should know who are those close to the bereaved parents, to whom they can turn for emotional or material support, and whose opinion and advice they value for what reasons. This information might be especially valuable because the therapist thus becomes aware of sources of influence apart from therapy, as well as the direction towards which these sources push the bereaved parents. Encouraging clients to proactively explore the consequences of change on their relationships with important others might further empower them to take responsibility for their change, weigh the consequences, and be prepared for them.

Through therapy, perinatally bereaved parents might become able to realize who can and is willing to support them, who is not, and decide which actions they want to take in order to receive the support they need, and how to remove sources causing additional distress. Research has shown that helping bereaved parents identify their social support group and encouraging them to reach out and seek that support, might be a catalytic step towards growth (Cacciatore et al., 2009; Prati & Pietrantoni, 2009; Taku et al., 2009; Thomadaki, 2012). Tedeschi and Calhoun (2004b) strongly urge clinicians to inform clients about support groups for bereaved parents, as others who have gone through a similar loss can be great sources of information, guidance, support, and comfort. Indeed, the beneficial effects of support groups on perinatal parental bereavement have been repeatedly documented (Cacciatore, 2007; Carlson et al., 2012; McCreight, 2007; Schwab, 1996).

Working with Cultural and Religious Influences

A therapist working with perinatally bereaved parents should become informed of their sociocultural context and the ways this shapes their grief experience. Tedeschi and Calhoun (2004b) suggested that the clinician should become familiar with the social rules and norms by which the bereaved parents abide, their religious faith and rituals, and the linguistic idioms on death and mourning used in their cultural milieu. All these are affecting the parents' course of bereavement. The social norms and rules might affect the availability of social support, opportunities for disclosure of emotions, and what the parent feels is permitted as part of a normal grieving process; thus, unless therapists can judiciously learn them, they cannot follow the client in this journey. While preferred language and the need for the therapist to honor them is a familiar idea for clinicians, the sensitivity and vulnerability of perinatally bereaved parents make this need even more imperative because therapists might be the only individuals validating parents' grief. For example, if a parent always talks about the baby by his/her name and the therapist continuously refers to the baby anonymously, the parent may feel that the therapist does not validate the existence of their child and as a result, withdraw from the therapeutic relationship.

To understand their clients' religious and spiritual assumptions, a clinician working with bereaved parents should adopt the viewpoint of *pragmatic religious constructivism*, which assumes that "... it is desirable for the clinician to enter, respectfully, into the client's religious worldview and help him or her utilize [...] spiritual understanding to recover, grow, and develop." (Calhoun, & Tedeschi, 1999, p. 110). Regardless of their own religious views and stance, the therapist must explore the parents' beliefs about the afterlife and the continued existence of the child, possibilities for contacting the child, and the role of God(s). The role of religion in an individual's adjustment to traumatic events has been well documented (Calhoun et al., 2010; Matthews & Marwit, 2006; McIntosh et al., 1993; Overcash et al., 1996; Pargament, 1990; Tedeschi, & Calhoun, 2006). Furthermore, religious and spiritual coping has been identified as a predictor of PTG (Calhoun, Cann et al., 2000; Calhoun et al., 2010; Shaw et al., 2005; Tedeschi & Calhoun, 2006; Znoj, 2006). Two functions of religious coping are specifically relevant to perinatally bereaved parents; first, religion can help parents find meaning or an explanation to an otherwise inconceivable event, and second, religion can offer comfort and solace through its claims about the afterlife (McIntosh et al., 1993; Tedeschi, & Calhoun, 2006).

Religion can function to preserve existing schemas (Joseph, & Linley, 2005) thus providing the means to attribute misfortune to one's own inappropriate behavior or the will of God rather than initiating the revision of existing schemas. Parents who use religious beliefs to explain the death of their baby might discontinue their search for the meaning of their experience and consequently experience limited growth. Some parents resort to the existence of a Divine Plan and of Heaven, while others believe in the spiritual existence of their children, which allows them an ongoing connection and a hope to reunite after death. Both of these views have been found to have a positive impact on mothers' grief resolution with only the latter contributing to their growth (Thomadaki, 2012).

Consequently, religious and spiritual issues are central to parental bereavement and can either enhance or impede the journey to growth. For example, until Pope Benedict XVI abolished it in 2007, the Catholic belief was that children who die perinatally do not go to hell but cannot go to heaven either because they are not baptized, thus bearing the Original Sin, they stay in limbo forever (Peelen, 2009). This representation of unwanted and sinful infants can be very painful for parents and deprive them of the possibility of a reunion in the afterlife. Similarly, according to the Christian dogma of the Greek Orthodox Church, unbaptized babies are not supposed to be buried in the Holy grounds of cemeteries. The death of these babies is seen as Divine intervention because a Divine Providence knows that if they grew older, they would become sinful, and thus, life was cut short before they committed their sins to protect their souls (Fanaras, 2008). When working therapeutically with a perinatally bereaved parent, a clinician should address these religious beliefs and try to alleviate unnecessary guilt and anguish that a parent may experience.

Beyond religious beliefs, it is important for therapists to explore parents' existential stances, such as the meaning of life. Parents may engage consciously in meaning-making processes that often lead to identifying values emanating from the experience of loss.

Tedeschi and Calhoun (2004b) underline that sometimes positive changes arising from the struggle with loss can act as memorials for the dead child. This might be a more intense need for parents who lose a baby perinatally, as their child did not have the opportunity to live and they need to commit to actions that create for those short lives a legacy that touches the lives of as many peoples as possible. This has been confirmed as a source of growth in perinatally bereaved mothers (Thomadaki, 2012). A therapist can help fulfill this need by suggesting memorials, charities, scholarships or other ways where the name and the legacy of their child would live.

Adopting a Growth Perspective

Tedeschi and Calhoun (2004b) recommend that the therapist adopt a growth perspective. The first step is for the therapist to be aware of the possibility of growth following the struggle of bereaved parents with their loss. The therapist should pay attention to themes related to growth in the parent's narrative, though not necessarily name them as such, to avoid forcing clients to address the concept of growth before they are ready. Therapists should use their clinical judgment as to when the time is right for parents to acknowledge the positive changes and explore them further. Using respectful language in this process is key to the maintenance of a good therapeutic rapport. It is strongly advised to suggest that it was the parents' struggle with the loss that has brought about some positive changes rather than the loss itself.

Finally, Calhoun and Tedeschi (2007; Tedeschi, & Calhoun, 2004a) describe how listening and being changed can lead therapists to *vicarious posttraumatic growth*. This was observed in the context of a qualitative study (Arnold et al., 2005), of 21 clinical or counseling psychologists. The most frequently reported positive consequences of observing and encouraging clients' PTG (90%) were experiencing changes in themselves, mostly increased sensitivity, empathy, compassion, insight, and tolerance. Enhanced spirituality and heightened awareness of their good fortunes were reported by more than half of the therapists, while nearly half shared that their clients' struggle with trauma had deepened their own appreciation of the strength and resilience of the human spirit. These results, although preliminary, indicate that working with traumatized individuals can be both hazardous for the therapist e.g., generating vicarious posttraumatic stress (McCann & Pearlman, 1990), and a very valuable experience generating positive changes in the therapist.

In sum, the models and suggestions presented in this chapter do not necessarily have strong empirical evidence to support them as treatment manuals, or models that could be adhered to and applied universally. Rather, it is an attempt to provide therapists with a concise overview of the unique characteristics and therapeutic needs of perinatally bereaved parents and inspire them to start considering growth as a possible therapeutic outcome after this type of traumatic loss. That therapists adopt a non-intervention approach might prove instrumental in empowering those parents by providing the support and companionship needed for the resolution of their loss.

References

Albuqueque, S., Narciso, I., & Pereira, M. (2018). Posttraumatic growth in bereaved parents: A multidimensional model of associated factors. *Psychological Trauma: Theory, Practice, and Policy*, *10*(2), 199–207. 10.1037/tra0000305

Allumbaugh, D. L., & Hoyt, W. T. (1999). Effectiveness of grief therapy: A meta-analysis. *Journal of Counseling Psychology*, *46*(3), 370–380. 10.1037/0022-0167.46.3.370

Arnold, D., Calhoun, L. G., Tedeschi, R., & Cann, A. (2005). Vicarious posttraumatic growth in psychotherapy. *Journal of Humanistic Psychology*, *45*(2), 239–263. 10.1177/0022167805274729

Bartl, H., Hagl, M., Kotoučová, M., Pfon, G., & Rosner, R. (2018). Does prolonged grief treatment foster posttraumatic growth? Secondary results from a treatment study with long-term follow-up and mediation analysis. *Psychology and Psychotherapy: Theory, Research, and Practice*, *91*(1), 27–41. 10.1111/papt.12140

Bogensperger, J., & Lueger- Schuster, B. (2014). Losing a child: Finding meaning in bereavement. *European Journal of Psychotraumatology*, *5*, Article 22910. 10.3402/ejpt.v5.22910

Braun, M. J., & Berg, D. H. (1994). Meaning reconstruction in the experience of parental bereavement. *Death Studies*, *18*(2), 105–129. 10.1080/07481189408252647

Büchi, S., Mörgeli, H., Schnyder, U., Jenewein, J., Hepp, U., Jina, E., Neuhaus, R., Fauchère, J. C., Bucher, H. U., & Sensky, T. (2007). Grief and post-traumatic growth in parents 2-6 years after the death of their extremely premature baby. *Psychotherapy and Psychosomatics*, *76*(2), 106–114. 10.1159/000097969

Cacciatore, J. (2007). Effects of support groups on posttraumatic stress responses in women experiencing stillbirth. *Omega: Journal of Death and Dying*, *55*(1), 71–90. 10.2190/M447-1X11-6566-8042

Cacciatore, J., Blood, C., & Kurker, S. (2018). From "Silent Birth" to voices heard: Volunteering, meaning, and posttraumatic growth after stillbirth. *Illness, Crisis & Loss*, *26*(1), 23–39. 10.1177/1054137317740799

Cacciatore, J., & Bushfield, S. (2008). Stillbirth: A sociopolitical issue. *Affilia*, *23*(4), 378–387. 10.1177/0886109908323972

Cacciatore, J., Lacasse, J. R., Lietz, C. A., & McPherson, J. (2018). A parent's tears: Primary results from the traumatic experiences and resiliency study. *Omega: Journal of Death and Dying*, *68*(3), 183–205. 10.2190/OM.68.3.a

Cacciatore, J., Schnebly, S., & Frøen, J. F. (2009). The effects of social support on maternal anxiety and depression after stillbirth. *Health and Social Care in the Community*, *17*(2), 167–176. 10.1111/j.1365-2524.2008.00814.x

Calhoun, L. G., Cann, A., & Tedeschi, R. G. (2010). The posttraumatic growth model: Sociocultural considerations. In T. Weiss & R. Berger (Eds.), *Posttraumatic growth and culturally competent practice: Lessons learned from around the globe* (pp. 1–14). Wiley.

Calhoun, L. G., Cann, A., Tedeschi, R. G., & McMillan, J. (2000). A correlational test of the relationship between posttraumatic growth, religion, and cognitive processing. *Journal of Traumatic Stress*, *13*(3), 521–527. 10.1023/A:1007745627077

Calhoun, L. G., & Tedeschi, R. G. (1989–90). Positive aspects of critical life problems: Recollections of grief. *Omega: The Journal of Death and Dying*, *20*(4), 265–272. 10.2190/QDY6-6PQC-KQWV-5U7K

Calhoun, L. G., & Tedeschi, R. G. (1998). Beyond recovery from trauma: Implications for clinical practice and research. *Journal of Social Issues*, *54*(2), 357–371. 10.1111/0022-4537.701998070

Calhoun, L. G., & Tedeschi, R. G. (1999). *Facilitating posttraumatic growth: A clinician's guide*. Lawrence Erlbaum.

Calhoun, L. G., & Tedeschi, R. G. (2007). Posttraumatic growth: The positive lessons of loss. In R. A. Neimeyer (Ed.), *Meaning reconstruction and the experience of loss* (pp. 157–172). American Psychological Association.

Calhoun, L. G., Tedeschi, R. G., Cann, A., & Hanks, E. A. (2010). Positive outcomes following bereavement: Paths to posttraumatic growth. *Psychologica Belgica*, *50*(1–2), 125–143. 10.5334/pb-50-1-2-125

Calhoun, L. G., Tedeschi, R. G., Fulmer, D., & Harlan, D. (4–8 August, 2000). *Parental grief: The relation of rumination, distress, and posttraumatic growth*. [Paper presentation]. Annual Meeting of the American Psychological Association, Washington DC, United States.

Carlson, R., Lammert, C., & O'Leary, J. M. (2012). The evolution of group and online support for families who have experienced perinatal or neonatal loss. *Illness, Crisis, and Loss*, *20*(3), 275– 293. 10.2190/IL.20.3.e

Corr, C. A. (1998–99). Enhancing the concept of disenfranchised grief. *Omega: Journal of Death and Dying*, *38*(1), 1–20. 10.2190/LD26-42A6-1EAV-3MDN
Currier, J. M., Holland, J. M., & Neimeyer, R. A. (2006). Sense-making, grief, and the experience of violent loss: Toward a meditational model. *Death Studies*, *30*(5), 403–428. 10.1080/07481180600614351
Davis, C. G., Wohl, M. J. A., & Verberg, N. (2007). Profiles of posttraumatic growth following an unjust loss. *Death Studies*, *31*(8), 693–712. 10.1080/07481180701490578
Davis, C. G., Wortman, C. B., Lehman, D. R., & Silver, R. C. (2000). Searching for meaning in loss: Are clinical assumptions correct? *Death Studies*, *24*(6), 497–540. 10.1080/07481180050121471
de Bernis, L., Kinney, M. V., Stones, W., Ten Hoope-Bender, P., Vivio, D., Leisher, S. H., Bhutta, Z. A., Gülmezoglu, M., Mathai, M., Belizán, J. M., Franco, L., McDougall, L., Zeitlin, J., Malata, A., Dickson, K. E., Lawn, J. E., Lancet Ending Preventable Stillbirths Series study group, & Lancet Ending Preventable Stillbirths Series Advisory Group (2016). Stillbirths: ending preventable deaths by 2030. *Lancet (London, England)*, *387*(10019), 703–716. 10.1016/S0140-6736(15)00954-X
Doka, K. (1989). *Disenfranchised grief: Recognizing hidden sorrow*. Lexington Books.
Engelkemeyer, S. M., & Marwit, S. J. (2008). Posttraumatic growth in bereaved parents. *Journal of Traumatic Stress*, *21*(3), 344–346. 10.1002/jts.20338
Fanaras, V. G. (2008). Θεολογικοί στοχασμοί για τα έμβρυα και τα νήπια που ο βίος τους τερματίζεται πρόωρα [Theological reflections for the embryos and babies whose lives are cut short]. In D. G. Magriplis (Ed.), *Όψεις του πολιτιστικού φαινομένου: Επιστημονικές προσεγγίσεις του θανάτου και της ζωής* (pp. 203–213). Εκδόσεις Σταμούλη.
Flenady, V., Wojcieszek, A. M., Middleton, P., Ellwood, D., Erwich, J. J., Coory, M., Khong, T. Y., Silver, R. M., Smith, G., Boyle, F. M., Lawn, J. E., Blencowe, H., Leisher, S. H., Gross, M. M., Horey, D., Farrales, L., Bloomfield, F., McCowan, L., Brown, S. J., Joseph, K. S., ... Lancet Stillbirths In High-Income Countries Investigator Group (2016). Stillbirths: recall to action in high-income countries. *Lancet (London, England)*, *387*(10019), 691–702. 10.1016/S0140-6736(15)01020-X
Frankl, V. E. (1969). *The will to meaning: Foundations and applications of logotherapy*. The World Publishing.
Frøen, J. F., Cacciatore, J., McClure, E. M., Kuti, O., Jokhio, A. H., Islam, M., Shiffman, J., & Lancet's Stillbirths Series steering committee (2011). Stillbirths: Why they matter. *Lancet (London, England)*, *377*(9774), 1353–1366. 10.1016/S0140-6736(10)62232-5
Gerrish, N. J., Steed, L. G., & Neimeyer, R. A. (2010). Meaning reconstruction in bereaved mothers: A pilot study using the biographical grid method. *Journal of Constructivist Psychology*, *23*(2), 118–142. 10.1080/10720530903563215
Heriot, M. J. (1996). Fetal rights versus the female body: Contested domains. *Medical Anthropology Quarterly*, *10*(2), 176–194. 10.1525/maq.1996.10.2.02a00050
Horton, R. (2013, December 11). *Stillbirths* [Video]. You Tube. https://www.youtube.com/watch?v=EOR079DuuZs
Janoff-Bulman, R. (1992). *Shattered assumptions: Towards a new psychology of trauma*. Free Press.
Jordan, J. R., & Neimeyer, R. A. (2003). Does grief counselling work? *Death Studies*, *27*(9), 765–786. 10.1080/713842360
Joseph, S. (2004). Client-centred therapy, post-traumatic stress disorder and post traumatic growth: Theoretical perspectives and practical implications. *Psychology and Psychotherapy: Theory, Research, & Practice*, *77*(1), 101–119. 10.1348/147608304322874281
Joseph, S., & Linley, P. A. (2005). Positive adjustment to threatening events: An organismic valuing theory of growth through adversity. *Review of General Psychology*, *9*(3), 262–280. 10.1037/1089-2680.9.3.262
Joseph, S., & Linley, P. A. (2006). Growth following adversity: Theoretical perspectives and implications for clinical practise. *Clinical Psychology Review*, *26*(8), 1041–1053. 10.1016/j.cpr.2005.12.006
Joseph, S., & Linley, P. A. (Eds.) (2008). *Trauma, recovery, and growth: Positive psychological perspectives on posttraumatic stress*. Wiley.
Karwoski, L., Garratt, G. M., & Ilardi, S. S. (2006). On the integration of cognitive-behavioral therapy for depression and positive psychology. *Journal of Cognitive Psychotherapy: An International Quarterly*, *20*(2), 159–170. 10.1891/088983906780639763

Keefe-Cooperman, K. (2004). A comparison of grief as related to miscarriage and termination for fetal abnormality. *Omega: Journal of Death and Dying*, *50*(4), 281–300. 10.2190/QFDW-LGEY-CYLM-N4LW
Klass, D. (1986–87). Marriage and divorce among bereaved parents in a self-help group. *Omega: Journal of Death and Dying*, *17*(3), 237–249. 10.2190/T8L3-UVD8-J2RD-TLLB
Kovit, L. (1978). Babies as social products: The social determinants of classification. *Social Science and Medicine*, *12*, 347–351. 10.1016/0271-7123(78)90088-3
Krosch, D., & Shakespeare-Finch, J. (2017). Grief, traumatic stress, and posttraumatic growth in women who have experienced pregnancy loss. *Psychological Trauma: Theory, Research, Practice, and Policy*, *9*(4), 425–433. 10.1037/tra0000183
Layne, L. L. (2003). Unhappy endings: A feminist reappraisal of the women's health movement from the vantage of pregnancy loss. *Social Science and Medicine*, *56*(9), 1881–1891. 10.1016/s0277-9536(02)00211-3
Lehman, D. R., Davis, C. G., Delongis, A., Wortman, C. B., Bluck, S., Mandel, D. R., & Ellard J. H. (1993). Positive and negative life changes following bereavement and their relations to adjustment. *Journal of Social and Clinical Psychology*, *12*(1), 90–112. 10.1521/jscp.1993.12.1.90
Lehman, D. R., Wortman, C. B., & Williams, A. F. (1987). Long-term effects of losing a spouse or child in a motor vehicle crash. *Journal of Personality and Social Psychology*, *52*(1), 218–231. 10.1037/0022-3514.52.1.218
Linley, P. A., & Joseph, S. (2004). Positive change following trauma and adversity: A review. *Journal of Traumatic Stress*, *17*(1), 11–21. 10.1023/B:JOTS.0000014671.27856.7e
Martinčeková, L., & Klatt, J. (2017). Mothers' grief, forgiveness, and posttraumatic growth after the loss of a child. *Omega – Journal of Death and Dying*, *75*(3), 248–265. 10.1177/003022281 6652803
Matthews, L. T., & Marwit, S. J. (2006). Meaning reconstruction in the context of religious coping: Rebuilding the shattered assumptive world. *Omega: Journal of Death and Dying*, *53*(1–2), 87–104. 10.2190/DKMM-B7KQ-6MPD-LJNA
May, R. (1981). *Freedom and destiny*. Norton.
McCann, I. L., & Pearlman, L. A. (1990). Vicarious traumatization: A framework for understanding the psychological effects of working with victims. *Journal of Traumatic Stress*, *3*(1), 131–149. 10.1007/BF00975140
McCreight, B. S. (2007). Narratives of pregnancy loss: The role of self-help groups in supporting parents. *Medical Sociology Online*, *2*, 3–16. Retrieved from http://uir.ulster.ac.uk/23313/1/MSOVol2Issue1Jun07.pdf
McIntosh, D. N., Silver, R. C., & Wortman, C. B. (1993). Religion's role in adjustment to a negative life event: Coping with the loss of a child. *Journal of Personality and Social Psychology*, *65*(4), 812–821. 10.1037/0022-3514.65.4.812
Michael, C., & Cooper, M. (2013). Post-traumatic growth following bereavement: A systematic review of the literature. *Counselling Psychology Review*, *28*, 18–33.
Miles, M. S., & Crandall, E. K. B. (1983). The search for meaning and its potential for affecting growth in bereaved parents. *Health Values*, *7*(1), 19–23.
Moore, M. M., Cerel, J., & Jobes, D. A. (2015). Fruits of trauma? Posttraumatic growth among suicide-bereaved parents. *Crisis*, *36*(4), 241–248. 10.1027/0227-5910/a000318
Morgan, L. M. (2002). "Properly disposed of": A history of embryo disposal and the changing claims on fetal remains. *Medical Anthropology*, *21*(5), 247–274. 10.1080/01459740214079
Moulton Milo, E. (1997). Maternal responses to the life and death of a child with developmental disability. *Death Studies*, *21*(5), 443–476. 10.1080/074811897201822
Neria, Y., & Litz, B. T. (2003). Bereavement by traumatic means: The complex synergy of trauma and grief. *Journal of Loss and Trauma*, *9*(1), 73–87. 10.1080/15325020490255322
Overcash, W. S., Calhoun, L. G., Cann, A., & Tedeschi, R. G. (1996). Coping with Crises: An examination of the impact of traumatic events on religious beliefs. *The Journal of Genetic Psychology*, *157*(4), 455–464. 10.1080/00221325.1996.9914878
Ozer, E. J., Best, S. R., Lipsey, T. L., & Weiss, D. S. (2003). Predictors of posttraumatic stress disorder and symptoms in adults: A meta-analysis. *Psychological Bulletin*, *129*(1), 52–73. 10.103 7/0033-2909.129.1.52

Pan, X., Liu, J., Li, L. W., & Kwok, J. (2016). Posttraumatic growth in aging individuals who have lost their only child in China. *Death Studies*, 40(7), 395–404. 10.1080/07481187.2016.1169234

Pargament, K. (1990). God help me: Toward a theoretical framework of coping for the psychology of religion. *Research in the Social Scientific Study of Religion*, 2, 195–224. 10.1007/BF00938065

Peelen, J. (2009). Reversing the past: Monuments for stillborn children. *Mortality*, *14*(2), 173–186. 10.1080/13576270902808043

Polatinsky, S., & Esprey, Y. (2000). An assessment of gender differences in the perception of benefit resulting from the loss of a child. *Journal of Traumatic Stress*, *13*(4), 709–718. 10.1023/A:1007870419116

Prati, G., & Pietrantoni, L. (2009). Optimism, social support, and coping strategies as factors contributing to posttraumatic growth: A meta-analysis. *Journal of Loss and Trauma*, *14*(5), 364–388. 10.1080/15325020902724271

Rädestad, I., Steineck, G., Nordin, C., & Sjögren, B. (1996). Psychological complications after stillbirth--Influence of memories and immediate management: Population based study. *British Medical Journal*, *312*(7045), 1505–1508. 10.1136/bmj.312.7045.1505

Riley, L. P., LaMontagne, L. L., Hepworth, J. T., & Murphy, B. A. (2007). Parental grief responses and personal growth following the death of a child. *Death Studies*, *31*(4), 277–299. 10.1080/07481180601152591

Rogers, C. R. (1951). *Client-centered therapy: Its current practice, implications, and theory.* Houghton Mifflin.

Royal College of Obstetricians and Gynaecologists (2010). *Guideline number 55: Late intrauterine fetal death and stillbirth*, first edition. Accessed in www.rcog.org.uk

Rubin, S. S., Malkinson, R., & Witztum, E. (2003). Trauma and bereavement: Conceptual and clinical issues revolving around relationships. *Death Studies*, *27*(8), 667–690. 10.1080/713842342

Sanders, C. M. (1980). A comparison of adult bereavement in the death of a spouse, child and parent. *Omega: The Journal of Death and Dying*, *10*(4), 302–322. 10.2190/X565-HW49-CHR0-FYB4

Schubert, C. F., Schmidt, U., Comtesse, H., Gall-Kleebach, D., & Rosner, R. (2019). Posttraumatic growth during cognitive behavioural therapy for posttraumatic stress disorder: Relationship to symptom change and introduction of significant other assessment. *Stress and Health*, *35*(5), 617–625. 10.1002/smi.2894

Schwab, R. (1996). Bereaved parents and support group participation. *Omega: Journal of Death & Dying*, *32*(1), 49–61. 10.2190/GE71-45VV-B37F-7D5T

Shaw, A., Joseph, S., & Linley, P. A. (2005). Religion, spirituality, and posttraumatic growth: a systematic review. *Mental Health, Religion, and Culture*, *8*(1), 1–11. 10.1080/1367467032000157981

Seligman, M. E. P., & Csikszentmihalyi, M. (2000). Positive psychology: An introduction. *American Psychologist*, *55*(1), 5–14. 10.1037/0003-066X.55.1.5

Smith, J. A., Flowers, P., & Larkin, M. (2009). *Interpretative phenomenological analysis: Theory, method, and research*. Sage.

Stroebe, M., & Schut, H. (2005). To continue or relinquish bonds: A review of consequences for the bereaved. *Death Studies*, *29*(6), 477–494. 10.1080/07481180590962659

Taku, K., Tedeschi, R. G., Cann, A., & Calhoun, L. G. (2009). The culture of disclosure: Effects of perceived reactions to disclosure on posttraumatic growth and distress in Japan. *Journal of Social and Clinical Psychology*, *29*(10), 1226–1243. 10.1521/jscp.2009.28.10.1226

Tedeschi, R. G., & Calhoun, L. G. (1996). The posttraumatic growth inventory: Measuring the positive legacy of trauma. *Journal of Traumatic Stress*, *9*(3), 455–472. 10.1002/jts.2490090305

Tedeschi, R. G., & Calhoun, L. G. (2004a). Posttraumatic growth: Conceptual foundations and empirical evidence. *Psychological Inquiry*, *15*(1), 1–18. 10.1207/s15327965pli1501_01

Tedeschi, R. G., & Calhoun, L. G. (2004b). *A clinician's guide: Helping bereaved parents*. Brunner-Routledge.

Tedeschi, R. G., & Calhoun, L. G. (2006). Time of change? The spiritual challenges of bereavement and loss. *Omega: Journal of Death and Dying*, *53*(1-2), 105–116. 10.2190/7MBU-UFV9-6TJ6-DP83

Tedeschi, R. G., Calhoun, L. G., & Groleau, J. M. (2015). Clinical applications of posttraumatic growth. In Joseph, S. (Ed.), *Positive psychology in practice: Promoting human flourishing in work, health, education, and everyday life* (2nd ed., pp. 503–518). Wiley. 10.1002/9781118996874.ch30

Tennen, H., & Affleck, G. (1999). Finding benefits in adversity. In C. R. Snyder (Ed.), *Coping: The psychology of what works* (pp. 279–304). Oxford University Press.
Thomadaki, O. O. (2012). How mothers experience personal growth after a perinatal loss [Unpublished doctoral dissertation]. City, University of London. https://openaccess.city.ac.uk/id/eprint/3008/1/Thomadaki%2C_Olga.pdf
Thomadaki, O. O. (2017). Bereavement, post-traumatic stress and post-traumatic growth: Through the lenses of positive psychology. *European Journal of Psychotraumatology*, *8*(sup4), 1351220. 10.1080/20008198.2017.1351220
Trulsson, O., & Rädestad, I. (2004). The silent child-mothers' experiences before, during, and after stillbirth. *Birth*, *31*(3), 189–195. 10.1111/j.0730-7659.2004.00304.x
Uren, T. H., & Wastell, C. A. (2002). Attachment and meaning-making in perinatal bereavement. *Death Studies*, *26*(4), 279–308. 10.1080/074811802753594682
Wagner, B., Knaevelsrud, C., & Maercker, A. (2007). Post-traumatic growth and optimism as outcomes of an internet-based intervention for complicated grief. *Cognitive Behaviour Therapy*, *36*(3), 156- 161. 10.1080/16506070701339713
Waugh, A., Kiemle, G., & Slade, P. (2018). What aspects of post-traumatic growth are experienced by bereaved parents? *European Journal of Psychotraumatology*, *9*(1), 1506230. 10.1080/20008198.2018.1506230
Wheeler, I. (2001). Parental bereavement: The crisis of meaning. *Death Studies*, *25*(1), 51–66. 10.1080/07481180126147
Xiu, D., McGee, S. L., & Maercker, A. (2018). Sense of coherence and posttraumatic growth: The moderating role of value orientation in Chinese and Swiss bereaved parents. *Journal of Loss and Trauma*, 23(3), 259–270. 10.1080/15325024.2018.1436120
Yalom, I. (1980). *Existential therapy*. Basic Books.
Znoj, H. (2006). Bereavement and posttraumatic growth. In L. G. Calhoun & R. G. Tedeschi (Eds.), *Handbook of posttraumatic growth: Research and practice* (pp. 176–196). Lawrence Erlbaum.
Znoj, H. J., & Keller, D. (2002). Mourning parents: Considering safeguards and their relations to health. *Death Studies*, 26(7), 545–565. 10.1080/074811802760191708
Zoellner, T., & Maercker, A. (2006). Posttraumatic growth and psychotherapy. In L. G. Calhoun & R. G. Tedeschi (Eds.), *Handbook of posttraumatic growth: Research and practice* (pp. 334–354). Lawrence Erlbaum.
Zoellner, T., Rabe, S., Karl, A., & Maercker, A. (2011). Post-traumatic growth as outcome of cognitive- behavioural therapy trial for motor vehicle survivors with PTSD. *Psychology and Psychotherapy: Theory, Research and Practice*, *84*(2), 201–213. 10.1348/147608310X520157

22

PARENTING AND GROWTH IN THE CONTEXT OF PEDIATRIC PALLIATIVE CARE

Susan Cadell and Jessica Furtado

Parenting is by definition about growth. Children begin as completely dependent beings and the role of parents is to nurture their growth into adulthood and independence. Along the way of shaping their children, parents are also developing and maturing. The role of parenting can be both stressful and beneficial to the parent.

The term "parent" in this chapter means anyone in that role including, but not limited to, birth, biological, step-, co-, adoptive, surrogate, foster, and grandparents. Parents may be in this role alone, in couples, or in a family configuration with more parental figures. The choice to include all those parents throughout this chapter is informed by feedback from research participants who preferred to be referred to as parents rather than as caregivers, even when their role involves providing medical care to their children (Levy et al., 2020).

The population of bereaved parents during and following their caregiving for a child's life-limiting illness is often overlooked and misunderstood. Parents expect to care for their children and nurture their growth beginning before birth and continuing well into adulthood. When children have a life-limiting illness, the parental role changes, as it does when parents are bereaved. Despite the adverse experiences of parents of children with life-limiting illness, they may continue to demonstrate also growth, throughout caregiving and after their child's death (Cadell et al., 2014; Waugh et al., 2018).

The current use of the term posttraumatic growth (PTG) grew out of work with grieving individuals. Tedeschi and Calhoun worked with grieving widows (Calhoun & Tedeschi, 2001). The realization that they were hearing about positive aspects that were unaccounted for in the literature led them to conceptualize PTG. An important aspect of the idea of growth in any context is that wisdom and strength coexist alongside ongoing distress related to grief or an adverse event. Henson and colleagues (2021, p. 1) posit that "growth is not the result of the event itself, but the struggle to deal with it." We assert that the key to understanding PTG as it relates to parenting in the face of serious illness and grief is to embrace the contrasts and complexity. This holds especially true in relation to the ongoing distress that co-exists with growth. We highlight the key sources of adversity and strength of parents.

For bereaved parents and many grieving individuals, grief never ends (Klass & Walter, 2001). The approach of starting with diagnosis and ending with grief underestimates the impact of the life-limiting illness on the lives of those who are grieving during and beyond the child's life.

DOI: 10.4324/9781032208688-28

Rather than recounting parents' experiences of caregiving and bereavement in chronological order, we simultaneously explore life and death as well as caregiving and bereavement, mirroring the ways in which parents have described living in a dual reality. Parents' lived experiences are illustrated by including quotes from narratives of parents' experiences of caregiving for a child with a life-limiting illness in a study by Cadell and colleagues (2014).

Trauma, Disruption, and Dialectics: Living in the In-Between

> ... on the one hand I'm aware of the fragility of life and the importance of life and the importance of living life to the fullest, and on the other hand I'm aware of the fear that comes with that, because I live it. I live it when my daughter says, "I have a headache, Mom." If you're a parent of a child with a life-threatening illness, that can trigger major emotions and for me, it does. I can re-visit trauma, this - these events, this way of life has impacted on me hugely. It has been traumatic. (Caregiving mother of a 12-year-old daughter with brain cancer)

PTG involves adversity or potential trauma, which disrupts the individual and instigates a process that includes positive change. The two potentially traumatic events that are most often discussed with respect to this population of parents are receiving the child's diagnosis and the child's death (Bally et al., 2018; Dutta et al., 2019). Both involve a threat to someone's life and fit psychiatric definitions of trauma exposure (American Psychological Association, 2013). Within both the growth and the trauma literature, "objective" clinical definitions of trauma have been deemed less important than the subjective experience that the event has on the individual (Picoraro et al., 2014; Rodríguez-Rey et al., 2018); therefore, it is important to consider these *potentially* traumatic events.

These significant events are likely to be part of the adversities that parents face during their involvement with the pediatric healthcare system, whose potentially traumatizing impact has been conceptualized by the umbrella term pediatric medical trauma. Additional examples of traumatizing events in this process may include receiving or witnessing invasive treatments or testing and overwhelming medical surroundings. These experiences cause posttraumatic stress symptoms in up to 30% of children and families and are associated with poorer medical and psychosocial outcomes (Price et al., 2016).

Janoff-Bulman (2010) defined trauma as the "shattering of assumptions" about one's self and their place in the world. Tedeschi and Calhoun's (2014) description of trauma as an "earthquake", means in the context of childhood serious illness, disrupting the foundational assumptions parents made about their child's life and their family's future. If a child's initial diagnosis is experienced by parents as an earthquake, shifting the firm grounding they had, their following experiences can be considered the aftershocks of the event.

While the majority of research has focused on parental caregiving of infants and children with a life-limiting illness (Bally et al., 2018; Dutta et al., 2019; Price et al., 2016; Winger et al., 2020), parental caregiving tasks can continue into adolescence and adulthood, presenting new challenges around autonomy. For example, mothers worried if their grown children would have the physical ability to manage their children's daily needs (Levy et al., 2020).

Parents who have experienced pediatric medical trauma can also demonstrate PTG (Picoraro et al., 2014). We prefer to discuss trauma in the context of growth rather than resilience as critiques of resilience, particularly from Black and Indigenous scholars, have highlighted the ways in which resilience relies on the individual while focusing less on accountability of structures and systems that cause vulnerability (Amo-Agyemang, 2021; Breda & D, 2018; Fast & Collin-Vézina, 2019; Humbert & Joseph, 2019; Thomas et al., 2016). PTG, in contrast, acknowledges the existence of trauma as well as its potential impact making both the source of adversity and those impacted a potential target for change.

The trauma or disruptions that parents experience can include events they perceive both as depreciation and growth. These parents exist within a "dual reality that alternated between two dominant experiences: the highs associated with focusing on their child's and their own survival, and the lows related to their fear of their child's death" (Bally et al., 2018, p. 92). Oscillating between these highs and lows can be destabilizing, particularly at times after diagnosis (Bally et al., 2018) and after death (Dutta et al., 2019); however, parents' experiences fluctuate throughout their child's life, death, and related grief.

Grief, Caregiving, and Losses

> And so we're always kind of day-by-day ... having the experience of not knowing if he's going to live to see his next birthday but grooming him for adulthood ... so it's kind of interesting. It's like half of my day is filled with elation and half of it is grief. It's a constant grieving process. But it's also really thrilling and exciting. (Caregiving adoptive mother of a 9-year-old son with multiple disabilities)

As this quote illustrates, for parents of children with a life-limiting illness, before bereavement exists grief, i.e., the emotional, physical, spiritual, and social reaction to loss (Breen et al., 2022). Grief can occur in relation to any kind of loss and is not limited to losses related to death. For parents of children with life-limiting illnesses, grief has been reported during caregiving as "pervasive" rather than beginning with death and bereavement (Collins et al., 2016). Grief has no timeline and can last for years (Rubin, 1999). Those who are grieving oscillate between being focused on the loss and being oriented toward the restoration of life (Stroebe & Schut, 2010). Grief following a death-related loss does not end the parents' relationship with their child; rather it transforms it (Mitchell et al., 2012), continuing their bonds (Klass, 2006; Klass et al., 1996; Klass & Steffen, 2017). Issues that parents experience in grief include caregiving challenges, caring for themselves, and maintaining connections with others. These challenges intertwine and are oftentimes, immersive rather than considered in isolation.

Caregiving Challenges

> Okay, it is not just important to my child that I have been involved in caregiving, it's ... he would not have survived otherwise (caregiving adoptive mother of a 17-year-old child with multiple disabilities related to being born prematurely, having cerebral palsy, lung disease, inability to swallow, and spinal cord injury)

Some children could not live without intensive medical caregiving from their parents. Koch and Jones (2018) identified five types of caregiving: (1) instrumental activities of daily living; (2) personal activities of daily living (habilitation); (3) information management; (4) medical administration; and (5) emotional support. While parents can typically expect their role to involve each of these caregiving types to some degree, particularly when children are younger, the caregiving demands within each of these categories tend to be much greater when managing life-limiting illness of seriously ill children, making it difficult for these parents to arrange or accept respite as they felt they understood their child's needs best (Collins et al., 2016).

Typically, when parents are expecting a child and imagining their future, they do not anticipate extensive medicalization of their lives, nor do they imagine they may outlive their child. A suspicion or diagnosis of a life-limiting illness defies the hopes that they had for their family and puts them into a reality that is now focused on life and death. Parents have described immense grief for what could have been (Collins et al., 2016). Fathers described a particularly difficult time with the news of their child's life-limiting diagnosis as they considered themselves the protectors of the family (Nicholas et al., 2016).

As providers for their families, parents who were working may be required to change their hours and schedule or find different work altogether to accommodate the scheduling required for healthcare. Some parents experienced this change in their professional lives as a loss of themselves (Collins et al., 2016). Forty-three percent of parents of children with life-limiting illnesses across North America described their income as inadequate to meet their family needs (Cadell et al., 2014). However, bereaved mothers reported that while they experienced challenges and losses related to caregiving, they found the strength to persevere in their love for their child (Levy et al., 2020). As the demands on parents accumulate, so does the parental realization that this is what their child needs from them.

Caring for Self

> I think they [Healthcare providers] need to be asking how are we coping - are we doing okay, do we need any help with anything? Can we get you somebody – a cup of coffee? We'll sit and chit chat, or whatever, and somebody else can watch him play in the family centre, or whatever. Just – I mean, it sounds so trivial and so small, but for sometimes it's – and when he was in the hospital, like wandering through the hallways and stuff at nighttime, like nobody ever asked, "Are you okay?" or anything like that. (caregiving parent of an HIV-positive, 9-year-old boy)

Caregiving parents are often thrust into the unfamiliar territory of the medical world. Being in the health care system may change identities - the child becomes a patient and the parents, visitors, or caregivers (Macdonald et al., 2012). Parents are moved into a passive position where the focus is on the child and their needs, without recognition of parents and familial needs, including siblings (Bally et al., 2018, 2021; Eaton Russell et al., 2018; Koch & Jones, 2018). Some parents must be engaged in advocacy for their children to get the treatment that they need.

Parents' experiences within the medical system vary and may have significant impacts on their coping (Dutta et al., 2019; Verberne et al., 2019). Some parents have excellent experiences and feel reassured by the care and attention they and their child receive; others feel overwhelmed and out of control in medical settings (Dutta et al., 2019). Relative to their relationships with healthcare providers, parents have raised concerns about the ways in which information is – and is not – shared (Bally et al., 2021). Parents are frustrated by having to share their stories repeatedly with multiple healthcare providers and teams (Dutta et al., 2019) whereas more effective palliative care services would limit this need and create a space to talk with parents (Bally et al., 2021).

Research has highlighted the importance of caregiver self-care, which is not always welcomed by caregivers who are already overburdened by child-focused caretaking tasks

(Koch & Jones, 2018; Levy et al., 2020). Despite embracing family-centered care within pediatric palliative care settings, support for parents remains limited (Clercq et al., 2017). Greater support in the form of social connections has the potential to enhance the possibility of growth in this context.

Maintaining Connections

Mom: It's very hard to get people to understand – I know at first, doing the walks and everything, my goal was so that people could understand, but five years down the road I realized ...

Dad: They don't – they'll never understand. They think it's something that's going to be cured like in a month or two, a year, and it's gonna be over

Mom: No matter how many times you say it – that's why going to the MPS [Hurler syndrome] conference, it's like "ahh," I'm like, you don't have to explain anything, all these parents know it all. It's like a family. (Parents of 10-year-old girl with MPS)

Parents report significant disruptions to their family dynamics and social bonds as they manage the demands of caregiving. As described by the above parents, they sometimes face the ironic position of their closest relationships not understanding their realities and yet having strangers "get it". The mother and father in the quote above are describing the experience of feeling the closeness and unspoken understanding that one might expect with family in a new context – not with relatives, but instead with other families who share the same caregiving experiences. Caregiving parents reported that they tend to prefer building community with others they can consider as peers (Koch & Jones, 2018).

Some parents report that they feel isolated from other families as those without children with life-limiting illnesses tend to not understand their realities. Thus, bereaved mothers report that the loss of their child is also experienced as a loss of connections to others, particularly when their grief is not recognized, validated, or supported (Levy et al., 2020). Caregiving parents report that managing offerings of care from others can be stressful in itself, especially for end-of-life care (Winger et al., 2020).

Caregiving parents explain that the medical complications of caring for their child may mean that they need to be in close proximity to their child, which they described as being "trapped" inside their home (Collins et al., 2016), feeling isolated and lacking freedom (Levy et al., 2020). This experience may have cultural components, as interviews with bereaved Asian parents found that caregiving was a collaborative effort with extended family (Dutta et al., 2020). That access to social networks contributes to PTG (Henson et al., 2021) highlights the importance of the ways in which individuals derive meanings from their experiences.

Meaning-Making and PTG

Studies have found that parents acknowledged changes in family dynamics while caring for children with life-limiting illnesses (Dutta et al., 2019, 2020). These changes included on one hand spending less time with other children and feeling guilty as a result (Dutta et al., 2019), and at the same time, some parents have found that the situation has brought them closer to their spouse, children, and extended family. One father summarized the growth he experienced, "I think when you go through a fire like that with someone … it'll bring you closer together – or I found it did. I felt it strengthened an already pretty strong relationship" (Nicholas et al., 2016, p. 139).

As parents are experiencing the aforementioned disruptions, they may also be engaging in meaning-making (Cadell et al., 2014; Collins et al., 2016; Dutta et al., 2020). Living in the devastation of uncertainty (Bally et al., 2018) is taxing for parents cognitively, emotionally, physically, and spiritually. Theories of PTG assert that parents engage in processes to reduce this load by attempting to make sense of the complex dialectic realities they face (Cadell et al., 2014). For most parents, rather than resolving issues, this means learning to accept and live with the ebbs and flows that come with their caregiving and bereavement experiences (Bally et al., 2018; Cadell et al., 2014; Dutta et al., 2019). This process of meaning-making may eventually lead to PTG.

PTG has been noted in parents of children of all ages, including following infant loss (Barr, 2011). Parents reported changes in themselves individually and in their couple relationships. For example, Cadell and colleagues (2014) studied 367 parents in the US and Canada who were caring for a child with a life-limiting illness and demonstrated growth in multiple domains. Using comparative structural equation models, the model that fits best demonstrated that personal well-being, as measured by self-esteem, optimism, spirituality, and depression, contributed to PTG, which was moderated by the meaning that parents found in caregiving. Three domains emerged in an investigation of PTG in parents of children with life-limiting illnesses: perceptions of self, interpersonal relationships, and transcendental relationships (Rodríguez Rey et al., 2016). A longitudinal examination of mothers and fathers of critically ill children indicated that they experienced at least medium levels of growth with evidence that engaging in processes that encourage positive thinking led to greater PTG (Rodríguez-Rey et al., 2018).

Meaning-making is understood to be the result of processes involving both avoidance and rumination (Brooks et al., 2019). While avoidance and rumination are typically considered posttraumatic stress symptoms (American Psychological Association, 2013), they also have functionality toward PTG (Calhoun & Tedeschi, 2014). For example, in pediatric palliative care, parents have reported that they tend to avoid thoughts and conversations about their child's death (Dutta et al., 2019; Verberne et al., 2019). As parents learn to manage daily life as caregivers for a seriously ill child, this type of active avoidance may be functional. Intrusive thoughts, though disturbing, such as those a parent might have about their child's death, also offer an opportunity for rumination as a form of meaning-making (Tedeschi & Calhoun, 2004). As parents navigated the dialectic between avoidance and rumination, they recognized that they require support in facilitating conversations with their children about death (Dutta et al., 2019).

As mothers learned to navigate the dialectic realities of their experiences, they reported understanding themselves in new ways, including new strengths as demonstrated by one mother who shared "I have learned so much about myself and my ability to be completely selfless for another person, even when she [the daughter] doesn't always want me. I am stronger than I ever imagined I could be." (Levy et al., 2020, p. 368). While much of the literature disproportionately includes mothers, fathers have also reported growth, especially increased closeness in their relationships (Nicholas et al., 2016). Fathers described moving forward while deeply in pain, social connections, spousal support, spirituality, positive outlook and hope, recognizing strength and growth, and shifting priorities.

Changes in parental roles can also impact the quality of the couple's relationship. Berger (2015) points out that, with increased familial stress less time is available to invest in the couple's relationship, and discusses the importance of dyadic coping, where individuals demonstrate mutual care and support, working together to manage stress. Effective dyadic coping alleviates stress and allows couples to deepen their relationships by building trust, intimacy, and well-being. Henson and colleagues (2021) confirmed this, highlighting the potential of shared experiences to add both stress and growth, particularly when couples are communicative and responsive to one another. Further, evidence suggests that PTG experienced by one person in the couple influences the social perceptions and expectations of the other, reinforcing behaviors consistent with growth.

When a child dies, meaning-making appears to be a dyadic process within the couple (Albuquerque et al., 2017). Spousal interdependency for emotional support was an important theme in a study of Asian bereaved parents of a child with a life-limiting illness (Dutta et al., 2020). Heterosexual couples who received a serious prenatal illness diagnosis, reported PTG with greater closeness in their relationship, as well as in relationships with others within and beyond the family (Black & Sandelowski, 2010). For bereaved parents of premature infants, mutually supporting one another's emotions contributed to concordant experiences of grief and were related to PTG individually (Büchi et al., 2009). Parents assigned meaning to their dyadic coping as emotional regulation reinforcing their sense of security (Koivula et al., 2019) and could engage in a process of meaning-making to move toward reconnecting with relationships.

Moving Forward: Reconnection and Integration

The lived experiences of parents who are caregiving and who are bereaved is a non-stepwise process of disruption and meaning-making that can facilitate reconnection and integration. Their narratives of memorial tattoos and advocacy efforts demonstrate how they weave together elements of growth at different stages of their caregiving and bereavement journeys.

Meaning-Making through Memorial Tattoos

One expression of growth in grief that has received very little attention in spite of being increasingly common is memorial tattoos that honor someone who has died (Cadell et al., 2020). A study (Cadell et al., 2020) explored the stories about the tattoos of 41 parents of children who had died. The children that the parents were honoring ranged in age from dying at birth to being in their 20s. They died of an overdose, suicide, accident, or illness. Parents' ages ranged from 20s to the oldest in his 80s who obtained his first tattoo in his 70s.

Two mothers in the sample had similar stories. Both their daughters died of cancer before the age of three and neither had tattoos before getting their memorial tattoos. While their stories shared similarities in the age and cause of their children's deaths, their tattoos were very different; yet both were narratives of growth.

Both women have two children in addition to the child who died. One woman's tattoo includes three hearts representing all her children, with wings on the heart that represent the child who died. The tattoo is very colorful and is designed with images of beads that the deceased child was given during treatment including a purple butterfly that represents the end of life. The tattoo is located in a private spot on the mother's hip, which she chose because "it's not for anybody else to see, I'm not looking to explain it to every person that walks by." The tattoo allowed her to feel a bond with her deceased daughter and connected her other children to their siblings.

The second mother had two tattoos honoring her daughter who died. The first and smaller tattoo is an infinity symbol with her daughter's name in it along with the words "Because love never dies ..." The second and larger tattoo depicts cherry blossoms, which she explains "are beautiful, they are vibrant, they only bloom for a very short time but when they do, they are just full of life and wonderful and that was my daughter." Her tattoos do not include her other two children. She explained to them that they were with her all the time. Both tattoos are on her shoulders because she wanted them to be visible. She commented, "they are reminders of my daughter, and they were symbols of her and I wanted people to be able to ask about them and people do all the time." The tattoos facilitate her keeping her daughter's memory alive in part because of the placement on her shoulders, "I didn't want it to be hidden away somewhere ... she, is already sort of hidden in our family because people can't see her like they see our two sons, so I thought it was important that it was some sort of a visual and 'out there' representation of her."

Tattoos can be worn to challenge stigma. The second mother's tattoos form part of her persona as a bereaved parent "with attitude", as she and her partner learned in support groups following their daughter's death. The tattoos allow her to have conversations with people and challenge silence about being a bereaved parent, "I am not going to let other people's discomfort with grief and lost children change how I feel and how I have to deal with it."

The tattoos have also helped her to continue to parent her child, "I need to be able to somehow still parent my child and include her in my life somehow, she has to be part of me." Both mothers felt a stronger bond to their deceased child through the tattoos and obtaining and wearing the tattoos challenged the stigma of grief regardless of the placement on the body and the visibility or privacy of the tattoos.

Meaning-Making through Advocacy

> I spoke to the doctor and he said, "Well ... the good part is that it's a disease with a medication out there." The bad part was it wasn't approved in Canada ... I kept searching on the internet and found the Canadian MDS Society; called them, talked to the lady that was in charge and she said, "Yeah, you know what, you have to fight real hard." Because she said there are a few kids in Canada who already are on the medication, but you have to make a lot of noise, you have to put your story out (there). (We) called the radio stations, newspapers and - our daughter needed a medication to slow down the progress of this disease – we started a walk that year too to raise awareness and even our MP did the walk! So he came to the walk, our pharmacist at the drug store came to the walk, and the geneticist came to the walk. (Caregiving parent of a 13 year old boy with Myelodysplastic Syndromes).

A consistent theme across research and practice in grief work is parents' finding meaning through advocacy, both when their child is alive as well as after their child has died. Parents shared a desire to participate in research and activities that they felt would improve the experience of other families, sometimes based on their own challenges within the system. For example, Merk and Merk (2013) wrote about being denied access to visiting their child as a family at the end of his life, which was one of the last opportunities they had together to do so. They considered that in order to move on they needed to bring the situation to the attention of hospital administrators and work with them to develop visiting practices that are more family-centered. This family developed a sense of meaning through their actions, and in doing so, improved the PICU (pediatric intensive care unit) experiences of other families.

Advocacy efforts in support of caregiving and bereaved families should come not only from parents but also from intentional healthcare practitioners. For groups that have been marginalized by discriminatory access to health systems, intentional engagement and awareness of cultural needs become even more important. For example, Indigenous mothers accessing the NICU (neonatal intensive care unit) described a need for strong relationships with medical providers, healthcare that recognized holistic wellness, and sensitivity to child protection matters, necessitating a trauma-informed approach (Wright et al., 2020). Race and other factors of intersectionality are important influences on the healthcare experience and need to be taken into account in order to improve the experiences of all, including the most marginalized, especially at the end of life (Davis & Gentlewarrior, 2015; Giesbrecht et al., 2018).

Bourque and colleagues (2020) followed eight parents who were highly involved in research after their child's death in the NICU. All overwhelmingly shared a desire to help others by improving the NICU experiences. Through this process, parents found that they were helped and were able to derive meaning from their experiences. Though PTG was not explicitly explored, the themes that emerged fit well with PTG.

In addition to memorial tattoos and advocacy work, parents develop multiple ways to make space for grief and loss within a cohesive story and find in their losses reconnection and reintegration into life. Others can help them in this ongoing journey to unlearn grief work as "getting over" and substitute it with "living through".

Conclusion

"The path to posttraumatic growth is not a simple one" (Cadell et al., 2014, p. 123). In this chapter parent experiences were explored in a non-linear timeline. The goal was to shift from viewing parents as a singular image to existing as holistic individuals within what is often a dual reality, each existing as a nuanced range of roles simultaneously. Binaries must be challenged; positive aspects of parenting, caregiving, and grieving do not replace the negative. Rather, they coexist as parents learn to live with uncertainty and duality. In this way, the chapter mirrors how parents exist in a complex experience where their current reality also includes the past with the present. Discussions with families of the past, present, and future seem to be worthwhile avenues (Levy et al., 2020). The adversity faced by parents of children with life-limiting illnesses is not connected exclusively to death but can be understood as cumulative experiences of grief and trauma. These experiences, as painful as they may be, can lead to growth.

References

Albuquerque, S., Buyukcan-Tetik, A., Stroebe, M. S., Schut, H. A. W., Narciso, I., Pereira, M., & Finkenauer, C. (2017). Meaning and coping orientation of bereaved parents: Individual and dyadic processes. *PLOS ONE*, *12*(6), e0178861. 10.1371/journal.pone.0178861

American Psychological Association. (2013). *Diagnostic and statistical manual of mental disorders: DSM-5TM*, 5th ed (pp. xliv, 947). American Psychiatric Publishing, Inc. 10.1176/appi.books.9780890425596

Amo-Agyemang, C. (2021). Unmasking resilience as governmentality: Towards an Afrocentric epistemology. *International Politics*, *58*(5), 679–703. 10.1057/s41311-021-00282-8

Bally, J. M., Burles, M., Smith, N. R., Holtslander, L., Mpofu, C., Hodgson-Viden, H., & Zimmer, M. (2021). Exploring opportunities for holistic family care of parental caregivers of children with life-threatening or life-limiting illnesses. *Qualitative Social Work*, *20*(5), 1356–1373. 10.1177/14 73325020967739
Bally, J. M., Smith, N. R., Holtslander, L., Duncan, V., Hodgson-Viden, H., Mpofu, C., & Zimmer, M. (2018). A metasynthesis: Uncovering what is known about the experiences of families with children who have life-limiting and life-threatening illnesses. *Journal of Pediatric Nursing*, *38*, 88–98. 10.1016/j.pedn.2017.11.004
Barr, P. (2011). Posttraumatic growth in parents of infants hospitalized in a neonatal intensive care unit. *Journal of Loss and Trauma*, *16*(2), 117–134. 10.1080/15325024.2010.519265
Berger, R. (2015). *Stress, trauma, and posttraumatic growth: Social context, environment, and identities*. Routledge. 10.4324/9780203118795
Black, B., & Sandelowski, M. (2010). Personal growth after severe fetal diagnosis. *Western Journal of Nursing Research*, *32*(8), 1011–1030. 10.1177/0193945910371215
Bourque, C. J., Dahan, S., Mantha, G., Reichherzer, M., & Janvier, A. (2020). My child's legacy: A mixed methods study of bereaved parents and providers' opinions about collaboration with NICU teams in quality improvement initiatives. *BMJ Open*, *10*(9), e034817. 10.1136/bmjopen-2019-034817
Breda, V., & D, A. (2018). A critical review of resilience theory and its relevance for social work. *Social Work*, *54*(1), 1–18. 10.15270/54-1-611
Breen, L. J., Kawashima, D., Joy, K., Cadell, S., Roth, D., Chow, A., & Macdonald, M. E. (2022). Grief literacy: A call to action for compassionate communities. *Death Studies*, *46*(2), 425–433. 10.1080/07481187.2020.1739780
Brooks, M., Graham-Kevan, N., Robinson, S., & Lowe, M. (2019). Trauma characteristics and post-traumatic growth: The mediating role of avoidance coping, intrusive thoughts, and social support. *Psychological Trauma: Theory, Research, Practice, and Policy*, *11*(2), 232–238. 10.1037/tra0000372
Büchi, S., Mörgeli, H., Schnyder, U., Jenewein, J., Glaser, A., Fauchère, J.-C., Bucher, H. U., & Sensky, T. (2009). Shared or discordant grief in couples 2–6 years after the death of their premature baby: Effects on suffering and posttraumatic growth. *Psychosomatics*, *50*(2), 123–130. 10.1176/appi.psy.50.2.123
Cadell, S., Hemsworth, D., Smit Quosai, T., Steele, R., Davies, E., Liben, S., Straatman, L., & Siden, H. (2014). Posttraumatic growth in parents caring for a child with a life-limiting illness: A structural equation model. *American Journal of Orthopsychiatry*, *84*(2), 123–133. 10.1037/h0099384
Cadell, S., Reid Lambert, M., Davidson, D., Greco, C., & Macdonald, M. E. (2020). Memorial tattoos: Advancing continuing bonds theory. *Death Studies*, *46*(1), 132–139. 10.1080/074811 87.2020.1716888
Calhoun, L. G., & Tedeschi, R. G. (2001). Posttraumatic growth: The positive lessons of loss. In *Meaning reconstruction & the experience of loss* (pp. 157–172). American Psychological Association. 10.1037/10397-008
Calhoun, L. G., & Tedeschi, R. G. (2014). *Handbook of posttraumatic growth: Research and practice*. Routledge.
Clercq, E. D., Rost, M., Pacurari, N., Elger, B. S., & Wangmo, T. (2017). Aligning guidelines and medical practice: Literature review on pediatric palliative care guidelines. *Palliative & Supportive Care*, *15*(4), 474–489. 10.1017/S1478951516000882
Collins, A., Hennessy-Anderson, N., Hosking, S., Hynson, J., Remedios, C., & Thomas, K. (2016). Lived experiences of parents caring for a child with a life-limiting condition in Australia: A qualitative study. *Palliative Medicine*, *30*(10), 950–959.
Davis, A., & Gentlewarrior, S. (2015). White privilege and clinical social work practice: Reflections and recommendations. *Journal of Progressive Human Services*, *26*(3), 191–208. 10.1080/1042 8232.2015.1063361
Dutta, O., Tan-Ho, G., Choo, P. Y., & Ho, A. H. Y. (2019). Lived experience of a child's chronic illness and death: A qualitative systematic review of the parental bereavement trajectory. *Death Studies*, *43*(9), 547–561. 10.1080/07481187.2018.1503621
Dutta, O., Tan-Ho, G., Choo, P. Y., Low, X. C., Chong, P. H., Ng, C., Ganapathy, S., & Ho, A. H. Y. (2020). Trauma to Transformation: The lived experience of bereaved parents of children with chronic life-threatening illnesses in Singapore. *BMC Palliative Care*, *19*(1), 46. 10.1186/ s12904–020-00555-8

Eaton Russell, C., Widger, K., Beaune, L., Neville, A., Cadell, S., Steele, R., Rapoport, A., Rugg, M., & Barrera, M. (2018). Siblings' voices: A prospective investigation of experiences with a dying child. *Death Studies*, *42*(3), 184–194. 10.1080/07481187.2017.1334009

Fast, E., & Collin-Vézina, D. (2019). Historical trauma, race-based trauma, and resilience of indigenous peoples: A literature review. *First Peoples Child & Family Review: An Interdisciplinary Journal Honouring the Voices, Perspectives, and Knowledges of First Peoples through Research, Critical Analyses, Stories, Standpoints and Media Reviews*, *14*(1), 166–181. 10.7202/1071294ar

Giesbrecht, M., Stajduhar, K. I., Mollison, A., Pauly, B., Reimer-Kirkham, S., McNeil, R., Wallace, B., Dosani, N., & Rose, C. (2018). Hospitals, clinics, and palliative care units: Place-based experiences of formal healthcare settings by people experiencing structural vulnerability at the end-of-life. *Health & Place*, *53*, 43–51. 10.1016/j.healthplace.2018.06.005

Henson, C., Truchot, D., & Canevello, A. (2021). What promotes post traumatic growth? A systematic review. *European Journal of Trauma & Dissociation*, *5*(4), 100195. 10.1016/j.ejtd.2020.100195

Humbert, C., & Joseph, J. (2019). Introduction: The politics of resilience: Problematising current approaches. *Resilience*, *7*(3), 215–223. 10.1080/21693293.2019.1613738

Janoff-Bulman, R. (2010). *Shattered assumptions*. Simon and Schuster.

Klass, D. (2006). Continuing conversation about continuing bonds. *Death Studies*, *30*(9), 843–858. 10.1080/07481180600886959

Klass, D., Silverman, P. R., & Nickman, S. L. (1996). *Continuing bonds: New understandings of grief*. Taylor & Francis.

Klass, D., & Steffen, E. M. (2017). *Continuing bonds in bereavement*. New Directions for Research and Practice, Londres, Routledge.

Klass, D., & Walter, T. (2001). Processes of grieving: How bonds are continued. In *Handbook of bereavement research: Consequences, coping, and care* (pp. 431–448). American Psychological Association. 10.1037/10436-018

Koch, K. D., & Jones, B. L. (2018). Supporting parent caregivers of children with life-limiting illness. *Children*, *5*(7), Article 7. 10.3390/children5070085

Koivula, K., Kokki, H., Korhonen, M., Laitila, A., & Honkalampi, K. (2019). Experienced dyadic emotion regulation and coping of parents with a seriously ill child. *Couple and Family Psychology: Research and Practice*, *8*(1), 45–61. 10.1037/cfp0000115

Levy, K., Grant, P. C., Tenzek, K. E., Depner, R. M., Pailler, M. E., & Beaupin, L. K. (2020). The experience of pediatric palliative caregiving: A qualitative analysis from the Photographs of Meaning Program. *American Journal of Hospice and Palliative Medicine®*, *37*(5), 364–370. 10.1177/1049909119879413

Macdonald, M. E., Liben, S., Carnevale, F. A., & Cohen, S. R. (2012). An office or a bedroom? Challenges for family-centered care in the pediatric intensive care unit. *Journal of Child Health Care*, *16*(3), 237–249. DOI: 10.1177/1367493511430678

Merk, L., & Merk, R. (2013). A parents' perspective on the pediatric intensive care unit: Our family's journey. *Pediatric Clinics*, *60*(3), 773–780. 10.1016/j.pcl.2013.02.012

Mitchell, L. M., Stephenson, P. H., Cadell, S., & Macdonald, M. E. (2012). Death and grief on-line: Virtual memorialization and changing concepts of childhood death and parental bereavement on the Internet. *Health Sociology Review*, *21*(4), 413–431. 10.5172/hesr.2012.21.4.413

Nicholas, D. B., Beaune, L., Barrera, M., Blumberg, J., & Belletrutti, M. (2016). Examining the experiences of fathers of children with a life-limiting illness. *Journal of Social Work in End-of-Life & Palliative Care*, *12*(1–2), 126–144. 10.1080/15524256.2016.1156601

Picoraro, J. A., Womer, J. W., Kazak, A. E., & Feudtner, C. (2014). Posttraumatic growth in parents and pediatric patients. *Journal of Palliative Medicine*, *17*(2), 209–218. 10.1089/jpm.2013.0280

Price, J., Kassam-Adams, N., Alderfer, M. A., Christofferson, J., & Kazak, A. E. (2016). Systematic review: A reevaluation and update of the Integrative (Trajectory) Model of Pediatric Medical Traumatic Stress. *Journal of Pediatric Psychology*, *41*(1), 86–97. 10.1093/jpepsy/jsv074

Rodríguez Rey, R., Alonso Tapia, J., Kassam-Adams, N., & Garrido Hernansaiz, H. (2016). The factor structure of the Posttraumatic Growth Inventory in parents of critically ill children. *Psicothema*, *28*(4), 495–503. 10.7334/psicothema2016.162

Rodríguez-Rey, R., Alonso-Tapia, J., & Colville, G. (2018). Prediction of parental posttraumatic stress, anxiety and depression after a child's critical hospitalization. *Journal of Critical Care*, *45*, 149–155. 10.1016/j.jcrc.2018.02.006

Rubin, S. S. (1999). The two-track model of bereavement: Overview, retrospect, and prospect. *Death Studies*, *23*(8), 681–714.

Stroebe, M., & Schut, H. (2010). The dual process model of coping with bereavement: A decade on. *OMEGA-Journal of Death and Dying*, *61*(4), 273–289. 10.2190/OM.61.4.b

Tedeschi, R. G., & Calhoun, L. G. (2004). Posttraumatic growth: Conceptual foundations and empirical evidence. *Psychological Inquiry*, *15*(1), 1–18. https://www.jstor.org/stable/20447194

Thomas, D., Mitchell, T., & Arseneau, C. (2016). Re-evaluating resilience: From individual vulnerabilities to the strength of cultures and collectivities among indigenous communities. *Resilience*, *4*(2), 116–129. 10.1080/21693293.2015.1094174

Verberne, L. M., Kars, M. C., Schouten-van Meeteren, A. Y. N., van den Bergh, E. M. M., Bosman, D. K., Colenbrander, D. A., Grootenhuis, M. A., & van Delden, J. J. M. (2019). Parental experiences and coping strategies when caring for a child receiving paediatric palliative care: A qualitative study. *European Journal of Pediatrics*, *178*(7), 1075–1085. 10.1007/s00431-019-03393-w

Waugh, A., Kiemle, G., & Slade, P. (2018). What aspects of post-traumatic growth are experienced by bereaved parents? A systematic review. *European Journal of Psychotraumatology*, *9*(1), 1506230. 10.1080/20008198.2018.1506230

Winger, A., Kvarme, L. G., Løyland, B., Kristiansen, C., Helseth, S., & Ravn, I. H. (2020). Family experiences with palliative care for children at home: A systematic literature review. *BMC Palliative Care*, *19*(1), 165. 10.1186/s12904-020-00672-4

Wright, A. L., Ballantyne, M., & Wahoush, O. (2020). Caring for Indigenous families in the neonatal intensive care unit. *Nursing Inquiry*, *27*(2), e12338. 10.1111/nin.12338

23

WALKING THROUGH DIFFERENT WORLDS

The Experience of Posttraumatic Growth in Childhood Cancer Survivors and Their Families

Marta Tremolada and Sabrina Bonichini

PTG in Children and Adolescents who Struggle with Pediatric Cancer and their Parents: Key Issues

Pediatric Cancer: Negative and Positive Sequelae

The incidence of malignant tumors in children and adolescents is increasing. According to the report from the International Union of Cancer Prevention and Control, the number of new pediatric cases of cancer in the world is about 175,000 per year, with the annual incidence increasing at the rate of 1.5% (Siegel et al., 2021). However, the mortality of these patients decreased significantly thanks to new advances and continued research to identify effective treatments (Howlader et al., 2021). Thus, the increase in the number of pediatric cancer survivors also means that a series of physical and psychological problems require researchers' and clinicians' attention.

Having cancer impacts child development, particularly during adolescence, which is a crucial phase of the transition from childhood to adulthood. This special stage passage may make young people experience difficulties in their age-related developmental tasks. Individuals who suffer from traumatic events like pediatric cancer may have negative psychological reactions such as post-traumatic stress disorder, depression, and anxiety (D'agostino et al., 2016; Friend et al., 2018). Pediatric cancer has been widely studied especially in relation to post-traumatic stress symptoms (PTS) in childhood cancer survivors, as well as in their parents. Results from these studies showed that in general survivors are not at increased risk of severe PTS or full post-traumatic stress disorder compared to the norms and to healthy populations (Bruce, 2006; Taïeb et al. 2003;). Parents, especially mothers, reported higher levels of PTS than childhood cancer survivors themselves (Kazak et al., 2004), and there seems to be an association between levels of PTS in mothers of pediatric oncology patients and higher levels of PTS in their children (Okado et al., 2016).

However, several studies have shown that pediatric cancer ex-patients may have in addition to negative psychological reactions, also positive psychological changes, of which post-traumatic growth (PTG) is the most representative (Barakat et al., 2006; Howard Sharp et al., 2016; Howard Sharp et al., 2015). Thus, in addition to negative psychosocial

DOI: 10.4324/9781032208688-29

consequences such as PTS, both childhood cancer survivors and their parents report PTG, defined as positive changes following a traumatic experience, typically in the domains of relating to others, new possibilities, personal strength, spiritual change, and appreciation of life (Tedeschi & Calhoun, 2004).

Pediatric Cancer and PTG

The majority of studies found that childhood cancer survivors exhibited elements of PTG, i.e., positive aspects of change following traumatic events, and in some cases greater than would be expected in a control population (Arpawong et al., 2013; Barakat et al., 2006; Gunst et al., 2016; Gianinazzi et al., 2016; Kamibeppu et al., 2010; Koutná et al., 2017; Yi & Kim, 2014; Zebrack et al., 2012). Findings emphasize that personal growth in pediatric cancer survivors can occur in different areas including spirituality and appreciation for life, intentionally or unintentionally, and imparting meaning through the cancer experience (Lee, 2008). The reported prevalence of PTG in survivors and their parents is between 80–90 % (Barakat et al., 2006). A PTG experience can help survivors who had malignant tumors during their pediatric age successfully resume their maturation in the continuation of their daily life (Gianinazzi et al., 2016).

Researchers have attempted to understand the multiple domains of positive growth in cancer survivors (Park et al.,1996; Park & Peterson, 2006) and have postulated that through the struggle with cancer, one can grow in spirituality (Connerty & Knott, 2013; Denney et al., 2011; Mehrabi et al., 2015), interrelationships (Chambers et al., 2012; Connerty & Knott, 2013; Sabiston et al., 2007; Tomich & Helgeson, 2002), resilience (Chambers et al., 2012; Mehrabi et al., 2015; Rinaldis et al., 2010), personal cognition and mentality such as priorities and worldview (Connerty & Knott, 2013; Helgeson, 2011; Mehrabi et al., 2015; Rinaldis et al., 2010; Sabiston et al., 2007) and social activity (Duran, 2013). Specifically related to pediatric cancer, an analysis of interviews with survivors showed that how adolescents and young adults survivors perceived the influence of the disease on their life concerned child's temperament, maturation and personal growth, increased resilience and sensitivity, perception of own life and events, personal working choices, academic, degree of enthusiasm and propensity towards the future (Tremolada et al., 2018).

Interviews with young adult cancer survivors illustrated that in agreement with the aforementioned findings, while the stress of facing pediatric cancer can become unbearable and result in psychological symptoms that could threaten patients' psychological health, it can also improve PTG (Tremolada et al., 2018). Adolescent and young adult survivors of pediatric cancer expressed their perception of how the disease has influenced their life positively and reported that they feel grateful for life. The following excerpt from an interview with a 21-year-old woman illustrates this point,

> They [the experiences] make you mature, because in my opinion if it did not happen to me, in the misfortune of what happened to me I have matured a lot, now I know what it really means to live, I will never say "How disgusting life" because before I was one of those classic girls who complained about everything.

A 20-year-old female adult survivor explained,

> Well, I think I've blocked a lot of my adolescence out, in the sense that, because it happened in a period of transition. I went to the secondary school, in the second year,

> I knew no-one, that is, in short, it was a bit tragic, in fact I have very bad memories of that period and up to the third year of school there was no way to unblock. They were not good years in terms of relationships [...] that is, I always felt a bit looked at by the other people.

A 20-year-old male said,

> I realized that I am what I am because I experienced what I experienced ... and making my retrospective appraisal I am convinced that, even if this thing [the illness] was physically and psychologically devastating, an experience to the limit, it gave me a lot in terms of thought analysis and reasoning ... forcing me to grow up on some things much faster than the majority of my peers.

Some patients stated that they were able to derive from the experience of illness considerable benefits, in terms of psychological well-being, and that they changed their life perspectives and priorities. For example, a 17-year-old said,

> Yes, before I was maybe let's say apart from the age, I was such a superficial boy and I was based only on momentary cravings, fashion and all things like that, but now I've started to appreciate every moment, every moment. In my opinion it is different, it has changed me [...] in fact I don't smoke, I don't drink [...] throwing money away like this has never interested me, not to mention the damage you do to yourself [...]. I have already risked a lot and struggled to overcome all the various problems and several times I thought I would not make it and I don't think about it at all.

Another 18-year-old woman said,

> surely the illness left me many things, but really many, in my opinion it really changed my way of seeing life in the sense [...] I started to give much more value to relationships, to human relationships things, to the detriment of much else, I create much less problems [...] I always say, in bad luck I was lucky, because I have recovered and in my opinion it makes you aware of many things and I say I am very happy to have this awareness.

Further exploration is needed to inform designing interventions to promote and stimulate personal positive growth in pediatric patients with malignant tumors and their families, as PTG emerged as very important for the quality of life and mental health of this population.

Association between Child and Parent PTG

Data on the correlation between parent-child PTG following pediatric cancer is very limited and findings are mixed. Michel et al. (2009) reported no parent-child association in perceiving positive changes following pediatric cancer. However, Yaskowich (2002) reported an association between parent-child PTG, with higher levels of PTG in children who are aware of PTG in their parents. Some studies provided indirect support for parent-child PTG associations by pointing to the role of the parent-child relationship and factors of parenting in child PTG following pediatric cancer (Howard Sharp et al., 2015; Howard Sharp et al., 2016). In fact, parents may shape the process and outcomes of child psychosocial adaptation, including both PTS and PTG, through the socialization of coping and emotions (Koutná & Blatný, 2020). They provide social support and simultaneously serve as coping models and sources of information for childhood cancer survivors (Wakefield et al., 2013).

Self- and Proxy-Reports in PTG Assessment

PTG research offers a possible perspective on adopting parents (significant others) as proxy reporters. The majority of PTG studies face criticism because of overreliance on self-report measures, and PTG research in pediatric oncology is no exception. The veracity of PTG reports obtained by self-report measures is often questioned, because it does not allow to distinguish actual positive changes from other concepts, such as positive illusions. To address this issue, some authors suggested corroboration of self-reports by reports of significant others (Park & Lechner, 2006) such that parent-proxy reports of PTG in their children could serve as a means for verifying child self-report. This approach was utilized in several studies focused on adults and their spouses or significant others (family members and close friends) and showed significantly high correlations (Blackie et al., 2015; Moore et al., 2011; Weiss, 2002). To the best of our knowledge, the agreement between child self-report and parent-proxy report of positive outcomes following the struggle with pediatric cancer has not been widely studied, so further investigation to clarify this association is needed.

Stable and Modifiable Factors Impacting PTG in Childhood Cancer Survivors

Childhood cancer survivors face several traumas and show different adaptations both to the illness and to its short and long-term sequelae that could be evident and maintained in their daily lives. Because PTG was identified in some but not all studies (Scrignaro et al. 2016; Turner-Sack et al., 2012) it is important to identify which stable factors (e.g., socio-demographic and illness-related variables) and modifiable factors (social support, coping styles, symptomatology presence) could influence PTG, which is a possible precursor of resilience and associated with well-being and adaptation to the daily life.

Stable and illness-related variables that could be predictive of childhood cancer survivors' personal growth include older age at diagnosis (Zannini et al., 2014) and at the time of assessment, gender, more aggressive treatment, and shorter time between diagnosis and recovery (Yi et al., 2015; Zebrack et al., 2012) and longer duration of treatment (Gianinazzi et al., 2016).

Age

Results indicated that ex-patients who were older at both time of diagnosis and assessment were more likely to experience PTG. Whereas in adults, age and PTG have typically been negatively correlated (Helgeson et al., 2006; Shand et al., 2015), findings about how PTG is affected by the age at which the trauma occurs in children and adolescents are inconsistent. In light of these inconsistencies, Meyerson and colleagues (2011) suggested that PTG is independent of age in children and adolescents who have experienced diverse types of trauma. However, small, significant, negative associations between PTG and time since both diagnosis and treatment were reported, indicating that more recent diagnosis or treatment completion was associated with greater PTG. These findings may reflect an increase in abstract thinking after the age of 11 or 12 (Piaget, 1971). The capacity for the cognitive processes necessary for the development of PTG, contemplation of philosophical concepts, meaning-making, and the development of personal values typically emerges during adolescence. Having cancer in adolescence could be very disruptive and requires particular strength to face and win against this traumatic illness. This situation could activate coping strategies and eventually PTG. The results of pediatric and adult mixed-trauma PTG research suggest that PTG may take a curvilinear trajectory, plateauing during adolescence or early adulthood (Meyerson et al., 2011).

Gender

Findings regarding gender are also inconsistent as in some studies, gender was not clearly related to PTG (Turner et al., 2018) whereas some Italian studies found significant gender differences (Tremolada et al., 2016a), with females more inclined to PTG. Probably, cultural differences may allow females more confidence in reporting their feelings or being more inclined to social and caring activities (at least in the Italian context). Another reason could be that as in the aforementioned study, PTSS was strongly associated with PTG, with females showing more PTSS symptoms and, in turn, higher PTG when they narrate their illness experiences. The same factors (older age, shorter time since off therapy, female gender, younger age at diagnosis) were predictors of the perception of life and self-perceptions, a scale included in the Personal Growth Inventory (CCSS, https://ccss.stjude.org/tools-documents/questionnaires.html), which is a sort of a new point of view on self and on life in general (Tremolada et al., 2016a).

Socio-economic status as defined by parental income, parental education level, and formal socio-economic measurements, were combined as measures of socio-economic status across studies. Results indicated that socio-economic status and PTG were unrelated.

Modifiable factors that may be associated with PTG include social support, coping styles, and symptomatology presence.

Social Support

A recent meta-analysis (Turner et al., 2018) has indicated medium, significant, positive associations between PTG and both social support and optimism whereas depression, pessimism, anxiety, and quality of life did not correlate with PTG. Consistent with past research, greater social support and optimism were associated with greater PTG in individuals affected by childhood or adolescent cancer (Duran, 2013; Ekim & Ocakci, 2015; Meyerson et al., 2011; Picoraro et al, 2014). Social support is an integral aspect of Tedeschi and Calhoun's PTG theoretical framework. Trauma could generate a personal growth experience in survivors' lives and self-perceptions if they had family sqpport that helped them throughout the cancer treatments and in their daily routine re-entry processes (Tremolada et al., 2016b). It has been argued that optimism is distinct from PTG and facilitates it by motivating coping styles and redirecting attention from uncontrollable threats to positive appraisals. Plausibly, a bidirectional relationship exists between PTG and social support and optimism such that an increase in PTG may lead to higher social support and optimism and vice versa.

The aforementioned interviews by Tremolada et al., (2018) illustrated the importance of social support as many survivors stated that although they were quite young at the time of diagnosis, they often had the opportunity to talk to their family members and ask them for important information and details about their long time at the hospital. Through these reconstructed stories, they were able to compensate and combine the memories imprinted in their brain relating to the traumatic event, with those narrated by the people who assisted them and who shared with them the entire path of the disease.

In addition to their family, adult, and young adolescent cancer survivors are more able to remember and narrate experiences related to their illness, when expressing a high level of satisfaction with the relationship established with the ward staff during the long period of hospitalization, consequently reporting higher levels of personal growth. Many declared feeling a deep sense of gratitude towards their "saviours", which definitely helps characterize these important and strong relations. A 19-year-old woman said,

> Especially in the period when I was physically ill, they [the doctors] were the lifeline, always ready, always with a smile on their face, always optimistic and positive .... All sick people should have such comfort and support ... It was priceless to have these really closed and precious persons.

Recovered patients who have established a good relationship with the hospital staff, based on trust and sincerity, are the ones who show higher PTG, tranquillity, and serenity in returning to the hospital and have lower levels of concerns with regard to a possible relapse. During visits to the ward, some of them were happy to meet the doctors and nurses, now considered members of the family, with whom they had shared many painful and stressful circumstances but also positive and happy moments, such as the time recovering. A 22-year-old woman said,

> I have always had a great time [at the hospital]. I grew up here, and I feel at home here now. In fact, back to those times when I was here almost every day, it once happened that my dad and I were looking for a parking place, and I told him, "Daddy, park there [pointing at the hospital]—in front of home".

Another boy said, "I can only admire ... I have had no problem with anybody here and I have wonderful memories of all the people, they all work perfectly ... doctors, nurses, volunteers, psychologists, everybody ... Thanks to them I am born again, physically, spiritually and psychologically.

The Impact of Time

Linley and Joseph (2004) suggested that links between PTG and rumination, intrusions, and avoidance coping were indicative of the cognitive processing necessary for PTG. For example, cognitive processing, rumination, reflection, meaning-making, and fluctuations in affect may plausibly peak during and soon after significant life events such as receiving a cancer diagnosis or completing a final treatment, and reflect the process of successfully dealing with the associated PTSS. Subsequently, natural decline in internal reactions, the passage of time, and competing environmental factors may contribute to decreases in PTG over time. However, results regarding the association between time since traumatic event and PTG are generally mixed, with negative (Barakat et al., 2006) or nonsignificant associations (Alisic et al., 2008; Milam et al., 2004).

Existence of PTSS

Recent studies identified a significant correlation between PTG and PTSS. By definition, the struggle with trauma is necessary for the development of PTG. For example, as a result of leukemia, a teen may experience intrusive memories and distress, as well as a greater appreciation for life and spiritual development. Joseph and Hefferon (2013) argue that as distinct constructs, post-traumatic stress triggers PTG, and in turn, PTG reduces post-traumatic stress. The results of a meta-analysis (Shakespeare-Finch et al., 2014) suggested that in adults, PTSS and PTG may follow a curvilinear pathway, depending on age and trauma type. Further research is recommended (Howard Sharp et al., 2015; Meyerson et al., 2011) to clarify the nature and trajectory of the complicated relationship between post-traumatic stress and PTG, both in pediatric contexts and during lifespan.

Figure 23.1 summarizes the factors related to the development of PTG in children and adolescents.

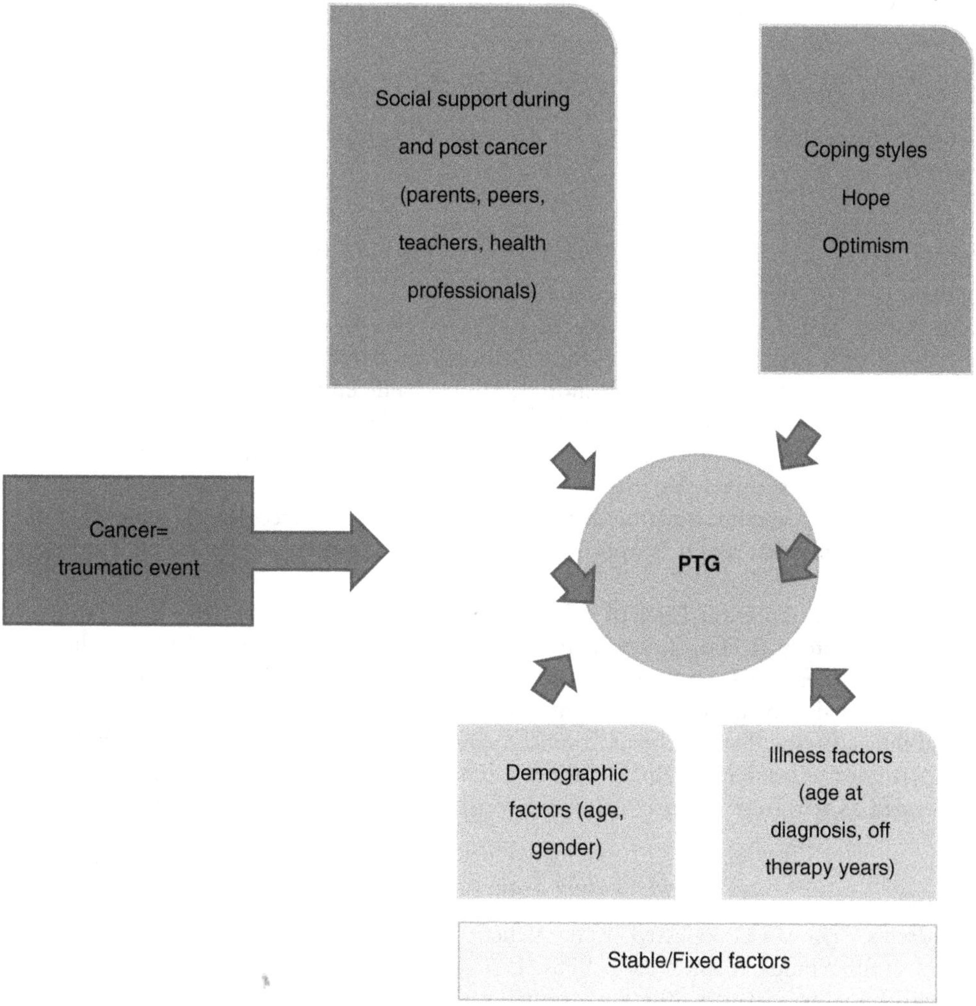

Figure 23.1 Stable and modifiable factors impacting PTG.

Instruments Used to Assess PTG: Self-Report Questionnaires, Qualitative and Narrative Approaches

The study of growth following adversity and trauma has focused largely on adults. While there is also a developing literature on children and adolescents, it is only relatively recently that empirical studies have been published focusing specifically on the topic of growth in children and adolescents following trauma, such as cancer. There are several reasons why formal assessment of PTG in children and adolescents can be useful both from a clinical and research point of view (Clay et al., 2009). First, measuring PTG at several points, prior to, during, and after interventions, provides an opportunity to monitor progress. The introduction of PTG within clinical work may help children, adolescents, and their caregivers look at their experience also in a positive light (Tedeschi & Kilmer, 2005), while usually the focus is primarily on negative aspects such as PTSS. The investment in PTG can predict better outcomes on other indices of post-traumatic stress, depression, and anxiety. Thus, there is a need for instruments for assessing PTG clinically and in research.

Child and Parent Self-Reported PTG Questionnaires

Various instruments exist currently for assessing PTG in children, adolescents, and their parents.

Post-Traumatic Growth Inventory (PTGI)

Milam et al. (2004) adapted Tedeschi and Calhoun's (1996) Posttraumatic Growth Inventory (PTGI) for use with adolescents who have experienced diverse traumas such as the death of a loved one, serious illness (cancer), or parental separation. Items were reworded and modified to produce a shorter, 16-item self-report scale (as opposed to the 21 items on the adult PTGI), covering the same five subscales as the adult measure: New possibilities, relating to others, personal strength, appreciation of life and spiritual change. Preliminary data showed that the modified scale has good internal consistency and reliability. Although encouraging, further construct validation is necessary as well as work to determine from what age it is appropriate because the instrument can be demanding for young children.

For assessing parental level of PTG (parent self-reported PTG), the Post-Traumatic Growth Inventory (PTGI; Tedeschi & Calhoun, 1996) can be used. PTGI is the most widely used measure for assessing positive changes following a traumatic experience in adults. It consists of 21 items, that cover PTG in the domains of relating to others, new possibilities, personal strength, spiritual change, and appreciation of life. The reliability of PTGI is good (Cronbach's alpha = 0.937). The constructs in this instrument have been confirmed as relatively robust, with good construct validity (Yi et al., 2015).

Benefit Finding Scale for Children (BFSC)

Children's PTG can be assessed by the Benefit Finding Scale for Children (BFSC; Michel et al., 2009; Phipps et al., 2007). BFSC is a widely used 10-item measure assessing the degree of positive changes following trauma on a 5-point Likert scale. It was administered to childhood cancer survivors, who reported their own positive changes following cancer survival (i.e., child self-reported PTG), and to their parents, who reported positive changes in their child (i.e., parent-proxy reported PTG). The reliability of BFSC was good (Cronbach's alpha for child self-report = 0.901; parent-proxy report = 0.847).

Posttraumatic Growth Assessment Scale

The post-traumatic Growth Assessment Scale includes five dimensions measured through 21 items. Each item is scored from 0 (no change at all), to 5 (change a lot) and the total score is from 0 to 105. Higher scores reflect higher PTG. The total score ≥ 54.23 is regarded as showing the existence of PTG. The Cronbach'α coefficient of the scale is good (α = 0.919).

Qualitative Methods

While the development of instruments allowed to support the PTG constructs in quantitative studies (Zoellner & Maercker, 2006) that showed the aforementioned five domains, the nature of quantitative methodology limits the development of a deeper understanding of each PTG domain and of how the process of growth and related factors mediate the positive changes in childhood and adolescent cancer survivors. A qualitative approach may help to enrich the comprehension of the PTG concept; specifically, the qualitative assessment of the positive impact of cancer in this population, using PTG as a theoretical framework, can help to better understand how they derive meaning-making from their cancer experience. For instance, Zamora and colleagues (2017) used phone interviews starting with a very general question (What positive effects has cancer had on your life?) that allowed them to individuate themes that were in line with the five PTG domains identified by Tedeschi and Calhoun (1996), and further expand these themes through the development of sub-themes. Another qualitative (narrative) method used in this field is the new version of the Nihira et al.'s (1994) Ecocultural Family Interview (EFI) developed by Tremolada et al. (2011), named Ecocultural Family Interview-Cancer (EFI-C) and administered to families with children with leukemia. The EFI-C explores the family's everyday life and scheduling and analyzes salient concerns regarding how that routine is organized. Rather than a formal question-answer interview, it has the sociolinguistic form of a casual conversation about daily life. The interview is a mix of conversation, probing questions by the interviewer, and preplanned questions. Participants use their own words and emphasis. In a recent study (Tremolada et al., 2018), a new version of this guided conversational method was adopted with adolescent and young adult cancer survivors for the purpose of gaining evidence about their illness and present quality of life. The interview starts with questions such as: 'Would you guide me through your daily life? 'What is your routine at this point/now?', 'How is everything going now?', 'Could you narrate your illness experience?', 'What about your positive and negative illness memories?', 'What about school or social experiences?'. Through the interview, participants narrate episodes about relationships with the medical staff in the clinic, family members, and others during the therapeutic process. Other questions relate to the impact of the malignant disease on the physical, social, and psychological aspects of their current life. While narratives may be unique to every adolescent and young adult cancer survivor, clear items and overall dimensions that can be reliably scored have been identified across interviews, including PTG. Using a coding book, the interview allows one to switch from a qualitative level to a quantitative one showing good reliability, with a Cohen's K = 0.75 (Tremolada et al., 2018).

Strategies for Intervention and Clinical Recommendations for Health Professionals

Interviews with survivors of pediatric cancer (Tremolada et al., 2018) suggest that to enable their personal growth, interventions should consider the aspects of memory, which are fundamental for facilitating the re-elaboration of their past experiences. Helping ex-patients recall episodes that characterized their experience, inviting and stimulating them to obtain more information and details about them, and giving them the opportunity to express feelings associated with the illness situation is important in facilitating their personal growth, an aspect closely linked to higher levels of psychological well-being and a better-perceived quality of life.

Adolescent and young adult cancer survivors who had established strong relationships with health professionals are more able to narrate their experiences and display a positive comprehension of the events with a pragmatic acceptance of follow-up procedures. Relationships with health professionals should therefore be monitored and improved, both during the cancer treatment and in the off-therapy period. The narrative technique allows adolescent and young adult cancer survivors to reorganize and shape their traumatic experiences (Tremolada et al., 2018). Jirek (2017) stressed that it is necessary to use narrative reconstruction and PTG interventions to promote empowerment and social justice and that social workers should help trauma survivors to reconstruct their life stories, create spaces for the less-welcomed narratives, and engage in efforts to address social problems and inequalities. It is illuminating to examine narratives when daily life has been disrupted due to a serious illness such as a tumor, requiring the narrators to recreate or reconstruct their life stories. A first example of this occurs after individuals experience trauma. Following such disruptions, the processes through which narratives are created, structured, and performed become most apparent.

That positive associations exist between PTG and both optimism and social support is valuable information for individuals, caregivers, and clinicians. One of the most important forms of social support for a child or adolescent with cancer is the relationship with family members. Ekim and Ocakci (2015) found that adolescents aged 12–18 with cancer experienced more support from family than from friends, whereas older adolescents drew greater support from friends than younger adolescents. They recommended that health professionals plan social support interventions for adolescents with cancer, including family, friends, and support groups.

Several studies have been published on interventions targeting social support. Kazak and colleagues (1999) evaluated a 1-day cognitive behavioral and family therapy-based therapeutic intervention for adolescent survivors of childhood cancer and their family members. The intervention was deemed helpful by all and facilitated alternative perspective-taking, peer support, and in-depth family discussion about cancer and its impact. At 6-month follow-up, posttraumatic stress and anxiety were reduced, although it was not possible to evaluate time as a confounding factor without a control group. Elad and colleagues (2003) evaluated an 8-day adventure jeep trip for young survivors of adolescent cancer. Content analysis of video footage and interviews conducted throughout the trip indicated that self-confidence, independence, and social contacts were improved. Importantly, at 1-year follow-up, social connection was maintained, with participants arranging outdoor adventure activities, social events, and discussion groups. Other important forms of social support for oncological populations may include camps for children with cancer, aerobic classes, age-appropriate support groups, online networks, survivor day picnics, family retreats, and facilitation of storytelling (Tedeschi & Calhoun, 2004; Zebrack & Landier, 2011). A systematic review of psychological therapies for children, adolescents, and adults affected by cancer indicated that group therapy, education, counseling, and cognitive behavioral therapy can be tentatively recommended for a range of medium- and long-term psychosocial outcomes (Newell et al., 2002).

Psychological treatment and psychotherapy may have important implications for the improvement of optimism, in addition to improved interpersonal relationships. Clay and colleagues (2009) argue that introducing PTG into clinical work with young people and their families may build self-esteem and encourage a solution-focused cognitive style. Services, programs, and enhanced social support have the potential to decrease PTSS and promote PTG in this population (Zebrack & Landier, 2011). Other possible interventions to give more significance to their illness experiences, especially in adolescents could be drawing, writing a diary of their experiences, mutual story-telling, social network experiences (telling their experience through a medical story), online meetings, Instagram pages of adolescents as a group, art therapy and meeting with schools. There is a pressing need for further research on the efficacy of such treatments.

Conclusions

Pediatric cancer is seen as a traumatic event that can influence children's and adolescents' lives, both negatively, with PTSS and other psycho-social consequences, but also positively, with PTG experience. This chapter stresses how a growing body of research is dedicated to the observation that some childhood cancer survivors experience PTG, namely a positive psychological change, resulting from struggling with the highly challenging life experience of cancer. Research on PTG in this population has prompted some interesting results and clinical suggestions, but this topic is still immature and new studies should be carried out on AYA (adolescents & young adults) cancer survivors, their parents, and their siblings, possibly adopting a multi-method and multi-informant approach.

References

Alisic, E., Van der Schoot, T., van Ginkel, J. R., & Kleber, R. J. (2008). Looking beyond posttraumatic stress disorder in children: Posttraumatic stress reactions, posttraumatic growth, and quality of life in a general population sample. *Journal of Clinical Psychiatry*, *69*(9), 1455–1461. 10.4088/JCP.v69n0913

Arpawong, T., Oland, A., Milam, J. E., Ruccione, K., & Meeske, K. A. (2013). Post-traumatic growth among an ethnically diverse sample of adolescent and young adult cancer survivors. *Psychooncology*, *22*(10), 2235–2244. 10.1002/pon.3286

Barakat, L. P., Alderfer, M. A., & Kazak, A. E. (2006). Posttraumatic growth in adolescent survivors of cancer and their mothers and fathers. *Journal of Pediatric Psychology*, *31*(4), 413–419. 10.1093/jpepsy/jsj058

Blackie, L. E. R., Jayawickreme, E., Helzer, E. G., Forgeard, M. J. C., Roepke, A. M. (2015). Investigating the veracity of self-perceived posttraumatic growth. *Social Psychology and Personality Science*, *6*(7), 788–796. 10.1177/1948550615587986

Bruce, M. (2006). A systematic and conceptual review of posttraumatic stress in childhood cancer survivors and their parents. *Psychology Review*, *26*(3), 233–256. 10.1016/j.cpr.2005.10.002

Chambers, S. K., Baade, P., Meng, X., Youl, P., Aitken, J., Dunn, J. (2012). Survivor identity after colorectal cancer: Antecedents, prevalence and outcomes. *Psychooncology*, *21*(9), 962–969.

Clay, R., Knibbs, J., & Joseph, S. (2009). Measurement of posttraumatic growth in young people: A review. *Clinical Child Psychology and Psychiatry*, *14*(3), 411–422. 10.1177/1359104509104049

Connerty, T. J., & Knott, V. (2013). Promoting positive change in the face of adversity: Experiences of cancer and post-traumatic growth. *European Journal of Cancer Care*, *22*(3), 334–344.
D'agostino, N. M., Edelstein, K., Zhang, N., Recklitis, C. J., Brinkman, T. M., Srivastava, D., & Krull, K. R. (2016). Comorbid symptoms of emotional distress in adult survivors of childhood cancer. *Cancer*, *122*(20), 3215–3224. 10.1002/cncr.30171
Denney, R. M., Aten, J. D., & Leavell, K. (2011). Posttraumatic spiritual growth: A phenomenological study of cancer survivors. *Mental Health, Religion and Culture*, *14*(4), 371–391.
Duran, B. (2013). Posttraumatic growth as experienced by childhood cancer survivors and their families: A narrative synthesis of qualitative and quantitative research. *Journal of Pediatric Oncology Nursing*, *30*(4), 179–197. 10.1177/1043454213487433
Ekim, A., & Ocakci, A. F. (2015). Relationship between posttraumatic growth and perceived social support for adolescents with cancer. *Journal of Hospice and Palliative Nursing*, *17*(5), 450–455. 10.1097/njh.0000000000000183
Elad, P., Yagil, Y., Cohen, L., & Meller, I. (2003). A jeep trip with young adult cancer survivors: Llessons to be learned. *Support Care Cancer*, *11*(4), 201–206. 10.1007/s00520-002-0426-4
Friend, A. J., Feltbower, R. G., Hughes, E. J., Dye, K. P., & Glaser, A. W. (2018). Mental health of long-term survivors of childhood and young adult cancer: A systematic review. *International Journal of Cancer*, *143*(6), 1279–1286. 10.1002/ijc.31337
Gianinazzi, M. E., Rueegg, C. S., Vetsch, J., Lüer, S., Kuehni, C. E., & Michel, G. (2016). Cancer's positive flip side: Posttraumatic growth after childhood cancer. *Support Care Cancer*, *24*(1), 195–203. 10.1007/s00520-015-2746-1
Gunst, D. C. M., Kaatsch, P., & Goldbeck, L. (2016). Seeing the good in the bad: Which factors are associated with posttraumatic growth in long-term survivors of adolescent cancer? *Support Care Cancer*, *24*(11), 4607–4615. 10.1007/s00520-016-3303-2
Helgeson, V. S. (2011). Survivor centrality among breast cancer survivors: Implications for well-being. *Psychooncology*, *20*, 517–524.
Helgeson, V. S., Reynolds, K. A., & Tomich, P. L. (2006). A meta-analytic review of benefit finding and growth. *Journal of Consulting and Clinical Psychology*, *74*(5), 797–816. 10.1037/0022-006X.74.5.797. PMID: 17032085.
Howard Sharp, K. M., Willard, V. W., Barnes, S., Tillery, R., Long, A., & Phipps, S. (2016). Emotion socialization in the context of 345 childhood cancer: Perceptions of parental support promotes post-traumatic growth. *Journal of Pediatric Psychology*, *42*(1), 95–103. 10.1093/jpepsy/jsw062
Howard Sharp, K. M., Willard, V. W., Okado, Y., Tillery, R., Barnes, S., Long, A., & Phipps, S. (2015). Profiles of cconnectedness: Processes of resilience and growth in children with cancer. *Journal of Pediatric Psychology*, *40*(9), 904–913. 10.1093/jpepsy/jsv036
Howlader, N., Noone, A. M., & Krapcho, M. (eds) (2021). SEER Cancer Statistics Review, 1975–2018, *National Cancer Institute*. Bethesda, MD, https://seer.cancer.gov/csr/1975_2018/, based on November 2020 SEER data submission, posted to the SEER web site, April 2021. http://www.jstor.org/stable/41488228
Jirek, S. L. (2017). Narrative reconstruction and post-traumatic growth among trauma survivors: The importance of narrative in social work research and practice. *Qualitative Social Work: Research and Practice*, *16*(2), 166–188. 10.1177/1473325016656046
Joseph, S., Hefferon, K. (2013). Post-traumatic growth: Eudaimonic happiness in the aftermath of adversity. In I. Boniwell, S. A. David & A. C. Ayers (Eds.), *Oxford Handbook of Happiness* (pp. 926–940). Oxford, England: Oxford University Press.
Kamibeppu, K., Sato, I., Honda, M., Ozono, S., Sakamoto, N., Iwai, T., Okamura, J., Asami, K., Maeda, N., Inada, H., Kakee, N., Horibe, K., & Ishida, Y. (2010). Mental health among young adult survivors of childhood cancer and their siblings including posttraumatic growth. *Journal of Cancer Survivorship*, *4*(4), 303–312. 10.1007/s11764-010-0124-z
Kazak, A. E., Alderfer, M. A., Rourke, M. T., Simms, S., Streisand, R., & Grossman, J. R. (2004). Posttraumatic stress disorder (PTSD) and posttraumatic stress symptoms (PTSS) in families of adolescent childhood cancer survivors. *Journal of Pediatric Psychology*, *29*(3), 211–219. 10.1093/jpepsy/jsh022
Kazak, A. E., Simms, S., Barakat, L., Hobbie, W., Foley, B., Golomb, V., & Best, M. (1999). Surviving cancer competently intervention program (SCCIP): A cognitive-behavioral and family therapy intervention for adolescent survivors of childhood cancer and their families. *Family Process*, *38*(2), 175–191. 10.1111/j.1545-5300.1999.00176.x

Koutná, V., & Blatny, M. (2020). Socialization of coping in pediatric oncology settings: Theoretical consideration on parent–child connections in posttraumatic growth. *Frontiers in Psychology, 11*, 554325. 10.3389/fpsyg.2020.554325
Koutná, V., Jelínek, M., Blatný, M., & Kepák, T. (2017). Predictors of posttraumatic stress and posttraumatic growth in childhood cancer survivors. *Cancers*, *9*(3), 26. 10.3390/cancers9030026
Lee, V. (2008). The existential plight of cancer: Meaning making as a concrete approach to the intangible search for meaning. *Support Care Cancer*, *16*(7), 779e–785e. 10.1007/s00520-007-0396-7
Linley, P. A., & Joseph, S. (2004). Positive change following trauma and adversity: A review. *Journal of Trauma Stress*, *17*(1), 11–21. 10.1023/B:JOTS.0000014671.27856.7e
Mehrabi, E., Hajian, S., Simbar, M., Houshyari, M., & Zayeri, F. (2015). Post-traumatic growth: A qualitative analysis of experiences regarding positive psychological changes among Iranian women with breast cancer. *Electron Physician*, 16, *7*(5), 1239–1246. 10.14661/1239
Meyerson, D. A., Grant, K. E., Carter, J. S., & Kilmer, R. P. (2011). Posttraumatic growth among children and adolescents: A systematic review. *Clinical Psychology Reviews*, *31*(6), 949–964. 10.1016/j.cpr.2011.06.003
Michel, G., Taylor, N., Absolom, K., & Eiser, C. (2009). Benefit finding in survivors of childhood cancer and their parents: Further empirical support for the benefit finding scale for children. *Child Care Health Development*, *36*(1), 123–129. 10.1111/j.1365-2214.2009.01034.x
Milam, J. E., Ritt-Olson, A., & Unger, J. B. (2004). Posttraumatic growth among adolescents. *Journal of Adolescent Research*, *19*(2), 192–204.
Moore, A. M., Gamblin, T. C., Geller, D. A., Youssef, M. N., Hoffman, K. E., Gemmell, L., Likumahuwa, S. M., Bovbjerg, D. H., Marsland, A., & Steel, J. L. (2011). A prospective study of posttraumatic growth as assessed by self-report and family caregiver in the context of advanced cancer. *Psychooncology*, *20*(5), 479–487. 10.1002/pon.1746
Newell, S. A., Sanson-Fisher, R. W., & Savolainen, N. J. (2002). Systematic review of psychological therapies for cancer patients: Overview and recommendations for future research. *Journal of the National Cancer Institute*, *94*(8), 558–584.
Nihira, K., Weisner, T. S., & Bernheimer, L. P. (1994). Ecocultural assessment in families of children with development delays: Construct and concurrent validities. *American Journal of Mental Retardation*, *98*(5), 551–566.
Okado, Y., Tillery, R., Howard Sharp, K., Long, A. M., & Phipps, S. (2016). Effects of time since diagnosis on the association between parent and child distress in families with pediatric cancer. *Child Health Care*, *45*(3), 303–322. 10.1080/02739615.2014.996883
Park, C. L., & Lechner, S. C. (2006). Measurement issues in assessing growth following stressful life experiences. In L. G. Calhoun & R. G. Tedeschi (Eds.), *Handbook of posttraumatic growth: Research & practice* (pp 47–67). Mahwah, NJ: Lawrence Erlbaum Associates Publishers.
Park, C. L., Cohen, L. H., & Murch, R. L. (1996). Assessment and prediction of stress-related growth. *Journal of Personality*, *64*(1), 71–105, 71e105. 10.1111/j.1467-6494.1996.tb00815.x
Park, N., & Peterson, C. (2006). Character strengths and happiness among young children: Content analysis of parental descriptions. *Journal of Happiness Studies*, *7*(3), 323–341. 10.1007/s10902-005-3648-6
Phipps, S., Long, A. M., & Ogden, J. (2007). Benefit Finding Scale for children: Preliminary findings from a childhood cancer population. *Journal of Pediatric Psychology*, *32*(10), 1264–1271. 10.1093/jpepsy/jsl052
Piaget, J. (1971). The theory of stages in cognitive development. In D. R. Green, M. P. Ford, & G. B. Flamer (Eds.), *Measurement and Piaget* (pp. 1–11). New York, NY, US: McGraw-Hill.
Picoraro, J. A., Womer, J. W., Kazak, A. E., & Feudtner, C. (2014). Posttraumatic growth in parents and pediatric patients. *Journal of Palliative Medicine*, *17*(2), 209–218. 10.1089/jpm.2013.0280
Rinaldis, M., Pakenham, K. I., & Lynch, B. M. (2010). Relationships between quality of life and finding benefits in a diagnosis of colorectal cancer. *British Journal of Psychology*, *101*(Pt. 2), 259–275.
Sabiston, C. M., McDonough, M. H., & Crocker, P. R. (2007). Psychosocial experiences of breast cancer survivors involved in a dragon boat program: Exploring links to positive psychological growth. *Journal of Sport & Exercise Psychology*, *29*(4), 419–438.
Scrignaro, M., Sani, F., Wakefield, J. R., Bianchi, E., Magrin, M. E., & Gangeri, L. (2016). Post-traumatic growth enhances social identification in liver transplant patients: A longitudinal study. *Journal of Psychosomatic Research*, *88*, 28–32. 10.1016/j.jpsychores.2016.07.004

Shakespeare-Finch, J., & Lurie-Beck, J. (2014). A meta-analytic clarification of the relationship between posttraumatic growth and symptoms of posttraumatic distress disorder. *Journal of Anxiety Disorder*, *28*(2), 223–229. 10.1016/j.janxdis.2013.10.005

Shand, L. K., Cowlishaw, S., Brooker, J. E., Burney, S., & Ricciardelli, L. A. (2015). Correlates of post-traumatic stress symptoms and growth in cancer patients: A systematic review and meta-analysis. *Psychooncology*, *24*(6), 624–634. 10.1002/pon.3719

Siegel, R. L., Miller, K. D., Fuchs, H. E., & Jemal A. (2021). Cancer Statistics. *CA: A Cancer Journal for Clinicians*, *71*(1), 7–33.

Taïeb, O., Moro, M. R., Baubet, T., Revah-Lévy, A., & Flament, M. F. (2003). Posttraumatic stress symptoms after childhood cancer. *Child and Adolescent Psychiatry*, *12*(6), 255–264. 10.1007/s00787-003-0352-0

Tedeschi, R. G., & Calhoun, L. G. (1996). The posttraumatic growth inventory: Measuring the positive legacy of trauma. *Journal of Traumatic Stress*, *9*(3), 455–471.

Tedeschi, R. G., & Calhoun, L. G. (2004). Posttraumatic growth: Conceptual foundations and empirical evidence. *Psychological Inquiry*, *15*(1), 1–18. 10.1207/s15327965pli1501_01

Tedeschi, R. G., & Kilmer, R. P. (2005). Assessing strengths, resilience, and growth to guide clinical interventions. *Professional Psychology: Research and Practice*, *36*(3), 230–237.

Tomich, P. L., & Helgeson, V. S. (2002). Five years later: A cross-sectional comparison of breast cancer survivors with healthy women. *Psychooncology*, *11*(2), 154–169.

Tremolada, M., Bonichini, S., Altoè, G. M., Pillon, M., Carli, M., & Weisner, T. S. (2011). Parental perceptions of health-related quality of life in children with leukemia in the second week after diagnosis: A quantitative model. *Supportive Care in* Cancer, *19*(5), 591–598. 10.1007/s00520-010-0854-5

Tremolada, M., Bonichini, S., Basso, G., & Pillon, M. (2016a). Post-traumatic stress symptoms and post-traumatic growth in 223 childhood cancer survivors: Predictive risk factors. *Frontiers in Psychology*, 7, 287–299. 10.3389/fpsyg.2016.00237

Tremolada, M., Bonichini, S., Basso, G., & Pillon, M. (2016b). Perceived social support and health related quality of life in AYA cancer survivors of childhood and controls. *Psycho-oncology*, *25*(12), 1408–1417. 10.1002/pon.4072

Tremolada, M., Bonichini, S., Basso, G., & Pillon, M. (2018). AYA Adolescent and young adult cancer survivors narrate their stories: Predictive model of their personal growth and their follow-up acceptance. *European Journal of Cancer Nursing*, *36*, 119–128. 10.1016/j.ejon.2018.09.001

Turner-Sack, A. M., Menna, R., & Setchell, S. R. (2012). Posttraumatic growth, coping strategies, and psychological distress in adolescent survivors of cancer. *Journal of Pediatric Oncology Nursing*, *29*(2), 70–79. 10.1177/1043454212439472

Turner, J. K., Hutchinson, A., & Wilson, C. (2018). Correlates of post-traumatic growth following childhood and adolescent cancer: A systematic review and meta-analysis. *Psychoncology*, *27*(4), 1100–1109. 10.1002/pon.4577

Wakefield, C. E., McLoone, J., Butow, P., Lenthen, K., & Cohn, R. J. (2013). Support after the completion of cancer treatment: Perspectives of Australian adolescents and their families. *Journal of Cancer Care*, *22*(4), 530–539. 10.1111/ecc.12059

Weiss, T. (2002). Posttraumatic growth in women with breast cancer and their husbands: An intersubjective validation study. *Journal of Psychosocial Oncology*, *20*(2), 65–80.

Yaskowich, K. M. (2002). Post-traumatic growth in children and adolescents with cancer, (Doctoral dissertation) University of Calgary, 341 2002. 10.11575/PRISM/20242

Yi, J., & Kim, M. A. (2014). Postcancer experiences of childhood cancer survivors: How is posttraumatic stress related to posttraumatic growth? *Journal of Trauma Stress*, *27*(4), 461–467. 10.1002/jts.21941

Yi, J., Zebrack, B., Kim, M. A., & Cousino, M. (2015). Posttraumatic growth outcomes and their correlates among young adult survivors of childhood cancer. *Journal of Pediatric Psychology*, *40*, 981–991.

Zamora, E. R., Yi, J., Akter, J., Kim, J., Warner, E. L., & Kirchhoff, A. C. (2017). 'Having cancer was awful but also something good came out': Post-traumatic growth among adult survivors of pediatric and adolescent cancer. *European Journal of Oncology Nursing*, *28*, 21–27.

Zannini, L., Cattaneo, C., Jankovic, M., & Masera G. (2014) Surviving childhood Leukemia in a Latin culture: An explorative study based on young adults' written narratives. *Journal of Psychosocial Oncology*, *32*(5), 576–601. 10.1080/07347332.2014.936648

Zebrack, B. J., & Landier, W. (2011). The perceived impact of cancer on quality of life for post-treatment survivors of childhood cancer. *Quality of Life Research*, *20*(10), 1595–1608.
Zebrack, B. J., Stuber, M. L., Meeske, K. A., Phipps, S., Krull, K. R., Liu, Q., Yasui, Y., Parry, C., Hamilton, R., Robison, L. L., & Zeltzer, L. K. (2012). Perceived positive impact of cancer among long-term survivors of childhood cancer: A report from the childhood cancer survivor study. *Psychooncology*, *21*(6), 630–639. 10.1002/pon.1959
Zoellner, T., & Maercker, A. (2006). Posttraumatic growth in clinical psychology – A critical review and introduction of a two component model. *Clinical Psychology Review*, *26*(5), 626e–653e.

PART 4C

PTG in Communities

24

POSTTRAUMATIC GROWTH DURING THE COVID-19 PANDEMIC

Dana Rose Garfin, Ana Laura Estevez, and Michelle Veronica Zernick

The COVID-19 pandemic has been an unprecedented traumatic event, embodying elements of both acute and chronic stressors (Garfin & Estes, 2022) with far-reaching implications for mental health and well-being. Research conducted early in the pandemic (Holman et al., 2020) and throughout (Ettman et al., 2020; Rudenstine et al., 2021) demonstrated that the crisis has been associated with increases in traumatic stress responses including anxiety, depression, and acute and posttraumatic stress (PTS: Cénat et al., 2021; Cooke et al., 2020). Yet posttraumatic growth (PTG), which often occurs in tandem with traumatic stress responses (Solomon & Dekel, 2007) has also been documented (Vazquez et al., 2021), in alignment with reports of people finding positive benefits associated with the COVID-19 pandemic (Kowalski et al., 2021). This chapter provides a brief overview of PTG during prior collective traumas and reviews the literature on PTG during COVID-19, including a critique of the current research and suggestions for future inquiry.

PTG during Prior Collective Traumas and Personal Illness

The COVID-19 pandemic has embodied aspects of acute traumatic events and personal illness; devastating sickness and death have occurred at the individual level, with many grieving the death of loved ones and others managing the debilitating effects of long-COVID (Garfin & Estes, 2022). The pandemic has also been a chronic, collective trauma, with psychological effects rippling throughout society for those both directly and indirectly exposed (Silver et al., 2021). Indirect, media-based exposure and secondary stressors (e.g., education disruption, financial loss) that occurred both as a result of widespread infection and associated mitigation efforts (e.g., restrictions on movement, business closures) have resulted in protracted exposure over the course of months and years. Moreover, the crisis has been compounded by co-occurring stressors including intense weather events, overwhelmed hospitals, social unrest, and economic recession, which have created a confluence of stressors associated with increased acute stress, ongoing worry, and symptoms of depression and traumatic stress (Holman et al., 2020; Silver et al., 2021).

DOI: 10.4324/9781032208688-31

PTG during Prior Collective Trauma

Prior research on collective traumas, such as terrorism (Rimé et al., 2010; Solomon & Dekel, 2007), natural disasters (Wlodarczyk et al., 2017), and infectious disease outbreaks (Rzeszutek et al., 2016; Rzeszutek & Gruszczyńska, 2021) suggests that both children and adults can experience PTG during community crises. For example, after a terrorist attack in Spain, adult participants reported giving greater importance to intrinsic motivations and increased gratitude for the "smaller things" in life (Nadeem et al., 2019; Rimé et al., 2010). Research with adult survivors of the 2010 8.8 magnitude earthquake in Chile found PTG can occur across multiple dimensions, including individual, spiritual, community, and societal growth (Wlodarczyk et al., 2017).

Some variability in reports of event-related PTG has been explained by key indices of adversity exposure. For example, direct objective exposure (e.g., damage to a home, injury, or threat to life), subjective exposure (e.g., self-reported reactions such as fear or worry), and indirect exposure (e.g., learning about the event from others, contact with media coverage, or living near the affected community) have been associated with PTG in children and adolescents (Bernstein & Pfefferbaum, 2018). In adults, the self-report intensity of direct, earthquake-related traumatic experience was positively associated with PTG, suggesting that the severity of adverse exposure may elicit greater experiences of growth (Wlodarczyk et al., 2017). Taken together, these examples suggest that despite the strong association between the COVID-19 pandemic and psychological distress, experiences of PTG and resilience may also be common, with pandemic-related exposures associated with increased experiences of growth.

PTG during Personal Illness

The experience of contracting and caring for those with COVID-19 may also be associated with PTG during the pandemic. PTG has been documented following the micro-level experience of illness including HIV (Lau et al., 2018), SARS (Cheng et al., 2006; Cheng & Wong, 2005) and cancer, and for those with Huntington's Disease and their caregivers (Luszczynska et al., 2012). Collectively, research on illness-related PTG has found that PTG can manifest as increased optimism (Cheng & Wong, 2005), self-confidence (Cheng et al., 2006), compassion for others (Lau et al., 2018), spirituality (Cheng et al., 2006; Cheng & Wong, 2005; Luszczynska et al., 2012), and a focus on the importance of family and friends (Lau et al., 2018). Moreover, cognitive representations (i.e., personal control, treatment control, and illness coherence) may be positively associated with illness-related PTG through factors including self-efficacy and hopefulness (Lau et al., 2018). Such findings suggest the experience of contracting and surviving COVID-19 may paradoxically also be associated with some positive psychological benefits including the experience of PTG.

PTG during COVID-19

The first two years of the COVID-19 pandemic ushered in a staggering amount of research regarding the mental health effects of the crisis, with systematic reviews documenting the relationship between the pandemic and various forms of psychological distress including anxiety, depression (Pashazadeh Kan et al., 2021; Xiong et al., 2020) and PTS (Salehi et al., 2021) in adults; high prevalence of mental health problems have been noted in children and adolescents as well (Ma et al., 2021). Yet as documented in previous accounts of growth associated with collective trauma exposure, an increasing body of literature suggests that PTG may be a common experience during COVID-19 as well (Na et al., 2021). Specifically, COVID-19-related PTG has been evidenced in healthcare (Zhang et al., 2021) and other frontline workers (Cui et al., 2021), tourism employees (Luu, 2022), and in clinical samples (Sun et al., 2021). These findings demonstrate the widespread phenomenon of COVID-19-related PTG that occurred despite the unprecedented disruption and adversity experienced worldwide.

Literature on PTG experienced during COVID-19 has evaluated growth using a variety of indicators, yielding a rich picture of the type of growth people experienced. Reports of PTG-related experiences were common: one online study (N=311) found that over 90% of respondents reported at least one type of growth experience (Jin et al., 2020). Common experiences across samples included greater appreciation of life (Asmundson et al., 2021; Jin et al., 2020; Na et al., 2021; Stallard et al., 2021), improved relations with others (Arnout & Al-sufyani, 2021; Jin et al., 2020; Stallard et al., 2021), changed priorities (Asmundson et al., 2021; Pietrzak et al., 2021), and increased personal strength (Arnout & Al-sufyani, 2021; Jin et al., 2020). Increased sense of gratitude was also common, as demonstrated in a sample of veterans (Pietrzak et al., 2021) and in a random sample of Saudi respondents (Arnout & Al-sufyani, 2021). Relatedly, some reported feeling a greater appreciation for friends, family, and healthcare workers (Asmundson et al., 2021). Other outcomes included greater spiritual connection (Arnout & Al-sufyani, 2021; Stallard et al., 2021), discovering and embracing new possibilities (Stallard et al., 2021), greater feelings of self-reliance (Asmundson et al., 2021), and feeling like it was possible to "rise above the trauma" (Foli et al., 2021).

Personal growth was also expressed as increased self-care and exploration of meaningful activities. For example, in a sample of 1175 New Zealand residents, many reported increased personal development that included self-care activities, developing new skills or habits, improved personal health due to healthier diets, increased physical exercise, and better sleep (Jenkins et al., 2021). Nurses working with COVID-19 patients also described increased self-care as a consequence of adapting to and managing stress (Foli et al., 2021). Personal growth was exemplified in a qualitative study of Italian adolescents of whom 33% reported positive experiences related to "discovering oneself", finding pleasure in spending time with oneself, and exploring meaningful hobbies such as reading, listening to music, art, and working out (Fioretti et al., 2020).

Populations Studied and Methods Implemented

Healthcare Workers

A substantial portion of the early research on PTG during COVID-19 focused on healthcare workers (Chen et al., 2021; Kalaitzaki, 2021; Kalaitzaki et al., 2021; Lee & Lee, 2020; Zhang et al., 2021). Despite reporting pandemic-related burnout and ambivalent feelings towards patients, during COVID-19 many nurses reported concurrent PTG, often related to finding positive meaning in their work (Li et al., 2022; Zhang et al., 2021). In-depth interviews with 18 COVID-19 hospital nurses in South Korea found that they reported new feelings of pride and satisfaction in their profession as they felt they were making a tangible contribution to the fight against COVID-19 (Lee & Lee, 2020). Early on, healthcare professionals often responded to the pandemic with increased levels of distress, which was, in some cases, replaced by personal growth as the pandemic continued (Kalaitzaki et al., 2021). Yet, longitudinal findings of frontline healthcare workers during COVID-19 indicated that high early burnout and emotional exhaustion contributed to lower PTG over time (Lyu et al., 2021), suggesting that efforts seeking to reduce burnout could help facilitate PTG and other growth-related outcomes.

The extent to which healthcare workers reported PTG during COVID-19 varied, with experiential and social factors associated with key differences (Chen et al., 2021). For example, 39.3% of a sample of 12,596 nurses reported PTG during the pandemic, with rates higher for participants who worked in COVID-19 designated hospitals or with COVID-19 patients compared to those who worked with other patients (Chen et al., 2021). Compared to non-frontline nurses, being a frontline nurse who interacted or offered treatment directly to patients diagnosed with COVID-19 was associated with reporting higher levels of PTG (Li et al., 2022). Similarly, a study of 1,790 clinical nurses, assessed in June 2020 in China, found a "moderately high" level of PTG among clinical nurses, with social support and self-efficacy positively associated with PTG (Zhang et al., 2021). A longitudinal study of psychotherapists, many transitioning to online services, found that PTG was associated with vicarious trauma exposure as well as more acceptance of online therapy at baseline (Doorn et al., 2021). Such data suggests that although potentially more stressful and challenging, more direct and secondary (vicarious) COVID-19-related experiences in healthcare workers may have elicited greater experiences of growth and resilience, particularly if such experiences were accompanied by self-confidence, self-efficacy, and social support rather than burnout.

General Populace

PTG has also been documented in the general populace; studies have been conducted in the United States (Na et al., 2021), Canada (Asmundson et al., 2021), Europe (Miragall et al., 2021), China (Cui et al., 2021), Turkey (Ikizer & Gul, 2021), and elsewhere, lending cross-cultural credibility to findings. Yet many of these studies relied on cross-sectional data and convenience sampling, limiting the strength of inferences. For example, an e-mail recruitment strategy was used to assess French residents (Miragall et al., 2021) as were online opt-in survey platforms (Jin et al., 2020) and snowball samples (Robles-Bello et al., 2020). One exception was a study from Spain that used a quota-based, stratified sampling strategy to recruit a representative sample (N=2,122) (Vazquez et al., 2021). That study found that primary beliefs in goodness, identification with humanity, and openness to the future were associated with PTG, while suspicious beliefs and lower primal beliefs about goodness were associated with posttraumatic impairment. Some studies were representative of the target population but did not report details of the recruitment method (Robles-Bello et al., 2020). While the use of convenience samples and cross-sectional data allowed for early findings to emerge to provide preliminary insights regarding PTG during an unprecedented global phenomenon, they may also have contributed to inconsistent findings across studies.

Several early studies found relatively low levels of PTG (Arnout & Al-sufyani, 2021; Feng et al., 2021; Jin et al., 2020) at the onset of the pandemic. This could be due to lower exposure to secondary stressors associated with the beginning phases of the pandemic (e.g., loss of a loved one, physical illness, financial strain), that subsequently emerged over time. Relatedly, as postulated by Robles-Bello et al. (2020), early in the pandemic, lower perceptions of personal risk and low compliance with restrictions in some communities may have led to less disruption and stress, and consequently, less growth through adversity. However, one study from Indonesia found that, despite reports of traumatic stress responses, those responses were not associated with stress-related growth (Kaloeti et al., 2021). However, the small (N=119) non-representative (86.6% women), non-probability-based sample may limit inferences whereas a large (N=29,118) study of Chinese adults assessed in early 2020 found positive associations between PTS and PTG (Zhao et al., 2021).

Clinical Samples

Despite evidence that PTG can often emerge post-illness, the research on PTG in clinical samples during COVID-19 is relatively nascent. Qualitative findings from participants recruited from a COVID-19 hospital in Shanghai, China (interviewed between April-July 2020) found that many reported common growth experiences including re-evaluating values and priorities, improved social relationships, and general personal growth (Sun et al., 2021). Likewise, in a sample of 140 recently discharged COVID-19 patients in Hunan, China, assessed by an online nurse-supervised questionnaire, patients reported finding new possibilities, identification of personal strengths, and enhanced relations with others (Yan et al., 2021). The study also found that those living in non-urban areas exhibited higher PTG compared to those in urban areas, suggesting contextual factors in the community may contribute to resilience. Finally, a qualitative study of 18 nurses diagnosed with COVID-19 found that although being diagnosed with COVID-19 was associated with negative experiences, such as fear or death, and stigma, it was also associated with positive experiences including PTG and engaging in more empathetic and prosocial nursing care (Aydin & Assistant, 2021).

One study assessed the trajectory of PTG in a sample of 422 individuals experiencing COVID-19-related bereavement (Chen & Tang, 2021). The study found four latent classes related to grief, PTS, and PTG, with heterogeneity between groups: *resilience* (low prolonged grief and PTS and high PTG; 10.7% of respondents), *growth* (low prolonged grief, PTS, and PTG; 20.1% of respondents), *moderate* (moderate scores on prolonged grief, PTS, and PTG; 42.2% of respondents), and *high* (high scores on prolonged grief, PTS, and PTG; 27% of respondents), with closeness to the deceased and whether the loss was of a partner predicting moderate and high PTG scores. Such findings suggest more severe experiences were associated with concurrent PTS and PTG, in alignment with prior studies of collective trauma that linked the severity of adversity exposure and PTS with PTG.

Caregivers

Caregivers of children were also studied with respect to COVID-19-related PTG. One study found that while many mothers were managing a variety of pandemic-related stressors (including remote work, reduced income, homeschooling, and COVID-19-related illness in the family), they also reported experiences of PTG. These included experiences commonly identified in other samples (e.g., improved relationships, a greater appreciation of life, positive spiritual change) as well as experiences unique to caregivers such as the adoption of a better work-family balance and the acquisition of new technology-related competencies that helped with children's education and socialization (Stallard et al., 2021). Some parents also viewed the opportunity to home-school as a positive outcome, reporting "this has been a wonderful experience." Importantly, the number of positive experiences was negatively correlated with anxiety and positively correlated with well-being, suggesting that growth experiences can occur in the absence of psychological distress.

Children, Youth, and Young Adults

Systematic reviews have documented the deleterious mental health impacts of the COVID-19 pandemic and related public health interventions (e.g., school closures) on children's mental health (Samji et al., 2021; Viner et al., 2022). The pandemic brought a host of stressors unique to younger individuals and alteration of key life narratives (Fioretti et al., 2020) such as online graduations and lack of opportunities to participate in team sports (Garfin & Estes, 2022). Yet qualitative analyses from a sample of Italian female adolescents (mean age=16.6) found that despite the identification of negative themes including "anguish and loss," some positive experiences were also reported (Fioretti et al., 2020). These positive aspects included being part of an extraordinary experience, discovering oneself, rediscovering family, and sharing life at a distance. Similar to findings from adults, a sample of 683 adolescents in China found heterogeneity in growth trajectories that suggests that distress and growth occurred concurrently during COVID-19 (Zhen & Zhou, 2021). Despite this overall heterogeneity, trajectories indicating growth tended to be associated with positive refocusing and reappraisal, suggesting those cognitive mechanisms could bolster adaptive responses even in the context of high distress.

Several studies focused on young adults and university students. For example, a longitudinal survey of 805 young adults in the U.S. (mean age = 24) found that, in general, PTG remained relatively low, with PTSD and COVID-19-related worry positively associated with PTG, and depression negatively associated with it (Hyun et al., 2021). Likewise, a convenience sample of 99 university students who completed an online survey in Poland found PTSD and PTG were positively associated (Tomaszek & Muchacka-cymerman, 2020). However, the non-representativeness of those samples (for example, 78% and 85% were women, respectively) limit broad inferences.

Older Adults

Despite being more at risk for COVID-19-related complications compared to younger individuals, limited work has focused specifically on older adults. In one sample of older adults (age 55 or older), who were senior students at the University of Experience (University of Barcelona), only 25% reported higher PTG after the forced lockdown in Spain (in March-April 2020). On average, the highest PTG subscale reported was "appreciation of life" and the lowest "spiritual change" (Celdran et al., 2021). Yet the cross-sectional nature and sample of this and other studies limit relevance to a gerontological sample more broadly. Interestingly, this study found both increases and decreases in loneliness were associated with the experience of PTG, suggesting that altered life circumstances, whether positive or negative, might lead individuals to experience growth during adverse life events.

Correlates of COVID-19 Related PTG

Research has documented a variety of indicators associated with COVID-19-related PTG, elucidating heterogeneity in responses. Some of these factors included demographic indicators (e.g., age, socioeconomic status, race/ethnicity), coping techniques (including cognitive strategies and styles), social support, and other psychosocial predictors.

Demographic Indicators

Gender

Across a variety of studies, women, on average, reported higher PTG than men. This was evident in a sample of hospitality workers (Luu, 2022), a nationally representative sample of U.S. military veterans (Na et al., 2021), a sample of 12,596 nurses in Japan (Chen et al., 2021), a sample of young adults (Hyun et al., 2021), and the populace more generally (Kalaitzaki, 2021). This may be because women tend to report higher distress symptoms including PTS, which often correlated with growth experiences during COVID-19 (Kalaitzaki, 2021) and following trauma generally. Yet the data linking gender and PTG have not been definitive; some studies found no effects of gender on PTG (Casali et al., 2021; Ikizer & Gul, 2021); others did not report the results of gender (Feng et al., 2021), including one study with a representative sample (Vazquez et al., 2021). Importantly, the non-representativeness of many early studies on the psychological effects of COVID-19 (which often included more women) could be a potential reason for these inconsistent findings (Robles-Bello et al., 2020).

AGE

The experience of PTG during COVID-19 has been documented in age-specific samples across the lifespan (Celdran et al., 2021; Fioretti et al., 2020; Samji et al., 2021; Tomaszek & Muchacka-cymerman, 2020; Viner et al., 2022; Zhen & Zhou, 2021). Parsing out which age groups are more likely to experience PTG during COVID-19 has been elusive, with some studies demonstrating non-linear relationships between PTG and age (e.g., middle age had the highest PTG) (Zhao et al., 2021) and others not finding a relationship between age and PTG (Casali et al., 2021). Yet in studies looking at healthcare workers (Kalaitzaki et al., 2021) and adult residents in the United States (Northfield & Johnston, 2021), age was negatively correlated with PTG, specifically in the dimensions of relating to others and being open to new possibilities. This could be because younger individuals may be more open to changing their cognitive schemas (Kalaitzaki et al., 2021), or due to the fact that in general age has been negatively correlated with traumatic stress responses throughout the COVID-19 pandemic (Holman et al., 2020), which in turn, could elicit the experience of PTG.

SOCIOECONOMIC STATUS

The relationship between the socioeconomic indicators of education and income and PTG during COVID-19 has also been inconsistent. Some studies have reported null effects (Hamam et al., 2021; Pietrzak et al., 2021), other studies reported positive correlations between income and PTG (Yildiz, 2021) and education and PTG (Cui et al., 2021; Zhang et al., 2021); yet others found negative relationships between education and PTG (Ikizer & Gul, 2021). Some research demonstrated non-linear effects; for example, Feng and collaborators (2021) reported that those with lower education (e.g., less than high school) or those with some college experience more PTG. In contrast, Zhao et al. (2021) found that those with a high school education had the highest PTG compared to those with less or those with more education. Lastly, several studies reported socioeconomic indicators as part of an assessment of demographic indicators (Chen et al., 2021; Vazquez et al., 2021), but did not detail the findings of specific relationships. More work on the relationship between socioeconomic status and PTG during COVID-19 is needed, particularly given the widely documented inequity in exposure to COVID-19-related stressors across different groups (Shigemoto, 2021).

RACE/ETHNICITY

Several studies reported differences in COVID-19-related PTG according to racial/ethnic group identification. For example, results from a study of 893 Canadian and U.S. adults found that, compared to individuals identifying as White, those identifying as African American/Black reported higher PTG (Asmundson et al., 2021). This finding was mirrored in a smaller sample, which found that participants identifying as non-White/European American reported higher PTG compared to those identifying as White/European American (Shigemoto, 2021). One explanation is that underrepresented minorities may have faced additional stressors such as health inequalities and discrimination, which were exacerbated by the COVID-19 pandemic, driving higher distress and in turn PTG. Yet this phenomenon did not extend to individuals identifying as Asians; both US-born and foreign-born Asians were less likely to report COVID-19-related PTG compared to White participants (Hyun et al., 2021). Hyun and collaborators (2021) postulated that Asian-specific racism and increased violence and hate crimes targeted at Asian communities may have made it particularly difficult to report finding benefits during the COVID-19 pandemic. These paradoxical findings regarding group differences should be clarified with future research.

Coping Techniques

PTG may be both a cause and a correlate of effective coping strategies during an ongoing, chronic stressor such as COVID-19. Indeed, PTG may be viewed both as a result of the experience of adversity and a type of cognitive coping strategy that occur as the result of surviving trauma; thus, as with prior research on PTG, research conducted in relation to COVID-19 found that coping and PTG often demonstrated significant correlations (Yan et al., 2021). Importantly, both adaptive and maladaptive coping strategies were associated with PTG (Kalaitzaki et al., 2021). For example, in a sample of healthcare workers in Greece, problem-focused coping (e.g., positive reframing) and emotion-focused coping (e.g., self-distraction) partially mediated the relationship between secondary traumatic trauma exposure and PTG, while maladaptive coping (e.g., denial) fully mediated the relationship (Kalaitzaki et al., 2021). This suggests that certain types of avoidance and emotion-focused coping may be beneficial in promoting some types of PTG (including personal strength and appreciation of life), at least in short term. This is in alignment with prior research that supports the efficacy of both avoidant and non-avoidant coping strategies, with some avoidant strategies associated with short-term positive coping and non-avoidant strategies predicting more positive adaption long term (Suls & Fletcher, 1985). In the context of COVID-19, this signals the need for longitudinal research to parse out the effectiveness of coping strategies over time.

During stressful and traumatic events, cognitive coping helps individuals understand and process the event and their "shattered assumptions" about the safety and security of the world around them (Janoff-Bulman, 1992; Tedeschi & Calhoun, 2004). Variability in the use of such cognitive process was associated with variability in PTG during COVID-19. For example, cognitive strategies such as positive refocusing and reappraisal were associated with growth, while deliberate rumination, catastrophizing, and "putting it in perspective" were associated with distress (Zhen & Zhou, 2021). Prior research suggests deliberate rumination or meaning-making tends to be associated with growth experiences and intrusive ruination tends to show more mixed effects (Tedeschi & Calhoun, 2004). Data collected during COVID-19 tend to support the relationship between deliberate rumination and PTG. For example, in the summer of 2020, in a sample of 685 Turkish adults, deliberate rumination (as opposed to intrusive rumination) was associated with COVID-19-related PTG (Ikizer & Gul, 2021). This suggests deliberately thinking about the meaning of COVID-19 with a focus on finding solutions may have contributed to growth experiences. Such findings were also evidenced in a sample of 918 Chinese college students where deliberate rumination enhanced the relationship between the experience of COVID-19-related PTG and resilience (Zeng et al., 2021). Finally, in a sample of tourism workers during the COVID-19 shutdown, deliberate rumination was positively associated with a positive stress mindset, particularly in the context of high family support, which in turn was associated with PTG (Luu, 2022). Taken together, these results suggest PTG may occur as part of cognitive coping strategies that include finding meaning and sense-making during adverse experiences (Silver et al., 1983; Updegraff et al., 2008), which can facilitate the process of PTG.

Social Support

Despite the consistent finding that PTG is associated with stress, adversity, and COVID-19-related distress responses, social support during COVID-19 appeared to buffer the negative psychological effects of the pandemic, leading to PTG. Various forms of social support were associated with PTG throughout the pandemic including support from family (Northfield & Johnston, 2021; Yan et al., 2021) and friends (Northfield & Johnston, 2021) and contacts more generally (Zhang et al., 2021). A cross-sectional study of 296 adults residing in the United States (assessed in August 2020) found that social support from both friends and family was associated with PTG, with perceived social support moderating the relationship between distress and PTG (Northfield & Johnston, 2021). Nurses working with COVID-19 patients reported social support from family, friends, and the public in general as being associated with PTG (Lee & Lee, 2020). Finally, in a sample of 4000 individuals from 21 countries, social connection (specifically compassion and social safeness) was associated with both PTS and PTG, whereas social disconnection was associated with only PTS (Matos et al., 2021). Marital status and having children, demographic indicators which could be a proxy for social support, were also associated with PTG, although the quality of that support and type, which are likely impactful, were not assessed (Li et al., 2022). These results suggest increasing social support could be a fruitful way to increase PTG during COVID-19 and future crises.

Other Psychosocial Factors

Other psychological factors positively associated with PTG during COVID-19 include self-efficacy (Lee & Lee, 2020; Zhang et al., 2021) and self-esteem (Yan et al., 2021), suggesting that one's perception of own ability to effectively manage the stress of the pandemic facilitated or allowed for growth to occur. The character trait of humanity, where individuals place a higher value on interpersonal relationships was also associated with PTG (Casali et al., 2021), aligning with research documenting improved interpersonal relationships as a key aspect of pandemic-related PTG. Emotional creativity, which relates to the originality of emotional experience and expression, was associated with PTG (Zhai et al., 2021). This personality trait could help with a more positive reframing of the negative experience of COVID-19. Finally, both anger (Yan et al., 2021) and extroversion were associated with PTG (Feng et al., 2021).

Limitations of the Research and Future Directions

The dynamic nature of the COVID-19 pandemic presented unique challenges for researchers. As with many disasters, investigators were tasked with balancing the need for rapid information with research rigor (Garfin & Silver, 2016; Silver & Garfin, 2016). Unfortunately, this resulted in many early studies of the psychological effects of the COVID-19 pandemic being defined by online surveys and convenience samples, many of which were not using probability-based methods, instead relying on the more biased methods of snowball sampling, word-of-mouth, and social media. This may have generated samples that disproportionately represent individuals who are more engaged and interested in the topic while missing vulnerable groups including those with low socioeconomic status, limited internet access, older individuals, and those with pre-COVID-19 mental health problems (Pierce et al., 2020) and potentially biased results, particularly for making prevalence-based estimates (Bradley et al., 2021).

Future research should target specific populations with the potential for both distress and growth and include a nuanced assessment of COVID-19 exposures. For example, most of the research on PTG during the COVID-19 pandemic has focused on workers, those in the healthcare industry, and the general public whereas less literature has addressed those dealing with a COVID-related personal loss or virus contraction. As many grapple with the effects of long-COVID, those experiencing persistent problems could also be a target population for future research on PTG (Sudre et al., 2021). Relatedly, few studies took a nuanced approach to exploring the relationship between specific COVID-19-related stressors and PTG, although research suggests these stressors varied greatly across respondents and were differentially associated with psychosocial outcomes (Garfin et al., 2021).

The timeframe of many studies also limits the knowledge of PTG during COVID-19. Many studies reviewed herein were conducted in the early phase of the COVID-19 pandemic, and not enough time may have been for the process of PTG to emerge (Asmundson et al., 2021; Vazquez et al., 2021). With some notable exceptions (e.g., Doorn et al., 2021; Lyu et al., 2021; Zhen & Zhou, 2021), the extant literature on PTG during COVID-19 was typically cross-sectional in design, limiting an examination of trajectory of responses, which can be important in evaluating responses over time as prior research on infectious disease outbreaks has shown (Rzeszutek & Gruszczyńska, 2021). Research using a longitudinal design must be conducted to understand the long-term effects of the COVID-19 pandemic on PTG over time, particularly as the COVID-19 pandemic waxes and wanes and new collective traumas emerge (Silver et al., 2021). As we emerge from the acute phase of the COVID-19 pandemic, studying PTG can help delineate when healing begins and the experience of PTG may emerge more predominantly, facilitating the experience of recovery and resilience that may strengthen people for future challenges.

Implications and Recommendations

During the COVID-19 pandemic, the experience of PTG was associated with increased psychological resilience (Chen & Tang, 2021; Zeng et al., 2021) as well as other benefits including reduced odds of suicidal ideation in a sample of veterans (Pietrzak et al., 2021). Given these benefits, clinicians, organizations, and policymakers should utilize research on PTG and related constructs to guide recovery efforts from COVID-19 and inform strategies to help guide adaption to future uncontrollable stressors and viral outbreaks, which scientists anticipate to increase in the future (Khetan, 2020).

Specifically, a review of PTG and resilience in workers during COVID-19 suggested that organizational programs and workshops could be implemented to develop adaptive coping strategies, e.g., deliberate rumination and positive reappraisal (Finstad et al., 2021). Qualitative data from nurses caring for COVID-19 patients yielded a set of proposed guidelines including implementing counseling programs for patients and nurses and increasing staffing to combat mental health ailments and facilitate growth experiences (Lee & Lee, 2020).

The current research about the effects of COVID-19 has delineated areas that should be considered by practitioners when designing interventions. Vazquez et al. (2021) recommend the implementation of interventions that promote positive cognitions about the goodness of the world and human nature as these cognitive-based interventions may have positive effects on PTG. Others note that interventions emphasizing self-compassion and increased resilience are among the most promising for reducing the risk of compassion fatigue among volunteers (Gonzalez-Mendez & Díaz, 2021). Effective coping strategies have also been identified as an area to target to enhance COVID-19-related growth experiences (Kalaitzaki et al., 2021; Zhang et al., 2021). Yet, Kalaitzaki et al. (2021) suggest that while a variety of strategies may help individuals to cope and adapt to stressful events, some may not fit the strict classification of positive coping strategies, e.g., avoidant techniques (Zhang et al., 2021). However, more research on such topics is needed as ineffective coping mechanisms may be related to illusory PTG, rather than sustained resilience and positive change (Asmundson et al., 2021). In addition to coping styles, since both social support and self-efficacy were positively correlated with PTG, interventions that target those factors as well should be designed and evaluated, particularly for nurses and other healthcare professionals who will be dealing with the trauma of COVID-19 as the pandemic shifts toward indemnify.

Workplace policies for healthcare professionals dealing with COVID-19 patients as well as other industries at high risk for exposure and COVID-19-related distress (Garfin et al., 2022) can also utilize findings about PTG to promote recovery and adaption in the wake of COVID-19. Indeed, an early commentary published in *JAMA* noted that involuntary, intrusive, and unresolved memories of traumatic experiences can lead to PTSD, while directed and deliberate reflection allows for growth, providing an opportunity to promote strategies for a more resilient workforce (Olson et al., 2020). Similarly, others have proposed real-world systematic infection control education as well as educational programs that focus on the mental and physical health of nurses and patients to promote COVID-19-related PTG (Lee & Lee, 2020). Future work should leverage these preliminary findings into guidelines and best practices to be used by clinicians, organizations, and policymakers.

Conclusions

In summary, despite the widespread adversity and distress associated with the COVID-19 pandemic, many also reported silver linings including PTG and other related psychosocial benefits. These positive experiences do not negate the social, psychological, and economic suffering associated with the protracted pandemic. However, they do provide insights into how individuals adapt and respond to adversity such as the COVID-19 pandemic, and offer useful information to guide evidence-based interventions that promote growth during times of crisis.

Acknowledgment

This work was supported by National Science Foundation RAPID Grants SES-2026337 and SES-2030139 NIMHD K01 MD013910.

References

Arnout, B. A., & Al-sufyani, H. H. (2021). Quantifying the impact of COVID-19 on the individuals in the Kingdom of Saudi Arabia: A cross-sectional descriptive study of the posttraumatic growth. *Journal of Public Affairs*, 21(4) e2659. 10.1002/pa.2659

Asmundson, G. J. G., Paluszek, M. M., & Taylor, S. (2021). Real versus illusory personal growth in response to COVID-19 pandemic stressors. *Journal of Anxiety Disorders*, *81*, 102418. 10.1016/J.JANXDIS.2021.102418

Aydin, R., & Assistant, R. N. (2021). Experiences of nurses diagnosed with COVID-19 in Turkey: A qualitative study. *International Nursing Review*, 1–11. 10.1111/inr.12735

Bernstein, M., & Pfefferbaum, B. (2018). Posttraumatic growth as a response to natural disasters in children and adolescents. *Current Psychiatry Reports*, *20*(37), 1–10. 10.1007/s11920-018-0900-4

Bradley, V. C., Kuriwaki, S., Isakov, M., Sejdinovic, D., Meng, X.-L., & Flaxman, S. (2021). Unrepresentative big surveys significantly overestimate US vaccine uptake. *Nature*, *600*, 695–700. 10.1038/s41586-021-04198-4

Casali, N., Feraco, T., & Meneghetti, C. (2021). Character strengths sustain mental health and post-traumatic growth during the COVID-19 pandemic. A longitudinal analysis. *Psychology and Health*, *0*(0), 1–17. 10.1080/08870446.2021.1952587

Celdran, M., Serrat, R., & Villar, F. (2021). Post-traumatic growth among older people after the forced lockdown for the COVID-19 pandemic. *The Spanish Journal of Psychology*, *24*, e43. 10.1017/SJP.2021.40

Cénat, J. M., Blais-Rochette, C., Kokou-Kpolou, C. K., Noorishad, P. G., Mukunzi, J. N., McIntee, S. E., Dalexis, R. D., Goulet, M. A., & Labelle, R. P. (2021). Prevalence of symptoms of depression, anxiety, insomnia, posttraumatic stress disorder, and psychological distress among populations affected by the COVID-19 pandemic: A systematic review and meta-analysis. *Psychiatry Research*, *295*, 113599. 10.1016/j.psychres.2020.113599

Chen, C., & Tang, S. (2021). Profiles of grief, post-traumatic stress, and post-traumatic growth among people bereaved due to COVID-19. *European Journal of Psychotraumatology*, *12*(1), 1947563. 10.1080/20008198.2021.1947563

Chen, R., Sun, C., Chen, J. J., Jen, H. J., Kang, X. L., Kao, C. C., & Chou, K. R. (2021). A large-scale survey on trauma, burnout, and posttraumatic growth among nurses during the COVID-19 pandemic. *International Journal of Mental Health Nursing*, *30*(1), 102–116. 10.1111/inm.12796

Cheng, S. K. W., Chong, G. H. C., Chang, S. S. Y., Wing, C., Wong, C. S. Y., Wong, M. T. P., & Wong, K. C. (2006). Adjustment to severe acute respiratory syndrome (SARS): Roles of appraisal and post-traumatic growth. *Psychology and Health*, *21*(3), 301–317. 10.1080/14768320500286450

Cheng, S. K. W., & Wong, C. W. (2005). Psychological intervention with sufferers from Severe Acute Respiratory Syndrome (SARS): Lessons learnt from empirical findings. *Clinical Psychology and Psychotherapy*, *12*(1), 80–86. https://10.1002/cpp.429

Cooke, J. E., Eirich, R., Racine, N., & Madigan, S. (2020). Prevalence of posttraumatic and general psychological stress during COVID-19: A rapid review and meta-analysis. *Psychiatry Research, 292*, 3–5. 10.1016/j.psychres.2020.113347

Cui, P. P., Wang, P. P., Wang, K., Ping, Z., Wang, P., & Chen, C. (2021). Post-traumatic growth and influencing factors among frontline nurses fighting against COVID-19. *Occupational and Environmental Medicine, 78*(2), 129–135. 10.1136/oemed-2020-106540

Doorn, K. A., Békés, V., Luo, X., Prout, T. A., & Hoffman, L. (2021). Therapists' resilience and posttraumatic growth during the COVID-19 pandemic. *Psychological Trauma: Theory, Research, Practice, and Policy, 14*(S1), S165–S173. 10.1037/TRA0001097

Ettman, C. K., Abdalla, S. M., Cohen, G. H., Sampson, L., Vivier, P. M., & Galea, S. (2020). Prevalence of depression symptoms in US adults before and during the COVID-19 pandemic. *JAMA Network Open*, 3(9), e2019686 10.1001/jamanetworkopen.2020.19686

Feng, L. Sen, jiao Dong, Z., qian Wu, X., Zhang, L., yu Yan, R., Ma, J., & Zeng, Y. (2021). COVID-19-related post-traumatic growth in the general public: A cross-sectional study from Yunnan, China. *Psychology, Health, & Medicine, 27*(4), 925–930. 10.1080/13548506.2021.1966700

Finstad, G. L., Giorgi, G., Lulli, L. G., Pandolfi, C., Foti, G., León-Perez, J. M., Cantero-Sánchez, F. J., & Mucci, N. (2021). Resilience, coping strategies and posttraumatic growth in the workplace following COVID-19: A narrative review on the positive aspects of trauma. *International Journal of Environmental Research and Public Health, 18*(18), 33–56. 10.3390/ijerph18189453

Fioretti, C., Palladino, B. E., & Nocentini, A. (2020). Positive and negative experiences of living in COVID-19 pandemic: Analysis of Italian adolescents' narratives. *Frontiers in Psychology, 11*, 599531. 10.3389/fpsyg.2020.599531

Foli, K. J., Forster, A., Cheng, C., Zhang, L., & Chiu, C. (2021). Voices from the COVID-19 frontline: Nurses' trauma and coping. *Journal of Advanced Nursing, 77*(9), 3853–3866. 10.1111/jan.14988

Garfin, D. R., Djokovic, L., Silver, R. C., & Holman, E. A. (2022). Acute stress, worry, and impairment in healthcare and non-healthcare essential workers during the COVID-19 pandemic. *Psychological Trauma: Theory, Research, Practice, and Policy.* 10.1037/tra0001224

Garfin, D. R., Fischhoff, B., Holman, E. A., & Silver, R. C. (2021). Risk perceptions and health behaviors as COVID-19 emerged in the United States: Results from a probability-based nationally representative sample. *Journal of Experimental Psychology: Applied, 27*(4), 584–598. 10.1037/xap0000374

Garfin, D. R., & Estes, K. (2022). The collective trauma and chronic stress of COVID-19: Risk and resilience. In M. Miller (Ed.), *The social science of the COVID-19 pandemic: A call to action for researchers.* Oxford University Press.

Garfin, D. R., & Silver, R. C. (2016). Responses to natural disasters. In H. S. Friedman (Ed.), *Encyclopedia of mental health* 2nded., (Vol. 4, pp. 35–46). Waltham, MA: Academic Press.

Gonzalez-Mendez, R., & Díaz, M. (2021). Volunteers' compassion fatigue, compassion satisfaction, and post-traumatic growth during the SARS-CoV-2 lockdown in Spain: Self-compassion and self-determination as predictors. *PLoS One, 16*(9). 10.1371/JOURNAL.PONE.0256854

Hamam, A. A., Milo, S., Mor, I., Shaked, E., Eliav, A. S., & Lahav, Y. (2021). Peritraumatic reactions during the COVID-19 pandemic – The contribution of posttraumatic growth attributed to prior trauma. *Journal of Psychiatric Research, 132*, 23–31. 10.1016/j.jpsychires.2020.09.029

Holman, E. A., Thompson, R. R., Garfin, D. R., & Silver, R. C. (2020). The unfolding COVID-19 pandemic: A probability-based, nationally representative study of mental health in the U.S. *Science Advances, 6*(42), eabd 5390, eabd5390. 10.1126/sciadv.abd5390

Hyun, S., Wong, G. T. F., Levy-Carrick, N. C., Charmaraman, L., Cozier, Y., Yip, T., & Hahm, H. C. & Liu, C. H. (2021). Psychosocial correlates of posttraumatic growth among U.S. young adults during the COVID-19 pandemic. *Psychiatry Research, 302.* 10.1016/J.PSYCHRES.2021.114035

Ikizer, G., & Gul, E. (2021). Post-traumatic stress, growth, and depreciation during the COVID-19 pandemic: Evidence from Turkey. *European Journal of Psychotraumatology, 12*(1). 10.1080/20008198.2021.1872966

Janoff-Bulman, R. (1992). *Shattered assumptions: Towards a new psychology of trauma.* Free Press.

Jenkins, M., Hoek, J., Jenkin, G., Gendall, P., Stanley, J., Beaglehole, B., Bell, C., Rapsey, C., & Every-Palmer, S. (2021). Silver linings of the COVID-19 lockdown in New Zealand. *PLoS One, 16*(4), e0249678. 10.1371/JOURNAL.PONE.0249678

Jin, M., Zhang, X., He, H., Zeng, L., & Yuan, Z. (2020). Psychological symptoms and post-traumatic growth among the general population in Wuhan, China during the COVID-19 pandemic A cross-sectional study. *Journal of Psychosocial Nursing*, *60*(4), 39–46. 10.3928/02793695-20211118-03

Kalaitzaki, A. (2021). Posttraumatic symptoms, posttraumatic growth, and internal resources among the general population in Greece: A nation-wide survey amid the first COVID-19 lockdown. *International Journal of Psychology: Journal International de Psychologie*, *56*(5), 766–771. 10.1002/IJOP.12750

Kalaitzaki, A., Tamiolaki, A., & Tsouvelas, G. (2021). From secondary traumatic stress to vicarious posttraumatic growth amid COVID-19 lockdown in Greece: The role of health care workers' coping strategies. *Psychological Trauma: Theory, Research, Practice, and Policy*, 14(2), 273–280. 10.1037/TRA0001078

Kaloeti, S., Ardhiani, L. N., & Stuck, M. (2021). The consequences of COVID-19 toward human growth: The role of traumatic event and coping strategies among Indonesian sample. *Frontiers in Psychology*, *12*, 685115. 10.3389/fpsyg.2021.685115

Khetan, A. K. (2020). COVID-19: Why declining biodiversity puts us at greater risk for emerging infectious diseases, and what we can do. *Journal of General Internal Medicine*, *35*(9), 2746–2747. 10.1007/s11606-020-05977-x

Kowalski, R. M., Carroll, H., & Britt, J. (2021). Finding the silver lining in the COVID-19 crisis. *Journal of Health Psychology*. 10.1177/1359105321999088

Lau, J. T. F., Wu, X., Wu, A. M. S., Wang, Z., & Mo, P. K. H. (2018). Relationships between illness perception and post-traumatic growth among newly diagnosed HIV-positive men who have sex with men in China. *AIDS and Behavior*, *22*(6), 1885–1898. 10.1007/s10461-017-1874-7

Lee, N., & Lee, H. J. (2020). South Korean nurses' experiences with patient care at a COVID-19-designated hospital: Growth after the frontline battle against an infectious disease pandemic. *International Journal of Environmental Research and Public Health*, *17*(23), 1–22. 10.3390/IJERPH17239015

Li, L., Mao, M., Wang, S., Yin, R., Yan, H., Jin, Y., & Cheng, Y. (2022). Posttraumatic growth in Chinese nurses and general public during the COVID-19 outbreak. *Psychology, Health and Medicine*, 27(2), 301–311. 10.1080/13548506.2021.1897148

Luszczynska, A., Durawa, A. B., Dudzinska, M., Kwiatkowska, M., Knysz, B., & Knoll, N. (2012). The effects of mortality reminders on posttraumatic growth and finding benefits among patients with life-threatening illness and their caregivers. *Psychology and Health*, *27*(10), 1227–1243. 10.1080/08870446.2012.665055

Luu, T. T. (2022). Family support and posttraumatic growth among tourism workers during the COVID-19 shutdown: The role of positive stress mindset. *Tourism Management*, *88*(1), 104399. 10.1016/j.tourman.2021.104399

Lyu, Y., Ni, S., & Lu, S. (2021). Positive functioning at work during COVID-posttraumatic growth, resilience, and emotional exhaustion in Chinese frontline healthcare workers. *International Journal of Applied Psychology*, *13* (4), 871–886. 10.1111/aphw.12276

Ma, L., Mazidi, M., Li, K., Li, Y., Chen, S., Kirwan, R., Zhou, H., Yan, N., Rahman, A., Wang, W., & Wang, Y. (2021). Prevalence of mental health problems among children and adolescents during the COVID-19 pandemic: A systematic review and meta-analysis. *Journal of Affective Disorders*, *293*, 78–89. 10.1016/j.jad.2021.06.021

Matos, M. , Mcewan, K., Kanovsky, M., Steindl, R., Ferreira, N., Id, M. L., Id, D. R., Asano, K., Brito-pons, G., Lucena-, P., Vilas, P., Ma, M. G., Oliveira, S., Leonardo, E., Id, D. S., Llobenes, L., Gumiy, N., Costa, M. I., Id, N. H., ...Gilbert, P. (2021). The role of social connection on the experience of COVID-19 related post-traumatic growth and stress. *PLoS One*, *16*(12), e0261384. 10.1371/journal.pone.0261384

Miragall, M., Vara, M. D., Galiana, L., Baños, R. M., Kruskal, J. B., Shanafelt, T., Mion, G., Hamann, P., Saleten, M., Plaud, B., & Baillard, C. (2021). Psychological impact of the COVID-19 pandemic and burnout severity in French residents: A national study. *The European Journal of Psychiatry*, *12*(8), 1198–1207.

Na, P. J., Tsai, J., Southwick, S. M., & Pietrzak, R. H. (2021). Factors associated with post-traumatic growth in response to the COVID-19 pandemic: Results from a national sample of U.S. military veterans. *Social Science and Medicine*, *289*, 114409. 10.1016/j.socscimed.2021.114409

Nadeem, T., Asad, N., Khan, M. M., Siddiqui, S., Hamid, S. N., & Pirani, S. (2019). Trauma and post traumatic growth in young survivors of a terrorist attack: An experiential account of supportive interventions in a tertiary care hospital in Pakistan. *Child Care in Practice*, 28(2), 210–218. 10.1080/13575279.2019.1664990

Northfield, E.-L., & Johnston, K. L. (2021). "I get by with a little help from my friends": Posttraumatic growth in the COVID-19 pandemic. *Traumatology*, *28*(1), 195–201. 10.1037/trm0000321

Olson K., Shanafelt T., & Southwick S. (2020). Pandemic-driven posttraumatic growth for organizations and individuals. *JAMA* 324(18), 1829–1830. 10.1001/jama.2020.20275

Pashazadeh Kan, F., Raoofi, S., Rafiei, S., Khani, S., Hosseinifard, H., Tajik, F., Raoofi, N., Ahmadi, S., Aghalou, S., Torabi, F., Dehnad, A., Rezaei, S., Hosseinipalangi, Z., & Ghashghaee, A. (2021). A systematic review of the prevalence of anxiety among the general population during the COVID-19 pandemic. *Journal of Affective Disorders*, *293*(April), 391–398. 10.1016/j.jad.2021.06.073

Pierce, M., Mcmanus, S., Jessop, C., John, A., Hotopf, M., Ford, T., Hatch, S., Wessely, S., & Abel, K. M. (2020). Says who? The significance of sampling in mental health surveys during COVID-19 effects of the COVID-19 pandemic on the mental health of prisoners. *The Lancet Psychiatry*, *7*(7), 567–568. 10.1016/S2215-0366(20)30237-6

Pietrzak, R. H., Tsai, J., & Southwick, S. M. (2021). Association of symptoms of posttraumatic stress disorder with posttraumatic psychological growth among US veterans during the COVID-19 pandemic. *JAMA Network Open*, *4*(4), e214972. 10.1001/jamanetworkopen.2021.4972

Rimé, B., Páez, D., Basabe, N., & Martínez, F. (2010). Social sharing of emotion, post-traumatic growth, and emotional climate: Follow-up of Spanish citizen's response to the collective trauma of March 11th terrorist attacks in Madrid. *European Journal of Social Psychology*, *40*(6), 1029–1045. 10.1002/ejsp.700

Robles-Bello, M. A., Sánchez-Teruel, D., & Naranjo, N. V. (2020). Variables protecting mental health in the Spanish population affected by the COVID-19 pandemic. *Current Psychology*, October 22, 1–12. 10.1007/s12144-020-01132-1.

Rudenstine, S., McNeal, K., Schulder, T., Ettman, C. K., Hernandez, M., Gvozdieva, K., & Galea, S. (2021). Depression and anxiety during the COVID-19 pandemic in an urban, low-income public university sample. *Journal of Traumatic Stress*, *34*(1), 12–22. 10.1002/jts.22600

Rzeszutek, M., & Gruszczyńska, E. (2021). Trajectories of posttraumatic growth following HIV infection: Does one PTG pattern exist? *Journal of Happiness Studies*, *23*, 1653–1668. 10.1007/s10902-021-00467-1

Rzeszutek, M., Oniszczenko, W., & Firląg-Burkacka, E. (2016). Gender differences in posttraumatic stress symptoms and the level of posttraumatic growth among a polish sample of HIV-positive individuals. *AIDS Care*, *28*(11), 1411–1415. 10.1080/09540121.2016.1182615

Salehi, M., Amanat, M., Mohammadi, M., Salmanian, M., Rezaei, N., Saghazadeh, A., & Garakani, A. (2021). The prevalence of post-traumatic stress disorder related symptoms in Coronavirus outbreaks: A systematic-review and meta-analysis. *Journal of Affective Disorders*, *282*, 527–538. 10.1016/j.jad.2020.12.188

Samji, H., Wu, J., Ladak, A., Vossen, C., Stewart, E., Dove, N., Long, D., & Snell, G. (2021). Review: Mental health impacts of the COVID-19 pandemic on children and youth – a systematic review. *Child and Adolescent Mental Health*. 10.1111/camh.12501

Shigemoto, Y. (2021). Association between daily rumination and posttraumatic growth during the COVID-19 pandemic: An experience sampling method. *Psychological Trauma: Theory, Research, Practice and Policy*, *14*(2), 229–236. doi.org/10.1037/TRA0001061

Silver, R. C., Boon, C., & Stones, M. H. (1983). Searching for meaning in misfortune: Making sense of incest. *Journal of Social Issues*, *39*(2), 81–101. 10.1111/j.1540-4560.1983.tb00142.x

Silver, R. C., Holman, E. A., & Garfin, D. R. (2021). Coping with cascading collective traumas in the United States. *Nature Human Behaviour*, *5*(1), 4–6. 10.1038/s41562-020-00981-x

Silver, R. C., & Garfin, D. R. (2016). Coping with disasters. In D. K. F. J. C. Norcross, & G. R. VandenBos (Eds.), *APA handbook of clinical psychology: Vol. 4. Psychopathology and health* (pp. 597–611). American Psychological Association.

Solomon, Z., & Dekel, R. (2007). Posttraumatic stress disorder and posttraumatic growth among Israeli ex-POWs. *Journal of Traumatic Stress*, *20*(3), 251–262. 10.1002/jts

Stallard, P., Pereira, A. I., & Barros, L. (2021). Post-traumatic growth during the COVID-19 pandemic in carers of children in Portugal and the UK: Cross-sectional online survey. *BJPsych Open*, *7*(1) E37. 10.1192/BJO.2021.1

Sudre, C. H., Murray, B., Varsavsky, T., Graham, M. S., Penfold, R. S., Bowyer, R. C., Pujol, J. C., Klaser, K., Antonelli, M., Canas, L. S., Molteni, E., Modat, M., Cardoso, M. J., May, A., Ganesh,

S., Davies, R., Nguyen, L. H., Drew, D. A., Astley, C. M., Joshi, A. D., Merino, J., Tsereteli, N., Fall, T., Gomez, M. F., Duncan, E. L., Menni, C., Williams, F. M. K., Franks, P. W., Chan, A. T., Wolf, J., Ourselin, S., Spector, T., & Steves, C. J. (2021). Attributes and predictors of long COVID. *Nature Medicine*, *27*, 626–631. 10.1038/s41591-021-01292-y

Suls, J., & Fletcher, B. (1985). The relative efficacy of avoidant and nonavoidant coping strategies: a meta-analysis. *Health Psychology*, *4*(3), 249–288. 10.1037/0278-6133.4.3.249

Sun, W., Chen, W. T., Zhang, Q., Ma, S., Huang, F., Zhang, L., & Lu, H. (2021). Post-traumatic growth experiences among COVID-19 confirmed cases in China: A qualitative study. *Clinical Nursing Research*, *30*(7), 1079–1087. 10.1177/10547738211016951

Tedeschi, R. G., & Calhoun, L. G. (2004). Posttraumatic growth: Conceptual foundations and empirical evidence. *Psychological Inquiry*, *15*(1), 1–18. 10.1207/s15327965pli1501

Tomaszek, K., & Muchacka-cymerman, A. (2020). Thinking about my existence during COVID-19, I feel anxiety and awe — The mediating role of existential anxiety and life satisfaction on the relationship between PTSD symptoms and post-traumatic growth. *International Journal of Environmental Research and Public Health*, *17*(19), 7062. 10.3390/ijerph17197062.

Updegraff, J. A., Silver, R. C., & Holman, E. A. (2008). Searching for and finding meaning in collective trauma: Results from a national longitudinal study of the 9/11 terrorist attacks. *Journal of Personality and Social Psychology*, *95*(3), 709–722. 10.1037/0022-3514.95.3.709

Vazquez, C., Valiente, C., García, F. E., Contreras, A., Peinado, V., Trucharte, A., & Bentall, R. P. (2021). Post-traumatic growth and stress-related responses during the COVID-19 pandemic in a national representative sample: The role of positive core beliefs about the world and others. *Journal of Happiness Studies*, *22*(7), 2915–2935. 10.1007/S10902-020-00352-3

Viner, R., Russell, S., Saulle, R., Croker, H., Stansfield, C., Packer, J., Nicholls, D., Goddings, A. L., Bonell, C., Hudson, L., Hope, S., Ward, J., Schwalbe, N., Morgan, A., & Minozzi, S. (2022). School closures during social lockdown and mental health, health behaviors, and well-being among children and adolescents during the first COVID-19 Wave: A systematic review. *JAMA Pediatric*, *176*(4), 400–409. 10.1001/jamapediatrics.2021.5840

Wlodarczyk, A., Basabe, N., Páez, D., Villagrán, L., & Reyes, C. (2017). Individual and collective posttraumatic growth in victims of natural disasters: A multidimensional perspective. *Journal of Loss and Trauma*, *22*(5), 371–384. 10.1080/15325024.2017.1297657

Xiong, J., Lipsitz, O., Nasri, F., Lui, L. M. W., Gill, H., Phan, L., Chen-Li, D., Iacobucci, M., Ho, R., Majeed, A., & McIntyre, R. S. (2020). Impact of COVID-19 pandemic on mental health in the general population: A systematic review. *Journal of Affective Disorders*, *277*, 55–64. 10.1016/j.jad.2020.08.001

Yan, S., Yang, J., Ye, M., Chen, S., Xie, C., Huang, J., & Liu, H. (2021). Post-traumatic growth and related influencing factors in discharged COVID-19 patients: A cross-sectional study. *Frontiers in Psychology*, *12*, 658307. 10.3389/fpsyg.2021.658307

Yildiz, E. (2021). Posttraumatic growth and positive determinants in nursing students after COVID-19 alarm status: A descriptive cross-sectional study. *Perspectives in Psychiatric Care*, *57*(4), 1876–1887. 10.1111/ppc.12761

Zeng, W., Wu, X., Xu, Y., Wu, J., Zeng, Y., & Shao, J. (2021). The impact of general self-efficacy on psychological resilience during the COVID-19 pandemic: The mediating role of posttraumatic growth and the moderating role of deliberate rumination. *Frontiers in Psychiatry*, *12*, 684354. 10.3389/fpsyg.2021.684354

Zhai, H., Li, Q., Hu, Y., Cui, Y., Wei, X., & Zhou, X. (2021). Emotional creativity improves posttraumatic growth and mental health during the COVID-19 pandemic. *Frontiers in Psychology*, *12*, 600798. 10.3389/fpsyg.2021.600798

Zhang, X. T., Shi, S. S., & Wang, Y. Q. R. L. (2021). The traumatic experience of clinical nurses during the COVID-19 pandemic: Which factors are related to post-traumatic trowth? *Risk Management and Healthcare Policy*, *14*, 2145–2151. 10.2147/RMHP.S307294

Zhao, Q., Sun, X., Xie, F., Chen, B., Wang, L., Hu, L., & Dai, Q. (2021). Impact of COVID-19 on psychological wellbeing. *International Journal of Clinical and Health Psychology*, *21*(3), 100252. 10.1016/j.ijchp.2021.100252

Zhen, R., & Zhou, X. (2021). Latent patterns of posttraumatic stress symptoms, depression, and posttraumatic growth among adolescents during the COVID-19. *Journal of Traumatic Stress*, *35*(1), 197–209. 10.1002/jts.22720

25

POSTTRAUMATIC GROWTH AND PSYCHOSOCIAL ADJUSTMENT OF SYRIAN REFUGEES IN TURKEY

Zeynep Şimşir Gökalp and H. İrem Özteke Kozan

Introduction

Over the course of the last decade, the number of displaced people reached record levels. Since 2009 this number has doubled worldwide such that at the end of 2021, 89.3 million forcibly displaced persons, 24.1 million refugees, 48 million internally displaced people, and 4.6 million asylum-seekers have been reported around the globe (The High Commissioner for Refugees [UNHCR], 2021a). Furthermore, the COVID-19 disaster increased the vulnerability of women, men, children, and boys who had been forcibly displaced. It restricted access to the homeland, risked livelihoods, and put in danger the lives of people who did not have equal access to health care (UNCHR, 2021b) creating one of the worst humanitarian crises worldwide.

Parallel to the increase in the number of people who were displaced worldwide last decade, the amount of refugees has rapidly increased in Turkey. One of the biggest reasons for this increase is the civil war that broke out in the Middle East. Turkey's neighbor Syria erupted in a civil war in 2011, forcing about 13.4 million people to migrate, of whom about 6.7 million were internationally displaced (UNHCR, 2021b). Many Syrians escaping the war scattered to Turkey, Lebanon, Jordan, Iraq, Egypt, and European countries with Turkey becoming one of the leading host countries for this population. As of 8 September 2022, there were 5,614,331 registered Syrian refugees worldwide; 65.1% of whom were registered by the government of Turkey, where the total number of Syrian refugees is 3,655,489 (UNCHR, 2022). The aforementioned trends are presented in Figure 25.1.

Syrian Refugees in Turkey

Turkey is preferred by the vast majority of Syrians who fled the war because it is the nearest neighbor and has adopted a humanist approach by implementing an "open-door policy" (Akar & Erdoğdu, 2019). Turkey has welcomed and provided temporary protection status to all the Syrians who started arriving in March 2011. This means that protection is given to foreigners who have been forced to migrate and have reached or crossed Turkey's

DOI: 10.4324/9781032208688-32

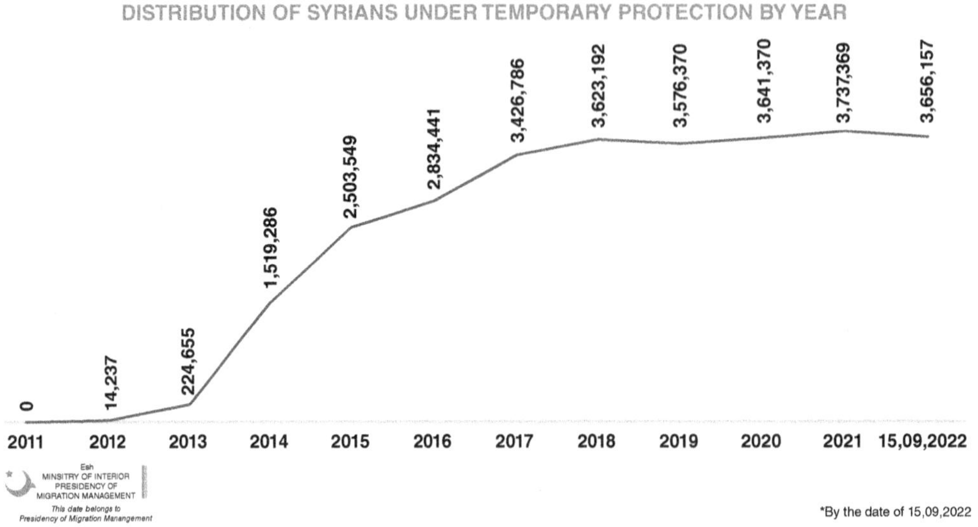

Figure 25.1 The trend of registered Syrian refugees in Turkey (Republic of Ministry of Interior Directorate General of Migration Management, 2022).

borders on a large scale to obtain urgent and temporary safeguards (Kaya & Eren, 2015). Syrians have secured the right to live in Turkey until a more permanent solution to their situation has been found, protection against forced return to Syria, and access to their most basic rights and needs, including access to health, schooling, social services, psychological support, and access to the labor market (UNCHR Help Turkey, 2021).

Of the Syrians under temporary protection status in Turkey, 51,774 live in temporary refugee camps, and 3,676,838 live in various provinces of Turkey, mostly in İstanbul, Adana, Hatay, Kilis, Gaziantep, Şanlıurfa, İzmir, Konya, and Bursa. The majority of Syrians are children, youth, and adults, respectively. 19,669,831 are males and 1,689,174 are females (Republic of Turkey Ministry of Interior Directorate General of Migration Management, 2022).

The initial influx of refugees was perceived to be a temporary phenomenon, and Syrian refugees were accepted as "guests." However, particularly after the influx in 2014–2015, the Turkish society began to realize that a significant proportion of these refugees should remain in Turkey (Akar & Erdoğdu, 2019) because the Syrian war deteriorated and expanded further with the emergence of ISIL (the Islamic State in Iraq and the Levant) and the intervention of Russia (Saraçoğlu & Bélanger, 2019). Therefore, the outlook for Syrian refugees has changed from short-term protection and humanitarian assistance to longer-term economic and social integration (Akar & Erdoğdu, 2019).

Considering that settlement of Syrians in Turkey became permanent, the Turkish government has taken significant measures in the fields of health care, education, access to the labor market, social benefits and support, and interpretation. Turkish authorities have decided that white-collar employees, especially those who teach in Temporary Education Centers under the control of the Ministry of National Education, will be accepted as Turkish citizens. In addition, to date, Syrians in Turkey sustain their life establishing or working registered/unregistered work in various sectors and adapting economically.

However, the issue of social and cultural adaptation is not as easy as economic adjustment and requires a longer process. It is estimated that one or two generations will have to pass for the Turkish people to accept Syrians and for Syrians to adapt to the social structure (Batalla & Tolay, 2018).

Challenges Faced by Syrian Refugees

Regardless of the purpose and intention, leaving one's country is a traumatic experience. Because immigration includes separations, losses, shifts, conflicts, and demands that seriously threaten or shatter the past ways of making sense of and defining oneself (Berger, 2004; Berger & Weiss, 2003). Many refugees are subject to multiple traumatic stressors before, during, and after immigration (Berger & Weiss, 2003; Boyle & Ali, 2010; Schick et al., 2018). They typically face challenges and obstacles related to lack of services, separation of families, social isolation, housing and health problems, adaptation problems, acculturation and prejudice, socioeconomic problems, and immigration policies (Akar & Erdoğdu, 2019; Schick et al., 2018). Most refugees are also hindered by cultural shock, language abilities, and a low level of education. Moreover, they face problems when seeking a career and a new home, (Wehrle et al., 2018).

The migration process of war refugees, beginning with the emigration from the home country through the adjustment to life in the country of resettlement is more complicated and long (Segal et al., 2006). Refugees exposed to the war experience its negative effects as well as the trauma of migration. War is a traumatic event that causes permanent damage to individuals and societies and causes people to leave their homeland (Martz & Lindy, 2010, Şimşir et al., 2021). People can be directly exposed to negative events such as injury, disability, and loss of family, friends, and relatives during the war. In addition, they may encounter problems such as job loss, lack of health care and services that are usually accessible (food, clean water, power, etc.), and the destruction of urban buildings (Martz, 2010). Consequently, unlike the traumatic events encountered personally, people exposed to war continually face an unstable atmosphere with multiple stressful experiences, leading them to move to another environment (Rosner & Powell, 2006).

Syrian migrants who are war refugees have been exposed to both war-related and migration-related traumatic events. Firstly, Syrian refugees have directly witnessed war before immigration. During the war, they had great difficulties in meeting their basic needs such as food, clean water, health care, and shelter (Ghumman et al., 2016). Many of them were subjected to direct violence, torture, and aggression during the war, were injured or lost their home, relatives, family members, jobs, as well as financial and social resources (Balcilar & Nugent, 2019; Ghumman et al., 2016; Şimşir et al., 2021). Secondly, Syrians, who had to leave their country due to the aforementioned difficult living conditions, faced both physical and psychological difficulties such as conflict, violence, loss, and missing their homeland during migration (Farhat et al., 2018; Ghumman et al., 2016). Thirdly, they have experienced many problems in their resettlement countries after immigration (e.g., Kaya et al., 2019; Şimşek, 2020). Specifically, it has been reported that Syrian refugees living in Turkey face the following difficulties: Absence of refugee status and citizenship (Şimşek, 2020), language barriers (Eryaman & Evran, 2019), cultural differences, prejudice, and discrimination and integration problems (Şafak-Ayvazoğlu et al., 2021; Şimşek, 2020), restricted access to health care (Assi et al., 2019), shelter and house problems (Akbasli & Mavi, 2021; Aydın Yıldırım & Gümüş Şekerci, 2020), financial problems, unemployment, and child labor (Bahcekapili & Cetin, 2015; Harunogullari, 2016), education problems (Şimşir & Dilmaç, 2018), and mental health problems (Acarturk et al., 2021; Kaya et al., 2019).

Aside from these challenges, the COVID-19 pandemic has further deteriorated the situation of Syrian refugees in Turkey (e.g., Budak & Bostan, 2020; Elçi et al., 2021; Özensoy, 2021). Syrian refugees may suffer from a lack of information about the COVID-19 pandemic, restricted access to personal protective equipment (Budak & Bostan, 2020), economic difficulties (Elçi et al., 2021), a loss of resources, and a sense of discrimination (Kurt et al., 2021), and mental health difficulties (Alpay et al., 2021; Kurt et al., 2021) during the pandemic. As a result, the adverse effects of migration have become more severe.

Mental Health Problems of Syrian Refugees

The experiences of trauma, suffering, and desperation most frequently characterize war refugee stories. These adverse experiences negatively impact the well-being of war refugees and increase mental health problems. Psychiatric conditions are reported to be substantially higher in refugees than in other populations (Davis & Davis, 2006). A meta-analysis conducted by Fazel et al. (2005) indicated that in Western countries, about one in ten adult refugees have posttraumatic stress disorder (PTSD), about one in 20 has severe depression and about one in 25 has a generalized anxiety disorder. Depression and PTSD are the most common psychiatric disorders seen among war refugees (Başoğlu et al. 2005; Kien et al., 2019; Momartin et al., 2004). Additionally, many war refugees suffer from various mental health problems including anxiety disorders (Silove et al., 2010), eating disorders (Aoun et al., 2013), emotional and behavioral problems (Kien et al., 2019), somatic complaints (Rometsch et al., 2020), and suicide (Amiri, 2022).

A growing body of literature has addressed the mental health problems of Syrian refugees in Turkey. For example, Alpak et al. (2015) reported a prevalence of 33.5 percent of PTSD among Syrian refugees who sought asylum in Turkey, indicating that it is a significant mental health problem in refugee camps. Sagaltici et al. (2020) identified determinants of PTSD severity among Syrian refugees living in a camp in Turkey. Based on face-to-face clinical interviews with 342 refugees, they reported that 31.0 percent ($n = 106$) met the criteria of the Diagnostic and Statistical Manual of Mental Disorders (DSM-IV-TR) for PTSD with CAPS (Clinician-Administered PTSD Scale) scores at the level of extreme and above among 86.8 percent of refugees with PTSD. PTSD symptom intensity was predicted by the female demographic, the total number of stressful experiences, and age. Specifically, a majority of female refugees were subjected to two or more types of distress. The prevalence and predictors of PTSD and depression in Syrian refugees living in an urban region in Turkey were evaluated by Kaya et al. (2019) who found that the rates of PTSD and depression among participants were 36.5 percent and 47.7 percent, respectively. Both PTSD and depression were predicted by female gender, physical disease, and a larger number of potentially stressful events.

Tekeli-Yesil et al. (2018) compared the prevalence of several mental health conditions among Syrian refugees living in Turkey and internally displaced persons in Syria. The study found that in both groups, mental problems were exceedingly widespread with major depression more widespread among refugees in Turkey than among internally displaced people. A recent study by McGrath et al. (2020) that examined the somatic responses of Syrian refugees in Istanbul, Turkey, showed that about 40% of the participants experienced moderate to severe somatic symptoms. Some studies reported problems of alcohol, substance, hookah, and cigarette addictions among Syrian refugees (İlhan et al., 2020; Taşdemir et al., 2020).

While adverse experiences relating to conflict and migration may be damaging to people of all ages, it has been recognized that children and adolescent refugees are much more prone to the development of mental disorders such as anxiety disorders, depression, and PTSD (Bhugra et al., 2011; Fazel et al., 2005). High scores of depression and anxiety were reported among Syrian child and adolescent refugees living outside of camps in Turkey (Kandemir et al., 2018). Similarly, Yayan et al. (2020) indicated that Syrian refugee children suffer from physical and psychosocial health problems such as high levels of PTSD, depression, and anxiety. Especially, mental health problems were found to be higher among children who lost their mothers during the war, lost their fathers, and were separated from their families. Finally, Gormez et al. (2018) showed that refugee children in Turkey experienced numerous stressful situations during the war and therefore, the prevalence of PTSD was 18.3 percent and that of anxiety-related conditions was as high as 69 percent.

In sum, war and subsequent migration have devastating short or long-term effects on people's lives. Hence, refugee mental health literature has commonly emphasized adversary results; however, the resilience, strengths, and possible beneficial effects of these experiences should not be overlooked (Berger & Weiss, 2003). Even though the empirical study of positive psychological consequences of the immigrant experience is in its infancy, over the past few years, PTG or adversarial development has grown into a commonly used and accepted term (Rosner & Powell, 2006; Şimşir Gökalp & Haktanir, 2022; Weiss & Berger, 2008;). We addressed the PTG processes of Syrian refugees in the following section.

Posttraumatic Growth Experiences of Syrian Refugees

PTG is characterized as positive psychological growth that is a consequence of managing very difficult life crises (Tedeschi et al., 1998; Tedeschi & Calhoun, 2004). Individuals who experience PTG move beyond the pre-traumatic adjustment and undergo personal transformation (Tedeschi & Calhoun, 2004). The manifestations of PTG were identified as a better appreciation for life, stronger interpersonal connections, a greater awareness of one's own strengths, reorganized priorities, and existential and spiritual development (Tedeschi et al., 1998, Tedeschi, 1999). These positive changes have been reported in a variety of populations who have been exposed to traumatic events such as cancer (Ochoa-Arnedo et al., 2021), the COVID-19 pandemic (Şimşir Gökalp et al., 2022), serious physical damage (Kampman et al., 2015), conflict (Simsir & Dilmac, 2021), earthquake (Taku et al., 2015), and bereavement (Engelkemeyer & Marwit, 2008). Recent studies have shown that PTG is prevalent among refugees who are living in different countries throughout the world (e.g., Abraham et al., 2018; Hussain & Bhushan, 2013; Kim & Lee, 2009).

Recent studies have commonly revealed PTG in Syrian refugees. For example, Wen et al. (2020) demonstrated that Syrian refugees living in Istanbul had a modest level of PTG (N= 768) and that a greater level of PTG is observed in refugees with moderate PTSD, younger, more educated, and with less somatic pain. Kangaslampi et al. (2022) conducted a study with Syrian and Iraqi refugees living in 11 provinces in Turkey. The findings indicated that refugees typically exhibit moderate to high levels of posttraumatic development, with PTG's most desirable aspects including realizing one is stronger than one believed, becoming able to achieve better things in life, increased religious belief, and understanding better that one can face obstacles. Additionally, a U-shaped association between PTSS and PTG levels was identified. In a study of Syrian refugees residing in Hatay, Turkey, Cengiz et al. (2019) reported that Syrian refugees with PTSD had greater PTG.

Survivors' early reactions to trauma are mostly influenced by their personal experiences, coping mechanisms, the availability of a support system, and religious commitment (Beck et al., 1979). Similarly, there are many factors that impact the PTG process of refugees (Chan et al., 2016). Exiting studies indicated that social support (Kheirallah et al., 2022; Özcan & Arslan, 2020; Şimşir et al., 2021), values (Simsir & Dilmac, 2021), coping strategies (Acar et al., 2021; Ersahin, 2022), some demographic variables (Wen et al. 2020), resilience (Cengiz et al., 2019) and religiosity (Ersahin, 2022; Özcan & Arslan, 2020) are important resources that increase the level of PTG among Syrian refugees. On the other hand, depressive symptoms (Özdemir et al., 2021), a history of accommodation in a medical institution for mental health treatment (Wen et al., 2020), and a background of severe traumatic experiences (Şahin et al., 2020) are adversely associated with PTG in refugees.

According to meta-synthesis research by Şimşir Gökalp and Haktanir (2022), PTG in refugees is a global phenomenon that may be displayed in both Eastern and Western civilizations. Correspondingly, current research revealed that Syrian refugees experience PTG although they face many challenging conditions and suffer from mental health issues. Addressing the psychological and social adjustment of refugees is essential to understanding the PTG and mental health of Syrian refugees.

Psychological and Social Adjustment of Syrian Refugees

Migration is becoming increasingly important for societies (Haase et al., 2019) due to social, economic, and political issues (Kaya & Keklik, 2021), and this migration process may be voluntary or forced (Kaya, 2021). Societies call for refugees to adapt to new settings; however, the adaptation requires mutual interaction between the host and the migrants (Kaya & Keklik, 2021). Ward and Kennedy (1999) configured refugees' adaptation process in two categories: Psychological (emotional) and socio-cultural (behavioral). Psychological adaptation refers to the migrant's well-being, whereas socio-cultural adaptation refers to achieving the abilities and daily tasks to fit into the host country's culture-based skills and behaviors.

Psychological and social adaptation of refugees is not a unilateral process and waiting for refugees to adapt to society puts on them pressure resulting in mental health problems. Atari-Khan et al. (2021) stated that experiencing terrifying violence and life stressors contribute to these mental health problems Because after moving to a new country, reference systems, i.e., how they perceive and interpret the world, of refugees change, they might lose familiar symbols of relationships, norms, or traditions (de Lucena et al., 2020).

The adjustment processes of refugees are affected by their pre-migration expectations (Yijälä & Jasinskaja-Lahti, 2010) attitudes, prejudices, and policies of host countries (Berry et al., 1987; Kuo & Roysircar, 2006) coping self-efficacy (von Haumeder et al., 2019), environmental and familial factors (Edwards & Lopez, 2006; von Haumeder et al., 2019; Paat, 2013) and personal factors such that age, gender, and coping styles (Berry et al., 1987). Moreover, acquiring a new language, mastering new behaviors, or connecting with new networks may influence the adaptation to a new country and this may result in acculturative stress (Tartakovsky, 2007).

The adjustment processes and problems of Syrian refugees who migrated all over the world have been subject in recent years to numerous studies that generally linked their adjustment problems to the factors that affect their adjustment processes (e.g., de Lucena et al., 2020; Martzoukou & Burnett, 2018; von Haumeder et al., 2019).

Syrian Refugees in Turkey and Adjustment Process

Researchers examined the psychological and social adjustment of Syrian refugees in Turkey. For example, Şafak-Ayvazoğlu et al. (2021) revealed that Syrian refugees‘ socio-cultural adaptation was affected by Turkish natives' positive or negative attitudes. Whereas positive attitudes toward migrants increase their well-being, negative attitudes may result in low socio-cultural adaptation. Similarly, Karataş et al. (2021) found that Syrian adolescents' same-ethnic and cross-ethnic friendships positively related to their well-being. In a recent study, Kaya and Keklik (2021) used a qualitative approach to investigate the adjustment processes of Syrian refugee university students in Turkey and revealed that social support, individual features, being a university student and social activities increase their adjustment processes.

The Social-Ecological Model of the Process of Psycho-Social Adjustment of Refugees

People need to interact with other people in their environment and that is a sign of development and growth. Paat (2013) advocated the application of Bronfenbrenner's social-ecological model (1974, 1977, 1979) to immigrants. The model is based on the associations between family and other ecological systems in the culture. It consists of five basic systems, i.e., a microsystem, mesosystem, exosystem, macrosystem, and chronosystem. Paat (2013) emphasized that particularly the microsystem, mesosystem, and exosystem have crucial value for immigrant children. At the microsystem, family dynamics play an important role in the assimilation of children into society. At the mesosystem level, families may monitor their children's peer relationships and want them to preserve their own ethnic rules in peer interactions. At the exosystem level, immigrants adapt better to society if there is support for them from neighborhoods. This theoretical framework may shed light on the adjustment process of immigrants considering the mutual understanding of interdependencies between migrants and society (Haase et al., 2019).

Families, peers, schools, and neighbors have a prominent role in the acculturation process of immigrants (El Hajj & Cook, 2018; McHale et al., 2011; Paat, 2013). Meda (2017) suggested that this model is important to understand how refugee children interact with other people in society during the migration process. The socio-ecological model also helps understand both the interactional and cognitive processes and the resilience of migrants (von Haumeder et al., 2019). For example, Edwards and Lopez (2006) found that family support is a significant predictor of life satisfaction among Mexican American migrants. Similarly, Gonzales et al. (2006) revealed that family conflict affects depressive symptoms among migrant adolescents. Related to the school context, Vedder and Horenczyk (2006) emphasized the importance of school among immigrant children and Walsh et al. (2010) revealed that family, teacher, and peer relations are very important in the risky behaviors of immigrant children.

Social-Ecological Approach and Syrian Refugees

Approaching the status of Syrian refugees living in Turkey from the perspective of a socio-ecological approach, we considered studies of teachers (Yaşar & Amaç, 2018), social support (Yildirim et al., 2020), mental health needs (Karaman & Ricard, 2016), and family factors (Eruyar et al., 2020). These studies generally aimed to reveal the needs, problems, and reaching mental health services or school settings of Syrian refugees and children. For example, Eruyar et al. (2020) found that Syrian refugee children's attachment relationships contribute to PTSD. Children securely attached to their families, also perceive their families as emotionally warmer. This illustrates how refugee children's mesosystem circle serves as a healing factor in psychosocial adjustment. However, the loss of family members is common among Syrian refugees (Balcilar & Nugent, 2019; Şimşir et al., 2021). Özer et al. (2013) reported that 74% of Syrian children living in a refugee camp lost their loved ones and thus may be maladaptive in their adjustment to society. Studies also showed that Syrian refugees have difficulties in peer relations (Alsayed & Wildes, 2018; Çiçekoğlu et al., 2019).

In sum, the social-ecological model of Bronfenbrenner (1974, 1977) is a crucial approach in the evaluation of the psychosocial adjustment of Syrian refugees. Peer, family, and neighborhood relationships shape their adjustment and acculturation Accepting refugee children, and avoiding prejudices facilitate overcoming their traumatic experiences and problems. Families' accepting children, preserving family bonds, and maintaining warm relationships help them strengthen their resilience and healthy neighborhood relationships fasten the adaptation process. Hence, studies and policies need to focus on adjusting these relationships to be more adaptive and resilient.

Psychological Adjustment and Coping Self-Efficacy (CSE)

Refugees' adjustment to the host country may be affected by their interpretation of trauma, their beliefs, and their coping self-efficacy (CSE). Benight and Bandura (2004) conceptualized the term "coping self-efficacy" based on social cognitive theory referring to people's self-beliefs regarding their capacity to manage their functioning following a traumatic event. Self-efficacy beliefs play an important role in humans' cognitive, emotional, and motivational processes and affect their functioning in different ways such as motivating themselves in difficult circumstances or vulnerability to depression. These beliefs also determine to what degree people are resilient to stressors (Benight & Bandura, 2004). Individuals' self-evaluative processes determine the CSE capacity, which involves being on alert for potential threats and providing posttraumatic recovery (Benight & Bandura, 2004).

Because forcible migration such as Syrian refugees' experience may be traumatic, their CSE levels might be an important predictor of their adaptation process. Syrian refugees' CSE has been studied in the last few years. For instance, von Haumeder et al. (2019) employed the concept of CSE for understanding the psychological adaptation of Syrian refugees in Germany and found that trauma-related CSE was negatively associated with PTSD. Qualitative findings grouped around five themes in psychological adaptation and included family, language, socioeconomic conditions, discrimination, and asylum procedures. Similarly, Chung and Shakra (2022) discovered that Syrian refugees' low CSE impacted on their psychological distress and that the war changed their beliefs about self and the world resulting in increased psychological symptoms.

Conclusions

In this chapter, we discussed Syrian refugees' PTG experiences and their psychological and social adaptation in Turkey. We mainly focused on their challenges and mental health problems and on their PTG experiences, and social and psychological adjustment. Syrian refugees in Turkey face challenges related to experiencing war-related trauma, separation, loss of family members, housing, educational and health problems, adaptation problems, acculturation, and prejudice. These challenges resulted in several mental health problems. Their adjustment process was affected by the host country's migration policies, positive or negative attitudes, and social support systems. All these factors are important for understanding the PTG experiences of Syrian refugees. Especially social and psychological adjustment of refugees serves as a protective factor and plays a major role in the PTG. Therefore, we suggest researchers conduct more studies to reveal PTG experiences and the adjustment process of refugees.

References

Abraham, R., Lien, L., & Hanssen, I. (2018). Coping, resilience and posttraumatic growth among Eritrean female refugees living in Norwegian asylum reception centers: A qualitative study. *International Journal of Social Psychiatry*, *64*(4), 359–366. 10.1177/0020764018765237

Acar, B., Acar, İ. H., Alhiraki, O. A., Fahham, O., Erim, Y., & Acarturk, C. (2021). The role of coping strategies in post-traumatic growth among Syrian refugees: A structural equation model. *International Journal of Environmental Research and Public Health*, *18*(16), 8829. 10.3390/ijerph18168829

Acarturk, C., McGrath, M., Roberts, B., Ilkkursun, Z., Cuijpers, P., Sijbrandij, M., Sondorp E., Ventevogel P., McKee M., Fuhr, D. C., & STRENGTHS consortium. (2021). Prevalence and predictors of common mental disorders among Syrian refugees in Istanbul, Turkey: A cross-sectional study. *Social Psychiatry and Psychiatric Epidemiology*. *56*(3), 475–484. 10.1007/s00127-020-01941-6

Akar, S., & Erdoğdu, M. M. (2019). Syrian refugees in Turkey and integration problem Ahead. *Journal of International Migration and Integration*, *20*(3), 925–940. 10.1007/s12134-018-0639-0

Akbasli, S., & Mavi, D. (2021). Conditions of Syrian asylum seeker students in a Turkish university. *International Journal of Inclusive Education*, *25*(7), 763–778. 10.1080/13603116.2019.1572796

Alpak, G., Unal, A., Bulbul, F., Sagaltici, E., Bez, Y., Altindag, A., Dalkilic, A., & Savas, H. A. (2015). Post-traumatic stress disorder among Syrian refugees in Turkey: A cross-sectional study. *International Journal of Psychiatry in Clinical Practice*, *19*(1), 45–50. 10.3109/13651501.2014.961930

Alpay, E. H., Kira, I. A., Shuwiekh, H. A. M., Ashby, J. S., Turkeli, A., & Alhuwailah, A. (2021). The effects of COVID-19 continuous traumatic stress on mental health: The case of Syrian refugees in Turkey. *Traumatology*, *41*(10), 7371–7382. 10.1007/s12144-021-01743-2.

Alsayed, A., & Wildes, V. J. (2018). Syrian refugee children: A study of strengths and difficulties. *Journal of Human Rights and Social Work*, *3*(2), 81–88. 10.1007/s41134-018-0057-4

Amiri, S. (2022). Prevalence of suicide in immigrants/refugees: A systematic review and meta-analysis. *Archives of Suicide Research*, 26(2), 370–405.10.1080/13811118.2020.1802379

Aoun, A., Garcia, F. D., Mounzer, C., Hlais, S., Grigioni, S., Honein, K., & Déchelotte, P. (2013). War stress may be another risk factor for eating disorders in civilians: A study in Lebanese university students. *General Hospital Psychiatry*, *35*(4), 393–397. 10.1016/j.genhosppsych.2013.02.007

Assi, R., Özger-İlhan, S., & İlhan, M. N. (2019). Health needs and access to health care: The case of Syrian refugees in Turkey. *Public Health*, *172*, 146–152. 10.1016/j.puhe.2019.05.004

Atari-Khan, R., Covington, A. H., Gerstein, L. H., Herz, H. A., Varner, B. R., Brasfield, C., Shurigar, B., Hinnenkamp, S. F., Devia, M., Barrera, S., & Deogracias-Schleich, A. (2021). Concepts of resilience among trauma-exposed Syrian refugees. *The Counseling Psychologist*, *49*(2), 233–268. 10.1177/0011000020970522

Aydın Yıldırım, T., & Gümüş Şekerci, Y. (2020). A door opening from Syria to Turkey; migration and the process of social acceptance and accommodation: Hatay and Karabuk provinces. *International Social Work*. *65*(2), 370–382. 10.1177/002087282093843

Bahcekapili, C., & Cetin, B. (2015). The impacts of forced migration on regional economies: The case of Syrian refugees in Turkey. *International Business Research*, *8*(9), 1–15. 10.5539/ibr.v8n9p1

Balcilar, M., & Nugent, J. B. (2019). The migration of fear: An analysis of migration choices of Syrian refugees. *The Quarterly Review of Economics and Finance*, *73*, 95–110. 10.1016/j.qref.2018.09.007

Başoğlu, M., Livanou, M., Crnobarić, C., Frančišković, T., Suljić, E., Đurić, D., & Vranešić, M. (2005). Psychiatric and cognitive effects of war in former Yugoslavia: Association of lack of redress for trauma and posttraumatic stress reactions. *JAMA*, *294*(5), 580–590. 10.1001/jama.294.5.580

Batalla, L., & Tolay, J. (2018). *Toward long-term solidarity with Syrian refugees? Turkey's policy response and challenges*. Atlantic Council.

Beck, A. T., Rush, J., Shaw, B., & Emery, G. (1979). *Cognitive therapy of depression*. Guildford Press.

Benight, C. C., & Bandura, A. (2004). Social cognitive theory of posttraumatic recovery: The role of perceived self-efficacy. *Behaviour Research and Therapy*, *42*(10), 1129–1148. 10.1016/j.brat.2003.08.008

Berger, R. (2004). *Immigrant women tell their stories*. Haworth Press.

Berger, R., & Weiss, T. (2003). Immigration and posttraumatic growth-a missing link. *Journal of Immigrant & Refugee Services*, *1*(2), 21–39. 10.1300/J191v01n02_02

Berry, J. W., Kim, U., Minde, T., & Mok, D. (1987). Comparative studies of acculturative stress. *International Migration Review*, *21*(3), 491–511. 10.1177/019791838702100З0

Bhugra D., Gupta S., Bhui K., Craig T., Dogra N., Ingleby J. D., Kirkbride J., Moussaoui D., Nazroo J., Qureshi A., & Stompe T. (2011). WPA guidance on mental health and mental health care in migrants. *World Psychiatry*, *10*(1), 2–10. 10.1002/j.2051-5545.2011.tb00002.x

Boyle, E. H., & Ali, A. (2010). Culture, structure, and the refugee experience in Somali immigrant family transformation. *International Migration*, *48*(1), 47–79. 10.1111/j.1468-2435.2009.00512.x

Bronfenbrenner, U. (1974). Developmental research, public policy, and the ecology of childhood. *Child Development*, *45*(1), 1–5. 10.2307/1127743

Bronfenbrenber, U. (1977). Toward an experimental ecology of human development. *American Psychologist*, *32*(7), 513–530. 10.1037/0003-066X.32.7.513

Bronfenbrenner, U. (1979). *The ecology of human development: Experiments by nature and design*. Harvard University Press

Budak, F., & Bostan, S. (2020). The effects of Covid-19 pandemic on Syrian refugees in Turkey: The case of Kilis. *Social Work in Public Health*, *35*(7), 579–589. 10.1080/19371918.2020.1806984

Cengiz, I., Ergün, D., & Cakici, E. (2019). Posttraumatic stress disorder, posttraumatic growth and psychological resilience in Syrian refugees: Hatay, Turkey. *Anadolu Psikiyatri Dergisi*, *20*(3), 269–276. 10.5455/apd.4862

Chan, K. J., Young, M. Y., & Sharif, N. (2016). Well-being after trauma: A review of posttraumatic growth among refugees. *Canadian Psychology/Psychologie canadienne*, *57*(4), 291–299. 10.1037/cap0000065

Chung, M. C., & Shakra, M. (2022). The association between trauma centrality and posttraumatic stress among Syrian refugees: The impact of cognitive distortions and trauma-coping self-efficacy. *Journal of Interpersonal Violence*, *37*(3-4), 1852–1877. 10.1177/0886260520926311

Çiçekoğlu, P., Durualp, E., & Kadan, G. (2019). Investigation of peer relations of preschool refugee and non-refugee children. *Archives of Psychiatric Nursing*, *33*(4), 319–324. 10.1016/j.apnu.2019.01.004

Davis, R. M., & Davis, H. (2006). PTSD symptom changes in refugees. *Torture: Quarterly Journal on Rehabilitation Of Torture Victims and Prevention of Torture*, *16*(1), 10–19.

de Lucena, M. S., Hoersting, R. C., & Modesto, J. G. (2020). The sociocultural and psychological adaptation of Syrian refugees in Brazil. *Psico*, *51*(3), e34372–e34372.

Edwards, L. M., & Lopez, S. J. (2006). Perceived family support, acculturation, and life satisfaction in Mexican American youth: A mixed-methods exploration. *Journal of Counseling Psychology*, *53*(3), 279–287.

Elçi, E., Kirisçioglu, E., & Üstübici, A. (2021). How COVID-19 financially hit urban refugees: Evidence from mixed-method research with citizens and Syrian refugees in Turkey. *Disasters*, 45(Suppl 1), S240–S263. 10.1111/disa.12498

El Hajj, D., & Cook, P. F. (2018). Acculturation and Arab immigrant health in Colorado: A socio-ecological perspective. *Nutrition & Food Science*, *48*(5), 796–806. 10.1108/NFS-10-2017-0207

Engelkemeyer, S. M., & Marwit, S. J. (2008). Posttraumatic growth in bereaved parents. *Journal of Traumatic Stress*, *21*(3), 344–346. 10.1002/jts.20338

Ersahin, Z. (2022). Post-traumatic growth among Syrian refugees in Turkey: The role of coping strategies and religiosity. *Current Psychology*, 41(4), 2398–2407.10.1007/s12144-020-00763-8

Eruyar, S., Maltby, J., & Vostanis, P. (2020). How do Syrian refugee children in Turkey perceive relational factors in the context of their mental health?. *Clinical Child Psychology and Psychiatry*, *25*(1), 260–272. 10.1177/1359104519882758

Eryaman, M. Y., & Evran, S. (2019). Syrian refugee students' lived experiences at temporary education centers in Turkey. In K. Arar, J. S. Brooks, & I. Bogotch. (Eds.), *Education, immigration and migration* (pp. 131–143). Emerald Publishing Limited. 10.1108/978-1-78756-044-420191009

Farhat, J. B., Blanchet, K., Bjertrup, P. J., Veizis, A., Perrin, C., Coulborn, R. M., Mayaud, P., & Cohuet, S. (2018). Syrian refugees in Greece: Experience with violence, mental health status, and access to information during the journey and while in Greece. *BMC Medicine*, *16*(1), 1–12. 10.1186/s12916-018-1028-4

Fazel, M., Wheeler, J., & Danesh, J. (2005). Prevalence of serious mental disorder in 7000 refugees resettled in western countries: A systematic review. *The Lancet*, *365*(9467), 1309–1314. 10.1016/S0140-6736(05)61027-6

Ghumman, U., McCord, C. E., & Chang, J. E. (2016). Posttraumatic stress disorder in Syrian refugees: A review. *Canadian Psychology/Psychologie Canadienne*, *57*(4), 246–253. 10.1037/cap0000069

Gonzales, N. A., Deardorff, J., Formoso, D., Barr, A., & Barrera Jr, M. (2006). Family mediators of the relation between acculturation and adolescent mental health. *Family Relations*, *55*(3), 318–330. 10.1111/j.1741-3729.2006.00405.x

Gormez, V., Kılıç, H. N., Orengul, A. C. et al. (2018). Psychopathology and associated risk factors among forcibly displaced Syrian children and adolescents. *Journal of Immigrant Minority Health*, *20*(3), 529–535. 10.1007/s10903-017-0680-7

Haase, A., Rohmann, A., & Hallmann, K. (2019). An ecological approach to psychological adjustment: A field survey among refugees in Germany. *International Journal of Intercultural Relations*, *68*, 44–54. 10.1016/j.ijintrel.2018.10.003

Harunogullari, M. (2016). Child labor among Syrian refugees and problems: Case of Kilis. *Journal of Migration*, *3*(1), 29–63.

Hussain, D., & Bhushan, B. (2013). Posttraumatic growth experiences among Tibetan refugees: A qualitative investigation. *Qualitative Research in Psychology*, *10*(2), 204–216. 10.1080/14780887.2011.616623

İlhan, M. N., Ertek, İ. E., Gözükara, M. G., Akil, Ö., Ursu, P., Ergüder, T., Polat, S., Şimşek, M. Y., Aktaş, M., Gazanfer, Ö. B., İlhan, S. Ö., & Kaptan, H. (2020). Substance use in refugee camps and local community: Şanlıurfa sample. *Noro Psikiyatri Arsivi*, *58*(2), 121–127. 10.29399/npa.24856

Kampman, H., Hefferon, K., Wilson, M., & Beale, J. (2015). "I can do things now that people thought were impossible, actually, things that I thought were impossible": A meta-synthesis of the qualitative findings on posttraumatic growth and severe physical injury. *Canadian Psychology/Psychologie Canadienne*, *56*(3), 283–294. 10.1037/cap0000031

Kandemir, H., Karataş, H., Çeri, V., Solmaz, F., Kandemir, S. B., & Solmaz, A. (2018). Prevalence of war-related adverse events, depression, and anxiety among Syrian refugee children settled in Turkey. *European Child & Adolescent Psychiatry*, *27*(11), 1513–1517. 10.1007/s00787-018-1178-0

Kangaslampi, S., Peltonen, K., & Hall, J. (2022). Posttraumatic growth and posttraumatic stress–a network analysis among Syrian and Iraqi refugees. *European Journal of Psychotraumatology*, *13*(2), 2117902. 10.1080/20008066.2022.2117902

Karaman, M., & Ricard, R. (2016). Meeting the mental health needs of Syrian refugees in Turkey. *The Professional Counselor*, *6*(4), 318–327. 10.15241/mk.6.4.318

Karataş, S., Crocetti, E., Schwartz, S. J., & Rubini, M. (2021). Psychological and social adjustment in refugee adolescents: The role of parents' and adolescents' friendships. *New Directions for Child and Adolescent Development*, *2021*(176), 123–139. 10.1002/cad.20395

Kaya, E., Kiliç, C., Çaman, Ö. K., & Üner, S. (2019). Posttraumatic stress and depression among Syrian refugees living in Turkey: Findings from an urban sample. *The Journal of Nervous and Mental Disease*, *207*(12), 995–1000. 10.1097/NMD.0000000000001104

Kaya, I., & Eren, E. Y. (2015). *Türkiye'deki Suriyelilerin hukuki durumu: Arada kalanların hakları ve yükümlülükleri*. SETA.

Kaya, Ö. S., & Keklik, İ. (2021). Adjustment experiences of Syrian immigrant university students in Turkey. *Current Psychology*. Advance Online Publication. 10.1007/s12144-020-01233-x

Kaya, Y. (2021). "If only they forgot that I was Syrian and an Arab, I am a human beings too." Syrian university students' experiences of being a foreigner: A phenomenological study. *International Journal of Intercultural Relations*, *83*, 43–54. 10.1016/j.ijintrel.2021.04.014

Kheirallah, K. A., Al-Zureikat, S. H., Al-Mistarehi, A. H., Alsulaiman, J. W., AlQudah, M., Khassawneh, A. H., Lorettu, L., Bellizzi, S., Mzayek, F., Elbarazi, I., & Serlin, I. A. (2022). The association of conflict-related trauma with markers of mental health among Syrian refugee women: The role of social support and post-traumatic growth. *International Journal of Women's Health*, *14*, 1251–1266. 10.2147/IJWH.S360465.

Kien, C., Sommer, I., Faustmann, A., Gibson, L., Schneider, M., Krczal, E., Jank, R., Klerings, I., Szelag, M., Kerschner, B., Brattström, P., & Gartlehner, G. (2019). Prevalence of mental disorders in young refugees and asylum seekers in European Countries: A systematic review. *European Child & Adolescent Psychiatry*, *28*(10), 1295–1310. 10.1007/s00787-018-1215-z

Kim, H. K., & Lee, O. J. (2009). A phenomenological study on the experience of North Korean refugees. *Nursing Science Quarterly*, *22*(1), 85–88. 10.1177/0894318408329242

Kuo, B. C., & Roysircar, G. (2006). An exploratory study of cross-cultural adaptation of adolescent Taiwanese unaccompanied sojourners in Canada. *International Journal of Intercultural Relations*, *30*(2), 159–183. 10.1016/j.ijintrel.2005.07.007

Kurt, G., Ilkkursun, Z., Javanbakht, A., Uygun, E., Karaoglan-Kahilogullari, A., & Acarturk, C. (2021). The psychological impacts of COVID-19 related stressors on Syrian refugees in Turkey: The role of resource loss, discrimination, and social support. *International Journal of Intercultural Relations*, *85*, 130–140. 10.1016/j.ijintrel.2021.09.009

Martz, E. (2010). *Trauma rehabilitation after war and conflict*. New York, NY: Springer.

Martz, E., & Lindy, J. (2010). Exploring the trauma membrane concept. In E. Martz (Ed.), *Trauma rehabilitation after war and conflict* (pp. 27–54). Springer.

Martzoukou, K., & Burnett, S. (2018). Exploring the everyday life information needs and the socio-cultural adaptation barriers of Syrian refugees in Scotland. *Journal of Documentation*, *74*(5), 1104–1132. 10.1108/JD-10-2017-0142

McGrath, M., Acarturk, C., Roberts, B., Ilkkursun, Z., Sondorp, E., Sijbrandij, M., Cuijpers, P., Ventevogel, P., McKee, M., & Fuhr, D. C. (2020). Somatic distress among Syrian refugees in Istanbul, Turkey: A cross-sectional study. *Journal of Psychosomatic Research*, *132*, 109993. 10.1016/j.jpsychores.2020.109993

McHale, S. M., Kim, J. Y., Kan, M., & Updegraff, K. A. (2011). Sleep in Mexican-American adolescents: Social ecological and well-being correlates. *Journal of Youth and Adolescence*, *40*(6), 666–679. 10.1007/s10964-010-9574-

Meda, L. (2017). *Refugee learner experiences. A case study of Zimbabwean refugee children*. Anchor Academic Publishing.

Momartin, S., Silove, D., Manicavasagar, V., & Steel, Z. (2004). Comorbidity of PTSD and depression: Associations with trauma exposure, symptom severity and functional impairment in Bosnian refugees resettled in Australia. *Journal of Affective Disorders*, *80*(2-3), 231–238. 10.1016/S0165-0327(03)00131-9

Ochoa-Arnedo, C., Casellas-Grau, A., Lleras, M., Medina, J. C., & Vives, J. (2021). Stress management or post-traumatic growth facilitation to diminish distress in cancer survivors? A randomized controlled trial. *The Journal of Positive Psychology*, *16*(21), 715–725. 10.1080/17439760.2020.1765005

Özcan, N. A., & Arslan, R. (2020). Travma sonrası stres ile travma sonrası büyüme arasındaki ilişkide sosyal desteğin ve maneviyatın aracı rolü. *Elektronik Sosyal Bilimler Dergisi*, *19*(73), 299–314.

Özdemir, P. G., Kırlı, U., & Asoglu, M. (2021). Investigation of the associations between post-traumatic growth, sleep quality and depression symptoms in Syrian refugees. *Eastern Journal of Medicine*, *26*(2), 265–272. 10.5505/ejm.2021.48108

Özensoy, A. U. (2021). Education experiences of Syrian refugee students in Mus during the COVID-19. *International Journal of Curriculum and Instruction*, *13*(1), 274–290.

Özer, S., Şirin, S., & Oppedal, B. (2013). Bahçeşehir study of Syrian refugee children in Turkey. https://www.fhi.no/globalassets/migrering/dokumenter/pdf/bahcesehir-study-report3.pdf

Paat, Y. F. (2013). Working with immigrant children and their families: An application of Bronfenbrenner's ecological systems theory. *Journal of Human Behavior in the Social Environment, 23*(8), 954–966. 10.1080/10911359.2013.800007

Republic of Ministry of Interior Directorate General of Migration Management (2022, 2 October). *Temporary protection.* https://en.goc.gov.tr/temporary-protection27

Republic Turkiye Ministry of Interior Presidency of Migration. (2022). https://en.goc.gov.tr/

Rometsch, C., Denkinger, J. K., Engelhardt, M., Windthorst, P., Graf, J., Gibbons, N., Pham, P., Zipfel, S., & Junne, F. (2020). Pain, somatic complaints, and subjective concepts of illness in traumatized female refugees who experienced extreme violence by the "Islamic State"(IS). *Journal of Psychosomatic Research, 130*, 109931. 10.1016/j.jpsychores.2020.109931

Rosner, R., & Powell, S. (2006). Posttraumatic growth after war. In L. G. Calhoun, & R. G. Tedeschi (Eds.), *Handbook of posttraumatic growth: Research and practice* (pp. 197–213). Psychology Press.

Sagaltici, E., Alpak, G., & Altindag, A. (2020). Traumatic life events and severity of posttraumatic stress disorder among Syrian refugees residing in a camp in Turkey. *Journal of Loss and Trauma, 25*(1), 47–60. 10.1080/15325024.2019.1654691

Saraçoğlu, C., & Bélanger, D. (2019). Syrian refugees and Turkey: Whose crisis. In C. Menjívar, M. Ruiz, & I. Ness, (Eds.), *The Oxford handbook of migration crises* (pp. 279–294). Oxford University Press.

Schick, M., Morina, N., Mistridis P., Schnyder, U., Bryant R. A., & Nickerson, A. (2018) Changes in post-migration living difficulties predict treatment outcome in traumatized refugees. *Frontiers in Psychiatry, 9*, 476. 10.3389/fpsyt.2018.00476

Segal, U. A., Mayadas, N. S., & Elliott, D. (2006). A framework for immigration. *Journal of Immigrant & Refugee Studies, 4*(1), 3–24. 10.1300/J500v04n01_02

Silove, D., Momartin, S., Marnane, C., Steel, Z., & Manicavasagar, V. (2010). Adult separation anxiety disorder among war-affected Bosnian refugees: Comorbidity with PTSD and associations with dimensions of trauma. *Journal of Traumatic Stress: Official Publication of the International Society for Traumatic Stress Studies, 23*(1), 169–172. 10.1002/jts.20490

Simsir, Z., & Dilmac, B. (2021). Experiences of posttraumatic growth in witnesses to the July 15 coup attempt in Turkey. *Illness, Crisis & Loss, 29*(3), 220–240. 10.1177/1054137318803848

Şafak-Ayvazoğlu, A., Kunuroglu, F., & Yağmur, K. (2021). Psychological and socio-cultural adaptation of Syrian refugees in Turkey. *International Journal of Intercultural Relations, 80*, 99–111. 10.1016/j.ijintrel.2020.11.003

Şahin, Ş., Altındağ, Ö., Elboga, G., Elçiçek, S., Akaltun, M. S., Altındağ, A., Gür, A., & Doğan, İ. (2020). The relations of traumatic life events with depression, loneliness, anxiety, posttraumatic growth, and pain in refugee university students. *Acta Medica Alanya, 4*(3), 264–269. 10.30565/medalanya.738966

Şimşek, D. (2020). Integration processes of Syrian refugees in Turkey:'Class-based integration'. *Journal of Refugee Studies, 33*(3), 537–554. 10.1093/jrs/fey057

Şimşir, Z., & Dilmaç, B. (2018). Yabancı uyruklu öğrencilerin eğitim gördüğü okullarda öğretmenlerin karşılaştığı sorunlar ve çözüm önerileri. *Elementary Education Online, 17*(3), 1116–1134. 10.17051/ilkonline.2018.419647

Şimşir, Z., Dilmaç, B., & Özteke Kozan, H. İ. (2021). Posttraumatic growth experiences of Syrian refugees after war. *Journal of Humanistic Psychology, 61*(1) 55–72. 0022167818801090

Şimşir Gökalp, Z., & Haktanir, A. (2022). Posttraumatic growth experiences of refugees: A meta-synthesis of qualitative studies. *Journal of Community Psychology*, 50, 1395–1410. 10.1002/jcop.22723

Şimşir Gökalp, Z., Koç, H., & Kozan, H. İ. Ö. (2022). Coping and post-traumatic growth among COVID-19 patients: A qualitative study. *Journal of Adult Development, 29*, 228–239. 10.1007/s10804-022-09398-4

Taku, K., Cann, A., Tedeschi, R. G., & Calhoun, L. G. (2015). Core beliefs shaken by an earthquake correlate with posttraumatic growth. *Psychological Trauma Theory, Research, Practice, and Policy, 7*(6), 563–569. 10.1037/tra0000054

Tartakovsky, E. (2007). A longitudinal study of acculturative stress and homesickness: High-school adolescents immigrating from Russia and Ukraine to Israel without parents. *Social Psychiatry and Psychiatric Epidemiology, 42*(6), 485–494. 10.1007/s00127-007-0184-1

Taşdemir, M., Küçükali, H., Uçar, A., & ve Sur, H. (2020). Exploring alcohol and substance addiction among Syrian Migrants in Turkey: A qualitative study integrating perspectives of addicts, their relatives, local and national institutions. *ADDICTA: The Turkish Journal on Addictions*, 7(4), 253–276. 10.5152/addicta.2020.20074

Tedeschi, R. G. (1999). Violence transformed: Posttraumatic growth in survivors and their societies. *Aggression and Violent Behavior*, *4*(3), 319–341. 10.1016/S1359-1789(98)00005-6

Tedeschi, R. G., & Calhoun, L. G. (2004). Posttraumatic growth: Conceptual foundations and empirical evidence. *Psychological Inquiry*, *15*(1), 1–18.

Tedeschi, R. G., Park, C. L., & Calhoun, L. G. (1998). Posttraumatic growth: Conceptual issues. In R. G. Tedeschi, C. L. Park, & L. G. Calhoun (Eds.), *Posttraumatic growth: Positive changes in the aftermath of crisis* (pp. 1–23). Erlbaum.

Tekeli-Yesil, S., Isik, E., Unal, Y., Aljomaa Almossa, F., Konsuk Unlu, H., & Aker, A. T. (2018). Determinants of mental disorders in Syrian refugees in Turkey versus ınternally displaced persons in Syria. *American Journal of Public Health*, *108*(7), 938–945. 10.2105/AJPH.2018.304405

UNCHR the UN Refugee Agency. (2021). *Turkey - 2021 plan summary*. https://reporting.unhcr.org/turkey-2021-plan-summary

United Nations High Commissioner for Refugees (2021a). *Refugee data finder*. https://www.unhcr.org/refugee-statistics/

United Nations High Commissioner for Refugees (2021b, March). *Syria emergency*. https://www.unhcr.org/syria-emergency.html

United Nations High Commissioner for Refugees (2022, 8 September). *Syria regional refugee response*. http://data2.unhcr.org/en/situations/syria

Vedder, P. H., & Horenczyk, G. (2006). Acculturation and the school. In D. L. Sam, & J. W. Berry (Eds.), *The Cambridge handbook of acculturation psychology* (pp. 419–438). Cambridge University Press. 10.1017/CBO9780511489891.031

von Haumeder, A., Ghafoori, B., & Retailleau, J. (2019). Psychological adaptation and post-traumatic stress disorder among Syrian refugees in Germany: A mixed-methods study investigating environmental factors. *European Journal of Psychotraumatology*, *10*(1), 1686801.10.1080/20008198.2019.1686801

Walsh, S. D., Harel-Fisch, Y., & Fogel-Grinvald, H. (2010). Parents, teachers and peer relations as predictors of risk behaviors and mental well-being among immigrant and Israeli born adolescents. *Social Science & Medicine*, *70*(7), 976–984. 10.1016/j.socscimed.2009.12.010

Ward, C., & Kennedy, A. (1999). The measurement of sociocultural adaptation. *International Journal of Intercultural Relations*, *23*(4), 659–677. 10.1016/S0147-1767(99)00014-0

Wehrle, K., Klehe, U. C., Kira, M., & Zikic, J. (2018). Can I come as I am? Refugees' vocational identity threats, coping, and growth. *Journal of Vocational Behavior*, *105*, 83–101. 10.1016/j.jvb.2017.10.010

Weiss, T., & Berger, R. (2008). Posttraumatic growth and immigration: Theory, research and practice implication. In S. Joseph, & P. A. Linley (Eds.), *Trauma, recovery and growth: Positive psychological perspective on posttraumatic stress*. Wiley.

Wen, K., McGrath, M., Acarturk, C., Ilkkursun, Z., Fuhr, D. C., Sondorp, E., Cuijpers, P., Sijbrandijd, M., & Roberts, B. (2020). Post-traumatic growth and its predictors among Syrian refugees in Istanbul: A mental health population survey. *Journal of Migration and Health*, *1–2*, 100010. 10.1016/j.jmh.2020.100010

Yaşar, M. R., & Amaç, Z. (2018). Teaching Syrian students in Turkish schools: Experiences of teachers. *Sustainable Multilingualism*, *13*(1), 225–238. 10.2478/sm-2018-0019

Yayan, E. H., Düken, M. E., Özdemir, A. A., & Çelebioğlu, A. (2020). Mental health problems of Syrian refugee children: Post-traumatic stress, depression and anxiety. *Journal of Pediatric Nursing*, *51*, e27–e32. 10.1016/j.pedn.2019.06.012

Yijälä, A., & Jasinskaja-Lahti, I. (2010). Pre-migration acculturation attitudes among potential ethnic migrants from Russia to Finland. *International Journal of Intercultural Relations*, *34*(4), 326–339. 10.1016/j.ijintrel.2009.09.002

Yildirim, H., Isik, K., Firat, T. Y., & Aylaz, R. (2020). Determining the correlation between social support and hopelessness of Syrian refugees living in Turkey. *Journal of Psychosocial Nursing and Mental Health Services*, *58*(7), 27–33. 10.3928/02793695-20200506-04

26

GROWING THROUGH ADVERSITY

The Case of Survivors of The *Gukurahundi* Genocide in Mathebeleland, Zimbabwe

Dumisani Maqeda Ngwenya

Zimbabwe, a former British colony known as Rhodesia before 1980, has a long history of violence dating back to pre-colonial times. However, one of the most violent episodes in the history of independent Zimbabwe occurred during the period between 1983 and 1987 and caused extreme suffering to a large number of its citizens. At that time the first black majority government of the Zimbabwe African National Union-Patriotic Front (ZANU-PF) (a political organization that has been the ruling party in Zimbabwe since independence in 1980) sent an especially trained army brigade to the Mathebeleland region (native spelling; the official colonialist spelling Matabeleland is wrong and meaningless) and parts of the Midlands Province, where the Ndebele (Bantu speaking people of southwestern Zimbabwe previously called Matabele) live. This caused the *Gukurahundi* genocide and resulted in approximately 20,000 civilians being killed and countless others maimed, disappeared, or raped (CCJP, 2007). The chapter discusses the atrocities, their impact, and how some of the affected communities have dealt with the resultant trauma and have managed to grow from it.

Historical Context of the Gukurahundi Atrocities

Prior to colonization by the British, the land bound by the Zambezi River to the north and the Limpopo River to the south included the southwestern part under the sovereignty of King Mzilikazi and later, his son King Lobhengula and the northeastern part that was held by various Shona chiefs but never as a unitary state (Beach, 1994; Ngwenya, 2018). After the defeat of both regions during the 1896 uprising—in which the Africans sought to stem the growing power and land grab by Cecil John Rhodes, before the Queen—the two states were brought together by the colonialists and christened Rhodesia, after Cecil John Rhodes. The fight against colonialism of the two states that were forcefully joined by their conquerors was united up to 1963. By the late 1950s and early 1960s, through a number of metamorphoses, the Zimbabwe African People's Union (ZAPU) led by Joshua Nkomo had become the champion for the liberation of the black majority in Zimbabwe (Ndlovu-Gatsheni, 2003). The political party brought together various tribal and ethnic groups that existed in then Rhodesia. In 1963 a split along tribal lines occurred in ZAPU, whereby a number of the

DOI: 10.4324/9781032208688-33

Shona-speaking leaders became disenchanted with the leadership of Nkomo who was from the Ndebele-speaking part of the country. These leaders pulled out of ZAPU and formed their own party, the Zimbabwe African National Union (ZANU) with Reverend Ndabaningi Sithole as its leader, later replaced by Robert Mugabe.

The London-brokered 1979 Lancaster House talks between the Rhodesian government and the liberation movements resulted in a ceasefire, and planned elections for 1980 after disarmament, demobilization, and reintegration of the three armies. ZAPU and ZANU had agreed to unite under the banner of the Patriotic Front supporting ending the white minority rule in Zimbabwe, South Africa, and Namibia. However, this unity was short-lived as Mugabe made a unilateral announcement, without prior notice to Nkomo that ZANU was going to stand alone for the elections and contest as ZANU-Patriotic Front, thus exacerbating the mutual suspicions and simmering tensions between the parties (Meredith, 2008).

Mugabe won the 1980 elections with 57 of the 100 seats, Nkomo won 20, all in Mathebeleland, 20 seats were reserved for whites (for 10 years) and three were won by the United African National Council (UANC) under Bishop Abel Muzorewa. Mugabe offered the largely ceremonial post of President to Nkomo who turned it down refusing to be "caught up in an official prison" (Meredith, 2008; Nkomo, 1984). Mugabe had always wanted a one-party state, and Nkomo and his ZAPU party became the only thing that blocked him from achieving this goal (Ngwenya, 2018).

While some armed former fighters on both sides wandered around terrorizing villagers during the period of disarmament, demobilization, and reintegration, after the elections Mugabe focused on the few bandits from the armed wing of the Zimbabwe People's Revolutionary Army (ZPRA), ignoring those from his own Zimbabwe African National Liberation Army (ZANLA). The tone and messaging began to change from "bandits" to "disgruntled dissidents" portrayed as unhappy with Mugabe's victory and wanting to overthrow his government. Enos Nkala (the only Ndebele in ZANU-PF leadership) introduced a tribal element to the accusations claiming that so-called dissidents were Ndebeles, calling for a second war of liberation and advocating shooting them. He also supported crushing Nkomo whom he called the "self-appointed Ndebele King" (Alexander et al., 2000), suggesting that Nkomo wanted to bring back pre-colonial era Ndebele domination of the Shona and invoking the hatred and resentment for the Ndebeles. The army's 5th Brigade, code-named *Gukurahundi*, was soon unleashing violence in the Mathebeleland region and some parts of Midlands Province (Ngwenya, 2018). This brigade, whose name means "the rain that washes away the chaff before the spring rain," was a secretly arranged private army of Mugabe, comprised mostly of Shona-speaking former ZANLA combatants and trained by South Koreans to deal with "internal security" (Todd, 2007). To the people of Mathebeleland and parts of the Midlands province, it came to mean they were the dirt that needed to be washed away.

Between 1980 and 1981, some ZPRA combatants who had joined the army were ill-treated by their ZANLA counterparts, sporadic fights occurred in some newly integrated battalions and at urban Assembly points. While these were soon contained, some ZPRA fighters who had fled the fighting went to their rural homes or to Botswana and South Africa. All these incidents worked well for Mugabe who, by 1982, had expelled Nkomo and other ZAPU officials from the unity government accusing them of using dissidents to try to assassinate him and causing havoc in Mathebeleland, accusations that were vehemently refuted by Nkomo and ZAPU who denied any links to the dissidents. Several top

ZAPU and ZPRA officials were arrested and detained, most without trial, and Nkomo fled to seek temporary asylum in Britain after a failed assassination attempt by the 5th Brigade (Meredith, 2008; Nkomo, 1984).

The 5th Brigade was carrying out mass beatings, killing, and torturing indiscriminately (Nkomo, 1984). Although claiming to target dissidents, evidence gathered by the Catholic Commission for Peace and Justice (CCJP) indicates otherwise. Within six weeks, some 2,000 civilians had been killed in Mathebeleland, many burnt alive inside huts, and thousands more tortured. The brigade forced people to kill their relatives, have sex with family members, and made husbands or sons watch their wives or mothers being raped. Victims were forced to dig their own graves, and onlookers were forced to dig mass graves, bury the dead, sing while being beaten, and dance on top of the freshly buried corpses. Pregnant women were often accused of carrying dissident babies and had their stomachs ripped open to reveal the "dissidents" they were carrying. Rape was common, and the soldiers would tell their victims (Ndebele women) they (the Shona soldiers) were creating a generation of Shona babies in Mathebeleland (Alexander et al., 2000; Alexander & McGregor, 1996; Ngwenya, 2018). While the exact number of those killed is unlikely to ever be known, it is generally estimated that up to 20,000 people lost their lives during this period (Eppel, 2006). In addition, some do not know the whereabouts of their family members who disappeared (Ngwenya, 2018) or were buried in mass graves usually in the absence of their relatives. Those who could bury their relatives were forced to do so in a hurry, and teachers and government workers were buried by their host communities because they worked away from their own home areas (CCJP, 2007). These practices left people unable to mourn their dead according to their cultural norms, and to observe traditional burial rites that normally last a day or two.

Since independence, in addition to *Gukurahundi*, the government has continued to perpetrate violence towards its citizens, especially those from opposition parties. This includes the violent farm invasions in the early 2000s, the destruction of urban dwellings during Operation Restore Order of 2005, which left 570 000 people internally displaced, and the continued repressive, marginalization, and dictatorial actions of the government. All these events continue to have the potential to traumatize individuals and communities.

Effects of Gukurahundi on the Population

The deliberate ploy by the Mugabe government to annihilate the SiNdebele-speaking people in Mathebeleland and parts of the Midlands Province left a general sense of collective anger, vulnerability, and mistrust in the President, ZANU-PF and the Shona people (Alexander & McGregor, 1996). These attitudes stem from the realization that "not only were they the targets of extermination, but that also everything that constituted their world, everything that made their life worth living—their work, their families and their children—was at the point of being wiped out too" (Zorbas, 2004, p. 30). The extreme nature of the *Gukurahundi* violence affected families and communities causing negative psychological and physiological impacts, economic hardships and marginalization, fear, and hatred.

Psychological and Physiological Impact

People were left with emotional wounds and physical injuries. As per one survivor, "This wound is huge and deep ... the liberation war was painful, but it had a purpose ... The war that followed was much worse. It was fearful, unforgettable, and unacknowledged" (CCJP, 2007, p. 96). Survivors of torture by the 5th Brigade carry permanent disabilities, partial lameness, paralysis, deafness, recurring backaches and headaches, impotence, infertility, and kidney damage (CCJP, 2007). The violence of the *Gukurahundi* also left emotional scars. According to the *Breaking the Silence* report (CCJP, 2007), at the time of their research in the 1990s, large numbers of the people in Tsholotsho district showed signs of psychological trauma, leading to recurring depression, dizzy spells, anxiety, and anger. Children were left with the trauma of having lost one or both parents and having witnessed extreme violence done to their loved ones. The cruel nature of the atrocities left people's grief unatoned for and the mourning process incomplete, creating what Brave Heart (1998) conceptualized as impaired mourning or impaired grief. Relatives of those for whom traditional burial rituals could not be observed encountered a spiritual and religious dilemma because the dead are supposed to be unhappy, and misfortune is believed to befall the living as punishment for neglecting to meet this expectation (Eppel, 2006). Furthermore, families whose loved ones disappeared face greater spiritual upheavals since,

> [t]he disappearance of the body implies that the soul can neither pass from the land of the living to the land of the dead. The wandering spirit continues to haunt the living in the form of the constant anxiety of the relatives who cannot mourn the disappeared and keep demanding a reckoning from society.
>
> *(Robben, 2000, p. 95)*

Economic Hardships and Marginalization

During the period of *Gukurahundi*, life came to a standstill in most of Mathebeleland contrary to the rest of the country for which the years 1980 to 1990 were seen as a golden decade of development and growth. Development stopped, people lost jobs, schools were closed and teachers were killed. Many able-bodied men and young people, who survived the killings, fled the country to South Africa, Botswana, and elsewhere, depriving the families and communities of their breadwinners, and compromising their future. Many school-age children did not go back to school, because people could not get death certificates and children could not get birth certificates, families were deprived of access to funds from bank accounts and pensions of the deceased since the government did not acknowledge these deaths and thus there was no official proof of their demise (Ngwenya, 2018). This problem still persists, legally limiting the ability of children to stay in school beyond seventh grade, get a job, or access any services that require proof of identity.

People in Mathebeleland often report economic and cultural marginalization, being sidelined from the mainstream politics of the country, and being deliberately discriminated against in sharing the national cake. They see their region as lagging behind in all aspects of developmental progress, and point to an unwritten law that individuals who belong to the Ndebele-speaking group should be disadvantaged on all fronts. The dominance of Shona-speaking people in almost all spheres of public life in Mathebeleland is often cited as an indication of this marginalization (Ndlovu-Gatsheni, 2003; Ngwenya, 2018). Shona-speaking Police officers and teachers who cannot speak or understand the languages and cultures of the people of Mathebeleland, are deployed even in remote parts of the region.

Fear and Hatred

The brutality and pervasiveness of the violence perpetrated by the 5th Brigade created a sense of permanent fear, distrust of government officials, and hatred for ZANU-PF and its leaders (chiefly, former president Robert Mugabe and his successor Emmerson Mnangagwa). Further, the politicization of the military and the strong link between ethnicity and political affiliation, promoted a negative perception of the military. Since *Gukurahundi* was a state-sanctioned pogrom, people in Mathebeleland perceive the military as Shona-dominated and the Shona language as the language of torture and oppression. Most of the people, especially the elderly, are still terrified of the army, and view the recurrence of the massacres as a distinct possibility. However, the younger generation is more driven by hatred than by fear and often opposes anything associated with ZANU-PF or the government. Hence, since the death of Joshua Nkomo in 1999 and the rise of the opposition, Mathebeleland has become a strong base for the opposition (Ngwenya, 2018).

Posttraumatic Growth in the Zimbabwean Context

The idea of deriving benefit from adversity is common in many of the world's religions and echoed in trauma studies (Jayawickreme & Blackie, 2016; Oginska-Bulik & Kobylarczyk, 2015; Werdel & Wicks, 2012). Many concepts have been used to refer to the possibility of positive changes after trauma as a potential source of transformation, evolution, and personal growth, most central among them is posttraumatic growth (PTG). However, as in Zimbabwe the adversity continues and the potential for trauma persists, Renos Papadopoulos' term Adversity-Activated Development (AAD) is preferable because the "Post" in posttraumatic growth suggests that the traumatic situation happened in the past, whereas AAD recognizes its ongoing nature.

Papadopoulos prefers the concept of adversity rather than trauma as the basis of his (AAD) model. He defines AAD as the positive developments that are a direct result of being exposed to adversity and posits that a notable number of individuals and groups have derived meaning from their suffering and have been able to transform these negative experiences in a positive way, gaining new strength and renewal. Furthermore, once they survive the initial life-threatening adversity, people may begin to appreciate life in a whole new way, re-examining their values and priorities, and beginning to live in a more conscious way with better quality. Therefore, AAD refers to positive, growth-focused developments, which result directly from the experiences of being exposed to adversity/trauma, as well as new elements, which did not exist prior to the adversity (Papadopoulos, 2007).

AAD in Survivors of Gukurahundi

The author of this chapter is a native of Mathebeleland and has worked with the communities affected by *Gukurahundi* for more than 20 years having carried out a 2-year action research project with a group of former ZPRA combatants designed to examine if communities affected by the violence of *Gukurahundi* could heal themselves in the absence of an official apology or healing program (Ngwenya, 2018). During this project, none of the participants displayed any signs of severe traumatic or pathological effects, even though most had experienced and witnessed violence firsthand.

It has been claimed that individuals who experience adverse circumstances are often unable to self-identify growth or development that might have occurred following the traumatic experience, and require external support and empathy from others to reconstruct meaning relative to their experiences (Jayawickreme & Blackie, 2016; Joseph, 2011). For the research participants, such an environment was provided through the Tree of Life (TOL) workshop which was part of the action component of the action research project.

The TOL Intervention Model

TOL is a group-based workshop that combines storytelling, empowerment, and healing of the spirit, and seeks to reconnect victims with their self and community by providing group therapy using nature as a means (Ngwenya, 2016). The TOL approach is very flexible and can be adapted to fit any context; it is relatively inexpensive and does not require highly trained professionals. TOL was originally designed to work with unemployed youths, was adapted in 2002 to the needs of Zimbabwean political refugees living in South Africa, and was later introduced in Zimbabwe in 2004. In both South Africa and Zimbabwe, its intended beneficiaries were mainly victims of political violence emanating from the violent farm invasions between 2000 and 2005, and from subsequent elections in Zimbabwe (Reeler et al., 2009; Templer, 2010). This approach has also been used in Australia with a young refugee from Liberia (Schweitzer et al., 2013).

The workshop included a two-and-a-half-day residential program held at a camping retreat away from the disruptions of everyday life. It was facilitated by two of the TOL staff members who had been victims of the early 2000s political violence in Zimbabwe. Participants comprised five ZPRA combatants and three student interns in their 20s associated with the ex-combatants' organization ZPRA Veterans Trust, whose parents and grandparents had been directly affected by *Gukurahundi*.

The process centered on a series of circles resembling the traditional village court; however, in this court, all were equal and participants utilized a "talking piece" such as a stone or any item that a speaker held while talking and then passed on to the next person to allow each other turns to speak. A central element in the TOL process is the use of a tree as an allegory for human suffering and the potential for agency and growth. A tree that is striving but has deformities such as cut-off or malformed branches, is used to assist participants reflect on their adverse circumstances (Ngwenya, 2018).

Over several circles, participants used sketches of trees to talk about different aspects of their lives. For instance, they discussed their roots (ancestry), trunk (childhood), leaves (important features of their lives), and fruit (family and future plans) and explored their connectivity and benefits from diversity. The "trauma circle" was the *most significant part of this process. During this stage, participants were given an opportunity to talk about their adverse experiences in a friendly, respectful, and loving environment. In the mornings, participants participated in a session in bodywork, consisting of breathing, balancing, stretching, and relaxation exercises to allow them to reconnect with their bodies, especially for those who had experienced physical torture.

At the end of the workshop, participants gathered around a living tree to discuss similarities between their lives and the tree that had been marred and scarred but was still alive and thriving. Through this process, and their reflection on the tree's "tribulations," participants were able to find meaning in their suffering and realize that there had been some positives that had resulted from it.

Participants' Reflections on ADD Following the TOL Experience

Participants' feedback reflects their newly found appreciation. The first epiphany came about when they realized that, just as the tree was striving in spite of its adverse circumstances, they too had succeeded despite their suffering. One participant stated,

> As long as the roots are not removed the tree will not die ... As long as it has roots it will always grow. This is one of the things I liked. If I am cut ... but then still you as a human being, how is your nature, it is to continue going forward; you must not go back and say 'I have been cut, and then stay there and limp'.

Another expressed,

> People would say 'but I am more than a tree, you see'. If you cut the tree and it continues to live, why can't I be the same? That's the way of trying to forego the past and continue focusing on the future, because the tree has a future, because it's still continuing to [live] isn't it? And to us this is a double advantage that we had, in the sense that we got to yield ourselves as individuals and also we obtained a vehicle or we acquired a vehicle which we can institute in our quest to develop this, this face, you see which we always have.

These comments marked the beginning of the process of participants' finding meaning and making sense of the suffering they had experienced. The fact that the tree was striving in spite of its previous adverse circumstances and still visible scars and distortions, represented a shift in how participants perceived life, moving from being victims to appreciating life in a new light. The realization was that even though their lives were full of challenges, they could make the choice not to continue living as victims. Just like the tree, their circumstances presented them with opportunities to find new ways of expressing their lives. As one participant put it,

> ... so the thing I am trying to say is 'Fine, all these things happened, but we should not glue ourselves to those things and say that all those things happened and my life ends here. No, you can still live within that situation'

Most participants realized that they had a measure of control over their lives and, as such, could live more meaningfully. Participants recognized the need for making meaning of their adverse circumstances, and referred to it as being "reconciled to oneself." A male participant said about the process,

> In our own hearts, we have **to be reconciled with ourselves**. Say, 'Yes, *Gukurahundi* it happened' (long pause) and of course it's not even in a thousand years will Mugabe come back and say sorry ... I think it is a departure point where we can look at another window where we can find a correct, *straight path to healing and personal empowerment*, because what we need at the end of the day is for our people to be healed, because as long as we remain with hurt we will not be able to forgive, whether forgiveness is necessary or not, but we may not be able to live with

history of the past that which is distorted, that tree trunk that got cut and probably bent on one side.

This process is similar to what Sherman et al. (2012) described in cancer patients,

> ... *the process of survivorship* continues by assuming an active role in self-healing, *gaining a new perspective and reconciling paradoxes*, creating *a new mindset* and moving to *a new normal, developing a new way of being in the world on one's own terms, and experiencing growth through adversity beyond survivorship* ... (p. 258, emphasis added).

About 18 months after the TOL workshop, a conversation with two of the student interns seemed to suggest a paradigm shift in their philosophy of life from seeing themselves as perpetual victims of their lives' circumstances to actively seeking to grow through their adverse circumstances. Rather than allowing the circumstances to get the better part of them, the two acknowledged them and were finding ways to live above them. According to one of them,

> We have to go on by ourselves; it's not about the other person, it's about you personally, so that you can move on because, *if you don't heal by yourself, you will always be living in the past; and if you hold on too much to the past, you tend not to grow as a person; it causes trauma to you because you will always be thinking about that event and blaming the event.* If only, if only, if only ... So, I think the Tree of Life helped me to have that view on life that you have to move on after you have been hurt (emphasis added).

Perhaps the following comments from the other student best illustrate this new perspective on life,

> Moving on is not necessarily forgetting what happened in the past, it is being strong to move on; that is healing. Healing for me is that; that wound which has been there shouldn't be a stumbling block to where you want to go; it should give you power to move on to the future. Yes, that thing happened to me, this thing happened like this to me. It should inspire and motivate me to move to the future rather than going back. Because sometimes we tend to focus too much on the wound or the scar— let me say on the scar— that it was like this here (pointing to a scar on himself), but then it's only a scar. That scar shouldn't pull you back; instead it should motivate you to forge to the future, to give you strength rather than pull you back.

It seems that, in line with Papadopoulos' Adversity-Activated Development model, participants felt that the workshop helped them discover the potential for growing every day through the adversities they faced. Further, their conclusions about how to deal with their everyday stressful situations mirror Meichenbaum's (2013) pathways to resilience and thriving. Specifically, six factors that he identifies as influencing how effectively people deal with trauma and adversity in their lives seem to be applicable to participants' coping strategies.

The Degree of Perceived Personal Control and the Extent to Which Individuals Focus Their Time and Energies on Tasks and Situations over Which They Have Some Impact and Influence

When individuals experiencing adversity feel that they have control over at least some of their life's circumstances and are able to make meaningful contributions that positively affect those situations, they are more likely to experience positive growth from the adverse situation. Participants revealed that having mastery over their circumstances or seeking to exert this mastery was an important aspect they learned at the workshop, which gave them the skills to deal with obstacles they encounter and helped their healing journey. One student described,

> If you have a victim mentality you will always have a bargaining chip, like, these people are the ones who did this to me. So, whilst you, you are not trying your best, you see, ... you won't try your best, you will be knowing that I am a victim, so you won't get to your full potential if you are a victim.

The student's perceptive insight agrees with Papadopoulos (2000) and Lamott (2005) who state that the attitude of self-entitlement and perpetuation of the victim mentality can be addictive and ultimately self-defeating as it prevents the development of the affected individual from victim to survivor. These participants indicated a determination to shake the lethargy and be proactive in the face of unfavorable circumstances.

The Degree to Which People Can Experience Positive Emotions and Self-Regulate Negative Emotions

Individuals who have a 3 to 1 ratio of positive versus negative experiences are more likely to be resilient. Individuals who tend to experience more positive than negative emotions by having mastery over their negative emotions stand a better chance of developing fortitude and self-agency. Having a positive attitude and focusing on the positive side of things were referred to constantly by the two students as important in assisting them to face their daily realities. They emphasized the need to not allow one's circumstances to dictate one's outlook on life. One posited,

> If you let a situation change who you are then you are destined to be bitter all your life. You will be bitter because every situation that comes will change you. At least if you are focused then no, you will keep on forging ahead step by step.

The Ability to Function with Cognitive Flexibility, Using Problem-Solving and Acceptance Skills, Depending on the Situation

Individuals who can accept their circumstances and figure out ways to deal with their adverse situations tend not to suffer from extreme traumatization. Participants indicated their ability to interact with their situations and, at least at that point, seemed to have found ways to address them. The most important dimension seemed to be their acceptance that life is full of obstacles and that what matters most is how one approaches these obstacles. Taking "each day as it comes" and "approaching each situation that you face with a positive mind," suggest a well-calculated effort to systematically encounter adversities. As one participant affirmed,

> Looking at the tree, how it is nurtured or how it nurtured itself, umm ... how it gets to adapt to the environment, all those things. I took it upon myself that, that tree resembles my life, how I've managed to go through all those things and found it helpful because this gave me the strength to keep on keeping on, because looking at the challenges that one might face, you might never in life get the chance for someone to come and apologise, ... but looking at this workshop that we had, I think it is, umm ... I think it was really helpful, a good benefit to me ... So, I took it upon myself that if the tree can survive under all those conditions, then I can also live under these conditions. That is how, I found this helpful to me.

The Ability to Be Involved in Activities That Follow Their Priorities and Values in Life That Reflect a Stake in the Future

One participant spoke about focusing at present on her education as a priority in order to secure future employment. This focus, she said, made her a "happier person." For another, being at the university and focusing on the prospects of a better future was a factor in dealing with the effects of a bad past,

> Every day you have to have your own goals, so I set my goals where I want to go. I know where I want to go each and every day. Sometimes, if I take one step back or when a situation makes me take a step back, I know where I want to go so that keeps me going.

The Ability to Face Life's Adversities and Trauma, Work through Them and Share Own Struggles with Others Instead of Denying or Avoiding Negative Emotions and Pain

In the context of the repressive regimes in Chile in the 1970s and early 1980s, Agger and Jensen (1996) found that some of those who had been tortured were unlikely to seek professional assistance but rather sought ways to self-heal by being involved in helping others who had also recently suffered torture. Their involvement in pro-social actions and self-disclosure in these groups facilitated the healing process and counteracted the feelings of being a victim. Sharing their experiences in a group setting allowed survivors to "de-privatize" their experiences, and to come to terms with them faster. Such sharing is a consciousness-raising process, which allowed survivors to see their traumatic experiences from a broader political perspective; thus giving context and meaning to their suffering. Similarly, the participants in the TOL group stressed the importance of viewing negative effects positively and believing that out of the bad good could eventually emerge, because "everything happens for a reason." For one participant, it was "about learning every day" because "*every negative aspect teaches you something about life*, so in the end, you will learn something that will help you in the future later." (Emphasis added).

The Perceived Availability of Social Relationships and the Ability to Access and Use Social Support

Political or ethnic violence, although perpetrated against individuals, is designed to break the social fabric and the social safety nets. When individuals experiencing these disruptions fail to access their traditional support systems, they may lose their ability to cope and overcome the disruptions as they might have, had the support systems been present (Farwell & Cole, 2002). Therefore, these "disruptions, along with those of interpersonal relationships, and the ability to regulate internal emotional states, co-exist with and give rise to intense trauma symptoms" (Staub et al., 2005, p. 299). The ability to have and access these relationships for support in times of hardship is crucial to victims' response to adverse circumstances. Participants appeared to be alluding to this concept by speaking of how sharing their painful experiences with others who understood it was important in their ability to cope. As one of them said,

> If I can share with the group what has happened to me, myself, it lessens the severity of the problem, because a problem shared is a problem relieved, so to say. It may not go away completely, but the fact that you now all know about my problem, I feel consoled. I don't know whether it happens to other people, unless if it is a secret I don't want you people to know. But if it is something that hurt me really and probably something that amputated my leg, it has to be known how I lost my leg, and for you people to be able to feel for me ... By this act of telling to other people, it reduces the severity of the problem that I carry.

This idea has been well collaborated by Herman (1992) who made clear that recovery cannot happen in isolation and can take place only within the context of relationships. Participants saw their supportive relationships and the ability to lean on them, whenever needed, as an important element of their wellbeing.

Conclusions

Clearly, there is a need to carry out more focused in-depth studies to gain a better understanding of the positive development and growth among the communities in Mathebeleland who are facing continued adverse circumstances. It would also be important to ascertain the applicability of the same to a larger and more representative population. Nevertheless, the above discussion offers preliminary insights into what might be pertaining to these communities. The aforementioned experiences closely mirror Papadopoulos' (2007) statement regarding the process of AAD "... a new epistemology (a way of understanding how one knows) emerges which is the sum total of all new perceptions that lead to the acquisition of a new way of understanding, speaking, relating about oneself, others and life itself" (p. 308). Participants in the described study appeared to have gained novel perspectives of comprehending their circumstances, and developed constructive mechanisms to live through their new realities positively. These conclusions can be applied to those who struggle with atrocities in diverse socio-political cultural contexts around the globe.

References

Agger, I., & Jensen, S. B. (1996). *Trauma and healing under state terrorism*. London: Zed.
Alexander, J., McGregor, J., & Ranger, T. (2000). *Violence and memory: One hundred years in the 'dark forests' of Matabeleland*. Oxford: James Curry.
Alexander, J., & McGregor, J. (1996). Democracy, development and political conflict: Rural institutions in Matabeleland North after independence. *International Conference on the Historical Dimensions of Democracy and Human Rights in Zimbabwe*. Harare, September, 1996.
Beach, D. (1994). *The Shona and their neighbours*. Oxford: Blackwell
Brave Heart, M. W. H. (1998). The return to the sacred path: Healing the historical trauma and historical unresolved grief response among the Lakota through a psychoeducational group intervention. *Smith College Studies in Social Work*, *68*(3), 287–305. 10.1080/00377319809517532
CCJP. (2007). *Gukurahundi in Zimbabwe: A report on the disturbances in Matabeleland and the Midlands 1980–1988*. Johannesburg: Jacana Media.
Eppel, S. (2006). 'Healing the dead': Exhumation and burial as truth-telling and peace-building activities in rural Zimbabwe. In T. A. Borer (Ed.), *Telling the truths: Truth telling and peace-building in post-conflict societies*. Notre Dame, IN: University of Notre Dame Press.
Farwell, N., & Cole, J. B. (2002). Community as context of healing: Psychosocial recovery of children affected by war and political violence. *International Journal of Mental Health*, *30*(4),19–41.
Herman, J. L. (1992). *Trauma and recovery: From domestic abuse to political terror*. London: Pandura.
Jayawickreme, E., & E.R. Blackie, L. E. R. (2016). *Exploring the psychological benefits of hardship: A critical reassessment of posttraumatic growth*. Cham: Springer.
Joseph, S. (2011). *What doesn't kill us: The new psychology of posttraumatic growth*. New York, NY: Basic Books.
Lamott, F. (2005). Trauma as a political tool. *Critical Public Health*, *15*(3), 219–228.
Meichenbaum, D. (2013). Ways to bolster resilience across the deployment cycle. *Military Psychologists' Desk Reference*, 325–355.
Meredith, M. (2008). *Mugabe: Power, plunder and the struggle for Zimbabwe*. Jeppestown: Jonathan Ball.
Ndlovu-Gatsheni, S. J. (2003). The post-colonial state and Matabeleland: Regional perceptions of civil-military relations, 1980–2002. In Williams, Rocky et al. (Eds.), *Ourselves to know: Civil military relations and defence transformation in Southern Africa* (pp. 17–38). Pretoria: Institute for Security Studies.
Ngwenya, D. (2016). "Our branches are broken": Using the Tree Of Life healing methodology with victims of *Gukurahundi* in Matabeleland, Zimbabwe. *Peace and Conflict Studies*, *23*(1), Article 2. https://nsuworks.nova.edu/pcs/vol23/iss1/2
Ngwenya, D. (2018). *Healing the wounds of Gukurahundi in Zimbabwe: A participatory action research project*. Cham: Springer.
Nkomo, J. (1984). *Nkomo: The story of my life*. London: Methuen.
Ogińska-Bulik, N., & Kobylarczyk, M. (2015). Relation between resiliency and post-traumatic growth in a group of paramedics: The mediating role of coping strategies. *International Journal of Occupational Medicine and Environmental Health*, *28*(4), 707–719. 10.13075/ijomeh.1896.00323
Papadopoulos, R. K. (2007). Refugees, trauma and adversity-activated development. *European Journal of Psychology and Counselling*, *9*(3), 301–312.
Reeler, T., Chitsike, K., Maizva, F., & Reeler, B. (2009). Tree of life: A community approach to empowering and healing survivors of torture in Zimbabwe. *Torture*, *19*(3), 180–193. http://www.ncbi.nlm.nih.gov/pubmed/20065537
Robben, A. C. G. M. (2000). The assault on basic trust: Disappearance, protest, and reburial. In A. C. G. M. Robben, & M. M. Suarez-Orozco (Eds.), *Cultures under siege: Collective violence and trauma*. Cambridge: Cambridge University Press,
Sherman, D. W., Rosedale M., & Haber S. (2012). Reclaiming life on one's own terms: A grounded theory of the process of breast cancer survivorship. *Oncology Nursing Forum*, *39*(3), 258–268.
Schweitzer, R. D., Vromans, L., Ranke, G., & Griffin, J. (2013). Narratives of healing: A case study of a young Liberian refugee settled in Australia. *The Arts in Psychology*, *41*(2014), 98–106.

Staub, E., Pearlman, L. A., Gubin, A., & Hagengimana, A. (2005). Healing, reconciliation, forgiving and the prevention of violence after genocide or mass killings: An intervention and its experimental evaluation in Rwanda. *Journal of Social and Clinical Psychology*, *24*(3), 297–334.
Templer, S. (2010). Integrity of process: How tree of life is taking root in Zimbabwe. *Africa Peace and Conflict Journal*, *3*(2), 106–112.
Todd, J. G. (2007). *Through the darkness: A life in Zimbabwe*. Cape Town: Zebra.
Werdel, M. B., & Wicks, R. J. (2012). *Primer on posttraumatic growth: An introduction and guide*. NJ: John Wiley & Sons.
Zorbas, E. (2004). Reconciliation in post-genocide Rwanda. *African Journal of Legal Studies*, *1*(1), 29–35.

PART 4D

PTG in Organizations

27

ORGANIZATIONAL POSTTRAUMATIC GROWTH

Beyond Crisis Management and Resilience

Benjamin N. B. Alexander, Bruce Greenbaum, and Abraham B. (Rami) Shani

While trauma has largely been examined at the individual level, organizations can also be traumatized. Organizations, such as firms or communities, are complex adaptive socio-technical systems (Eijnatten et al., 2008; Emery & Trist, 1965; Mitki et al., 2019; Pasmore et al., 2019) that are socially constructed (Miller & Page, 2007). Formal and informal, for-profit, non-profit and governmental, multi-national and locally-oriented, organizations are ubiquitous across societies. Organizational trauma is an experience of significant adversity involving the disruption of core organizational functions. A wide variety of precipitants can trigger organizational trauma including natural disasters, technological failures, leadership crises, and more. Organizational posttraumatic growth (OPTG) refers to a phenomenon wherein an organization achieves a higher level of well-being in the aftermath of significant adversity. While some organizations do not recover from trauma and fail, others experience OPTG. For example, following a structural collapse affecting its main facility, the B&O Railroad Museum in Baltimore Maryland, ultimately achieved a higher level of performance than before (Christianson et al., 2009). Toyota, likewise, developed new mechanisms to manage its supply chain in the aftermath of the 2011 Tohuku earthquake and tsunami (Batth, 2021).

The study of organizational trauma and OPTG is a recent endeavor in the management literature. While related to other discourses such as resilience and crisis management that also address serious adverse organizational phenomena, OPTG is distinct. Resilience research, while also concerned with adversity, is more concerned with preparedness by which disruption can be avoided and crisis management examines the restoration of functioning. OPTG however examines the potential for thriving following adversity. Maitlis (2012) explained that "resilience can thus be seen to differ from posttraumatic growth in that it emphasizes stability in the context of trauma, rather than a trajectory of increased positive functioning" (p. 913). Recent work directly examining these phenomena has examined the source and experience of organizational trauma and organizational responses (Alexander et al., 2021; Hormann, 2007; Hormann & Vivian, 2005; Nava, 2022).

This chapter provides an overview of these phenomena through the lens of organization theory. It explores OPTG in a diverse set of organizations including a large automobile company (Toyota), a museum (B&O Railroad Museum), a consulting firm branch, a

DOI: 10.4324/9781032208688-35

collectivist community (Kibbutz Shefayim), and California restaurants during COVID-19. While each of these represents complex cases, we have summarized them in short vignettes in Table 27.1 to provide a foundation for the examples we provide in later sections. The chapter first elaborates on organizations and the phenomenon of trauma at the organizational level. Then, it examines how organizations respond to trauma and two ways in which growth can be conceptualized.

Organizations

This section elaborates on OPTG by situating it in organization theory. Scholars of organization theory, organization design, and strategy have developed a wide variety of organization theories over the last century. Since its inception in the 1950s, the socio-technical systems (STS) perspective has become an increasingly popular organization and management theory (i.e., Pasmore et al., 2019), organization design theory (i.e., Mitki et al., 2019), and a planned change approach (i.e., Hanna, 1988). In elaborating on the OPTG phenomenon, we view organizations as complex social entities that function within a highly interdependent and complex local ecosystem and broader context. Organizations take shape in particular environmental contexts (Emery & Trist, 1965). The COVID-19 pandemic made salient many aspects of the multifaceted interface between organizations, their environments, and humanity. The environment for most organizations can be viewed as one with a distinct VUCA (Volatile, Uncertain, Complex, and Ambiguous) characteristic and nature.

Organizations, as complex adaptive sociotechnical systems, are communities of meaning, with rich tapestries of cultural rules, structural configurations, processes, technologies, roles, and interactions (i.e., Eijnatten et al., 2008; Emery & Trist, 1965; Pasmore et al., 2019). Complex adaptive systems are composed of many interacting agents (or subsystems), each with its own strategy for adapting to the environment and pursuing its goals (Axelrod & Cohen, 1999; Miller & Page, 2007). Every organization is made up of a *social subsystem* (the people) using tools, techniques, and knowledge (*the technical subsystem*) to produce a product or a service valued by the *environmental subsystem* (of which customers form a part). The success of an organization depends upon the interactions and compatibility between its three subsystems. Drawing heavily on open systems, Emery (1959) and Trist (1963) explored the nature of technical systems, social systems, and the work relationship structures that bring the two systems together within a specific environmental context. Thus, while every organization is perceived as a sociotechnical system, not every organization is designed using STS principles, methods, processes, and philosophy (Shani et al., 1992). From an STS perspective, major events or changes in one of the subsystems are likely to affect the other subsystems and as such will impact the overall performance of the organization.

Organizational Trauma

Organizational trauma is a process in which serious adverse events disrupt organizational subsystems. Triggering events such as earthquakes, pandemics, product failures, the sudden absence of an organizational leader, or sabotage can undermine an organization's capacity to fulfill core functions (Alexander et al., 2021; Hormann, 2018; Hormann & Vivian, 2017). For a collective trauma to occur, individuals must be interdependent, "bound in

Table 27.1 Mini-Cases on OPTG

B&O Railroad Museum Collapse (Christianson et al., 2009)

The museum, which began as part of the United States' first railroad, housed an extensive collective of artifacts in a historic landmark building. Amidst financial strain, it had been planning a fair to celebrate a historic milestone and drive attendance. However, not long before the fair, a record snowstorm collapsed the roof and damaged other systems and collections. The fair, into which the museum had already invested nearly $1 million, had to be canceled.

The museum's board of directors decided to rebuild the museum. This required significant financial resources, well beyond what the museum had at that point. In addition to insurance payouts, government support, and private support, the museum built a train restoration and repair facility. Building repair work proceeded.

After several months and after much of the work had been completed, a significant portion of the building was declared structurally unsound. "Staff realized that the museum could take advantage of the temporary cessation of operations not just to restore what had existed before, but also to re-think what would make the museum appeal to a wider public" (p. 849). The eventually reopened museum was bigger, sought to appeal to families as well as a niche railroad crowd, and was more accessible.

Consultancy Branch Office Illness (Kahn et al., 2013)

This mini-case is summarized from Kahn et al.'s (2013) example. When one of the senior consultants at a branch office of a consultancy had a heart attack, it set off a crisis at the firm. The branch office included a stable group of two senior consultants, additional junior consultants, and administrative staff. The relational patterns among these coworkers had been fixed in a manner that offered the organizational members little autonomy. However, the prior patterns were no longer feasible following the senior consultant's illness. "Chaos ensues as members dramatically shift routines" (p. 381).

Over the next months, the relational patterns among members changed several times. While previously, the two senior consultants had been equally capable, this was no longer the case. Reestablishing the relational system required defining new patterns, new levels of cohesion, and flexibility. The office eventually reached a new status quo that incorporated the senior consultant's chronic heart condition.

Kibbutz Shefayim Renewal and Theft (Alexander et al., 2021)

Kibbutz Shefayim is a collectivist community located on the Mediterranean coast near Herzliya, Israel. One of the oldest kibbutzim (Hebrew plural for "kibbutz") in Israel, Shefayim has progressed from an agricultural-based community to a diversified organization with retail, commercial, recreational, and tourism-related business interests. Over its 90-plus-year history, Shefayim became one of the country's most economically successful kibbutzim. In the early 2000s, Shefayim management uncovered significant financial improprieties related to an effort to avoid corporate taxes on income generated by several of the kibbutz's recreation and tourism businesses. Two members of Shefayim's former management team were arrested and ultimately convicted of stealing 16.5 million shekels (approximately US $4 million) from the kibbutz over a six-year period from 1996 to 2002 (the "theft").

The theft stunned the kibbutz and traumatized the organization in a variety of ways. It 1.) Shattered the social relationship bonds that were critical components of kibbutz life; 2.) Burdened the kibbutz with the threat of significant legal and financial penalties after news of the theft was made public; and 3.) Challenged the management structure of the kibbutz after the theft exposed weaknesses in the kibbutz's policies and oversight procedures.

The kibbutz and its new leadership team dedicated significant time, energy, and resources to addressing the theft within the kibbutz and rebuilding the connections among kibbutz members. Additionally, the aftermath of the theft enabled the kibbutz to institute a variety of organizational and financial policies and structures that positioned the kibbutz for long-term success. Further, the kibbutz made significant efforts to grow its membership and increase the social activities offered to kibbutz residents that reenergized the kibbutz while restoring many of the longstanding traditions that were being lost around the time of the theft. Ultimately, the actions taken helped restore trust in the kibbutz's leadership, which may have suffered the most after the full extent of the theft's effects on the organization was realized. Today, Shefayim is thriving and surpassed all performance metrics achieved prior to the theft.

(*Continued*)

Table 27.1 (Continued)

Toyota Motor Corp. Fukushima Disaster
In March 2011, Toyota Motor Corp. was the largest global automaker but experienced a traumatic disruption in manufacturing and its global supply chain as a result of an earthquake and tsunami. Four of Toyota's manufacturing facilities in Japan's Tohoku region were damaged in the tsunami. Additionally, more than two-thirds of Toyota's suppliers in the Tohoku region experienced significant disruptions for months after the tsunami. At the time of the disaster, Toyota produced more than 60% of its vehicles in Japan, with only 25% of its global vehicle sales occurring in Japan (Forbes, 2011). Market share in North America was expected to decline by 0.5% in 2012 and potentially fall to 80% of projected growth in 2013.
In response to the breakdown in the supply chain, Toyota worked to reopen its manufacturing facilities as quickly as possible – with two of the four facilities reopening within a month of the tsunami. Additionally, Toyota began asking more of its suppliers. ; specifically, requiring that suppliers stockpile products in advance of any future disruptions. While Toyota still pays less per unit for the higher volume of parts produced by its suppliers, the suppliers receive financial support from Toyota annually. Given the additional costs that would be incurred by suppliers for stockpiling parts, Toyota compensates its suppliers by returning a portion of the cost cuts it demands from suppliers each year during the life cycle of any car model in annual cost-down programs (Holderith, 2021).
Toyota continues to thrive more than a decade after the tsunami. In fact, the demands made on its suppliers in 2012 served Toyota well when facing the global supply chain breakdowns caused by the Covid-19 pandemic. Global semiconductor shortages have paralyzed much of the global auto industry over the past two years; however, Toyota has suffered much less than its competitors as a result of these enhanced relationships with its suppliers.

relationships and in communities by covenants, beliefs, and values" (Hormann, 2018, p. 94). While organizational members may also be traumatized, the concept of organizational trauma refers to a breakdown in the organization itself.

Organizational researchers have examined a broad set of adverse experiences. Both event-based and processual conceptualizations of adversity are salient in this research (Williams et al., 2017). Our view of trauma and OPTG are largely processual, in that trauma unfolds around a significantly adverse event or multiple events and persists as the organization responds, perhaps leading to growth. Organizational trauma is rooted in context (Roux-Dufort, 2007) and unfolds over time. In characterizing trauma as a process, we consider temporal and communal aspects that generalize across traumas with various triggering events (summarized in Table 27.2).

Temporality

Whereas some traumas may unfold from an abrupt trigger, others may be cumulative. "[A] dversity is heterogeneous; some challenges are triggered quickly, evolve rapidly, and are short in duration, whereas other challenges emerge slowly, evolve more gradually, and are extended over time" (Williams et al., 2017, p. 753). Traumas experienced through *abrupt* triggers (e.g., Hwang & Lichtenthal, 2000) such as an industrial accident, a snowstorm, or a tsunami, are distinguished by the perceived discontinuity between the periods preceding and following a triggering event. The disruptive adversity becomes visible around some "fault line between the past and the future" (Roux-Dufort, 2007, p. 109). To be clear, we are not re-conceptualizing traumas as singular events. Rather, some traumas may be

Table 27.2 Key Characteristics of Organizational Traumas

Aspects	*Description*		*Examples*
Temporal- Abrupt precipitating event	Demarcation of meaning; Discontinuity between periods	The initial impact on one organizational subsystem spreads to others	Toyota Motor Corp. Fukushima Disaster B&O Railroad Museum Collapse (initial collapse) Consultancy Branch Office Illness
Temporal- Cumulative or repeated precipitating events	Ongoing adverse experiences resulting in a perceived disruption; Multiple disruptions	Multiple subsystems impacted, perhaps exerting extreme pressure on one multiple subsystems impacted	Kibbutz Shefayim Renewal and Theft B&O Railroad Museum Collapse (initial collapse and later structural compromise) California Restaurants through COVID-19
Communal- Relationship between org members	Breakdown in social bonds; Destruction of sense of community	Social subsystem compromised as a primary or secondary effect of precipitants	Kibbutz Shefayim Renewal and Theft Consultancy Branch Office Illness

characterized by abrupt onset, clearly demarcated by a disruptive event. For example, Kahn et al. (2013) described how a leader's illness led to a breakdown of a branch of a consulting firm. The Tohoku Tsunami paralyzed Toyota's operations in that region and those of many of the firm's suppliers. The triggering or precipitating event is a demarcation of meaning within an ongoing organizational life (Roux-Dufort, 2007). The disruption resulting from an abrupt trigger is likely to start with a single subsystem, in the case of the consulting branch, the social subsystem, but eventually impacts the other systems due to their interdependence.

Unlike abrupt organizational traumas, the perception of *cumulative* organizational traumas involves either a gradual build toward disruption or repeated independently disruptive events. Gradual cumulative traumas entail multiple fractures which, while endurable in isolation, over time, lead to some fundamental breakdown in an organization (Hwang & Lichtenthal, 2000). For example, Kibbutz Shefayim in Israel was traumatized by the accumulated strain of its shifting financial model and theft perpetrated by a trusted member. At the individual level, the concept of trauma dose has been used to describe the multilateral impacts of complex traumas (e.g., Kira, 2001; Kira et al., 2008). Similarly, we might think of an organizational trauma dose in considering the accumulated impact of cumulative trauma. At the organization level at Kibbutz Shefayim, the precipitating experiences evolved to impact multiple subsystems, interacting over time to render a critical disruption within the social subsystem rather than originating and spreading from a single subsystem.

In addition, cumulative traumas may entail an organization's experience with multiple, repeated disruptions. For example, as multiple waves of the COVID-19 pandemic surged in California from 2020 through early 2022, restaurants have opened and closed different dining environments at multiple points in time. Considering the STS perspective, precipitating events directly compromise a single subsystem as occurs with an abrupt trigger. However, because triggers are repeated, the impact on other subsystems from whichever subsystem faced the initial disruption may exacerbate the total disruption until the organization has adequately responded or failed. Again, this suggests the value of considering an organizational trauma dose. In the aforementioned California restaurant example, whereas some restaurants developed ample new revenue streams (e.g., take-out, Zoom experiences, expanded outdoor dining in parklets) or other new processes amidst waves of COVID-19, others were ultimately forced to close.

Communal Aspects

Whereas characteristics relating to temporality describe how the disruption's onset is perceived, "communal" characterizes the content of the disruption. In communal trauma, the breakdown relates to relationships between organizational members and the organization, a breakdown in the "basic tissues of social life that damages the bonds attaching people together and impairs the prevailing sense of communality" (Erikson, 1976, p. 154). From an STS perspective, communal trauma entails a breakdown in the social subsystem, which may then spread to technological and environmental subsystems. In addition, communal trauma may originate in other subsystems. Erikson (1976) and Gill (2007) consider this a secondary trauma, for example, the social breakdown that persisted in New Orleans after Hurricane Katrina. Kahn et al. (2013) also capture communal trauma in their relational systems perspective crises. They describe how chaos resulted from the illness of a lead consultant in a small branch office. The disruption pertains to the way members engage with each other, their work, and other organizations. In this case, the onset of trauma was abrupt; however, communal trauma may also be a cumulative process, as occurred in the case of Kibbutz Shefayim, where the theft intersected with broader internal and external challenges that frayed social networks (Alexander et al., 2021; Mitki et al., 2008).

How Organizations Respond to Trauma

Organizational responses to traumas may foster OPTG or exacerbate a breakdown, perhaps even leading to organizational failure. While large bodies of scholarship have examined efforts to restore organizational functioning following crises or efforts to foster resilience, there is limited work on how responses to trauma can foster OPTG. In this section, we characterize the cognitive, relational, and structural responses we observed at Kibbutz Shefayim (Alexander et al., 2021) and in other cases, and consider how these relate to the role of organizational learning (e.g., Christianson et al., 2009; Nava, 2022; Williams et al., 2017). The cognitive, relational, and structural responses can be viewed as existing or new organizational capabilities that aided the organizational responses to the trauma and as such also served as triggers for the system's growth. These responses are summarized in Table 27.3.

We found evidence of both acceptance and positive reappraisals at Kibbutz Shefayim, by which the organization reframed the triggering event as an opportunity. This aligns with thinking on individual-level posttraumatic growth (PTG), which centers on the role of cognitive accommodation to trauma (e.g., Tedeschi & Calhoun, 1995, 2004). Some scholars have theorized that resilience may impede learning, pointing to an important area for further study. "If resilient individuals are 'immune' to these sense-making triggers in the face of challenges, they may fail to attend to and act on signals indicating the need to make

Table 27.3 Response to Organizational Traumas

Response Type	*Description*	*Examples*
Cognitive	Collective framing of trauma	Positive reappraisal – See trauma as an opportunity for acceptance – Recognition of trauma
Relational	Social capital building	Internally focused activities (i.e., among members) Externally focused activities
Structural	Reassessment and revision of organizational subsystems and their relationships to each other	Governance improvements, membership composition

changes to improve individual, group, or venture performance" (Williams et al., 2017, p. 756). However, acceptance and positive reappraisals may lead to relational and structural responses by encouraging learning and the opportunity for learning may be furthered in cumulative traumas (Christianson et al., 2009). For example, the B&O Railroad Museum's trauma was ongoing, with multiple triggers. The roof's initial collapse under heavy snow was followed by further disruptive incidents related to structural instability. Across these disruptions, the organization strengthened its capacity to learn and respond constructively.

Relational responses we observed involved both internally focused and externally focused efforts to build social capital (Alexander et al., 2021) and were also related to findings on social support at the individual level; for example, at Kibbutz Shefayim, leaders created forums for members to engage with each other and developed relationships with experts outside the organization who could help make sense of and navigate the trauma and at Toyota, the firm undertook a review of its relationships with different suppliers. Such responses to trauma may facilitate constructive cognitive responses (Maitlis, 2012) as well as entail emotional processing through which sense-making can occur (Berger & Weiss, 2008; Kahn, 2001; Kahn et al., 2013).

Organizations' structural responses to trauma have less of a corollary at the individual level than cognitive and relational responses to trauma. These entail changes to what the organization does and how it does it. In the language of STS, structural responses entail changes in organizational subsystems and how these subsystems interact. At Kibbutz Shefayim, we observed the implementation of new governance processes as well as new approaches to membership. While these changes may be the outcome of cognitive responses, i.e., the change imagined in a positive reappraisal, they may also yield new cognitive responses and further learning based on which additional cognitive, relational, and structural responses occur. Broadly, we hold with scholarship that views these types of responses as dynamically intertwined in a process by which organizations may ultimately grow through trauma (Nava, 2022).

Conceptualizing Growth

The characteristics of trauma interact with organizational characteristics, organizational responses, and the environment in an ongoing manner to shape outcomes over time.

Growth is more nuanced than a positive change in organizational performance assessed in financial or non-financial, quantitative or qualitative terms. However, our view departs from individual-level inventories of PTG, such as the Posttraumatic Growth Inventory (PTGI), which assesses growth as personal strength, new possibilities, relating to others, appreciation of life, and spiritual change (Tedeschi & Calhoun, 1996). In keeping with the STS perspective, we focus on how growth relates to organizational subsystems and avoid anthropomorphizing.

"After the crisis there are, of course, systematic tensions between the temptation to restore the status quo and the need to see the crisis as an opportunity for organizational change" (Roux-Dufort, 2007, p. 111). Broadly, one can separate two types of growth: (1) OPTG may involve achieving a higher level of performance based on a similar vision wherein subsystems are re-established, *or* (2) Through the effective pursuit of a different vision and different meanings, what Kahn et al. (2013) termed a "healthy transformation." These two paths are summarized in Table 27.4.

OPTG through the re-establishment of subsystems and elevated performance is exemplified in Toyota's emergence from the Fukushima disaster. Largely, the organization achieved higher levels of performance in the aftermath of the tsunami by improving its understanding of its supply chain and refining its relationships with key suppliers. Organizational subsystems were not fundamentally different but were instrumentally improved. Importantly, along this path for growth, performance in the post-trauma periods exceeds that of the pre-trauma period when assessed by quantitative and qualitative criteria germane to organizational objectives.

On the other hand, OPTG occurring through transformation entails a shift in an organization's self-concept and the effective pursuit of the new vision. The B&O Railroad Museum's roof collapse may serve as an example. For example, Christianson et al. (2009) posit that "The museum that finally reopened ... was considerably changed ..." (p. 849), having, among other things, expanded its space, adjusted its audience focus, and changed its financial model; Kibbutz Shefayim, emerging from trauma, established new frames for social bonds between its members. Along this path to growth, the organization's vision and its self-concept were fundamentally different and the content and relationship between organizational subsystems transformed. Comparing performance over time may be less applicable because the transformation implicates different dimensions of performance. Therefore, assessing growth entails a careful selection of indicators relevant to the changed organization.

Table 27.4 Two Paths for Growth in Organizational Posttraumatic Growth

Growth Type	*Description*	*Measurement Foci*
Re-establishment of subsystems	Elevated performance based on the pre-trauma vision	Financial and non-financial measures linked to organizational goals
Transformation; Revised content and interdependencies between subsystems	A shift in an organization's self-concept and its effective pursuit of a new vision	Organizational identification Financial and non-financial measures linked to organizational goals

Summary and Future Research and Conclusion

In this chapter, we examined the phenomenon of OPTG, a nascent area of organizational research. This work extends individual-level research to the organizational level, synthesizing and extending extant scholarship. We first expounded on the view of organizations offered by sociotechnical systems theory, which we draw throughout. Leveraging several mini-cases, we elaborated on what organizational trauma is by clarifying both its temporal and communal aspects. We then detailed findings on how organizations respond to trauma through cognitive, relational, and structural means, responses that are dynamically linked and may over time lead to learning and growth. Finally, we distinguished between two types of growth organizations may achieve following trauma.

In describing the aforementioned facets of this important and promising research domain, we hope to provide a foundation for further scholarship on OPTG and effective organizational responses to various types of traumas. This research requires a systematic study of OPTG. Practically, this reflection process will allow the system to learn from what worked well, what did not work, and what can be designed and facilitated to improve organizational responses to trauma.

Future research should identify capabilities that can help organizations navigate trauma and learning mechanisms that can be designed to improve the speed and depth of learning and adaptation cycles. The concept of agile-based organization design evolved within the broader discourse on complex adaptive sociotechnical systems that can learn and adapt. Agility represents a dynamic capability that enables timely and effective responses to rapidly changing environments and shifting stakeholder demands (Winter, 2003). Research that examines the key features of an agile organization, such as work systems, structures, management processes, human resources systems, and information systems with a focus on developing the capability to enhance the OPTG processes and outcomes would be of great added value. The field of organization development and change examines a wide array of generic change capabilities and advances ways to acquire them including hiring individuals with change management skills, training existing managers and employees to acquire them, developing an organization effectiveness function to support managers and employees, and cultivating a learning-by-doing culture (i.e., Cummings & Worley, 2015).

Beyond organizational capabilities and learning, there are numerous questions that might direct further exploration of OPTG, organizational capabilities, and learning. Future research might address types of traumas, the role of uncertainty, and contextual factors related to other institutions or organizations' industries. Further work on these topics will yield theoretical insights and practical guidance with which organizations may raise prospects for OPTG.

References

Alexander, B. N., Greenbaum, B. E., Shani, A. B., Mitki, Y., & Horesh, A. (2021). Organizational posttraumatic growth: Thriving after adversity. *The Journal of Applied Behavioral Science*, *57*(1), 30–56.

Axelrod, R., & Cohen, M. D. (1999). *Harnessing complexity: Organizational implications of scientific frontier*. New York, NY: Free Press.

Batth, V. (2021). Toyota Motor Corporation: Just in time (JIT) management strategy or beyond?. *Journal of Case Research*, *12*(1), 18–27.

Berger, R., & Weiss, T. (2008). The posttraumatic growth model: An expansion to the family system. *Traumatology*, *15*(1), 63–74.

Christianson, M. K., Farkas, M. T., Sutcliffe, K. M., & Weick, K. E. (2009). Learning through rare events: Significant interruptions at the Baltimore & Ohio railroad museum. *Organization Science*, *20*(5), 846–860. http://www.jstor.org/stable/25614699

Cummings, T. G., & Worley, C. G. (2015). *Organization development and change*. New York, NY: CENGAGE Learning

Emery, F. E. (1959). *The characteristics of sociotechnical systems: A critical review of theories and facts about the effects of technological change on the internal structure of work organizations*. Document #527, London: Tavistock Institute of Human Relations, Human Resources Centre.

Emery, F. E., & Trist, E. (1965). The causal texture of organizational environments. *Human Relations*, *18* (1), 21–32. 10.1177/001872676501800103

Eijnatten, F., Shani, A. B. (Rami), & Leary, M. (2008). Socio-technical systems: Designing and managing sustainable organizations. In T. Cumming (Ed.), *Handbook of organization development and change* (pp. 227–310), Thousand Oaks, CA: Sage.

Erikson, K. (1976). *Everything in its path*. New York, NY: Simon and Schuster.

Forbes. 2011. Japan quake, tsunami take heavy toll on Toyota. Retrieved from https://www.forbes.com/sites/greatspeculations/2011/04/08/japan-quake-tsunami-take-heavy-toll-on-toyota/?sh=6f61491661b4

Gill, D. A. (2007). Secondary trauma or secondary disaster? Insights from Hurricane Katrina. *Sociological Spectrum*, *27*(6), 613–632.

Hanna, D. P. (1988). *Designing organizations for high performance*. Reading, MA: Addison Wesley.

Holderith, P. (2021). Toyota unhurt by global chip shortage after learning from Fukushima nuclear disaster. Retrieved from https://www.thedrive.com/news/39697/toyota-unhurt-by-global-chip-shortage-after-learning-from-fukushima-nuclear-disaster#:~:text=Following%20the%20Fukushima%20nuclear%20disaster,ask%20more%20of%20its%20suppliers

Hormann, S. D. L. (2007). Organizational trauma: A phenomenological study of leaders in traumatized organizations (Doctoral dissertation). Antioch University, Ohio.

Hormann, S. (2018). Exploring resilience: In the face of trauma. *Humanistic Management Journal*, *3*(1), 91–104. 10.1007/s41463-018-0035-0

Hormann, S., & Vivian, P. (2005). Toward an understanding of traumatized organizations and how to intervene in them. *Traumatology*, *11*(3), 159–169.

Hormann, S., & Vivian, P. (2017). Intervening in organizational trauma: A tale of three organizations. *Leading and managing in the social sector* (pp. 175–189). Cham: Springer.

Hwang, P., & Lichtenthal, J. D. (2000). Anatomy of organizational crises. *Journal of Contingencies and Crisis Management*, *8*(3), 129–140.

Kahn, W. A. (2001). Holding environments at work. *The Journal of Applied Behavioral Science*, *37*(3), 260–279.

Kahn, W. A., Barton, M. A., & Fellows, S. (2013). Organizational crises and the disturbance of relational systems. *Academy of Management Review*, *38*(3), 377–396.

Kira, I. A. (2001). Taxonomy of trauma and trauma assessment. *Traumatology*, *7*(2), 73–86.

Kira, I. A., Lewandowski, L., Templin, T., Ramaswamy, V., Ozkan, B., & Mohanesh, J. (2008). Measuring cumulative trauma dose, types, and profiles using a development-based taxonomy of traumas. *Traumatology*, *14*(2), 62–87.

Maitlis, S. (2012). Posttraumatic growth: A missed opportunity for positive organizational scholarship. In K. Cameron, & G. Spreitzer (Eds.), *The Oxford handbook of positive organizational scholarship* (pp. 902–923). Oxford University Press.

Miller, J. H., & Page, S. E., (2007). *Complex adaptive systems: An introduction to computational models of social life*. Princeton, NJ: Princeton University Press.

Mitki, Y., Shani, A. B. (Rami), & Stjernberg, T. (2008). Leadership, development and learning mechanisms: System transformation as a balancing act. *Leadership & Organization Development Journal*, *29*(1), 68–84.

Mitki, Y., Shani, A. B. (Rami), & Greenbaum, B. (2019). Developing new capabilities: Longitudinal study of sociotechnical system redesign. *Journal of Change Management*, *19*(3), 167–182.

Nava, L. (2022). Rise from ashes: A dynamic framework of organizational learning and resilience in disaster response. *Business and Society Review*, *127* (S1), 299–318.

Pasmore, W. A., Winby, T., Mohrman, S. A., & Vanasse, R. (2019). Reflections: Sociotechnical systems design and organization change. *Journal of Change Management*, *19*(2), 67–85.

Roux-Dufort, C. (2007). Is crisis management (only) a management of exceptions? *Journal of Contingencies & Crisis Management*, *15*(2), 105–114.
Shani, A. B. (Rami), Grant, R., & Krishnan, R. (1992). Advanced manufacturing systems and organizational choice: A sociotechnical system approach. *California Management Review*, *34*(4), 91–111.
Tedeschi, R. G., & Calhoun, L. G. (1995). *Trauma and transformation*. Sage.
Tedeschi, R. G., & Calhoun, L. G. (1996). The posttraumatic growth inventory: Measuring the positive legacy of trauma. *Journal of Traumatic Stress*, *9*(3), 455–472. 10.1002/jts.2490090305
Tedeschi, R. G., & Calhoun, L. G. (2004). Posttraumatic growth: Conceptual foundations and empirical evidence. *Psychological Inquiry*, *15*(1), 1–18.
Trist, E. L. (1963). On sociotechnical systems. In W. A. Pasmore, & J. J. Sherwood (Eds.), *Sociotechnical systems: A sourcebook* (pp. 43–57). La Jolla, CA: University Associates.
Williams, T. A., Gruber, D. A., Sutcliffe, K. M., Shepherd, D. A., & Zhao, E. Y. (2017). Organizational response to adversity: Fusing crisis management and resilience research streams. *Academy of Management Annals*, *11*(2), 733–769.
Winter, S. G. (2003). Understanding dynamic capabilities. *Strategic Management Journal*, *24*(10), 991–995.

PART 5

PTG in the Context of Diverse Stressors

28
POSTTRAUMATIC GROWTH IN THE CONTEXT OF ILLNESS

Allison Marziliano, Anne Moyer, and Malwina Tuman

In general, trauma is an outcome of a life crisis and struggle (Menger et al., 2020). The traumatic nature of illnesses is distinct from other situations that induce trauma such as war or natural disasters, in that illnesses are located within the body and are medicalized (Kangas et al., 2002; Menger et al., 2020). Illnesses vary on a number of dimensions and thus can be experienced as more versus less traumatic. The well-known common sense model of illness specifies that the schemas, i.e., mental representations of illness that people hold, involve perceptions regarding the illness' identity (i.e., its label and its symptoms), its time course, consequences, causes and its controllability and likelihood of cure (Leventhal et al., 1980). Because people's unique schemas regarding the same illness may vary along these dimensions, there are likely to be individual differences in the extent to which illness experiences are traumatizing. Further, even within an individual, some parts of the illness could be considered traumatic while others are not.

Potentially Traumatizing Aspects of Illness

There are particular aspects of many types of physical and mental illnesses that could be potentially traumatizing. These include their life-threatening nature, their impact on quality of life, the side effects of their treatment, changes in roles, and the stigma attached to them.

Illnesses' Life-Threatening Nature

For some illnesses, a diagnosis represents an existential threat to life, as their prognosis may be poor even with treatment. For example, under an earlier version of the American Psychiatric Association's Diagnostic and Statistical Manual, DSM-IV-TR (American Psychiatric Association, 2000), individuals diagnosed with a life-threatening illness, almost by definition, could be diagnosed with posttraumatic stress disorder (PTSD), based on the criterion that a traumatic event must involve a threat to one's life or physical integrity, and one must experience fear, helplessness, or horror (Cordova, 2020). In its current version, DSM-V (American Psychiatric Association, 2013), the stipulation requiring the experience

DOI: 10.4324/9781032208688-37

of fear, helplessness, and horror has been removed and to qualify as trauma-inducing, medical incidents or conditions must involve sudden, catastrophic experiences (Shand et al., 2015). This change likely alters the types of illness connected to a formal diagnosis of PTSD. For instance, cancer that was commonly considered to involve trauma, no longer fits within these criteria, as it involves threats that unfold slowly over time, occur internally, are persistent, and relate to future fears (Cordova, 2020). Nonetheless, the life-threatening nature of some illnesses may still be interpreted as a dire, shocking, and existentially challenging notion that could be experienced as traumatizing, regardless of whether individuals experiencing them are likely to be formally diagnosed with PTSD.

Illness' Impact on Quality of Life

Some illnesses are accompanied by symptoms that are mentally or physically debilitating, or compromise quality of life, an adversity that has been viewed as potentially traumatizing. For instance, coronary artery disease brings limitations to physical functioning and concomitant mental distress (Leung et al., 2012), traumatic brain injury brings cognitive, emotional, physical, and behavioral challenges (Rogan et al., 2013), and psychosis brings fearful and destabilizing feelings (Slade et al., 2019).

Treatment-Related Side Effects

In addition to the adversity connected with the illnesses themselves, some conditions involve treatment that could be experienced as traumatizing due to the resulting side effects, discomfort, pain, or disfigurement. For instance, surgical removal of the breast as a treatment for breast cancer can create devastating alterations in body image (Soo & Sherman, 2015) and surgical treatment for prostate cancer can involve incontinence and impotence (Walsh et al., 2018), although ironically, such treatments do not involve relief from symptoms, as cancer patients may be asymptomatic when diagnosed. Similarly, pharmaceutical treatment for mental conditions such as depression may bring challenging consequences such as lowered libido (Balon, 2007).

Change in Roles

Physical and mental conditions can produce disability that may limit one's cherished professional and personal roles, which form aspects of one's core identity. The loss of a job, an occupation, or a career, can be traumatizing as can the loss of one's ability to function as one once did as a spouse, parent, family member, or friend (Catt et al., 2017).

Stigma

Some illnesses involve stigma, i.e., devaluing attributions by others, which may be a traumatizing experience. For example, lung cancer and HIV are conditions that may be viewed as behaviorally dependent and are thus particularly prone to be stigmatizing (Johnson et al., 2019). Mental illness carries a stigma as it may be erroneously linked to violent behavior (Pescosolido et al., 2019). Stigma linked to physical and mental disability can lead to marginalization and inequitable access to housing, employment, and health care (Jackson-Best & Edwards, 2018).

Illness and PTG

Over the last several decades, an ample body of research demonstrated that life-altering traumatic events, including illness and health-related trauma, can foster positive personal change such as positive shifts in self-perception, improvement in interpersonal relationships, and a deeper appreciation of life (Joseph & Linley, 2005; Park et al., 1996; Tedeschi & Calhoun, 1996; Tedeschi et al., 2018). These changes are referred to as PTG, and can occur concurrently with, or in the aftermath of trauma. Although there are many types of illnesses, only a few have been studied with respect to their traumatic nature and the potential for resulting PTG. These include cancer, which has been studied most commonly, HIV/AIDS, multiple sclerosis, myocardial infarction, rheumatoid arthritis, brain injury, stroke, diabetes, arm lymphedema, and kidney disease (Barskova & Oesterreich, 2009; Hefferon et al., 2009). Studies indicate that a sizable proportion of individuals with illness experience PTG; for example, 53–84% of women with breast cancer (Morrill et al., 2008; Sears et al., 2003), and 60–95% of cancer survivors (Nenova et al., 2013) reported PTG.

Some diseases seem particularly pertinent for studying PTG. For example, the nature, treatment, and meaning of cancer fit well with the aforementioned characteristics of trauma as it is life-threatening, treatments can involve disabling and disfiguring side effects, it carries stigma, and can compromise roles while the disease itself, depending on the success of treatment, may or may not be debilitating. Similarly, HIV/AIDS carries a stigma (Lau et al., 2018), was once more deadly (and still is in places without access to treatment), and may alter the way one negotiates romantic and sexual relationships. Illnesses of a more chronic nature such as diabetes or multiple sclerosis, while life-limiting to some extent, may be traumatic in their ongoing and pervasive requirement for monitoring, managing, and maintenance. Importantly, due to variations in the potentially traumatic nature of different illnesses, the potential for and routes to PTG may be disease-specific (Barskova & Oesterreich, 2009).

Factors Associated with PTG across Illnesses

A growing body of literature focuses on exploring factors related, either positively or negatively, to PTG across a range of different illnesses. Some of these factors are modifiable whereas others are not.

Non-Modifiable, Demographic, and Clinical Factors Related to PTG

Non-modifiable factors related to PTG include demographic characteristics, such as race, and clinical characteristics, such as severity of cancer. Younger age has consistently been associated with greater PTG in studies of patients with breast cancer (Paredes & Pereira, 2018; Tanyi et al., 2015), and prostate cancer (Tanyi et al., 2015). Another demographic factor related to higher PTG is the non-White race. Lower income (Pollard & Kennedy, 2007) and higher education (Danhauer et al., 2013), although somewhat modifiable, are also positively related to PTG.

In regard to clinical characteristics, greater PTG has been shown to be related to a longer time since diagnosis in women recently diagnosed with breast cancer (Danhauer et al., 2013), as well as longer survival in lung cancer patients (Dougall et al., 2017). In breast and prostate cancer patients, greater PTG was related to greater severity of cancer

(Tanyi et al., 2015). In other studies involving cancer patients, clinical variables such as cancer site, cancer surgery, and cancer recurrence were all unrelated to PTG (Casellas-Grau et al., 2017).

Modifiable Factors Related to PTG

The modifiable factors could be broadly categorized as mental health factors, behavior-based, religiosity/spirituality and meaning, outlook, social support, sense of control, and physical health.

Mental Health Factors

The umbrella term mental health can encompass a range of different constructs, including psychological distress, stress, posttraumatic stress, depressive or anxious symptoms, and helplessness. The relationship between PTG and psychological distress, posttraumatic stress, global stress, or illness-specific stress is varied, with some studies showing a positive relationship (Barakat et al., 2006; Pollard & Kennedy, 2007) and others showing a negative relationship (Groarke et al., 2017; Rogan et al., 2013). Further support for the variable relationship between PTG and posttraumatic stress was provided in a systematic review and meta-analysis examining these constructs in cancer patients or survivors (Marziliano et al., 2020). A similar pattern emerges regarding the relationship between PTG and depressive or anxious symptoms. A systematic review of cancer studies (Casellas-Grau et al., 2017) pointed to an inverse relationship between PTG and depressive or anxious symptoms; yet, in another work with women with breast cancer, higher anxiety was related to greater PTG (Groarke et al., 2017), and in a study of patients with coronary artery disease, higher depressive symptoms were related to greater PTG (Leung et al., 2010). In patients with inflammatory bowel disease, there was a negative association between helplessness and PTG (Hamama-Raz et al., 2021). In a meta-analysis of individuals with cancer or HIV/AIDS (Sawyer et al., 2010), PTG was related to increased positive mental health.

Potential explanations for both positive and negative relationships between PTG and mental health have been proposed. Some argue that elevated negative mental health factors such as distress or depression are a necessary initial step in causing one to re-think and re-order priorities and rebuild values that were shattered by the trauma (Janoff-Bulman, 2006). Findings of studies that have shown an inverse relationship between negative mental health outcomes and PTG (Yi & Kim, 2014) can be explained by the idea that negative mental health outcomes are so debilitating, burdensome, and mentally taxing causing PTG to diminish in their presence.

Behavior-Based Factors

Behavior-based predictors of PTG include coping and acceptance. Greater use of adaptive coping, approach-related coping, problem-focused coping, and behavioral or cognitive coping strategies was associated with greater PTG across multiple diseases, including acquired brain injury (Rogan et al., 2013), cancer (Scrignaro et al., 2011; Svetina & Nastran, 2012), spinal cord injuries (January et al., 2015), and other life-threatening illnesses (Barskova & Oesterreich, 2009). Similarly, acceptance was positively related to PTG in a sample of 200 patients with inflammatory bowel disease (Hamama-Raz et al., 2021). It is possible that a third factor is causing one to both engage in better-coping strategies and experience PTG.

Religiosity/Spirituality and Meaning

Greater spirituality or having a religion (Park et al., 2016) was related to greater PTG in patients with cancer (Casellas-Grau et al., 2017; Danhauer et al., 2013; Paredes & Pereira, 2018). By contrast, in HIV-positive men who have sex with men (Lau et al., 2018), attribution to God's will and to chance or luck were negative correlates of PTG. Meaning-making or meaning-focused coping has also been shown to be related to PTG in patients with cancer (Casellas-Grau et al., 2017; Thombre et al., 2010) or serious mental illness (Mazor et al., 2018).

Outlook

In patients with traumatic brain injury 1–5 years post-injury, those with a more positive outlook reported more frequent PTG consistent behaviors, such as showing care toward family and friends and appreciation of life (Pais-Hrit et al., 2020). PTG was also found to be positively related to hope (Casellas-Grau et al., 2017) and optimism (Casellas-Grau et al., 2017; Park et al., 2016), but negatively related to perceived burden (Zhang et al., 2019).

Social Support

Greater social support and greater social and family well-being are consistently related to greater PTG (Dougall et al., 2017), including in patients with life-threatening illnesses (Barskova & Oesterreich, 2009), coronary artery disease (Leung et al., 2010), and breast and lung cancer (Park et al., 2016), as well as long-term cancer survivors (Danhauer et al., 2013; Schroevers et al., 2010). It is possible that having the support of friends and family during a trauma such as an illness allows one to have the capacity to experience PTG.

Sense of Control

Greater PTG is associated with stronger beliefs about control of the illness or treatment-related side effects (Rogan et al., 2013).

Physical Health

Better subjective physical health (Sawyer et al., 2010) and better physical health-related quality of life (Dougall et al., 2017) have both been related to greater PTG.

Cultivating PTG after a Traumatic Experience

In addition to research focused on factors that are naturally associated with PTG, there is also literature on interventions designed to increase PTG after illness or its treatment. Tedeschi et al. (2015) describe critical issues that ought to be considered prior to implementing PTG-related interventions. First, although many people who experience traumas derive positive changes from the struggle with stressful events, PTG is not a universal or necessary outcome needed for full trauma recovery. If positive changes do occur in the aftermath of trauma, it does not imply that the negative event itself was desired in the first place, or that the trauma-related distress is lessened by the experience of growth. Furthermore, achieving PTG may take a different amount of time for different people, and for some this process takes months or even years (Calhoun & Tedeschi, 2012). PTG has been conceptualized as both an outcome and a process (Tedeschi & Calhoun, 2004) and research suggests that there is no consistent pattern of PTG that can describe the trajectory of adaptation for all, including those who experienced similar types of traumatizing events. Given the heterogeneity of psychosocial profiles with the PTG experience, and the multitude of factors related to PTG and its manifestations, interventions should be introduced with great attention to each individual's needs, and only after they have been able to fully adapt to the aftermath of the trauma (Tedeschi et al., 2015).

Cultivating PTG after Illness or Health-Related Trauma in Adult Populations

Although PTG has been extensively examined in the context of illness and health-related trauma (see Barskova & Oesterreich, 2009, for review), research examining psychosocial interventions promoting PTG in populations affected by illness and adverse health events is scarce. For example, a meta-analysis of psychosocial interventions in people who experienced hardship identified 12 randomized controlled trials examining PTG (Roepke, 2015). Notably, none of the interventions included in this quantitative synthesis was designed to promote PTG as the primary outcome, and only two were peer-reviewed studies that examined PTG specifically in the context of illness or health trauma (as opposed to similar, yet distinct constructs, such as benefit-finding, stress-related growth, or thriving).

The few intervention studies conducted with illness and health-related trauma populations that included PTG as an outcome offer promise. These interventions are widely variable and include couples-based skills training (Heinrichs et al., 2012), support groups (Ramos et al., 2018; Sherr et al., 2011), psycho-spiritual integrative therapy (Garlick et al., 2011), illness education and training in coping techniques (Sherr et al., 2011), cardiac rehabilitation programs (Chan et al., 2006), cognitive behavior therapy (Zoellner et al., 2011) and positive psychology exercises (Karagiorgou et al., 2018). These interventions have been examined most commonly with cancer populations (Garlick et al., 2011; Heinrichs et al., 2012; Pat-Horenczyk et al., 2015; Ramos et al., 2018), and less frequently with other populations, such as individuals living with HIV (Sherr et al., 2011), coronary heart disease patients (Chan et al., 2006), motor vehicle accident survivors (Zoellner et al., 2011), and survivors of brain injury (Karagiorgou et al., 2018). Due to the relative paucity of knowledge about interventions to promote PTG, it is challenging to categorize and classify these interventions by illness type, theoretical orientation, treatment type, or intervention modality, and be able to draw conclusions about what approaches work best for whom. This area manifests a gap in research and warrants further empirical examination.

Cultivating PTG after Illness or Health-Related Trauma in Pediatric Populations

The experience of severe pediatric illness can be highly traumatic for the child, parents, and other family members (Kazak et al., 2006). A systematic review examining PTG in pediatric illness identified seven studies that examined PTG in children following a medical trauma (Meyerson et al., 2011). The majority of the studies were cross-sectional, and none was an intervention study, which shows that, similar to the adult population, pediatric PTG intervention research is limited. Given that PTG has been reported by pediatric patients experiencing illness (e.g., Gunst et al., 2016), interventions facilitating PTG may offer promise for this population and represent a call for research in what has been a largely overlooked area thus far.

One explanation related to the limited work in this area is the changing definition of what constitutes trauma across different versions of the DSM. Because some of the illnesses that have been studied in relation to PTG are not considered traumatic under the current taxonomy, there may be a relative scarcity of intervention research in those areas.

The COVID-19 Pandemic as a Collective Health-Related Trauma

Extensive research has documented adverse consequences of the major global public health crisis caused by the COVID-19 pandemic, which impacts physical health and psychological functioning including insomnia, increased stress, psychological distress, posttraumatic stress symptoms, anxiety, and depression (Krishnamoorthy et al., 2020). Adverse psychological consequences of COVID-19 are predicted to last for months to years. Restoring psychological well-being and gaining a better understanding of the potential of experiencing PTG among individuals affected by COVID-19 will be an important part of the recovery from the collective trauma of the pandemic. Incorporating PTG facilitation may aid in catalyzing positive psychological change, healing, and recovery from the psychological fallout of the pandemic.

Conclusions

Several thoughts emerge from this review of the literature on PTG and illness. First, to date, the overwhelming majority of the research on PTG and illness has been in the area of cancer. It would be an important contribution to the PTG literature to include additional chronic and acute illnesses. Second, interventions focused mainly on augmenting PTG appear to be lacking and, given the association between greater PTG and several positive outcomes, increasing PTG is an area that warrants further attention. Third, more longitudinal studies evaluating PTG at multiple time points along the illness trajectory would provide a better understanding of the process associated with PTG in the context of illness. Fourth, understanding and facilitating PTG during and in the aftermath of the COVID-19 pandemic is a relatively new area ripe for research. In sum, the potential for positive changes related to illness, and specifically PTG represents a critical area of continued research.

References

American Psychiatric Association (2000). *Diagnostic and statistical manual of mental disorders* IV-TR (4th ed.). Arlington, VA: American Psychiatric Association

American Psychiatric Association (2013). *Diagnostic and statistical manual of mental disorders* (5th ed.). Arlington, VA: American Psychiatric Association.

Balon, R. (2007). Depression, antidepressants and human sexuality. *Primary Psychiatry, 14*(2), 42–44.

Barakat, L. P., Alderfer, M. A., & Kazak, A. E. (2006). Posttraumatic growth in adolescent survivors of cancer and their mothers and fathers. *Journal of Pediatric Psychology, 31*(4), 413–419. 10.1093/jpepsy/jsj058

Barskova, T., & Oesterreich, R. (2009). Post-traumatic growth in people living with a serious medical condition and its relations to physical and mental health: A systematic review. *Disability and Rehabilitation*, *31*(21), 1709–1733. 10.1080/09638280902738441

Calhoun, L. G., & Tedeschi, R. G. (2012). *Posttraumatic growth in clinical practice*. Routledge.

Casellas-Grau, A., Ochoa, C., & Ruini, C. (2017). Psychological and clinical correlates of post-traumatic growth in cancer: A systematic and critical review. *Psycho-Oncology*, *26*(12), 2007–2018. 10.1002/pon.4426

Catt, S., Starkings, R., Shilling, V., & Fallowfield, L. (2017). Patient-reported outcome measures of the impact of cancer on patients' everyday lives: A systematic review. *Journal of Cancer Survivorship*, *11*(2), 211–232. 10.1007/s11764-016-0580-1

Chan, I., Lai, J., & Wong, K. (2006). Resilience is associated with better recovery in Chinese people diagnosed with coronary heart disease. *Psychology & Health*, *21*(3), 335–349. 10.1080/14768320500215137

Cordova, M. (2020). Cancer-related posttraumatic stress disorder: Assessment and treatment considerations. *Psychiatric Times*, *37*(7). https://www.psychiatrictimes.com/view/cancer-related-posttraumatic-stress-disorder-assessment-and-treatment-considerations

Danhauer, S. C., Case, L. D., Tedeschi, R., Russell, G., Vishnevsky, T., Triplett, K., Ip, E. H., & Avis, N. E. (2013). Predictors of posttraumatic growth in women with breast cancer. *Psycho-Oncology*, *22*(12), 2676–2683. 10.1002/pon.3298

Dougall, A. L., Swanson, J., Kyutoku, Y., Belani, C. P., & Baum, A. (2017). Posttraumatic symptoms, quality of life, and survival among lung cancer patients. *Journal of Applied Biobehavioral Research*, *22*(3), 1–23. 10.1111/jabr.12065

Garlick, M., Wall, K., Corwin, D., & Koopman, C. (2011). Psycho-spiritual integrative therapy for women with primary breast cancer. *Journal of Clinical Psychology in Medical Settings*, *18*(1), 78–90. 10.1007/s10880-011-9224-9

Groarke, A., Curtis, R., Groarke, J. M., Hogan, M. J., Gibbons, A., & Kerin, M. (2017). Post-traumatic growth in breast cancer: How and when do distress and stress contribute? *Psycho-Oncology*, *26*(7), 967–974. 10.1002/pon.4243

Gunst, D. C. M., Kaatsch, P., & Goldbeck, L. (2016). Seeing the good in the bad: Which factors are associated with posttraumatic growth in long-term survivors of adolescent cancer? *Supportive Care in Cancer: Official Journal of the Multinational Association of Supportive Care in Cancer*, *24*(11), 4607–4615. 10.1007/s00520-016-3303-2

Hamama-Raz, Y., Nativ, S., & Hamama, L. (2021). Post-traumatic growth in inflammatory bowel disease patients: The role of illness cognitions and physical quality of life. *Journal of Crohn's & Colitis*, *15*(6), 1060–1067. 10.1093/ecco-jcc/jjaa247

Hefferon, K., Grealy, M., & Mutrie, N. (2009). Post-traumatic growth and life threatening physical illness: A systematic review of the qualitative literature. *British Journal of Health Psychology*, *14*(2), 343–378. 10.1348/135910708X332936

Heinrichs, N., Zimmermann, T., Huber, B., Herschbach, P., Russell, D. W., & Baucom, D. H. (2012). Cancer distress reduction with a couple-based skills training: A randomized controlled trial. *Annals of Behavioral Medicine: A Publication of the Society of Behavioral Medicine*, *43*(2), 239–252. 10.1007/s12160-011-9314-9

Jackson-Best, F., & Edwards, N. (2018). Stigma and intersectionality: A systematic review of systematic reviews across HIV/AIDS, mental illness, and physical disability. *BMC Public Health*, *18*, 919. 10.1186/s12889-018-5861-3

Janoff-Bulman, R. (2006). Schema-change perspectives on posttraumatic growth. In L. G. Calhoun, & R. G. Tedeschi (Eds.), *Handbook of post traumatic growth* (pp. 81–99). Erlbaum.

January, A. M., Zebracki, K., Chlan, K. M., & Vogel, L. C. (2015). Understanding post-traumatic growth following pediatric-onset spinal cord injury: The critical role of coping strategies for facilitating positive psychological outcomes. *Developmental Medicine and Child Neurology*, *57*(12), 1143–1149. 10.1111/dmcn.12820

Johnson, L. A., Schreier, A. M., Swanson, M., Moye, J. P., & Ridner, S. (2019). Stigma and quality of life in patients with advanced lung cancer. *Oncology Nursing Forum*, *46*(3), 318–328. 10.1188/19.ONF.318-328

Joseph, S., & Linley, P. A. (2005). Positive adjustment to threatening events: An organismic valuing theory of growth through adversity. *Review of General Psychology*, *9*(3), 262–280. 10.1037%2F1089-2680.9.3.262

Kangas, M., Henry, J. L., & Bryant, R. A. (2002). Posttraumatic stress disorder following cancer: A conceptual and empirical review. *Clinical Psychology Review*, *22*(4), 499–524. 10.1016/s0272-7358(01)00118-0

Karagiorgou, O., Evans, J. J., & Cullen, B. (2018). Post-traumatic growth in adult survivors of brain injury: A qualitative study of participants completing a pilot trial of brief positive psychotherapy. *Disability and Rehabilitation*, *40*(6), 655–659. 10.1080/09638288.2016.1274337

Kazak, A. E., Kassam-Adams, N., Schneider, S., Zelikovsky, N., Alderfer, M. A., & Rourke, M. (2006). An integrative model of pediatric medical traumatic stress. *Journal of Pediatric Psychology*, *31*(4), 343–355. 10.1093/jpepsy/jsj054

Krishnamoorthy, Y., Nagarajan, R., Saya, G. K., & Menon, V. (2020). Prevalence of psychological morbidities among general population, healthcare workers and COVID-19 patients amidst the COVID-19 pandemic: A systematic review and meta-analysis. *Psychiatry Research*, *293*, 113382. 10.1016/j.psychres.2020.113382

Lau, J. T. F., Wu, X., Wu, A. M. S., Wang, Z., & Mo, P. K. H. (2018). Relationships between illness perception and post-traumatic growth among newly diagnosed HIV-positive men who have sex with men in China. *AIDS and Behavior*, *22*, 1885–1898. 10.1007/s10461-017-1874-7

Leung, Y. W., Alter, D. A., Prior, P. L., Stewart, D. E., Irvine, J., & Grace, S. L. (2012). Posttraumatic growth in coronary artery disease outpatients: Relationship to degree of trauma and health service use. *Journal of Psychosomatic Research*, *72*(4), 293–299. 10.1016/j.jpsychores.2011.12.011

Leung, Y. W., Gravely-Witte, S., Macpherson, A., Irvine, J., Stewart, D. E., & Grace, S. L. (2010). Post-traumatic growth among cardiac outpatients: Degree comparison with other chronic illness samples and correlates. *Journal of Health Psychology*, *15*(7), 1049–1063. 10.1177/1359105309360577

Leventhal, H., Meyer, D., & Nerenz, D. (1980). The common sense model of illness danger. In S. Rachman (Ed.), *Medical psychology*, Vol. 2 (pp. 7–30). New York, NY: Pergamon Press.

Marziliano, A., Tuman, M., & Moyer, A. (2020). The relationship between post-traumatic stress and post-traumatic growth in cancer patients and survivors: A systematic review and meta-analysis. *Psycho-Oncology*, *29*(4), 604–616. 10.1002/pon.5314

Mazor, Y., Gelkopf, M., & Roe, D. (2018). Posttraumatic growth among people with serious mental illness, psychosis and posttraumatic stress symptoms. *Comprehensive Psychiatry*, *81*(6), 1–9. 10.1016/j.comppsych.2017.10.009

Menger, F., Patterson, J., OHara, J., & Sharp, L. (2020). Research priorities on post-traumatic growth: Where next for the benefit of cancer survivors? *Psycho-Oncology*, *29*(11), 1968–1970. 10.1002/pon.5490

Meyerson, D. A., Grant, K. E., Carter, J. S., & Kilmer, R. P. (2011). Posttraumatic growth among children and adolescents: A systematic review. *Clinical Psychology Review*, *31*(6), 949–964. 10.1016/j.cpr.2011.06.003

Morrill, E. F., Brewer, N. T., O'Neill, S. C., Lillie, S. E., Dees, C., Carey, L. A., & Rimer, B. K. (2008). The interaction of post-traumatic growth and post-traumatic stress symptoms in predicting depressive symptoms and quality of life. *Psychooncology*, *17*(9), 948–953. 10.1002/pon.1313

Nenova, M., DuHamel, K., Zemon, V., Rini, C., & Redd, W. H. (2013). Posttraumatic growth, social support, and social constraint in hematopoietic stem cell transplant survivors. *Psychooncology*, *22*(1), 195–202. 10.1002/pon.2073

Pais-Hrit, C., Wong, D., Gould, K. R., & Ponsford, J. (2020). Behavioural and functional correlates of post-traumatic growth following traumatic brain injury. *Neuropsychological Rehabilitation*, *30*(7), 1205–1223. 10.1080/09602011.2019.1569536

Paredes, A. C., & Pereira, M. G. (2018). Spirituality, distress and posttraumatic growth in breast cancer patients. *Journal of Religion and Health*, *57*(5), 1606–1617. 10.1007/s10943-017-0452-7

Park, C. L., Cohen, L. H., & Murch, R. L. (1996). Assessment and prediction of stress-related growth. *Journal of Personality*, *64*(1), 71–105. 10.1111/j.1467-6494.1996.tb00815.x

Park, J. H., Jung, Y. S., & Jung, Y. (2016). Factors influencing posttraumatic growth in survivors of breast cancer. *Journal of Korean Academy of Nursing*, *46*(3), 454–462. 10.4040/jkan.2016.46.3.454

Pat-Horenczyk, R., Perry, S., Hamama-Raz, Y., Ziv, Y., Schramm-Yavin, S., & Stemmer, S. M. (2015). Posttraumatic growth in breast cancer survivors: Constructive and illusory aspects. *Journal of Traumatic Stress*, *28*(3), 214–222. 10.1002/jts.22014

Pescosolido, B. A., Manago, B., & Monahan, J. (2019). Evolving public views on the likelihood of violence from people with mental illness: Stigma and its consequences. *Health Affairs (Project Hope)*, *38*(10), 1735–1743. 10.1377/hlthaff.2019.00702

Pollard, C., & Kennedy, P. (2007). A longitudinal analysis of emotional impact, coping strategies and post-traumatic psychological growth following spinal cord injury: A 10-year review. *British Journal of Health Psychology*, *12*(3), 347–362. 10.1348/135910707X197046

Ramos, C., Costa, P. A., Rudnicki, T., Marôco, A. L., Leal, I., Guimarães, R., Fougo, J. L., & Tedeschi, R. G. (2018). The effectiveness of a group intervention to facilitate posttraumatic growth among women with breast cancer. *Psycho-Oncology*, *27*(1), 258–264. 10.1002/pon.4501

Roepke, A. M. (2015). Psychosocial interventions and posttraumatic growth: A meta-analysis. *Journal of Consulting and Clinical Psychology*, *83*(1), 129–142. 10.1037/a0036872

Rogan, C., Fortune, D. G., & Prentice, G. (2013). Post-traumatic growth, illness perceptions and coping in people with acquired brain injury. *Neuropsychological Rehabilitation*, *23*(5), 639–657. 10.1080/09602011.2013.799076

Sawyer, A., Ayers, S., & Field, A. P. (2010). Posttraumatic growth and adjustment among individuals with cancer or HIV/AIDS: A meta-analysis. *Clinical Psychology Review*, *30*(4), 436–447. 10.1016/j.cpr.2010.02.004

Schroevers, M. J., Helgeson, V. S., Sanderman, R., & Ranchor, A. V. (2010). Type of social support matters for prediction of posttraumatic growth among cancer survivors. *Psycho-Oncology*, *19*(1), 46–53. 10.1002/pon.1501

Scrignaro, M., Barni, S., & Magrin, M. E. (2011). The combined contribution of social support and coping strategies in predicting post-traumatic growth: A longitudinal study on cancer patients. *Psycho-Oncology*, *20*(8), 823–831. 10.1002/pon.1782

Sears, S. R., Stanton, A. L., & Danoff-Burg, S. (2003). The yellow-brick road and the emerald city: Benefit finding, positive reappraisal coping and posttraumatic growth in women with early stage breast cancer. *Health Psychology*, *22*(5), 487–497. 10.1037/02786133.22.5.487

Shand, L. K., Brooker, J. E., Burney, S., Fletcher, J., & Ricciardelli, L. A. (2015). Symptoms of posttraumatic stress in Australian women with ovarian cancer. *Psycho-Oncology*, *24*(2), 190–196. 10.1002/pon.3627

Sherr, L., Nagra, N., Kulubya, G., Catalan, J., Clucas, C., & Harding, R. (2011). HIV infection associated post-traumatic stress disorder and post-traumatic growth—A systematic review. *Psychology, Health & Medicine*, *16*(5), 612–629. 10.1080/13548506.2011.579991

Slade, M., Rennick-Egglestone, S., Blackie, L., Llewellyn-Beardsley, J., Franklin, D., Hui, A., Thornicroft, G., McGranahan, R., Pollock, K., Priebe, S., Ramsay, A., Roe, D., & Deakin, E. (2019). Post-traumatic growth in mental health recovery: Qualitative study of narratives. *BMJ Open*, *9*(6), e029342. 10.1136/bmjopen-2019-029342

Soo, H., & Sherman, K. A. (2015). Rumination, psychological distress and post-traumatic growth in women diagnosed with breast cancer. *Psycho-Oncology*, *24*(1), 70–79. 10.1002/pon.3596

Svetina, M., & Nastran, K. (2012). Family relationships and post-traumatic growth in breast cancer patients. *Psychiatria Danubina*, *24*(3), 298–306.

Tanyi, Z., Szluha, K., Nemes, L., Kovács, S., & Bugán, A. (2015). Positive consequences of cancer: Exploring relationships among posttraumatic growth, adult attachment, and quality of life. *Tumori*, *101*(2), 223–231. 10.5301/tj.5000244

Tedeschi, R. G., & Calhoun, L. G. (1996). The posttraumatic growth inventory: Measuring the positive legacy of trauma. *Journal of Traumatic Stress*, *9*(3), 455–471. 10.1007/BF02103658

Tedeschi, R. G., & Calhoun, L. G. (2004). Posttraumatic growth: Conceptual foundations and empirical evidence. *Psychological Inquiry*, *15*(1), 1–18.

Tedeschi, R. G., Calhoun, L. G., & Groleau, J. M. (2015). Clinical applications of posttraumatic growth. In S. Joseph (Ed.), *Positive psychology in practice* (pp. 503–518). John Wiley & Sons, Ltd. 10.1002/9781118996874.ch30

Tedeschi, R. G., Shakespeare-Finch, J., Taku, K., & Calhoun, L. G. (2018). *Posttraumatic growth: Theory, research, and applications*. New York, NY: Routledge.

Thombre, A., Sherman, A. C., & Simonton, S. (2010). Posttraumatic growth among cancer patients in India. *Journal of Behavioral Medicine*, *33*(1), 15–23. 10.1007/s10865-009-9229-0

Walsh, D. M. J., Morrison, T. G., Conway, R. J., Rogers, E., Sullivan, F. J., & Groarke, A. (2018). A model to predict psychological- and health-related adjustment in men with prostate cancer: The role of post traumatic growth, physical post traumatic growth, resilience and mindfulness. *Frontiers in Psychology*, *9*, 136. 10.3389/fpsyg.2018.00136

Yi, J., & Kim, M. A. (2014). Postcancer experiences of childhood cancer survivors: How is posttraumatic stress related to posttraumatic growth? *Journal of Traumatic Stress*, *27*(4), 461–467. 10.1002/jts.21941

Zhang, C., Gao, R., Tai, J., Li, Y., Chen, S., Chen, L., Cao, X., Wang, L., Jia, M., & Li, F. (2019). The relationship between self-perceived burden and posttraumatic growth among colorectal cancer patients: The mediating effects of resilience. *BioMed Research International*, *2019*, 6840743. 10.1155/2019/6840743

Zoellner, T., Rabe, S., Karl, A., & Maercker, A. (2011). Post-traumatic growth as outcome of a cognitive-behavioural therapy trial for motor vehicle accident survivors with PTSD. *Psychology and Psychotherapy*, *84*(2), 201–213. 10.1348/147608310X520157

29

POSTTRAUMATIC GROWTH AND CARDIOVASCULAR DISEASES

Amy Ai and Beren Crim Sabuncu

Cardiovascular diseases (CVD) have a significant public health impact as the leading cause of death worldwide (Bozkurt et al., 2021; Mendis et al., 2011). It was estimated that by 2030, over 23 million people will die from CVD each year. Deaths caused by CVDs are higher in low- and middle-income countries causing over 80% of all global deaths in those countries (Mendis et al., 2011). Over the past decades, the mortality rate of CVD has declined due to improved treatments and assessments primarily in developed countries (Bozkurt et al., 2021), which signifies a rising survival rate of severe CVD conditions and/or relevant life-threatening events.

To date, epidemiological and clinical research on CVD patients has focused primarily on pathological outcomes. For example, extant studies have linked psychopathology, especially comorbid CVD and mental health problems such as depression and anxiety, with poor outcomes including mortality and poor functioning (Bozkurt et al., 2021; Daskalopoulou et al., 2016; Davidson et al, 2018; Dornelas & Sears, 2018; Lichtman et al., 2008, 2014; Meijer et al., 2011; Shen et al., 2011; Sin et al., 2015; Stoney et al., 2018; Wu & Kling, 2016). To improve the quality of disease management for CVD patients, health providers should be attentive to potential positive consequences of illness in a new era of patient-centered care.

One such consequence is posttraumatic growth (PTG), which is defined as the experience of positive change following the trauma and life-altering events that can occur in the struggle with highly challenging life crises (Calhoun & Tedeschi, 2006). Specifically, these gains may pertain to the reconstruction of one's worldviews, including the concept of self, relationships with others, life philosophies, and behavioral patterns. The concept of PTG has entered mainstream research in health and medicine (Ai et al., 2011). Life-threatening trauma, such as severe CVD, may shatter existing schemas and give rise to a subsequent alteration of perspectives and priorities in life (Linley & Joseph, 2004). Seemingly paradoxical, PTG is considered to be a desirable adaptation to adversity (Ai et al., 2011; Janoff-Bulman, 2004; Joseph & Linley, 2005). Addressing this positive outcome, which can also present as health-productive behavior patterns, may be important in managing chronic conditions, such as CVD, in medical and behavioral healthcare.

CVD is constituted of a class of diseases that involve the heart or blood vessels. The list includes heart diseases (HD) such as coronary heart disease (CHD), which can lead to

 DOI: 10.4324/9781032208688-38

angina (sudden chest pain) and myocardial infarction (MI or a heart attack), stroke, congestive heart failure (CHF), hypertensive heart disease, rheumatic heart disease, cardiomyopathy, arrhythmia (abnormal heart beats), congenital heart disease, valvular heart disease, carditis, aortic aneurysms, peripheral artery disease, thromboembolic disease, and venous thrombosis (Mendis et al., 2011). Because the concept of PTG is relevant to one's worldview changes and induced by stressful events or frightening experiences, not all types of CVD may corroborate these challenging circumstances. Accordingly, the current chapter focuses on a few severe CVD conditions, such as MI, advanced CHD, acute coronary symptoms (ACS), cardiopulmonary resuscitation (CPR) for cardiac arrest, open-heart surgeries (OHS), other HD-related procedures, and stroke, all of which might also result in positive changes in patients' lives.

The evidence for the current work was selected from a review of studies around the globe on the topic; exclusion criteria included extremely small samples, inadequate design, insufficient analytical strategies, or if the sample consisted of CVDs patients' caregivers as well as those that did not provide journal information, suggesting self-published pieces without undergoing a peer-review process as this group of literature tends to lack a sound research design.

MI

About two decades ago, Affleck's et al. (1987) study was the first to reveal that personal growth predicted lower mortality rates eight years after MI, in a very small sample. Nevertheless, since this pioneering report, there has been a paucity of studies with high-quality designs, which have investigated personal growth and its predictors in different types of CHD patients.

The earliest studies on PTG among CVD patients focused on MI. MI is diagnosed if one or more of the coronary arteries that supply the heart muscle become blocked. The *medical* event can be caused by a spasm of the artery or by atherosclerosis with acute clot formation. The event is often associated with its sudden occurrence of severe chest pain, leading to fear of death, depression, and anxiety (López-Medina et al., 2016; Meijer et al., 2011; Wu & Kling, 2016). A few decades ago MI tended to imply a life sentence because of its high mortality rate. Thus, the life-altering episode met the criteria for posttraumatic stress disorder (PTSD; Spindler & Pederson, 2005). Because it was a deadly emergency, MI has been the diagnosis that has attracted more empirical attention in its relation to PTG than other CVD conditions, including a systematic review of five studies (Hegarty et al., 2021).

One qualitative study reported PTG among 60% of patients with MI three months after discharge (Petrie et al., 1999). A few quantitative studies have documented that 65–71.2% of female MI patients experienced the positive effects of illness in Norway (Norekvål et al., 2008), Auckland, New Zealand (Petrie et al., 1999), Tel Aviv, Israel (Bluvstein et al., 2013) and the United States and United Kingdom (Sheikh, 2004), though the assessment tools varied across studies. PTG in the context of MI was shown to be positively associated with both posttraumatic stress symptoms (PTSS) and quality of life (Bluvstein et al., 2013) as well as the dimension of relationship to others and satisfaction with life (Ogińska-Bulik, 2014), as adaptive outcomes.

Other studies on MI have focused on predictors of PTG such as coping strategies, personalities, and social support (Hegarty et al., 2021). For example, personal growth was found to be associated positively with cognitive coping in the Netherlands (Costa & McCrae, 1992; Garnefski et al., 2008) and in Poland (Garnefski et al., 2001; Łosiak &

Nikiel, 2014). A similar finding on problem-focused coping was shown in Turkey (Senol-Durak & Ayvasik, 2010). PTG was further related positively to extraversion, openness-to-experience, conscientiousness, and agreeableness, but negatively to neuroticism (Javed & Dawood, 2016; Sheikh, 2004). Finally, MI patients who received more social support also reported higher growth in Pakistan and Turkey (Javed & Dawood, 2016; Senol-Durak & Ayvasik, 2010) and in Iran (Rahimi et al., 2016).

On the positive side, all five studies in the aforementioned systematic review were cross-sectional and mostly used validated instruments for growth, including PTG Inventory (PTGI by Tedeschi & Calhoun 1996), Benefit Finding Scale (BFS by Tomich & Helgeson, 2002), and Personal Growth (PG by Garnefski et al., 2001). A methodological short-come, however, lies in their cross-sectional design. Most importantly, these studies were limited by a lack of adequate controls for confounding health and medical factors. Perhaps for this reason, barely any of these publications were in high-impact medical, cardiac, or behavioral health journals, which could limit the impact of findings on cardiac health practice. Due to the inconsistent patterns of findings and the quality of the research design, no conclusion can be drawn from the five studies to inform cardiac and behavioral health interventions (Hegarty et al., 2021). Yet, this first small review in the UK offers some lessons and recommendations. The authors also underscored MI- or CHD-specific confounding variables such as time from diagnosis or event, number of MIs experienced, and medical or psychosocial intervention received (Hegarty et al., 2021). A new Greek study of 78 men, used the validated PTGI instrument (Tedeschi & Calhoun 1996), a cardiac function measure (of left ventricular ejection fraction, LVEF), and had a medical index (Maria et al., 2021). Planning, positive reinterpretation, and active coping were shown to be the strongest predictors for PTG. This study might be a small step to incentivize more PTG studies in MI patients to have a more effective influence on medical teams who save the lives of these patients.

Various Non-MI-Related HD Conditions

Because of the small number of studies and the overlapping patients in cardiac samples, the review of the next set of studies aggregates miscellaneous HD conditions, especially CHD.

CHD, also called coronary artery disease (CAD) and ischemic heart disease (IHD), is caused by the buildup of plaque, a waxy substance, inside the lining of larger coronary arteries. Similar to the design in the above five MI studies (Hegarty et al., 2021), a small-scale survey related to PTG with optimism and problem-focused coping in Pakistan (Masood & Rafique, 2013). Despite no PTG-based gender difference, men were more optimistic than women. Likewise, a cross-national study on HD patients ($N = 82$ in the UK, 28 in the US) demonstrated a positive association between extroversion and growth, but the relationship was partially moderated by problem-focused coping (Sheikh, 2004). The role of social support was unclear in this sample. However, in a large-scale cardiac outpatient survey ($N = 1237$) in Canada, social support was related to PTG, alongside positive illness perceptions, functional status, depressive symptoms, having lower income, and being younger and non-white (Leung et al., 2010).

Another report from the same group took an unusual approach to assess the link between PTG and healthcare utilization one year after discharge from hospitals (Leung et al., 2012). In addition to the large sample size ($N = 1717$), an advantage of this study was the utilization of morbidity data retrieved retrospectively from administrative reports.

After adjusting predicted risk and sociodemographic variables, greater PTG was associated with more physician visits ($p = 0.006$) and cardiac rehabilitation program enrollment ($p = 0.001$), though it was not related to urgent healthcare use. Interestingly, PTG was significantly linked with greater predicted risk of recurrent events ($p < 0.001$), but not with the actual rate of recurrent events ($p = 0.117$). Because PTG and utilization were cross-sectionally assessed, no causality can be drawn from these large-scale surveys regardless of sample sizes.

The Canadian study was published in a well-established international journal in health psychology, suggesting that the quality of design and credibility of findings were considerably better than in the above MI studies. However, one shortfall is the lack of mental health and medical indices controls. Because PTG often relates to distress (e.g., PTSS), including these factors can help explain the evident associations.

A U.S. study on CHF patients found that private religious practices, but not other faith factors pertaining to religion or spirituality (e.g., positive religious coping), predicted personal growth, whereas negative religious coping or spiritual struggle was inversely related to personal growth (Park et al., 2008). The merits of this study include a prospective design and adjusting the New York Heart Association Classification (NYHA Classification; no effect). It, nevertheless, did not control for depression as a key mental-health comorbidity confounder. Another U.S. study on CHF employed a cross-sectional design with their convenience sample, in which they collected data on perceived personal growth, symptom status, uncertainty, medical indices, and demographic characteristics (Overbaugh & Parshall, 2017). Controlling for participants' age, sex, ethnicity, disease severity, time since diagnosis, symptom burden, and uncertainty, results suggest community-residing patients with CHF report moderate personal growth. The authors noted that if they used another scale that emphasized growth through uncertainty, instead of the PTGI, they might show a stronger relationship between uncertainty and personal growth.

A single study explored PTG in adolescent survivors of CPR in Iran (Bagheri et al., 2020). CPR is an emergency lifesaving procedure performed immediately when cardiac arrest occurs (i.e., the heart stops beating). The usual cause of sudden cardiac arrest is an abnormal heart rhythm (arrhythmia) in the lower chamber of the heart (ventricle); thus, it can occur at young ages. Although a heart attack and CHD can sometimes trigger an electrical disturbance that leads to sudden cardiac arrest, the latter is not equivalent to the former. This new study found that 87.1% of survivors suffered from PTSD at the cutoff point of ≥ 33 on the Impact of Event Scale-Revised (IES-R; Weiss & Marmat, 1997). Multivariate linear regression documented a significant negative association of PTG with PTSD, and a significant positive link of PTG with time passed since CPR, and with physical disability caused by CPR. Despite large samples in the first two CHD studies in China (Zhang et al., 2018; Zhang & Song, 2018) and valuable information in the above Chinese and Iranian studies (Bagheri et al., 2020), like some aforenoted MI studies, the authors have drawn inadequate conclusions on causality and mediation based on cross-sample studies.

Stroke

Several newer projects have addressed growth after stroke. A cross-sectional survey indicated findings like those shown in CHD patients in Korea ($N = 165$; Jeong & Kim, 2019). Without referencing a control for illness conditions using medical indices, the researchers found that hope, meaning in life, and social support were positively associated with PTG.

However, in another study, social support scores were negatively but not significantly correlated with PTG at three-month post-operation (N = 65; Hu et al., 2020). Further, PTG was positively and significantly related to the stroke-related stigma associated with "internalized stigma" among patients at three-month after the medical event in China, after adjusting for functional outcomes (Hu et al., 2020). Total scores of stigma and depression scales were unrelated to total scores of PTG.

A prospective study conducted within 14 months post-stroke with a small sample (*N* = 43) in the United Kingdom (Kelly et al., 2018), documented PTG in Wave-1 (four to five months after stroke) and showed a significant increase in Wave-2 (i.e., over the next six months). This is single longitudinal evidence to support the finding linking post-trauma time with PTG in cross-sectional studies on CVD patients (Garnefski et al., 2008; Javed & Dawood, 2016; Łosiak & Nikiel, 2014; Rahimi et al., 2016; Senol-Durak & Ayvasik, 2010). Furthermore, active and denial coping and rumination in Wave-1 were shown to predict PTG in Wave-2, and younger patients reported greater growth. Acceptance coping was unrelated to PTG, whereas neither active coping nor rumination mediated the effect of social support on PTP as expected. Yet, rumination mediated the relationship between PTSS (Wave-1) and PTG (Wave-2). The small sample of this follow-up study made multivariate analysis with medical controls not possible.

A cross-sectional study conducted with a small sample (*N* = 52) recruited from a cardiovascular outpatient clinic examined the relationship between PTG, PTSD, and other trauma-related factors in cardiac outpatients (Magid et al., 2019). As the recruitment was carried out in a cardiac outpatient clinic, the participants had varying presenting cardiovascular problems including chronic cardiovascular disease or sudden cardiac events such as cardiac arrest or acute coronary syndrome. There was a significant relationship between elevated PTSD symptomology and PTG in their sample. Further, they found that there was a connection between the type of trauma exposure and PTGI factors. Specifically, past loss and abandonment experiences related to endorsement of the New Possibilities Factor of PTGI, natural disaster experiences were related to Spirituality, and witnessing trauma was predictive of Relating to Others endorsement. The study had several limitations. Their sample was a small convenience sample (*N* = 52), which limits their findings' generalizability. Further, medical indices were not included and therefore were not controlled for. Lastly, their study was cross-sectional as many others in this topic are, but longitudinal designs are necessary to observe the long-lasting effects of trauma experiences of cardiac procedures as these relate to PTG. Overall, the inconsistent findings of studies with various designs make it difficult to draw clear conclusions.

Cardiac Procedures

A few surveys have addressed PTG in patients undergoing cardiac procedures including OHS and other HD-related procedures. Although lifesaving, these procedures, especially OHS, are highly stressful (Ai et al., 2013). Two studies investigated CHD patients undergoing percutaneous coronary intervention (PCI), namely minimally invasive procedures used to open clogged coronary arteries, in China. One study of 360 individuals revealed that PTG was associated positively with attention to positive information and both purposeful and invasive rumination (using the Event Related Rumination Inventory or ERRI by Cann et al., 2011) but negatively with attention to negative information (Zhang et al., 2018).

Another report showed a high level of PTSS and a medium level of PTG in patients receiving interventional therapy (N = 337; Zhang & Song, 2018). PCI patients reported greater PTG, if they received more social support, and experienced low levels of impact of the event (as measured by the impact of event scale-R or IES-R by Weiss & Marmar, 1997) and social support moderated the role of event impact. Using PTGI (Tedeschi & Calhoun, 1996), a small-scale study found that PTG was positively related to PTSS that was, in turn, negatively associated with well-being and health-related quality of life (HRQOL) among MI survivors who received acute coronary artery bypass graft (CABG) surgery (N = 82; Bluvstein et al., 2013). PTG also moderated the relationship between PTSS and most mental health outcomes.

Recently, a survey of a large sample (*N* = 304) reported monitoring the pre-to-1-year-post OHS change in spiritual well-being as perceived by nonemergency CVD patients in the United States (Kearns et al., 2020). Only those who reported an increase of change (48.4% of the sample) also experienced PTG, in contrast to those who reported a decrease (40.8%) showing no such gains. Despite its advantage of using a longitudinal design, the study did not involve the measure of medical conditions.

Another prospective survey capitalized on mental and physical health in preoperative surveys and peri-operative medical indices from the *Society of Thoracic Surgeons* (STS) national database in studying patients undergoing non-urgent cardiac surgery (e.g., valve repair and replacement, CABG) in the United States (Ai et al., 2013). Attrition analysis showed no differences in age, cardiac indices, depression, or any faith factors between those who completed the 30-month postoperative follow-up (N = 262) and those who did not (N = 167), though the final sample (N = 262) had fewer medical comorbidities and were more likely to have a living partner. After controlling for key demographics, medical indices, and pre-OHS mental health and protective factors, preoperative positive religious/spiritual coping was found to predict growth 2.5 years later. Interestingly, none of the medical, surgical, or cardiac indices, character strengths (optimistic expectations), perceived social support, and other religious or spiritual factors in pre-OHS surveys were related to growth. With a sound design, the study was published in an influential journal of behavioral medicine and indicates the significance of adjusting critical confounders to avoid spurious associations in PTG research.

Summary and Conclusions

Overall, several dozen studies indicated a promising beginning in the area of CVD-related PTG. Most cited work used a validated measure of growth, such as PTGI (Garnefski et al., 2008; Javed & Dawood, 2016; Łosiak & Nikiel, 2014; Rahimi et al., 2016; Senol-Durak & Ayvasik, 2010). Most publications were presented in health-related professional journals, especially clinical psychology and nursing. Some studies have examined PTG with conventional CVD-related outcomes, including mental health (e.g., PTSS, depression, and illness perception), quality of life, functioning, and stress impact. As for predictors, the assessment in most studies (e.g., personality traits, coping strategies, cognitive thinking styles, and perceived social support) appears to be aligned with the need and focus within the above professions or disciplines. The information provided may thus offer some implications for the practice of the related professionals.

Nevertheless, limitations in research design are also obvious. It was wise for the MI-review author not to draw a conclusion based on five studies without a high-standard design. The same conclusion is applicable to other CVD studies.

First, the missing adequate control raises the question of whether the findings are related to a given CVD condition. Only a few studies have adjusted CVD-related medical indices.

This problem could contribute to spurious positive or negative associations in certain previous studies. For example, after adjusting for critical medical indices, mental health, and strength measures, social support did not predict either PTG or mental health in a prospective study of OHS patients (Ai et al., 2013). Although support may be generally beneficial to mental health as established in the literature, patients with poorer CAD conditions also receive more support. Thus, beyond the above suggestions, it will be critical to include medical indices used by cardiologists and physicians.

Second, only a few studies have employed prospective designs with sizable samples. Also, quite a few international studies in this area used causal language and concluded on mediation effects by merely using structural equation modeling with a cross-sectional design. These can be misleading for related professionals. Ten years ago, Maxwell et al. (2011) warned against using cross-sectional studies to test mediation and to make causal conclusions.

Third, as noted by the MI-review author, it is important to include the duration since the CVD event and the occurrence time of the event because PTG development is contingent on cognitive processing that demands time, as noted in the study on stroke (Hegarty et al., 2021). Also, unlike cancers that often become chronic conditions, CVD events tend to occur without the patients' expectations. These factors thus matter in this type of disease as acute trauma.

Finally, at the core of the deadly or disabling events of major CVD is the threat that raises an existential concern. Various theoretical and philosophical scholars in recent centuries including Kierkegaard, Sartre, and Tillich have highlighted existential concerns as a core human issue (Weems & Berman, 2012). However, such concerns may not be included in the assessment of professionals, and only two studies addressed related concepts. It should be noted that spirituality is considered a character strength rather than constrain by certain religions (Peterson & Seligman, 2004). For example, after the terrorist attack on 9/11 researchers asserted that the unprecedented catastrophe led to uncontrollable losses and existential challenges to core beliefs that stirred *uncertainty, cognitive-emotional disturbances,* and a sense of *human limitations* in collective trauma (Ai et al., 2009). To address this central concern in patients undergoing life-altering trauma, it is important to have a validated scale. Recently, Ai and colleagues (2021) published a tool book with dozens of spirituality assessments contributed by multidisciplinary scholars from four continents. These validated psychological instruments could help advance this area of PTG research.

As there is a paucity in PTG literature and further, dissymmetry across literature based on the use of medical indices and psychosocial co-occurrences, the recommendations for the field and for all related professionals are bound to be limited in scope. Future investigations should take higher standards such as prospective design, a large sample size, multivariate analysis with adequate medical and mental health controls, and attrition analysis to present solid evidence to convince medical and cardiac health providers. Researchers should also consider involving illness-related psychopathological factors, such as distress levels, illness perceptions, and anxiety. Further investigation should include illness-related psychopathological factors, such as distress levels, illness perceptions, and anxiety. Studying these factors will provide appropriate information for effective methods and timing of intervention. The use of medical indices to control for co-occurring and preexisting conditions that might affect PTG in CVD patients, the use of longitudinal designs to observe PTG experiences post-op, and the use of scales for measuring psychopathological factors are necessary for future studies examining PTG in CVD patients. Adequate control of objective medical indices will increase the opportunity for future publications and attention to cardiologists as key providers for CVD patients. From a methodological perspective, the pitfalls must be recognized to inform future advances in this important area.

Based on the studies above, it appears that certain psychosocial factors such as optimism, problem-focused coping, positive illness perceptions, attention to positive information, faith, and social support might be related to PTG in CVD patients. However, these findings remain preliminary and await more solid empirical evidence. While we cannot conclusively state that encouraging these psychosocial behaviors will result in PTG until the field addresses the discrepancies in this literature, both practitioners and patients might benefit from focusing on activities and thought processes that foster these psychosocial behaviors.

Acknowledgment

We gratefully acknowledge awards from the National Institutes of Health (R03 AG015686-01, R03 AG060212-01A1) for Amy L. Ai, PhD

References

Affleck, G., Tennen, H., Croog, S., & Levine, S. (1987). Causal attribution, perceived benefits and morbidity after a heart attack: An 8 year study. *Journal of Consulting and Clinical Psychology*, *55*(1), 29–35. 10.1037/0022-006X.55.1.29

Ai, A. L., Hall, D., Pargament, K., & Tice, T. N. (2013). Posttraumatic growth in patients who survived cardiac surgery: The predictive and mediating roles of faith-based factors. *Journal of Behavioral Medicine*, *36*(2), 186–198. 10.1007/s10865-012-9412-6

Ai, A. L., Tice, T. N., & Kelsey, C. L. (2009). Coping after 9/11: Deep interconnectedness and struggle in posttraumatic stress and growth. In M. J. Morgan (Ed.), *The impact of 9/11 on psychology and education. The day that changed everything*? New York, NY: Palgrave Macmillan. 10.1057/9780230101593_9

Ai, A. L., Tice, T. N., Lemieux, C. M., & Huang, B. (2011). Modeling the post-9/11 meaning-laden paradox: From deep connection and deep struggle to posttraumatic stress and growth. *Archive for the Psychology of Religion/Archiv Für Religionspsychologie*, *33*(2), 173–204. 10.1163/157361211X57573

Ai, A. L., Wink P., Paloutzian, P. F., & Harris, K. (Eds.) (2021). *Assessing spirituality in a diversified world*. Cham: Springer International Publishing AG.

Bagheri, S. H. S., Iranmanesh, S., Rayyani, M., Dehghan, M., Tirgari, B., & Hosseini, S. H. (2020). Post-traumatic stress and growth among CPR survivors in the southeast of Iran. *International Journal of Adolescent Medicine and Health*, *32*(3). 10.1515/ijamh-2017-0138

Bluvstein, I., Moravchick, L., Sheps, D., Schreiber, S., & Bloch, M. (2013). Posttraumatic growth, posttraumatic stress symptoms and mental health among coronary heart disease survivors. *Journal of Clinical Psychology in Medical Settings*, *20*(2), 164–172. 10.1007/s10880-012-9318-z

Bozkurt, B., Hershberger, R. E., Butler, J., Grady, K. L., Heidenreich, P. A., Isler, M. L., Kirklin, J. K., & Weintraub, W. S. (2021). ACC/AHA key data elements and definitions for heart failure: A report of the American College of Cardiology/American Heart Association task force on clinical data standards (Writing Committee to Develop Clinical Data Standards for Heart Failure). *Circulation: Cardiovascular Quality and Outcomes*, *14*(4), e000102. 10.1161/HCQ.0000000000000102

Calhoun, L. G., & Tedeschi, R. G. (2006). The foundations of posttraumatic growth: An expanded framework. In L. G. Calhoun, & R. G. Tedeschi (Eds.), *Handbook of posttraumatic growth: Research & practice* (pp. 3–23). Lawrence Erlbaum Associates Publishers.

Cann, A., Calhoun, L. G., Tedeschi, R. G., Triplett, K. N., Vishnevsky, T., & Lindstrom, C. M. (2011). Assessing posttraumatic cognitive processes: The event related rumination inventory. *Anxiety, Stress, and Coping*, *24*(2), 137–156. 10.1080/10615806.2010.529901

Costa Jr, P. T., & McCrae, R. R. (1992). Four ways five factors are basic. *Personality and Individual Differences*, *13*(6), 653–665. 10.1016/0191-8869(92)90236-I

Daskalopoulou, M., George, J., Walters, K. Osborn, D. P., Batty, G. D., Stogiannis, D., Rapsomaniki, E., Pujades-Rodriguez, M., Denaxas, S., Udumyan, R., Kivimaki, M., & Hemingway, H. (2016). Depression as a risk factor for the initial presentation of twelve cardiac, cerebrovascular, and peripheral arterial diseases: Data linkage study of 1.9 million women and men. *PLoS One*, *11*(4), e0153838–e0153838. 10.1371/journal.pone.0153838

Davidson, K. W., Alcántara, C., & Miller, G. E. (2018). Selected psychological comorbidities in coronary heart disease: Challenges and grand opportunities. *American Psychologist*, *73*(8), 1019–1030. 10.1037/amp0000239

Dornelas, E. A., & Sears, S. F. (2018). Living with heart despite recurrent challenges: Psychological care for adults with advanced cardiac disease. *The American Psychologist*, *73*(8), 1007–1018. 10.1037/amp0000318

Garnefski, N., Kraaij, V., Schroevers, M. J., & Somsen, G. A. (2008). Post-traumatic growth after a myocardial infarction: A matter of personality, psychological health, or cognitive coping? *Journal of Clinical Psychology in Medical Settings*, *15*(4), 270–277. 10.1007/s10880-008-9136-5

Garnefski, N., Kraaij, V., & Spinhoven, P. (2001). Negative life events, cognitive emotion regulation and emotional problems. *Personality and Individual Differences*, *30*(8), 1311–1327. 10.1016/S0191-8869(00)00113-6

Hegarty, G., Storey, L., Dempster, M., & Rogers, D. (2021). Correlates of post-traumatic growth following a myocardial infarction: A systematic review. *Journal of Clinical Psychology in Medical Settings*, *28*(2), 394–404. 10.1007/s10880-020-09727-3

Hu, R., Wang, X., Liu, Z., Hou, J., Liu, Y., Tu, J., Jia, M., Liu, Y., & Zhou, H. (2020). Stigma, depression, and post-traumatic growth among Chinese stroke survivors: A longitudinal study examining patterns and correlations. *Topics in Stroke Rehabilitation*, *29*(1), 16–29. 10.1080/10749357.2020.1864965

Janoff-Bulman, R. (2004). Posttraumatic growth: Three explanatory models. *Psychological Inquiry*, *15*(1), 30–34.

Javed, A., & Dawood, S. (2016). Psychosocial predictors of post-traumatic growth in patients after myocardial infarction. *Pakistan Journal of Psychological Research: PJPR*, *31*(2), 365–381.

Jeong, Y.-J., & Kim, H. S. (2019). Post-traumatic growth among stroke patients: Impact of hope, meaning in life, and social support. *Korean Journal of Adult Nursing*, *31*(6), 605–617. 10.7475/kjan.2019.31.6.605

Joseph, S., & Linley, P. A. (2005). Positive adjustment to threatening events: An organismic valuing theory of growth through adversity. *Review of General Psychology*, *9*(3), 262–280.

Kearns, N. T., Becker, J., McMinn, K., Bennett, M. M., Powers, M. B., Warren, A. M., & Edgerton, J. (2020). Increased spiritual well-being following cardiovascular surgery influences one-year perceived posttraumatic growth. *Psychology of Religion and Spirituality*, *12*(3), 288–293. 10.1037/rel0000291

Kelly, G., Morris, R., & Shetty, H. (2018). Predictors of post-traumatic growth in stroke survivors. *Disability and Rehabilitation* *40*(24), 2916–2924. 10.1080/09638288.2017.1363300

Leung, Y. W., Alter, D. A., Prior, P. L., Stewart, D. E., Irvine, J., & Grace, S. L. (2012). Posttraumatic growth in coronary artery disease outpatients: Relationship to degree of trauma and health service use. *Journal of Psychosomatic Research*, 72(4), 293–299. 10.1016/j.jpsychores.2011.12.011

Leung, Y. W., Gravely-Witte, S., Macpherson, A., Irvine, J., Stewart, D. E., & Grace, S. L. (2010). Post-traumatic growth among cardiac outpatients: Degree comparison with other chronic illness samples and correlates. *Journal of Health Psychology*, *15*(7), 1049–1063. 10.1177/1359105309360577

Lichtman, J. H., Bigger, J. T., Jr., Blumenthal, J. A., Frasure-Smith, N., Kaufmann, P. G., Lespérance, F., Mark, D. B., Sheps, D. S., Taylor, C. B., & Froelicher, E. S. (2008). Depression and coronary heart disease: Recommendations for screening, referral, and treatment: A science advisory from the American Heart Association Prevention Committee of the Council on Cardiovascular Nursing, Council on Clinical Cardiology, Council on Epidemiology and Prevention, and Interdisciplinary Council on Quality of Care and Outcomes Research: Endorsed by the American Psychiatric Association. *Circulation*, *118*(17),1768–1775. 10.1161/CIRCULATIONAHA.108.190769

Lichtman, J. H., Froelicher, E. S., Blumenthal, J. A., Carney, R. M., Doering, L. V., Frasure-Smith, N., Freedland, K. E., Jaffe, A. S., Leifheit-Limson, E. C., Sheps, D. S., Vaccarino, V/, & Wulsin, L. (2014). Depression as a risk factor for poor prognosis among patients with acute coronary syndrome: Systematic review and recommendations: A scientific statement from the American Heart Association. *Circulation*, *129*(12), 1350–1369. 10.1161/CIR.0000000000000019

Linley, P. A., & Joseph, S. (2004). Positive change following trauma and adversity: A review. *Journal of Traumatic Stress*, *17*(1), 11–21. 10.1023/B:JOTS.0000014671.27856.7e

López-Medina, I. M., Gil-García, E., Sánchez-Criado, V., & PancorboHidalgo, P. L. (2016). Patients' experiences of sexual activity following myocardial ischemia. *Clinical Nursing Research*, *25*(1), 45–66. 10.1177/1054773814534440

Łosiak, W., & Nikiel, J. (2014). Posttraumatic growth in patients after myocardial infarction: The role of cognitive coping and experience of life threat. *Health Psychology Report*, *2*(4), 256–262. 10.5114/hpr.2014.45894

Magid, K., El-Gabalawy, R., Maran, A., & Serber, E. R. (2019). An examination of the association between post-traumatic growth and stress symptomatology in cardiac outpatients. *Journal of Clinical Psychology in Medical Settings*, *26*(3), 271–281. 10.1007/s10880-018-9585-4

Maria, G. C., Christos, A. P., Theodoros, D. K., Ioannis, A. N., & Charalambos, I. K. (2021). Adjustment mechanisms in the acute phase of myocardial infarction in men. *Psychological Reports*. 10.1177/00332941211040425

Masood, S. M., & Rafique, R. (2013). Correlates of posttraumatic growth in patients diagnosed with coronary heart disease. *Pakistan Journal of Clinical Psychology*, *12*(2), 3–18.

Maxwell, S. E., Cole, D. A., & Mitchell, M. A. (2011). Bias in cross-sectional analyses of longitudinal mediation: Partial and complete mediation under an autoregressive model, *Multivariate Behavioral Research*, *46* (5), 816–841. 10.1080/00273171.2011.606716.

Meijer, A., Conradi, H. J., Bos, E. H., Thombs, B. D., van Melle, J. P., & de Jonge, P. (2011) Prognostic association of depression following myocardial infarction with mortality and cardiovascular events: A meta-analysis of 25 years of research. *General Hospital Psychiatry*, *33* (3), 203–216. 10.1016/j.genhosppsych.2011.02.007.

Mendis, S., Puska, P., Norrving, B., & World Health Organization. (2011). *Global atlas on cardiovascular disease prevention and control*. World Health Organization.

Norekvål, T. M., Moons, P., Hanestad, B. R., Nordrehaug, J. E., Wentzel-Larsen, T., & Fridlund, B. (2008). The other side of the coin: Perceived positive effects of illness in women following acute myocardial infarction. *European Journal of Cardiovascular Nursing*, *7*(1), 80–87. 10.1016/j.ejcnurse.2007.09.004

Ogińska-Bulik, N. (2014). Satisfaction with life and posttraumatic growth in persons after myocardial infarction. *Health Psychology Report*, *2*(2), 105–114. 10.5114/hpr.2014.43917

Overbaugh, K. J., & Parshall, M. B. (2017). Personal growth, symptoms, and uncertainty in community-residing adults with heart failure. *Heart & Lung*, *46*(1), 54–60. 10.1016/j.hrtlng.2016.09.002

Park, C. L., Aldwin, C. M., Fenster, J. R., & Snyder, L. B. (2008). Pathways to posttraumatic growth versus posttraumatic stress: Coping and emotional reactions following the September 11, 2001, terrorist attacks. *American Journal of Orthopsychiatry*, *78*(3), 300–312. 10.1037/a0014054.

Peterson, C., & Seligman, M. E. P. (2004). *Character strengths and virtues: A handbook and classification*. American Psychological Association; Oxford University Press.

Petrie, K. J., Buick, D. L., Weinman, J., & Booth, R. J. (1999). Positive effects of illness reported by myocardial infarction and breast cancer patients. *Journal of Psychosomatic Research*, *47*(6), 537–543. 10.1016/S0022-3999(99)00054-9

Rahimi, R., Heidarzadeh, M., & Shoaee, R. (2016). The relationship between posttraumatic growth and social support in patients with myocardial infarction. *Canadian Journal of Cardiovascular Nursing*, *26*(2), 19–24. PMID: 27382668.

Senol-Durak, E., & Ayvasik, H. B. (2010). Factors associated with posttraumatic growth among myocardial infarction patients: Perceived social support, perception of the event and coping. *Journal of Clinical Psychology in Medical Settings*, *17*(2), 150–158. 10.1007/s10880-010-9192-5

Sheikh, A. I. (2004). Posttraumatic growth in the context of heart disease. *Journal of Clinical Psychology in Medical Settings*, *11*(4), 265–273. 10.1023/B:JOCS.0000045346.76242.73

Shen, B. J., Eisenberg, S. A., Maeda, U., Farrell, K. A., Schwarz, E. R., Penedo, F. J., Bauerlein, E. J., & Mallon, S. (2011) Depression and anxiety predict decline in physical health functioning in patients with heart failure. *Annals of Behavioral Medicine: A Publication of the Society of Behavioral Medicine*, *41* (3), 373–382. 10.1007/s12160-010-9251-z

Sin, N. L., Yaffe, K., & Whooley, M. A. (2015). Depressive symptoms, cardiovascular disease severity, and functional status in older adults with coronary heart disease: The heart and soul study. *Journal of the American Geriatrics Society*, *63* (1), 8–15. 10.1111/jgs.13188

Spindler, H., & Pedersen, S. S. (2005). Posttraumatic stress disorder in the wake of heart disease: Prevalence, risk factors, and future research directions. *Psychosomatic Medicine*, *67*(5), 715–723. 10.1097/01.psy.0000174995.96183.9b. PMID: 16204429.

Stoney, C. M., Kaufmann, P. G., & Czajkowski, S. M. (2018) Cardiovascular disease: Psychological, social, and behavioral influences: Introduction to the special issue. *The American Psychologist*, *73* (8), 949–954. 10.1037/amp0000359. PMID: 30394774.

Tedeschi, R. G., & Calhoun, L. G. (1996). The posttraumatic growth inventory: Measuring the positive legacy of trauma. *Journal of Traumatic Stress*, *9*(3), 455–472. 10.1002/jts.2490090305

Tomich, P. L., & Helgeson, V. S. (2002). Five years later: A cross-sectional comparison of breast cancer survivors with healthy women. *Psycho-Oncology: Journal of the Psychological, Social and Behavioral Dimensions of Cancer*, *11*(2), 154–169. 10.1002/pon.570

Weems, C. F., & Berman, S. L. (2012). Existential anxiety. In R. Levesque (Ed.), *Encyclopedia of adolescence* (Part 5, pp. 890–895). New York, NY: Springer.

Weiss, D. S., & Marmar, C. R. (1997). The impact of event scale—Revised. In J. P. Wilson, & T. M. Keane (Eds.), *Assessing psychological trauma and PTSD* (pp. 399–411). The Guilford Press.

Wu, Q., & Kling, J. M. (2016). Depression and the risk of myocardial infarction and coronary death: A meta-analysis of prospective cohort studies. *Medicine (Baltimore)*, *95*(6), e2815. 10.1097/MD.0000000000002815

Zhang A., & Song J. (2018). Effects of social support and impact of event on posttraumatic growth of patients after percutaneous coronary intervention. *Chinese Journal of Practical Nursing*, *36*, 88–93.

Zhang, Y., Zhou, S., Liu, T., Gao, L., & Zhang, A. (2018). Effects of attention to positive and negative and rumination on post traumatic growth in patients with coronary artery disease undergoing interventional therapy. *Chinese Journal of Practical Nursing*, *36*, 1370–1375.

30

SOCIAL PERSPECTIVE TOWARD THE POSTTRAUMATIC GROWTH OF POTENTIALLY COVID-19-INFECTED INDIVIDUALS

Perceived Stigma and Social Identity

Wenjie Duan, Ye Tao, and Along He

The term perceived stigma was coined by Canadian sociologist Erving Goffman to refer to a grossly discredited attribute that turns the holder into "a tainted, discounted person" (Goffman, 1963, p. 3). Gilbert et al. (1998) perceived a stigmatized individual as someone whose social identity is derogated in a specific social context, i.e., an individual may be stigmatized because she or he belongs to a group that is devalued in a particular society (Berjot & Gillet, 2011).

Stigma is a Greek term dating back to the 17th century that refers to physical signs, such as burns or cuts, indicating that a person is being avoided because of a negative or degrading condition (Adiukwu et al., 2020). Rather than purely physical signs and demonstrations (Adiukwu et al., 2020), perceived stigma is associated with an increased rate of developing mental health problems and negatively affects the physical and mental well-being of people (Copel & Al-Mamari, 2015). Link and Phelan (2001) described stigma as the co-occurrence of labeling, stereotyping, separating, and status loss. Perceived stigma occurs when individuals exhibit significant social differences from the norm. They are labeled based on their emotional or physical symptoms or unrepresentative attributes and characteristics, thus threatening their social identity (Major & O'Brien, 2005).

Manifestations of stigma may include fear, rejection, avoidance, prejudice, and discrimination by individuals or the public against people with physical and mental health disorders (Adiukwu et al., 2020; Copel & Al-Mamari, 2015). In the public health context, perceived stigma refers to the association of an area or group of people with a particular negative characteristic of an infectious disease (Parcesepe & Cabassa, 2013). Disease-related stigma is affected by the characteristics of a disease such as its severity and infectiousness (Crandall, 1991).

With the increasing number of COVID-19 infections and fatalities, people have become afraid of coming in contact with people, places, or objects that are potentially, though not

DOI: 10.4324/9781032208688-39

necessarily, infected with the virus, thereby leading to COVID-19-related stigma (Bagcchi, 2020; Lin, 2020). To evaluate the severity of stigma perception among potentially COVID-19-infected individuals, several studies were conducted in Hubei Province, China, during the virus outbreak. To study stigma as perceived by individuals and the public, Li et al. (2021) developed a 10-item COVID-19-related stigma scale on the basis of the existing courtesy stigma scale (Liu et al., 2014) and the revised HIV stigma scale (Berger et al., 2001). This scale is comprised of two five items theory-driven subscales, namely, courtesy stigma (e.g., "Outcasts") and affiliate stigma (e.g., "Discriminated"). Results of the scale validate the good fit of its 10-item two-factor structure, with all items loading significantly on their target factors. The composite reliability and criterion-related validity of each subscale indicated their good internal consistency, reliability, and validity. The measurement invariance of the scale across gender was supported, and its psychometric properties were deemed acceptable.

Duan et al. (2021) confirmed the stability of the bi-dimensional construction through network analysis and identified "*plague*" (because the COVID-19 pandemic broke out in Wuhan/Hubei area, most people regard its residents as carriers of the plague) and "*no strong point*" (individuals of the same areas feel that people will no longer see their strong point) as the most important stigma characteristics. These findings indicate that the COVID-19 pandemic and its associated stigma potentially place individuals infected with it under double pressure, which leads to unprecedented adversity. Because perceived stigma can lead to suicidal thoughts and attempts, which can be more dangerous than COVID-19 itself (Gunawan et al., 2020), vigilance is critical.

The WHO director-general recognized the adverse consequences of this situation and stated that a significant challenge related to COVID-19 is the proliferation of rumors, fears, and stigma (World Health Organization, 2020). COVID-19-related stigma generates potentially deleterious outcomes for the affected population (Stangl et al., 2019), including delayed screening and treatment seeking, increased susceptibility to mental illness (e.g., depression, low self-efficacy, and self-esteem), and exacerbated social inequalities resulting from negative stereotypes and prejudice (e.g., arresting quarantine violators). This also resulted in a steady increase in unemployment and impeded social progress and development (Clissold et al., 2020; Logie & Turan, 2020).

Using a Social Identity Approach to Understand Posttraumatic Growth (PTG) Following the Struggle with Perceived Stigma

While stigmatized individuals may suffer from chronic stress, which can generate additional negative effects on their physical and mental health, the idea that "What doesn't kill you makes you stronger" resonates with many individuals and has been associated with a compelling cultural narrative that claims adversity as a source of strength and opportunity for PTG (Jayawickreme et al., 2020). However, only a few empirical studies have demonstrated positive changes among individuals facing COVID-19 (Cui et al., 2021; Pietrzak et al., 2021; Zhao et al., 2021).

PTG, which refers to the positive changes experienced by an individual after a crisis, manifests itself in various ways, such as increased gratitude for life, improved sense of personal power, change in priorities, and heightened feelings of presence and psychological well-being (Tedeschi & Calhoun, 2004). In some cases, an individual's perception of PTG may ultimately contribute to personality change (Jayawickreme et al., 2020). Consistent with the dynamic personality perspective, people's perceptions toward PTG may change the way they narrate their life experiences (e.g., explain past events based on their self-concept) and use their understanding and feelings of prior experiences to describe who they are and who they want to be (Pasupathi et al., 2007). This change in narrative identity may lead to personality changes that may promote greater adjustment and well-being. For instance, a great number of people have gone through a divorce, and the way they interpret and narrate such experience is critical to their perceived identity, well-being, and development and therefore predicts their health and well-being benefits (Adler et al., 2016).

In the context of the COVID-19 pandemic, the PTG dimensions that involve the social level (e.g., changes in relationships with others) of those who perceive COVID-19-related stigma may change, such as renewing self-awareness and social identity, cultivating a stronger sense of trust, and obtaining stronger social support (Ellena et al., 2021; Muldoon et al., 2019). Such consequences have also been reported in other infectious-disease-related stigma studies, such as HIV-related stigma (Logie, 2020). In their cross-sectional study, Murphy and Hevey (2013) provided evidence for the relationship between HIV-related perceived stigma and PTG. Findings from 56 males and 18 females suggested that the mode of perceived stigma transmission is associated with PTG and that a higher perceived stigma can directly or indirectly lead to higher PTG levels (Earnshaw et al., 2015). To induce PTG, adverse events must be disturbing enough to deconstruct an individual's assumptions about the world (Janoff-Bulman, 2004). In a potentially less traumatic diagnosis scenario, additional stress from a perceived stigma may make an event traumatic enough to arouse PTG (Garrido-Hernansaiz et al., 2017).

Social Identity Approach

The mechanism behind the relationship between perceived stigma and PTG can be explained by the social identity approach (Turner, 1981), which focuses on the role of group membership in developing one's self-concept and in guiding his or her feelings, thoughts, and actions in their social life (Read, 2015). An essential part of people's self-concept is perceived identification, which originates from their perception of their membership in certain groups and the affective meaning attached to such membership (Phinney, 1992). Individuals' cognition and beliefs about themselves are shaped by the interaction between their personal motivations and the surrounding environment (Tajfel, 1974; Turner, 1981). When trying to understand their environment, individuals expect to develop a positive self-concept that drives them to incorporate valuable personal and social identity characteristics into their identities (Hogg & Abrams, 1988).

Given the intersection between perceived identity and perceived stigma, an individual's group consciousness may greatly affect his or her responses when encountering negative experiences (Read, 2015). Specifically, individuals with a strong sense of social consciousness may strengthen their ties to their teams and develop behaviors that allow them to deal with the stigmatization they are facing (Steele et al., 2002). Thus, if the stigmatized individual identifies with a stigmatized group identity and tends to seek social support and use coping resources, such group identity can buffer the negative effects of discrimination on the self-esteem perceived or experienced by this individual (Read, 2015).

Perceived Social Identity as a Resource

According to the social identity approach, perceived identity can be a key psychological resource similar to a sense of social connectedness, social support, meaning, and efficacy for several reasons (Haslam et al., 2018). First, perceived identity generates a sense of social connectedness, i.e., being psychologically close to other people (Haslam et al., 2018). Numerous studies suggest the profound health implications of such awareness (Cruwys et al., 2014; Haslam et al., 2016; Saeri et al., 2017). An illustrative example of how social identity provides a sense of connectedness is the annual pilgrimage to Mecca in which more than two million Muslims take part every year during major religious festivals. In this context, the more people identify with the crowds participating in the pilgrimage, the more they feel one with their fellow pilgrims, and the more they feel supported by these pilgrims, and safer. (Alnabulsi & Drury, 2014).

Second, given that people tend to offer and receive support from those with whom they perceive as having a shared perceived identity (Haslam et al., 2004), perceived identity provides a foundation for people to benefit from multiple forms of social support and is important in buffering potentially stressful life events (Haslam et al., 2008). Similarly, in the context of international aid, the extent to which people provide social support to disaster victims heavily depends on how they identify with these victims. For example, British people are more likely to provide disaster aid in Italy when they perceive themselves as European than British (Levine & Thompson, 2004).

Third, perceived identity provides a sense of meaning, permanence, and stability that protect people from existential anxiety. For example, results of a BBC prison study show that prisoners achieved high levels of perceived identity over time, which in turn reduced their depressive symptoms (Reicher & Haslam, 2006). In line with this finding, Sani et al. (2010) found higher levels of identification and lower levels of psychiatric disorders and perceived stress among a sample of guards stationed in Italian prisons.

Fourth, shared perceived identity can provide people with a sense of control over their lives and power over their worlds (Turner, 2005). When threatened, group members attempt to restore their perceived group identity through social creation or social competition. Perceived identity actively creates a group's unique history and allows individuals to see their world from the perspective of a spectator (Drury & Reicher, 2005). This is particularly vital for people with clinical conditions (e.g., dementia, autism, and anxiety) who might otherwise succumb to feelings of helplessness and powerlessness (Clare et al., 2008; Crabtree et al., 2010) but can be motivated to "fight back" by an emerging sense of shared perceived identity. Greenaway et al. (2015) confirmed this idea in their analysis of World Values Survey data, which covered 62,000 people from 47 countries. They found that people report a stronger sense of personal control when they highly identify with their communities and countries.

Considerable evidence shows that perceived identity helps stigmatized minorities cope with perceived stigma and experienced negativity to restore their health and increase their sense of belonging, control, and agency over their lives (Haslam et al., 2021). For example, earthquake victims reported positive outcomes, including PTG that may be indicative of their successful identity restoration. These positive results are directly predicted by an individual's degree of identification with their damaged residential area and the degree to which they believe that their community is capable of overcoming challenges (Jetten et al., 2017).

Similar conclusions were documented among southern Italians who face discrimination by their northern compatriots (Latrofa et al., 2009; Mcnamara et al., 2013), immigrant groups (Jasinskaja-Lahtil, 2016), multi-ethnic groups (Giamo et al., 2012), people with body piercings (Jetten et al., 2001), obese people (Curll & Brown, 2020), and homosexuals (Cárdenas et al., 2018). Individuals are more likely to cope successfully with a perceived stigma when they can join forces with other members of their minority groups to work through their difficulties together rather than alone because by acting on their shared perceived identity, they can take advantage of the psychological resources provided by their group members (Haslam et al., 2018).

Further evidence suggests that one can have a positive experience of change despite—and sometimes because of—one's efforts to come to terms with a significant negative life event (Haslam et al., 2018). Moreover, Joseph (2011) argued that PTG involves a process of perceived identity change that "cuts to the heart of the way we exist in the world" (p. 147). Group members can provide trauma victims (e.g., Vietnam veterans or survivors of institutional abuse) with psychological and material resources (e.g., social support, a sense of purpose, and opportunities for collective self-actualization) that underpin positive forms of self-development (Haslam et al., 2018). People with acquired brain injury (ABI) can pursue a strategy of social creativity that serves as a basis for PTG (Haslam et al., 2018). Specifically, in cases where the identity of the ABI patient cannot be concealed, adjustment and growth can be facilitated by promoting positive social comparisons that may induce people to make downward social comparisons with severely injured others and avoid upward social comparisons with non-ABI patients (Jonessup et al., 2011). Such positive social comparisons may occasionally provide the basis for PTG (Haslam et al., 2018).

Perceived Stigma, Social Identity, and PTG

According to the social identity approach, individuals are motivated to recover their positive social identity when jeopardized by destructive events, e.g., low social status, stigmatization, team failure, or loss of important group relationships (Turner, 1981). Given the intersection between perceived stigma and perceived identity, an individual's perceived identification may considerably influence his or her reactions to encountering stigma. Specifically, individuals with low perceived identity may tend to distance themselves from a stigmatized group in the hope to protect themselves from the associated negative attitudes and thereby preserve their mental health and resources (Read, 2015). This strategy may manifest as a "passing" behavior, in which individuals attempt to conceal their compromised group membership by portraying themselves as individuals with multiple group memberships (Barreto et al., 2003). Conversely, individuals with high perceived identity may tend to increase their connection to a stigmatized group and develop action plans to respond or co-respond to the stigmatization they experience (Branscombe et al., 2012; Branscombe & Ellemers, 1998). Individuals who successfully cope with crises are more likely to report that they have acquired a new identity as a survivor and thus develop a strong sense of personal identity. This kind of perceived identity revival can serve as the basis for PTG (Muldoon et al., 2019).

An initial study in Hubei (Duan et al., 2021; Duan et al., 2021) revealed that the perceived identity change among potentially COVID-19-infected individuals can be a catalyst for PTG through enhanced identity meaning and group connection. One study showed that perceived identity significantly mediated the influence of perceived stigma on PTG such that greater perceived identity was associated with greater PTG regardless of perceived stigma (Duan et al., 2021). Specifically, compared with individuals with a low level of perceived stigma, those with a high level of perceived stigma greatly benefited from perceived identity enhancement, which can help them overcome discrimination and achieve

PTG. This finding provides a social perspective toward the role of perceived identity in stigmatized groups and in promoting PTG in the context of the COVID-19 epidemic, thereby highlighting the importance of improving perceived identity when treating individuals with perceived stigma.

Duan et al. (2020) identified three significantly different stigma profiles, namely, "Denier (35.98%)," "Confused moderate (48.13%)," and "Perceiver (15.89%)," that reflect low, moderate, and high levels of courtesy stigma (i.e., the perception of stigma among people who are associated with COVID-19) and affiliate stigma (i.e., internalization and psychological responses of courtesy stigma among associates). This study was conducted during the peak of the COVID-19 pandemic in China (i.e., January 31 to February 8, 2020), during which the Hubei population was living in a social atmosphere of targeting them by courtesy stigma. These residents may have internalized the socially stigmatized interpretations generated around Hubei identity, thereby leading to internal self-devaluation (Frost, 2011).

Using data collected after the lifting of restrictions in Hubei, Duan et al.'s (2021) further examination of the aforementioned profiles identified two significantly different profiles, namely, "Denier (35.77%)" and "Confused moderate (64.23%)," reflecting low and high perceived courtesy and affiliate stigma, respectively. In this study, a lower number of "Perceivers" was reported compared with the findings in the earlier study (Duan et al., 2020), whereas a greater proportion of participants were categorized as "Confused moderates." These findings suggest that along with the progression of the COVID-19 pandemic, both courtesy stigma and affiliate stigma decreased, thereby leading to PTG.

Duan et al. (2021) also examined the mediating role of perceived identity in the relationship between perceived stigma and PTG among different stigmatized groups. They found that the positive effect of courtesy stigma on PTG in the "Confused Moderate" group is partially mediated by social identity. However, in the "Denier" group, only the direct effects of courtesy stigma and affiliate stigma on PTG were significant, i.e., the mediating effect of social identity on the relationship among courtesy stigma, affiliate stigma, and PTG was not significant in the "Denier" group.

Overall, perceiving a valuable social identity or acquiring a new social identity can help stigmatized groups achieve PTG. This study offers a social perspective on the associations among courtesy stigma, affiliate stigma, social identity, and PTG in the COVID-19 context suggesting that perceived stigma should be avoided, reduced, and prevented at the time of the pandemic to prevent the emergence of more serious problems such as racial discrimination (Gronholm et al., 2021). These findings may guide policymakers and social workers in formulating practices and interventions that are widely applicable to stigmatized groups facing traumatic events.

Conclusions

This chapter provides theoretical and empirical evidence that maintaining a worthy social identity or acquiring a new one is a protective factor that can reduce perceived stigma and increase PTG in the context of collective trauma (Muldoon et al., 2019). Focusing on PTG in COVID-19-affected individuals in the "post-pandemic" era can benefit all those struggling with the virus (Tamiolaki & Kalaitzaki, 2020). Measures are required to prevent and reduce COVID-19-related stigma, enhance perceived identity, and protect people from the negative effects of the pandemic. Such measures should include increasing public awareness and providing psychological assistance to alleviate unnecessary emotional reactions, such as anxiety and panic (Bagcchi, 2020). Additionally, maintaining daily life and connection with family and friends helps people gain a sense of control and emotional support (Duan et al., 2020). Given that people tend to seek consensus, being surrounded by like-minded people and sharing their emotions can be a positive experience that may limit the threat of social distance and reduce feelings of isolation (Jaspal & Nerlich, 2020). Finally, the media, as a platform for improving public attitudes and promoting social cohesion, can be an important channel for reducing stigma (Duan et al., 2020). People should be advised to obtain scientific information from official websites, reliable television channels, and journals. Isolated people should be encouraged to share their isolation experiences online via pictures, videos, and live broadcasts (Duan et al., 2020) to promote the perceived identity of stigmatized people, protect them from internalized stigma, and facilitate their PTG (Corrigan & Watson, 2002).

References

Adiukwu, F., Bytyçi, D. G., Hayek, S. E., Gonzalez-Diaz, J. M., Larnaout, A., Grandinetti, P., Nofal, M., Pereira-Sanchez, V., Ransing, R., & Shalbafan, M. (2020). Global perspective and ways to combat stigma associated with COVID-19. *Indian Journal of Psychological Medicine*, *42*(6), 569–574. 10.1177/0253717620964932

Adler, J. M., Lodi-Smith, J., Philippe, F. L., & Houle, I. (2016). The incremental validity of narrative identity in predicting well-being: A review of the field and recommendations for the future. *Personality Social Psychology Review*, *20*(2), 142–175. 10.1177/1088868315585068

Alnabulsi, H., & Drury, J. (2014). Social identification moderates the effect of crowd density on safety at the Hajj. *Proceedings of the National Academy of Sciences*, *111*(25), 9091–9096. 10.1073/pnas.1404953111/-/DCSupplemental

Bagcchi, S. (2020). Stigma during the COVID-19 pandemic. *Lancet Infectious Diseases*, *20*(7), 782. 10.1016/S1473-3099(20)30498-9

Barreto, M., Spears, R., Ellemers, N., & Shahinper, K. (2003). Who wants to know? The effect of audience on identity expression among minority group members. *British Journal of Social Psychology*, *42*(2), 299–318. 10.1348/014466603322127265

Berger, B. E., Ferrans, C. E., & Lashley, F. R. (2001). Measuring stigma in people with HIV: Psychometric assessment of the HIV stigma scale. *Research in Nursing Health*, *24*(6), 518–529. 10.1002/nur.10011

Berjot, S., & Gillet, N. (2011). Stress and coping with discrimination and stigmatization. *Frontiers in Psychology*, *2*(33). 10.3389/fpsyg.2011.00033

Branscombe, N. R., Fernández, S., Gómez, A., & Cronin, T. (2012). Moving toward or away from a group identity: Different strategies for coping with pervasive discrimination. In S. A. Haslam (Ed.), *The social cure: Identity, health and well-being* (pp. 115–131). New York, NY: Psychology Press.

Branscombe, N. R., & Ellemers, N. (1998). Coping with group-based discrimination: Individualistic versus group-level strategies. *Prejudice: The target's perspective* (pp. 243–266), Academic Press. 10.1016/B978-012679130-3/50046-6

Cárdenas, M., Barrientos, J., Meyer, I., Gómez, F., Guzmán, M., & Bahamondes, J. (2018). Direct and indirect effects of perceived stigma on posttraumatic growth in gay men and lesbian women in Chile. *Journal of Traumatic Stress*, *31*(1), 5–13. 10.1002/jts.22256

Clare, L., Rowlands, J. M., & Quin, R. (2008). Collective strength: The impact of developing a shared social identity in early-stage dementia. *Dementia*, *7*(1), 9–30. 10.1177/1471301207085365

Clissold, E., Nylander, D., Watson, C., & Ventriglio, A. (2020). Pandemics and prejudice. *International Journal of Social Psychiatry*, *66*(5), 421–423. 10.1177/0020764020937873

Copel, L. C., & Al-Mamari, K. (2015). Stigma in mental health: A concept analysis. [Paper presentation]. 43rd Biennial Convention, Las Vegas, Nevada, USA. http://hdl.handle.net/10755/603232

Corrigan, P. W., & Watson, A. C. (2002). The paradox of self-stigma and mental illness. *Clinical Psychology: Science Practice*, *9*(1), 35. 10.1093/clipsy.9.1.35

Crabtree, J. W., Haslam, S. A., Postmes, T., & Haslam, C. (2010). Mental health support groups, stigma, and self-esteem: Positive and negative implications of group identification. *Journal of Social Issues*, *66*(3), 553–569. 10.1111/j.1540-4560.2010.01662.x

Crandall, C. S. (1991). Multiple stigma and AIDS: Illness stigma and attitudes toward homosexuals and IV drug users in AIDS-related stigmatization. *Journal of Community Applied Social Psychology*, *1*(2), 165–172. 10.1002/casp.2450010210

Cruwys, T., Haslam, S. A., Dingle, G. A., Haslam, C., & Jetten, J. (2014). Depression and social identity: An integrative review. *Personality Social Psychology Review*, *18*(3), 215–238. 10.1177/1088868314523839

Cui, P. P., Wang, P. P., Wang, K., Ping, Z., Wang, P., & Chen, C. (2021). Post-traumatic growth and influencing factors among frontline nurses fighting against COVID-19. *Occupational and Environmental Medicine*, *78*(2), 129–135. 10.1136/oemed-2020-106540

Curll, S. L., & Brown, P. M. (2020). Weight stigma and psychological distress: A moderated mediation model of social identification and internalised bias. *Body Image*, *35*, 207–216. 10.1016/j.bodyim.2020.09.006

Drury, J., & Reicher, S. (2005). Explaining enduring empowerment: A comparative study of collective action and psychological outcomes. *European Journal of Social Psychology*, *35*(1), 35–58. 10.1002/ejsp.231

Duan, W., Bu, H., & Chen, Z. (2020). COVID-19-related stigma profiles and risk factors among people who are at high risk of contagion. *Social Science & Medicine*, *266*, 113425. 10.1016/j.socscimed.2020.113425

Duan, W., He, A., & Bu, H. (2021). Social identity and post-traumatic growth in different COVID-19-related stigma groups (under review). School of Social and Public Administration, East China University of Science and Technology

Duan, W., Tao, Y., & Zhang, X. J. (2021). Perceived stigma and post-traumatic growth among potentially COVID-19-infected individuals inside and outside Wuhan: The mediator role of identity (under review). School of Social and Public Administration, East China University of Science and Technology

Duan, W., Wang, J., & Wang, Z. (2021). The network analysis of a brief measure of Perceived Courtesy and Affiliate Stigma on COVID-19 (under review). School of Social and Public Administration, East China University of Science and Technology

Earnshaw, V. A., Bogart, L. M., Dovidio, J. F., & Williams, D. R. (2015). Stigma and racial/ethnic HIV disparities: Moving toward resilience. *Stigma and Health*, *1*(*S*), 60–74. 10.1037/2376-6972.1.S.60

Ellena, A. M., Aresi, G., Marta, E., & Pozzi, M. (2021). Post-traumatic growth dimensions differently mediate the relationship between national identity and interpersonal trust among young adults: A study on COVID-19 crisis in Italy. *Frontiers in Psychology*, *11*, 576610. 10.3389/fpsyg.2020.576610

Frost, D. M. (2011). Social stigma and its consequences for the socially stigmatized. *Social Personality Psychology Compass*, *5*(11), 824–839. 10.1111/j.1751-9004.2011.00394.x

Garrido-Hernansaiz, H., Murphy, P. J., & Alonso-Tapia, J. (2017). Predictors of resilience and posttraumatic growth among people living with HIV: A longitudinal study. *AIDS and Behavior*, *21*(11), 3260–3270. 10.1007/s10461-017-1870-y

Giamo, L. S., Schmitt, M. T., & Outten, H. R. (2012). Perceived discrimination, group identification, and life satisfaction among multiracial people: A test of the rejection-identification model. *Cultural Diversity Ethnic Minority Psychology*, *18*(4), 319–328. 10.1037/a0029729

Gilbert, D. T., Fiske, S. T., & Lindzey, G. (1998). *The handbook of social psychology*. Oxford University Press.

Goffman, E. (1963). *Stigma: Notes on the management of spoiled identity, social theory*. New York, NY: Simon & Schuster.

Greenaway, K. H., Haslam, S. A., Cruwys, T., Branscombe, N. R., Ysseldyk, R., & Heldreth, C. (2015). From "we" to "me": Group identification enhances perceived personal control with consequences for health and well-being. *Journal of Personality Social Psychology*, *109*(1), 53–74. 10.1037/pspi0000019

Gronholm, P., Nosé, M., Van Brakel, W., Eaton, J., Ebenso, B., Fiekert, K., Hanna, F., Milenova, M., Sunkel, C., Barbui, C., & Thornicroft, G. (2021). Reducing stigma and discrimination associated with COVID-19: Early stage pandemic rapid review and practical recommendations. *Epidemiology and Psychiatric Sciences*, *30*(e15), 1–10. 10.1017/S2045796021000056

Gunawan, J., Aungsuroch, Y., & Marzilli, C. (2020). 'New Normal'in Covid-19 era: A nursing perspective from Thailand. *Journal of the American Medical Directors Association*, *21*(10), 1514–1515. 10.1016/j.jamda.2020.07.021

Haslam, C., Cruwys, T., Haslam, S. A., Dingle, G., & Chang, M. X.-L. (2016). Groups 4 health: Evidence that a social-identity intervention that builds and strengthens social group membership improves mental health. *Journal of Affective Disorders*, *194*, 188–195. 10.1016/j.jad.2016.01.010

Haslam, C., Haslam, S. A., Jetten, J., Cruwys, T., & Steffens, N. K. (2021). Life change, social identity, and health. *Annual Review of Psychology*, *72*, 635–661. 10.1146/annurev-psych-06012 0-111721

Haslam, C., Holme, A., Haslam, S. A., Iyer, A., Jetten, J., & Williams, W. H. (2008). Maintaining group memberships: Social identity continuity predicts well-being after stroke. *Neuropsychological Rehabilitation*, *18*(5-6), 671–691. 10.1080/09602010701643449

Haslam, C., Jetten, J., Cruwys, T., Dingle, G. A., & Haslam, S. A. (2018). *The new psychology of health: Unlocking the social cure*. London: Routledge.

Haslam, S. A., Jetten, J., O'Brien, A., & Jacobs, E. (2004). Social identity, social influence and reactions to potentially stressful tasks: Support for the self-categorization model of stress. *Stress Health: Journal of the International Society for the Investigation of Stress*, *20*(1), 3–9. 10.1002/smi.995

Hogg, M. A., & Abrams, D. (1988). Comments on the motivational status of self-esteem in social identity and intergroup discrimination. *European Journal of Social Psychology*, *18*(4), 317–334. 10.1002/ejsp.2420180403

Janoff-Bulman, R. (2004). Posttraumatic growth: Three explanatory models. *Psychological Inquiry*, 15(1), 30–34.

Jasinskaja-Lahtil. (2016). Perceived discrimination, social support networks, and psychological well-being among three immigrant groups. *Journal of Cross-Cultural Psychology*, *37*(3), 293–311. 10.1177/0022022106286925

Jaspal, R., & Nerlich, B. (2020). Social representations, identity threat, and coping amid COVID-19. *Psychological Trauma: Theory, Research, Practice, Policy*, *12*(S1), S249. 10.1037/tra0000773

Jayawickreme, E., Infurna, F. J., Alajak, K., Blackie, L., & Zonneveld, R. (2020). Post-traumatic growth as positive personality change: Challenges, opportunities and recommendations. *Journal of Personality*, *89*(1), 145–165. 10.1111/jopy.12591

Jetten, J., Branscombe, N. R., Schmitt, M. T., & Spears, R. (2001). Rebels with a cause: Group identification as a response to perceived discrimination from the mainstream. *Personality & Social Psychology Bulletin*, 27(9), 1204–1213. 10.1177/0146167201279012

Jetten, J., Haslam, S. A., Cruwys, T., Greenaway, K. H., Haslam, C., & Steffens, N. K. (2017). Advancing the social identity approach to health and well-being: Progressing the social cure research agenda. *European Journal of Social Psychology*, *47*(7), 789–802. 10.1002/ejsp.2333

Jonessup, J. M., Haslamsupa, A., Jettensupa, J., Williamssupa, H., Morrissupc, R., & Saroyansupa, S. (2011). That which doesn't kill us can make us stronger (and more satisfied with life): The contribution of personal and social changes to well-being after acquired brain injury. *Psychology Health*, *26*(3), 353–369. 10.1080/08870440903440699

Joseph, S. (2011). *What doesn't kill us: The new psychology of posttraumatic growth*. New York, NY: Basic Books.

Latrofa, M., Vaes, J., Pastore, M., & Ca Dinu, M. (2009). "United we stand, divided we fall"! The protective function of self-stereotyping for stigmatised members' psychological well-being. *Applied Psychology*, *58*(1), 84–104. 10.1111/j.1464-0597.2008.00383.x

Levine, M., & Thompson, K. (2004). Identity, place, and bystander intervention: Social categories and helping after natural disasters. *The Journal of Social Psychology*, *144*(3), 229–245. 10.3200/SOCP.144.3.229-245

Li, T., Bu, H., & Duan, W. (2021). A brief measure of perceived courtesy and affiliate stigma on COVID-19: A study with a sample from China. *Personality and Individual Differences*, *180*, 110993. 10.1016/j.paid.2021.110993

Lin, C. Y. (2020). Social reaction toward the 2019 novel coronavirus (COVID-19). *Social Health Behavior*, *3*(1), 1–2. 10.4103/SHB.SHB_11_20
Link, B. G., & Phelan, J. C. (2001). Conceptualizing stigma. *Annual Review of Sociology*, *27*(1), 363–385. 10.1146/annurev.soc.27.1.363
Liu, H., Xu, Y., Sun, Y., & Dumenci, L. (2014). Measuring HIV stigma at the family level: Psychometric assessment of the Chinese Courtesy Stigma Scales (CCSSs). *PLoS One*, *9*(3), e92855. 10.1371/journal.pone.0092855
Logie, C. (2020). Lessons learned from HIV can inform our approach to COVID-19 stigma. *Journal of the International AIDS Society*, *23*(5), e25504. 10.1002/jia2.25504
Logie, C. H., & Turan, J. M. (2020). How do we balance tensions between COVID-19 public health responses and stigma mitigation? Learning from HIV research. *AIDS Behavior*, *24*(7), 2003–2006. 10.1007/s10461-020-02856-8
Major, B., & O'Brien, L. T. (2005). The social psychology of stigma. *Annual Review of Psychology*, *56*, 393–421. 10.1146/annurev.psych.56.091103.070137
Mcnamara, N., Stevenson, C., & Muldoon, O. T. (2013). Community identity as resource and context: A mixed method investigation of coping and collective action in a disadvantaged community. *European Journal of Social Psychology*, *43*(5), 393–403. 10.1002/ejsp.1953
Muldoon, O., Haslam, S., Haslam, C., Cruwys, T., Kearns, M., & Jetten, J. (2019). The social psychology of responses to trauma: Social identity pathways associated with divergent traumatic responses. *European Review of Social Psychology*, *30*(1), 311–348. 10.1080/10463283.2020.1711628
Murphy, P. J., & Hevey, D. (2013). The relationship between internalised HIV-related stigma and posttraumatic growth. *AIDS and Behavior*, *17*(5), 1809–1818. 10.1007/s10461-013-0482-4
Parcesepe, A. M., & Cabassa, L. J. (2013). Public stigma of mental illness in the United States: A systematic literature review. *Administration and Policy in Mental Health and Mental Health Services Research*, *40*(5), 384–399. 10.1007/s10488-012-0430-z
Pasupathi, M., Mansour, E., & Brubaker, J. R. (2007). Developing a life story: Constructing relations between self and experience in autobiographical narratives. *Human Development*, *50*(2–3), 85–110. 10.1159/000100939
Phinney, J. S. (1992). The multigroup ethnic identity measure: A new scale for use with diverse groups. *Journal of Adolescent Research*, 7(2), 156–176. 10.1177/074355489272003
Pietrzak, R. H., Tsai, J., & Southwick, S. M. (2021). Association of symptoms of posttraumatic stress disorder with posttraumatic psychological growth among US veterans during the COVID-19 Pandemic. *JAMA Network Open*, *4*(4), e214972. 10.1001/jamanetworkopen.2021.4972
Read, S. A. (2015). Dilemmas of stigma, support seeking, and identity performance in physical disability: A social identity approach. *University of Exeter* (1780277513). http://hdl.handle.net/10871/18844
Reicher, S., & Haslam, S. A. (2006). Rethinking the psychology of tyranny: The BBC prison study. *British Journal of Social Psychology*, *45*(1), 1–40. 10.1348/014466605X48998
Saeri, A. K., Cruwys, T., Barlow, F. K., Stronge, S., & Sibley, C. G. (2017). Social connectedness improves public mental health: Investigating bidirectional relationships in the New Zealand attitudes and values survey. *Australian New Zealand Journal of Psychiatry*, *52*(4), 365–374. 10.1177/0004867417723990
Sani, F., Elena, M. M., Scrignaro, M., & McCollum, R. (2010). In-group identification mediates the effects of subjective in-group status on mental health. *British Journal of Social Psychology*, *49*(4), 883–893. 10.1348/014466610X517414
Stangl, A. L., Earnshaw, V. A., Logie, C. H., van Brakel, W., Simbayi, L. C., Barré, I. & Dovidio, J. F. (2019). The health stigma and discrimination framework: A global, crosscutting framework to inform research, intervention development, and policy on health-related stigmas. *BMC Medicine*, *17*(1), 1–13. 10.1186/s12916-019-1271-3
Steele, C. M., Spencer, S. J., & Aronson, J. (2002). Contending with group image: The psychology of stereotype and social identity threat. In M. P. Zanna (Ed.), *Advances in experimental social psychology*, *34* (379-440). Academic Press. 10.1016/S0065-2601(02)80009-0
Tajfel, H. (1974). Social identity and intergroup behaviour. *Social Science Information*, *13*(2), 65–93. 10.1177/0272431608325418
Tamiolaki, A., & Kalaitzaki, A. E. (2020). "That which does not kill us, makes us stronger": COVID-19 and posttraumatic growth. *Psychiatry Research*, *289*, 113044. 10.1016/j.psychres.2020.113044

Tedeschi, R. G., & Calhoun, L. G. (2004). Target article: Posttraumatic growth: Conceptual foundations and empirical evidence". *Psychological Inquiry*, *15*(1), 1–18. 10.1207/s15327965pli1501_01
Turner, J. C. (1981). Towards a cognitive redefinition of the social group. *Current Psychology of Cognition*, *1*(2), 93–118. 10.1136/bmj.2.5808.244
Turner, J. C. (2005). Explaining the nature of power: A three-process theory. *European Journal of Social Psychology*, *35*(1), 1–22. 10.1002/ejsp.244
World Health Organization. (2020). International Federation of Red Cross and Red Crescent Societies, United Nations Children's Fund. *Social stigma associated with COVID-19*. Geneva: World Health Organization, 2020 [cited 2020 Mar 28]. Available from: https://www.who.int/docs/default-source/coronaviruse/covid19-stigma-guide.pdf?sfvrsn=226180f4_2
Zhao, Q., Sun, X., Xie, F., Chen, B., Wan, L., Wang, L., Hu, L., & Dai, Q. (2021). Impacts of COVID-19 on psychological wellbeing. *International Journal of Clinical and Health Psychology*, *21*(3), 1–13. 10.1016/j.ijchp.2021.100252

31

POSTTRAUMATIC GROWTH EXPERIENCES AMONG PEOPLE LIVING WITH HIV

India Amos

Human Immunodeficiency Virus (HIV) and Acquired Immune Deficiency Syndrome (AIDS)

Human bodies contain white blood cells known as CD4 cells, which are central to responding to infections in the body; thus, a CD4 cell count offers an indication of the health of a person's immune system with a count between 500 and 1500 being indicative of a robust immune system. In the event of HIV acquisition, CD4 cells in the body become a target and are used as a host for HIV to replicate itself. Over time and without medication, a person's CD4 cell count is reduced significantly as a result of HIV, thus substantially weakening the body's defense against infection. Consequently, it becomes more difficult for the immune system to respond effectively to illness, and therefore, the likelihood of developing certain infections that can cause serious illness is increased. A CD4 cell count of below 200 signals a severely compromised immune system. If someone living with HIV becomes seriously ill and develops one or more opportunistic infections or diseases, they may be given a diagnosis of AIDS; this can be considered the most advanced stage of HIV and is most likely to develop in individuals whose HIV has not been effectively treated over a period of years.

While at present, there is no cure for HIV, effective testing and treatment can mean that a person living with HIV will never be diagnosed with an AIDS-related infection. However, due to the challenges of sustaining lifelong treatment facing millions of people living with HIV globally, a cure is irrefutably necessary (Ismail et al., 2021). The progression of HIV can be stopped through a daily prescription of antiretroviral therapy (ART) or what used to be known as highly active antiretroviral therapy (HAART). ART prevents the replication of HIV in the body and therefore helps repair and support the immune system to effectively respond to illness. The treatment works to reduce the amount of HIV that can be measured in the blood, known as viral load. Over time, in response to ART, viral load can be reduced to undetectable levels, and CD4 cells can increase and subsequently strengthen the immune system (Eisinger et al., 2019).

It has been estimated that at the end of 2020, 37.7 million people across the world were living with HIV, with reports of up to a million people dying from HIV-related causes and

DOI: 10.4324/9781032208688-40

1.5 million people acquiring HIV in that same year (World Health Organisation, 2021). The normalization of HIV via biomedicalization has resulted in a changing narrative, moving into "the age of treatment"' (Moyer, 2015), and in 2020, 28.2 million people with HIV (75%) were accessing ART globally (UNAIDS). However, "too many people with HIV or at risk of HIV still do not have access to prevention, care, and treatment" (HIV, n.d.), and with no cure available for HIV infection, it continues to be a serious global public health concern.

The course of HIV can be unpredictable (Breet et al., 2014) with adverse side effects from the pharmacological treatment and the combination of ART regimens, including gastrointestinal effects, fatigue, skin rash, and headache (Holtzman et al., 2013; Montessori et al., 2004), all of which affect a person's quality of life. Though there have been significant improvements in the reduction of severe side effects from first-line HIV drugs, fear of medication-related side effects is still a leading psychosocial barrier to commencing HIV treatment (Lessard et al., 2018).

It is argued that viral suppression should not be considered the ultimate treatment goal (Lazarus et al., 2016). In addition to the 90-90-90 targets set by the Joint United Nations Programme on HIV/AIDS (UNAIDS), i.e., that 90% of those living with HIV know their status, 90% of those diagnosed with HIV receive ART, and 90% of people in treatment be virally suppressed, it has been argued that a 'fourth 90' be added that emphasizes the equal importance of health-related quality of life for people living with HIV (Lazarus et al., 2016). While the prevention of new HIV infections remains the central focus, it has been argued that the social, psychological, spiritual, and environmental health of people living with HIV is left largely unaddressed (Bourne et al., 2022).

Living with HIV: Trauma and Related Stigma

"I want you all to see what this disease looks like. It looks like me and it looks like you. The first letter in HIV stands for human and I want you all to never forget that" (Falchuk & Our Lady, 2019).

Clinically, trauma is defined as experiencing, viewing, or being made aware of actual or threatened death, serious bodily injury, sexual violence, or other threats to personal integrity and safety (American Psychiatric Association, 2013), potentially leading to posttraumatic stress disorder (PTSD). Being diagnosed with HIV can be considered as a criterion A trauma for a PTSD diagnosis, i.e., exposure to a life-threatening traumatic situation. Global estimates of the prevalence of PTSD among people living with HIV is 28%, far exceeding that of the general population estimate of 3.9%. Consequently, the prevalence of PTSD among people living with HIV worldwide is likely to be higher than reported due to the lack of research in low- and middle-income countries (LMIC; Tang et al., 2020).

Calhoun and Tedeschi (1999) broadened the clinical definition of trauma, to describe events that are "seismic ... shaking or shattering foundations" (p. 16), meaning that a traumatic event is subjectively experienced as life-altering because of its stressful and challenging nature. For many, being diagnosed with HIV provokes a fundamental transformation in the physical, emotional, social, and spiritual aspects of life (Peltzer et al., 2016; Sherr et al., 2011). Stressors associated with living with HIV are well documented (Sanjuán et al., 2013) and highlight the exceptionality of HIV when compared to other life-threatening illnesses. While a diagnosis of cancer may also meet criterion A trauma for a

PTSD diagnosis, fewer people with cancer present with PTSD. For example, cancer diagnosis-related PTSD was documented in 6%–15% of patients (Abbey et al., 2015) compared to 30% of women living with HIV (Machtinger et al., 2012) probably due to the difference between the socio-cultural connotation of living with HIV (Neigh et al., 2016).

HIV can be felt like a social more than a medical diagnosis due to the negative judgment and stigmatizing responses, which have been cited as the most challenging aspect of living with HIV since the start of the epidemic in the mid to late 1970s (Walker, 2019). HIV-related stigma is defined as "negative beliefs, feelings and attitudes towards people living with HIV, groups associated with people living with HIV and other key populations at higher risk of HIV infection" (UNAIDS, 2020, p. 7). People living with HIV are aware that their HIV status is a "socially devalued attribute that renders them vulnerable to prejudice and discrimination" (Chaudoir et al., 2012, p. 2383), and an overwhelming majority of people living with HIV report experiencing discrimination or social rejection (Nachega et al., 2012). Frequent misunderstandings and inaccurate beliefs can drive HIV-related stigma (Berman et al., 2021) via mechanisms of anticipated, enacted, and internalized stigma (Earnshaw & Chaudoir, 2009), and media portrayals of individuals with HIV are reported to further compound a public narrative of fear (Fife, 2005).

HIV-related stigma is considered a layered experience, as a disproportionate number of people living with, or at the highest risk of acquiring HIV, are members of multiple stigmatized groups including sexual, racial, ethnic, and gender minorities, such as gay men, female sex workers, men who have sex with men, transgender women, and people who inject drugs (Stall & Mills, 2006). Correlates of the increased risk of contracting HIV for minority groups are structural and psychosocial factors including poverty and racism (Dale et al., 2021), hence problematizing the notion of "post" trauma (Ginwright, 2015; Ortega-Williams et al., 2021) and calling attention to the intersectional oppressions that further contribute to the psychological burden of living with HIV (Watkins-Hays, 2014).

Due to the advancements in HIV prevention and treatment, the prognosis and life expectancy for people diagnosed with HIV in the global north have dramatically changed. Yet, HIV-related stigma continues to have a significant and detrimental impact on a variety of health-related outcomes (Rueda et al., 2016) including stress responses (Link & Phelan, 2006), higher rates of depression (Meyer, 2003), lower levels of medication adherence (Katz et al., 2013), and reduced health and social care services utilization (Rice et al., 2017). Moreover, the distress felt because of HIV-related stigma has been found to affect the viral load, where high levels of stress were associated with a lower CD4 count, indicating an accelerated HIV progression because of stigma (Weinstein & Li, 2016).

The normalization of HIV, resulting from biomedicalization, has shifted the HIV care paradigm dramatically, and global health policy now refers to HIV as a manageable long-term health condition (McGrath et al., 2014). For example, in the United Kingdom, people diagnosed with HIV are encouraged to begin ART immediately (Lundgren et al., 2015). Someone diagnosed with HIV whose initial response to ART is good and acts to reduce their viral load to an undetectable level within the first year of starting treatment can expect to live equal to, if not longer than, a person in the general population (May et al., 2014). In lower middle-income countries, where the majority of people with HIV live, low education, socioeconomic factors, and limited access to healthcare prevent reaching the target of 90% of people living with HIV being on ART (Ismail et al., 2021). Therefore, the transferability of such life-expectancy research cannot be generalized to places where access to ART is limited.

Whilst this serves to reinforce that HIV is a disease embedded in social and economic inequality (Pellowski et al., 2013), the biomedical discourse has been largely supported by healthcare professionals, activists, and patient groups alike, as it is seen to encourage the uptake of ART and serves to reduce HIV-related stigma. However, this shift in the paradigm of HIV care has also been viewed as potentially undermining the continued social and psychological effects of living with HIV (Moyer & Hardon, 2014). Given reports of the gap between the normalized narrative of HIV medicine, policy, and practice, and the lived experience of HIV, where "'normal' conditions outside the clinic continue as before" (Moyer & Hardon, 2014, p. 264), research has consequently questioned the capacity of people living with HIV, irrespective of their access to ART, to enact the normalcy that such optimistic developments in HIV science promote (Mazanderani & Paparini, 2015).

Living with HIV and Psychological Growth

The shifting paradigm of HIV care in the global north has also had a significant influence on shifting the focus of HIV research away from an underlying assumption that people living with HIV are absorbed by their HIV status and the associated distress toward investigating positive psychological experiences and outcomes for this population group. Research has highlighted that people may experience both positive and negative changes as a consequence of struggling with trauma (Cann et al., 2010), and in addition to the posttraumatic stress experienced as a result of HIV that has long been studied, in the last 20 years, there has been increasing research on posttraumatic growth (PTG) experiences among people living with HIV (Milam, 2006).

Tedeschi and Calhoun (2004) defined PTG as a "positive psychological change experienced as a result of the struggle with highly challenging life circumstances" (p. 1) and listed five domains of PTG: personal strength, appreciation of life, relating to others, new possibilities, and spiritual development. A systematic review of the literature examining PTG and life-threatening physical illness (Hefferon et al., 2009) identified four key themes, namely, reappraisal of life and priorities, trauma equals the development of self, existential re-evaluation, and a new awareness of the body, thus extending the findings beyond the original five domains of PTG, and concluded that physical illness-related PTG experiences have unique features that distinguish them. As with other conditions, "Pain and growth can occur simultaneously following an HIV diagnosis, and even with the presence of PTSD symptoms, posttraumatic growth is possible" (Zeligman, 2018, p. 26).

As the term suggests, the focus of PTG is on enduring positive changes people experience following an event considered to be traumatic with "A higher level of functioning than which existed prior to the event" (Linley & Joseph, 2004, p. 11) reported. Yet there is no consensus on when such growth may be initiated among people living with HIV. PTG may not be as readily experienced among this population as it is by people with other long-term health conditions. This may be because emotional processing among people living with HIV could be hindered by the pervasiveness of HIV-related stigma fueled by a lack of knowledge about transmission and the perception of individual accountability (Lechner & Weaver, 2009), which inhibits sharing one's status with others. Yet, the discovery of meaning has been associated with a less rapid decline of CD4 cells among bereaved men who are HIV-seropositive, hence contributing to the deceleration of HIV progression (Bower et al., 1998). Studies investigating PTG among people living with HIV have found that growth is experienced in multidimensional ways. However, considering the historical and contemporary reports from people that reiterate the ongoing stressors of living with HIV, PTG is not necessarily triggered at the point of diagnosis (Rzeszutek & Gruszczyńska, 2018).

Reports of PTG experienced by people living with HIV include a re-evaluation of life, changes in relationships, spirituality and religiosity, and physical health restoration.

PTG and HIV literature commonly recounted that an HIV diagnosis has been reported to initiate a significant alteration to individual life journeys with rethinking of values and what matters to individuals (Ciambrone, 2001). Schwartzberg (1994), who researched positive changes among gay men living with HIV in the US at a time when treatment was limited and someone diagnosed with HIV was likely to die, reported a "here and now" focus that reflected a transformation in the understanding and appreciation of time, and the attempt to live each day more fully:

> I'm much more aware of time passing, how I spend time, and taking time for myself to let myself live. I've always been so scheduled and on a timetable, pushing hard-that's been the story of my life. HIV has introduced the other side, which is take time to enjoy this moment, this day, don't push so hard doing all these things you don't want to be doing.
>
> *(Lucas; Schwartzberg, 1994, p. 598)*

The transformation included what was considered important as well as what was now considered less important:

> After I accepted that I had AIDS, what happened was everything in life that I thought was important became so unimportant. So, AIDS, really, it's kind of like a gift, in a weird kind of way, because it really made me understand and realize a lot of things about life that maybe I wouldn't have seen so quickly.
>
> *(Siegel & Schrimshaw, 2000, p. 1548)*

When access to treatment became more likely for people diagnosed with HIV, Cadell and Sullivan (2006) reported a personal philosophy to 'live intensely' (p. 50). In one of the most recent studies investigating PTG among gay men living with HIV in Buenos Aires, Argentina (Radusky et al., 2022), participants still reported a temporal change appearing to describe a time before the diagnosis and a time after, in some cases interpreting their diagnosis as a new opportunity or rebirth: "Since one has a second chance to live […] it would be very foolish of me to waste it" (P1; Radusky et al., 2022, p. 97). Ogińska-Bulik and Kraska (2017) found positive changes in the appreciation of life to be the most frequently cited domain of PTG among respondents living with HIV in Poland. Cognitive processing of an HIV diagnosis was seen to bring about an increased level of acceptance and rediscovery of life values. Similarly, interviews about positive changes experienced by African women living with HIV in the UK (Dibb & Kamalesh, 2012) highlighted that alongside acknowledgment of the negative effects of their HIV diagnosis, meaning and value in life were discovered in a way that had not been felt prior to diagnosis:

> Now I can think more about my life, because of HIV. Back then, when I was not, I was not thinking about it. I could live, just like that, but now I am more careful … I think about my life, I take my life as very important … Living with HIV … I managed to value my life.
>
> *(Elizabeth; Dibb & Kamalesh, 2012)*

A new way of seeing the world included new possibilities for employment. For some people, it meant making choices in a more conscious manner, and the ability to change things that needed changing. For example, Serena, a participant in Lennon-Dearing's (2020) research, spoke of her experience with HIV as her having "turned a negative situation into a really great positive situation" (p. 6) by using her platform as a contestant in beauty pageants for raising HIV awareness.

It has been claimed that positive changes in life appreciation might be more likely to be realized for those who exhibit a stronger and more optimistic belief about their ability to manage (Evans et al., 2013), which is consistent with research investigating PTG following natural disasters and military combat (Benight & Bandura, 2004). Doyal and Anderson (2005) explored the significance of being female for the experience of HIV. Similar to previous findings, re-evaluation of their lives was a predominant theme in the women's personal narratives, and it was suggested that self-belief lends itself to living differently: "What I used to take for granted I don't take for granted anymore. If I'm doing something I always think oh maybe this is the last time I will be doing this. Let me do it properly" (Doyal & Anderson, 2005, p. 1734).

Changes in Relationships

Whether it is the deepening of familial relationships or the making of new connections, changes to people's interpersonal relationships are frequently central in the accounts of PTG among those living with HIV. Tedeschi and Calhoun (1995) claimed that a key component of PTG is more compassion when relating to others, and the fostering of stronger bonds with loved ones: "I learned to nurture relationships. It's given me life-long friendships that are real friendships: real, deep and meaningful. I couldn't have had those relationships before" (Marley; Valls, 2019, p. 108). For native Hawaiian women interviewed about their lived experience of HIV (Mueller et al., 2003), acting with *aloha*, i.e., heartfelt expressions was more readily offered within interpersonal relationships. Mueller et al. (2003) reported that the centrality of emotional bonds in social relationships was the most common theme emerging from women's accounts:

> For me it has brought out the best, I found out I am not so hard core, that I actually have a loving heart. Although I am very firm, I have tender space, I didn't let people get near before, it took me a while to release the wall I had built … being HIV+ does that for me.
>
> *(Participant H-7; Mueller et al., 2003, p. 7)*

A participant in Cadell and Sullivan's (2006) research advised "straightening out" and "making peace" (p. 51) for those with relationships that were not optimal with friends with whom there was an issue that needed addressing. Relationships with the self also seem to be affected. For many, this seemed to come about via their service to others in the form of volunteer work, activism, and/or advocacy. Altruistic behavior was seen to become a fundamental part of people's life and assisted in elevating self-esteem and a sense of purpose, similar to survivors of collective trauma, such as a war, who have often made an effort to make sense of their experiences through altruistic action (Frazier et al., 2013). The capability of what has been referred to as "heightened versions of moral sense" (Prior et al., 2021, p. 117) has been conceptualized in the literature as a consistently found component of PTG (Puvimanasinghe et al., 2014). In addition, Tedeschi and Calhoun's (2004) concept of PTG refers to higher levels of self-reliance and a greater ability to accept life's flow of events as a development of personal strength. This is captured in this excerpt from Emily, who came to find personal meaning in HIV by becoming involved in activism:

> And then I got mad ... And when I got mad, I started makin' things happen. I became an activist. I started screaming, I started confronting people. Literally. And my journey began, and next thing I know ... I'm doing international AIDS work, and doing a lot of advocacy work for people with AIDS.
>
> *(Emily; Massey et al., 1998)*

The researchers reported on the role of activism as essential to Emily's thriving; later Emily reflected on how her service to others was inextricably linked with self-service:

> Well, I didn't realize that my initial reason for doing it was to help people ... I didn't realize that in the midst of all of this, that the very thing that I thought I was doin' for everyone else saved me. That the more I talked about it, the more ... empowered I got, and the more ... hope I had. And the more feeling of a purpose I had.
>
> *(Emily; Massey et al., 1998)*

In Tedeschi and Calhoun's (2004) model, sharing of the experience of trauma and the subsequent access to and utilization of social support fosters PTG. Because HIV-related stigma is known to reduce the likelihood of people living with HIV telling their status to others and seeking help (Kamen et al., 2016), there is a great deal less research examining the impact of social support on the development of PTG among people living with HIV. However, Emlet et al. (2017) found social support and community engagement to be positively associated with resilience in older gay and bisexual men living with HIV. Social support, particularly emotional support from significant others, including friends, family, and partners, plays a vital role in facilitating PTG (Kamen et al., 2016). Care and reassurance felt within companionship can enhance emotion regulation (Nenova et al., 2013), and as William, a participant in Valls' (2019) research, stated, can change the course of someone's life journey:

> My relationships changed – I ended the ones that I had for the wrong reasons. I did a group at an HIV support network for black, gay men. So that turned my life into a new direction. I had never had an interaction like that with friends prior to my diagnosis.
>
> *(William; Valls, 2019, p. 109)*

Spirituality and Religion

Religion and spirituality are commonly cited as being important to people living with HIV (Davis et al., 2021), and changes in people's spiritual connections have been established as a pivotal component of PTG experiences for this population group (Ogińska-Bulik & Kraska, 2017). Some diversity in the definition of spirituality and religion is evident in the literature (see Hill & Pargament, 2008 for an overview). Whilst the discovery of spiritual meaning is a unique experience for each person, emotional well-being has been found to positively correlate with religious and/or spiritual involvement (Doolittle et al., 2018). PTG experiences in this domain have included turning to religion, as described by Kyle:

> I know that I'm not getting away from this. It's here, inside, and how I choose to deal with it is key. I've never had a very strong sense that I could get rid of this [HIV], heal myself that way, but I do have a strong sense that I can heal myself spiritually and emotionally.
>
> *(Schwartzberg, 1994, p. 596)*

A re-evaluation of spiritual beliefs, an enhanced connection with spirituality, and the presence of forgiveness in one's life have also been reported (Ironson et al., 2006), all of which have been found to be associated with higher levels of PTG. Participants in studies by Lennon-Dearing (2020) and Kremer et al. (2009) detailed intensification of spirituality and stated that it had taken them many years to come to terms with their HIV diagnosis. When they felt having reached acceptance, a new path as an HIV educator that was inextricably linked with their religiosity was uncovered:

> I got HIV because it is my purpose of being. I had to understand what it is like so I can help the community on a different level and help create social change. I didn't know that I had these powers inside of me, that I can be a dynamic leader and be an inspiration to others.
>
> *(Susan; Kremer et al., 2009, p. 373)*

> God has given me a purpose. My hopes and dreams in life are to continue to share my story to help others. I want to raise awareness of HIV and AIDS. If I can help one other person realize they are worthy of love, then I feel I have done what God has intended me to do.
>
> *(Suzie; Lennon-Dearing, 2020, p. 6)*

Understanding how spirituality and religion influence health and quality of life has been the subject of much research (Panzini et al., 2017), and the need for increased recognition by healthcare providers of an individual's religious and spiritual beliefs has been reported (Grill et al., 2020).

Physical Health Restoration

Health restoration is seen to be a central focus for people living with HIV who are experiencing PTG (Littlewood et al., 2008). This is not unlike the experience reported by participants identified as experiencing PTG while living with breast cancer, when a new awareness of and relationship to the body emerged (Hefferon, 2012), which, in turn, "increased awareness of health and conscious health behaviour changes" (p. 1239). A renewed importance of the body, leading to improvements in diet and exercise, was evident in people with lipodystrophy syndrome taking ART who sought a referral for dietary help in addition to their psychological support needs, "My doctor referred me to see the psychologist and the dietitian. One for the head, one for the body. It's helped" (Power et al., 2003, p. 139).

Participants were interviewed in a qualitative study of people living with HIV who take drugs when an HIV diagnosis prompted treatment for substance misuse as well as HIV. In addition to adhering to ART (Luszczynska et al., 2007), people also reported better physical self-care through stopping drug-taking and reducing alcohol misuse:

> I've always said that although it's not something, you know, that you'd wish for, becoming HIV is, ah, I think the major, the major part in why I stopped using [drugs], because I don't know if I would have stopped if I hadn't become positive.
>
> *(Participant; Siegel & Schrimshaw, 2000, p. 1547)*

Individuals who had experienced rock bottom because of substance misuse, and repeatedly tried unsuccessfully to give up their drug use prior to their diagnosis, later reflected that their HIV diagnosis was the motivation they needed to "get clean and stay clean" (Siegel & Schrimshaw 2000, p. 1547). In some cases, personal health status was deemed to be improved beyond that experienced before a detectable presence of HIV was discovered:

> Physically ... right now I feel like I could do a hundred push-ups, like ... I dance a lot ... I haven't done that in twenty years, so ... I feel good! I feel real good. On a scale from 1 to 10—probably 9.99.
>
> *(Alezandro; Mosack et al., 2005, p. 594)*

Conclusion

Because people living with HIV may experience PTG, the evidence suggests that PTG is a worthy intervention focus. PTG could be considered a particularly important and ideal outcome for people living with HIV given the presence of an abundance of illness-related stressors. Social and emotional support networks have been found to play a vital role in facilitating the psychological and physical benefits associated with PTG (Tedeschi & Calhoun, 2004).

References

Abbey, G., Thompson, S. B., Hickish, T., & Heathcote, D. (2015). A meta-analysis of prevalence rates and moderating factors for cancer-related post-traumatic stress disorder. *Psycho-Oncology*, *24*(4), 371–381.

American Psychiatric Association. (2013). *Diagnostic and statistical manual of mental disorders* (5th ed.). American Psychiatric Publishing.

Benight, C. C., & Bandura, A. (2004). Social cognitive theory of posttraumatic recovery: The role of perceived self-efficacy. *Behaviour Research and Therapy*, 42(10), 1129–1148.

Berman, M., Eaton, L. A., Watson, R. J., Maksut, J. L., Rucinski, K. B., & Earnshaw, V. A. (2021). Perpetuated HIV microaggressions: A novel scale to measure subtle discrimination against people living with HIV. *AIDS Education and Prevention*, *33*(1), 1–15.

Breet, E., Kagee, A., & Seedat, S. (2014). HIV-related stigma and symptoms of post-traumatic stress disorder and depression in HIV-infected individuals: Does social support play a mediating or moderating role? *AIDS Care*, *26*(8), 947–951.

Bourne, K., Croston, M., & Namiba, A. (2022). What are the current factors that impact on health-related quality of life for women living with HIV? *British Journal of Nursing*, *31*(1), S16–S22.

Bower, J. E., Kemeny, M. E., Taylor, S. E., & Fahey, J. L. (1998). Cognitive processing, discovery of meaning, CD4 decline, and AIDS-related mortality among bereaved HIV-seropositive men. *Journal of Consulting and Clinical Psychology*, *66*(6), 979–986.

Cadell, S., & Sullivan, R. (2006). Posttraumatic growth and HIV bereavement: Where does it start and when does it end? *Traumatology*, *12*(1), 45–59.

Calhoun, L. G., & Tedeschi, R. G. (1999). *Facilitating posttraumatic growth: A clinician's guide.* Lawrence Erlbaum Associates.
Cann, A., Calhoun, L. G., Tedeschi, R. G., & Solomon, D. T. (2010). Posttraumatic growth and depreciation as independent experiences and predictors of well-being. *Journal of Loss and Trauma, 15*(3), 151–166.
Chaudoir, S. R., Norton, W. E., Earnshaw, V. A., Moneyham, L., Mugavero, M. J., & Hiers, K. M. (2012). Coping with HIV stigma: Do proactive coping and spiritual peace buffer the effect of stigma on depression? *AIDS and Behavior, 16*(8), 2382–2391.
Ciambrone, D. E. (2001). Illness and other assaults on self: The relative impact of HIV/AIDS on women's lives. *Sociology of Health & Illness, 23*(4), 517–540.
Dale, S. K., Reid, R., & Safren, S. A. (2021). Factors associated with resilience among Black women living with HIV and histories of trauma. *Journal of Health Psychology, 26*(5), 758–766.
Davis, C. W., Hook, J. N., Hodge, A. S., DeBlaere, C., Davis, D. E., Van Tongeren, D. R., & Vosvick, M. (2021). Religious relief: Exploring the role of religion and spirituality among a broad range of people living with HIV. *Spirituality in Clinical Practice.* Advance online publication. 10.1037/scp0000252
Dibb, B., & Kamalesh, T. (2012). Exploring positive adjustment in HIV positive African women living in the UK. *AIDS Care, 24*(2), 143–148.
Doolittle, B. R., Justice, A. C., & Fiellin, D. A. (2018). Religion, spirituality, and HIV clinical outcomes: A systematic review of the literature. *AIDS and Behavior, 22*(6), 1792–1801.
Doyal, L., & Anderson, J. (2005). 'My fear is to fall in love again ...' How HIV-positive African women survive in London. *Social Science & Medicine, 60*(8), 1729–1738.
Earnshaw, V. A., & Chaudoir, S. R. (2009). From conceptualizing to measuring HIV stigma: A review of HIV stigma mechanism measures. *AIDS and Behavior, 13*(6), 1160–1177.
Eisinger, R. W., Dieffenbach, C. W., & Fauci, A. S. (2019). HIV viral load and transmissibility of HIV infection: Undetectable equals untransmittable. *JAMA*, 321(5), 451– 452. 10.1001/jama.2018.21167
Emlet, C. A., Shiu, C., Kim, H. J., & Fredriksen-Goldsen, K. (2017). Bouncing back: Resilience and mastery among HIV-positive older gay and bisexual men. *The Gerontologist, 57*(suppl_1), S40–S49.
Evans, S. D., Williams, B. E., & Leu, C. S. (2013). Correlates of posttraumatic growth among African Americans living with HIV/AIDS in Mississippi. *Online Journal of Rural and Urban Research, 3*(1).
Falchuk., B., & Our Lady J. (Writer). (July 23, 2019). Love's in need of love today (Season 2, Episode 6). In R. Murphy, & B. Falchuk (Creator), *Pose color force Brad Falchuk television.* Ryan Murphy Television Touchstone.
Fife, B. L. (2005). The role of constructed meaning in adaptation to the onset of life-threatening illness. *Social Science & Medicine, 61*(10), 2132–2143.
Frazier, P., Greer, C., Gabrielsen, S., Tennen, H., Park, C., & Tomich, P. (2013). The relation between trauma exposure and prosocial behavior. *Psychological Trauma: Theory, Research, Practice, and Policy, 5*(3), 286–294.
Ginwright, S. (2015). *Hope and healing in urban education: How urban activists and teachers are reclaiming matters of the heart.* Routledge.
Grill, K. B., Wang, J., Cheng, Y. I., & Lyon, M. E. (2020). The role of religiousness and spirituality in health-related quality of life of persons living with HIV: A latent class analysis. *Psychology of Religion and Spirituality, 12*(4), 494–504.
Hefferon, K. (2012). Bringing back the body into positive psychology: The theory of corporeal posttraumatic growth in breast cancer survivorship. *Psychology, 3*, 1238–1242.
Hefferon, K., Grealy, M., & Mutrie, N. (2009). Post-traumatic growth and life threatening physical illness: A systematic review of the qualitative literature. *British Journal of Health Psychology, 14*(2), 343–378.
Hill, P. C., & Pargament, K. I. (2008). Advances in the conceptualization and measurement of religion and spirituality: Implications for physical and mental health research. *American Psychologist, 58*(1), 64–74.
HIV (n.d.). *The Global HIV/AIDS Epidemic.* Retrieved 25 January 2022, from https://www.hiv.gov/
Holtzman, C., Armon, C., Tedaldi, E., Chmiel, J. S., Buchacz, K., Wood, K., Brooks, J. T., & the HOPS Investigators (2013). Polypharmacy and risk of antiretroviral drug interactions among the aging HIV-infected population. *Journal of General Internal Medicine, 28*(10), 1302–1310.

Ironson, G., Stuetzle, R., & Fletcher, M. A. (2006). An increase in religiousness/spirituality occurs after HIV diagnosis and predicts slower disease progression over 4 years in people with HIV. *Journal of General Internal Medicine*, *21*(5), S62–S68.

Ismail, S. D., Pankrac, J., Ndashimye, E., Prodger, J. L., Abrahams, M. R., Mann, J. F., Redd, A. D., & Arts, E. J. (2021). Addressing an HIV cure in LMIC. *Retrovirology*, *18*(1), 1–19.

Kamen, C., Vorasarun, C., Canning, T., Kienitz, E., Weiss, C., Flores, S., Etter, D., Lee, S., & Gore-Felton, C. (2016). The impact of stigma and social support on development of post-traumatic growth among persons living with HIV. *Journal of Clinical Psychology in Medical Settings*, *23*(2), 126–134.

Katz, I. T., Ryu, A. E., Onuegbu, A. G., Psaros, C., Weiser, S. D., Bangsberg, D. R., & Tsai, A. C. (2013). Impact of HIV-related stigma on treatment adherence: Systematic review and meta-synthesis. *Journal of the International AIDS Society*, *16*(3 Suppl 2), 18640. 10.7448/IAS.16.3.18640

Kremer, H., Ironson, G., & Kaplan, L. (2009). The fork in the road: HIV as a potential positive turning point and the role of spirituality. *AIDS Care*, 21(3), 368–377.

Lazarus, J. V., Safreed-Harmon, K., Barton, S. E., Costagliola, D., Dedes, N., del Amo Valero, J., Gatell, J. M., Baptista-Leite, R., Mendão, L., Porter, K., Vella, S., & Rockstroh, J. K. (2016). Beyond viral suppression of HIV–the new quality of life frontier. *BMC Medicine*, *14*(1), 1–5.

Lechner, S. C., & Weaver, K. E. (2009). Lessons learned about benefit finding among individuals with cancer or HIV/AIDS. In C. L. Park, S. C. Lechner, M. H. Antoni, & A. L. Stanton (Eds.), *Medical illness and positive life change: Can crisis lead to personal transformation?* (pp. 107–124). American Psychological Association.

Lennon-Dearing, R. (2020). "HIV is a gift": Posttraumatic growth in women with HIV. *Illness, Crisis & Loss*, 0(0), 1–16.

Lessard, D., Toupin, I., Engler, K., Lènàrt, A., I-Score Consulting Team, & Lebouché, B. (2018). HIV-positive patients' perceptions of antiretroviral therapy adherence in relation to subjective time: Imprinting, domino effects, and future shadowing. *Journal of the International Association of Providers of AIDS Care (JIAPAC)*, 17, 1–8.

Link, B. G., & Phelan, J. C. (2006). Stigma and its public health implications, *Lancet*, 367, 528–529. 10.1016/S0140-6736(06)68184-1

Linley, P. A., & Joseph, S. (2004). Positive change following trauma and adversity: A review. *Journal of Traumatic Stress: Official Publication of the International Society for Traumatic Stress Studies*, *17*(1), 11–21.

Littlewood, R. A., Vanable, P. A., Carey, M. P., & Blair, D. C. (2008). The association of benefit finding to psychosocial and health behavior adaptation among HIV+ men and women. *Journal of Behavioral Medicine*, 31(2), 145–155.

Lundgren, J. D., Babiker, A. G., Gordin, F., Emery, S., Grund, B., Sharma, S., Avihingsanon, A., Cooper, D. A., Fätkenheuer, G., Llibre, J. M., Molina, J-M., Munderi, P., Schechter, M., Wood, R., Kliongman, K. L., Collins, S., Lane, H. C., Phillips, A. N., & Neaton, J. D. (2015). Initiation of antiretroviral therapy in early asymptomatic HIV infection. *The New England Journal of Medicine*, *373*(9), 795–807.

Luszczynska, A., Sarkar, Y., & Knoll, N. (2007). Received social support, self-efficacy, and finding benefits in disease as predictors of physical functioning and adherence to antiretroviral therapy. *Patient Education and Counseling*, *66*(1), 37–42.

Machtinger, E. L., Wilson, T. C., Haberer, J. E., & Weiss, D. S. (2012). Psychological trauma and PTSD in HIV-positive women: A meta-analysis. *AIDS Behavior*, *16*, 2091–2100.

Massey, S., Cameron, A., Ouellette, S., & Fine, M. (1998). Qualitative approaches to the study of thriving: What can be learned? *Journal of Social Issues*, *54*(2), 337–355.

May, M. T., Gompels, M., Delpech, V., Porter, K., Orkin, C., Kegg, S., Hay, P., Johnson, M., Palfreeman, A., Gilson, R., Chadwick, D., Martin, F., Hill, T., Walsh., J., Post, F., Fisher, M., Ainsworth, J., Jose, J., Leen, C., & Sabin, C. (2014). Impact on life expectancy of HIV-1 positive individuals of CD4+ cell count and viral load response to antiretroviral therapy. *AIDS*, *28*(8), 1193–1202.

Mazanderani, F., & Paparini, S. (2015). The stories we tell: Qualitative research interviews, talking technologies and the 'normalisation' of life with HIV. *Social Science & Medicine*, *131*, 66–73. 10.1016/j.socscimed.2015.02.041

McGrath, J. W., Winchester, M. S., Kaawa-Mafigiri, D., Walakira, E., Namutiibwa, F., Birungi, J., Ssendegye, G., Nalwoga, A., Kyarikunda, E., Kisakye, S., Ayebazibwe, N., & Rwabukwali, C. B. (2014). Challenging the paradigm: Anthropological perspectives on HIV as a chronic disease. *Medical Anthropology*, 33(4), 303–317.

Meyer, I. H. (2003). Prejudice, social stress, and mental health in lesbian, gay, and bisexual populations: Conceptual issues and research evidence. *Psychological Bulletin*, 129(5), 674–697.

Milam, J. (2006). Posttraumatic growth and HIV disease progression. *Journal of Consulting and Clinical Psychology*, *74*(5), 817–827.

Montessori, V., Press, N., Harris, M., Akagi, L., & Montaner, J. S. (2004). Adverse effects of antiretroviral therapy for HIV infection. *Canadian Medical Association Journal*, *170*(2), 229–238.

Mosack, K. E., Abbott, M., Singer, M., Weeks, M. R., & Rohena, L. (2005). If I didn't have HIV, I'd be dead now: Illness narratives of drug users living with HIV/AIDS. *Qualitative Health Research*, *15*(5), 586–605.

Moyer, E. (2015). The anthropology of life after AIDS: Epistemological continuities in the age of antiretroviral treatment. *Annual Review of Anthropology*, *44*, 259–275.

Moyer, E., & Hardon, A. (2014). A disease unlike any other? Why HIV remains exceptional in the age of treatment. *Medical Anthropology*, 33(4), 263–269.

Mueller, C. W., Orimoto, L., & Kaopua, L. S. (2003). Psychosocial adjustment of Native Hawaiian women living with HIV/AIDS: The central role of affective bonds. *Pacific Health Dialog*, 10(2), 3–9.

Nachega, J. B., Morroni, C., Zuniga, J. M., Sherer, R., Beyrer, C., Solomon, S., Schecther, M., & Rockstroh, J. (2012). HIV-related stigma, isolation, discrimination, and serostatus disclosure: A global survey of 2035 HIV-infected adults. *Journal of the International Association of Physicians in AIDS Care*, *11*(3), 172–178.

Neigh, G. N., Rhodes, S. T., Valdez, A., & Jovanovic, T. (2016). PTSD co-morbid with HIV: Separate but equal, or two parts of a whole. *Neurobiology of Disease*, *92*, 116–123. 10.1016/j.nbd.2015.11.012

Nenova, M., DuHamel, K., Zemon, V., Rini, C., & Redd, W. H. (2013). Posttraumatic growth, social support, and social constraint in hematopoietic stem cell transplant survivors. *Psycho-oncology*, 22(1), 195–202.

Ogińska-Bulik, N., & Kraska, K. (2017). Posttraumatic stress disorder and posttraumatic growth in HIV-infected patients–the role of coping strategies. *Health Psychology Report*, *5*(4), 323–332.

Ortega-Williams, A., Beltrán, R., Schultz, K., Ru-Glo Henderson, Z., Colón, L., & Teyra, C. (2021). An integrated historical trauma and posttraumatic growth framework: A cross-cultural exploration. *Journal of Trauma & Dissociation*, *22*(2), 220–240.

Panzini, R. G., Mosqueiro, B. P., Zimpel, R. R., Bandeira, D. R., Rocha, N. S., & Fleck, M. P. (2017). Quality-of-life and spirituality. *International Review of Psychiatry*, *29*(3), 263–282.

Pellowski, J. A., Kalichman, S. C., Matthews, K. A., & Adler, N. (2013). A pandemic of the poor: Social disadvantage and the U.S. HIV epidemic. *American Psychologist*, *68*(4), 197–209. 10.1037/a0032694

Peltzer, J., Domian, E., & Teel, C. (2016). Infected lives: Lived experiences of young African American HIV-positive women. *Western Journal of Nursing Research*, 38(2), 216–230.

Power, R., Tate, H. L., McGill, S., & Taylor, C. (2003). A qualitative study of the psychosocial implications of lipodystrophy syndrome on HIV positive individuals. *Sexually Transmitted Infections*, *79*(2), 137–141. 10.1136/sti.79.2.137

Prior, K., Carvalheiro, M., Lawler, S., Stapinski, L. A., Newton, N. C., Mooney-Somers, J., Basto-Pereira, M., & Barrett, E. (2021). Early trauma and associations with altruistic attitudes and behaviours among young adults. *Child Abuse & Neglect*, *117*, 10.1016/j.chiabu.2021.105091

Puvimanasinghe, T., Denson, L. A., Augoustinos, M., & Somasundaram, D. (2014). "Giving back to society what society gave us": Altruism, coping, and meaning making by two refugee communities in South Australia. *Australian Psychologist*, *49*(5), 313–321.

Radusky, P. D., Zalazar, V., & Arístegui, I. (2022). Crecimiento postraumático en hombres gays con VIH en Buenos Aires, Argentina. *Psicología y Salud*, *32*(1), 93–104.

Rice, W. S., Burnham, K., Mugavero, M. J., Raper, J. L., Atkins, G. C., & Turan, B. (2017). Association between internalized HIV-related stigma and HIV care visit adherence. *Journal of Acquired Immune Deficiency Syndromes (1999)*, *76*(5), 482–487.

Rueda, S., Mitra, S., Chen, S., Gogolishvili, D., Globerman, J., Chambers, L., Wilson, M., Logie, C. H., Shi, Q., Morassaei, S., & Rourke, S. B. (2016). Examining the associations between HIV-related stigma and health outcomes in people living with HIV/AIDS: A series of meta-analyses. *BMJ Open*, *6*(7), e011453.

Rzeszutek, M., & Gruszczyńska, E. (2018). Posttraumatic growth among people living with HIV: A systematic review. *Journal of Psychosomatic Research*, *114*, 81–91.

Sanjuán, P., Molero, F., Fuster, M. J., & Nouvilas, E. (2013). Coping with HIV related stigma and well-being. *Journal of Happiness Studies*, *14*(2), 709–722.

Schwartzberg, S. S. (1994). Vitality and growth in HIV-infected gay men. *Social Science & Medicine*, *38*(4), 593–602.

Sherr, L., Clucas, C., Harding, R., Sibley, E., & Catalan, J. (2011). HIV and depression–a systematic review of interventions. *Psychology, Health & Medicine*, *16*(5), 493–527.

Siegel, K., & Schrimshaw, E. W. (2000). Perceiving benefits in adversity: Stress-related growth in women living with HIV/AIDS. *Social Science & Medicine*, *51*(10), 1543–1554.

Stall, R., & Mills, T. C. (2006). A quarter century of AIDS. *American Journal of Public Health*, *96*(6), 959–961.

Tang, C., Goldsamt, L., Meng, J., Xiao, X., Zhang, L., Williams, A. B., & Wang, H. (2020). Global estimate of the prevalence of post-traumatic stress disorder among adults living with HIV: A systematic review and meta-analysis. *BMJ Open*, *10*(4), e032435.

Tedeschi, R. G., & Calhoun, L. G. (1995). *Trauma and transformation: Growing in the aftermath of suffering*. Sage.

Tedeschi, R. G., & Calhoun, L. G. (2004). Posttraumatic growth: Conceptual foundations and empirical evidence. *Psychological Inquiry*, *15*(1), 1–18.

UNAIDS (2020). *Evidence for eliminating HIV-related stigma and discrimination: Joint United Nations programme on HIV/AIDS (UNAIDS)*. Available: https://www.unaids.org/en/resources/documents/2020/eliminating-discrimination-guidance

Valls, L. (2019). *The lived experience of posttraumatic growth in gay men after an HIV diagnosis: An interpretative phenomenological analysis* (Doctoral dissertation, Middlesex University/New School of Psychotherapy and Counselling).

Walker, L. (2019). 'There's no pill to help you deal with the guilt and shame': Contemporary experiences of HIV in the United Kingdom. *Health*, *23*(1), 97–113.

Watkins-Hayes, C. (2014). Intersectionality and the sociology of HIV/AIDS: Past, present, and future research directions. *Annual Review of Sociology*, *40*(1), 431–457. 10.1146/annurev-soc-071312-145621

Weinstein, T. L., & Li, X. (2016). The relationship between stress and clinical outcomes for persons living with HIV/AIDS: A systematic review of the global literature. *AIDS Care*, *28*(2), 160–169.

World Health Organisation (2021). HIV/AIDS. Retrieved 14 December 2021, from https://www.who.int/news-room/fact-sheets/detail/hiv-aids

Zeligman, M. (2018). Medical trauma: Assessing trauma and growth following an HIV diagnosis. *The Journal of Humanistic Counseling*, *57*(1), 14–30.

32

POSTTRAUMATIC GROWTH IN ACQUIRED BRAIN INJURY

A Narrative Review

Lowri Wilkie, Pamela Arroyo, Andrew Kemp, and Zoe Fisher

David was a British expat, living a happy life on the sunny coast of Spain with his wife and dogs. One morning, whilst doing work around their new Spanish home, David suddenly fell from a ladder, hitting his head on the concrete floor. David suffered a severe traumatic brain injury, which left him with memory loss, communication difficulties, chronic fatigue, low self-esteem and a range of other physical, cognitive, social, and emotional difficulties. He and his wife moved back to the UK, but he was isolated and felt like an outsider. Old interests which shaped his personality such as fishing, reading novels, and watching live bands had dissipated due to social anxiety and attention deficits. His emotional outbursts caused heated arguments with his wife. His confidence was at an all-time low, he felt a constant sense of shame and was in a downward spiral of depression.

David turned to his doctor for help and was referred to a neurorehabilitation service for brain injury survivors. He attended educational, psychotherapeutic, and nature-based rehabilitation programs with other survivors; he described feeling part of a community of individuals who understood him. He joined a local choir and started singing with them twice a week, attended a walking group, improved his fitness and dropped to a healthier weight.

David describes himself now as being a completely different person than he was before his injury. His life has slowed down, he enjoys going for long walks and watching nature, and he spends time noticing the seasons, animals, and flowers. He feels a deep sense of presence. He feels happier and finds true meaning through helping others. He is training to be a peer mentor and soon will lead groups, supporting new brain injury survivors starting their neurorehabilitation journey. He works every day to put a smile on other people's faces, and although he still carries problems, he feels he is a better person than before. He described feeling as though he is finally a part of a whole, instead of being on the outside looking in.

Suffering an ABI is often a life-shattering event. David's description of the negative impact his injury initially had on his well-being is commonly heard by clinicians working in this field. However, this story is also a source of hope that the aftermath of a brain injury does not have to end in distress or acceptance of a sub-optimal existence. For some, it has the potential to promote wellbeing and be the source of true human flourishing.

DOI: 10.4324/9781032208688-41

The Impact of Acquired Brain Injury

Acquired Brain Injury (ABI) is any type of brain damage that occurs after birth. It can be caused by infection, disease, lack of oxygen or an external force on the head. The causes of ABI include Traumatic Brain Injury (TBI), caused by a physical force to the head, resulting in damage to brain tissue, and Non-Traumatic Brain Injury (Non-TBI), which results from a stroke, brain tumor, hypoxia and meningitis. ABI is a leading global cause of disability in young people and can lead to permanent physical, cognitive, psychological and social difficulties (James et al., 2019; NICE, 2019). ABI is a chronic condition and over 40% of survivors hospitalized with ABI suffer long-term disability and require neurorehabilitation to integrate back into the community and everyday life (Corrigan et al., 2010). The consequences of ABI can unexpectedly and significantly disrupt one's life, impacting survivor's autonomy, social relationships, and the ability to resume their roles at work, at home and in the community. It is common for an ABI to be described as a traumatic event (Grace et al., 2015; Lyon et al., 2020; Powell et al., 2012) as survivors often face psychological distress and significantly increased rates of depression and suicide (Glenn et al., 2009; Jorge et al., 2004; Osborn et al., 2014; Teasdale & Engberg, 2001).

The process of adaptation following brain injury involves resolving discrepancies in relation to one's social identity, interpersonal relationships, and personal identity, a process described by the "Y-Shaped" model (Gracey et al., 2009). It is common for survivors to report a 'loss of self' with regard to their current identity, as well as how they see themselves in the future (Ownsworth & Haslam, 2014). Survivors of ABI frequently encounter social stigmatization, misunderstanding, and negative attitudes from the general public (McLellan et al., 2010). Fear of stigma can result in withdrawal from social groups and relationships. For example, a qualitative study following individuals with ABI (Nochi, 1998) found that a loss of self was experienced in relation to the self and in the eyes of others. Participants reported a fear of being defined as 'disabled', being mistakenly categorized as having a learning disability or mental illness. Those who adopt a stigmatized identity struggle to maintain social relationships and social identities (Gracey et al., 2009). Therefore, a focus on building new personal and social identities is important for growth following ABI. As the individual starts to resolve these discrepancies, new meanings, values and identities are formed (Gracey et al., 2009).

It has been proposed that trauma and identity have a reciprocal relationship, such that trauma can alter the survivor's identity, while identity can influence the impact that the trauma has on psychological functioning (Berman et al., 2020). The extent to which an experienced trauma is related to one's identity, i.e., the 'event centrality' is associated with one's reactions to the trauma (Fitzgerald et al., 2016). In cases where highly adverse events become central to one's identity, the associated negative emotions may impact subsequent life events via worries, rumination, or avoidance (Berntsen & Rubin, 2006). As ABI contributes to neurobiological, neuropsychological, and psycho-social changes, it will likely become central to the survivor's identity and therefore have high event centrality (Yeates et al., 2008). For example, research shows that stroke survivors tend to redefine their identity after their injury, and that this re-definition significantly exceeds normal levels of identity change typically experienced in personal development (Kuenemund et al., 2016).

Characteristics of Posttraumatic Growth in Acquired Brain Injury

Posttraumatic growth (PTG) refers to "positive change that the individual experiences as a result of the struggle with a traumatic event" (Calhoun & Tedeschi, 1999, p. 11). Identified core domains of PTG include a greater appreciation of life, a changed sense of priorities, warmer and more intimate relationships with others, a greater sense of personal strength, and recognition of new possibilities or paths for one's life and spiritual development. One longitudinal study (mean follow-up = 11.5 years) of 563 ABI survivors found that up to 50% of the sample experienced components of positive psychological growth, according to the Positive Changes in Outlook Questionnaire (Hawley & Joseph, 2008). A prospective study of 95 ABI survivors found that one-third of the sample experienced an improved quality of life rating post-injury compared to pre-injury (Gould & Ponsford, 2014). This evidence suggests that an estimated 30-50% of survivors seem to experience adaptive and positive adjustment following their injury. Although this estimate is based on a limited number of studies, due to their relatively large samples and prospective designs their findings are likely to be robust.

PTG is both a process and an outcome, it develops over time, commencing early in the first-year post-ABI (Silva et al., 2011) and can take ten years post-ABI or longer to be achieved (Goldberg et al., 2019; Powell et al., 2007). A recent study reported that positive attitudes around ABI develop gradually over time since injury, reflecting the accumulation of experiences which promote growth and optimism (Lefkovits et al., 2020). Moreover, time since injury has been found to be a predictor of PTG, whereby the longer the time since injury, the higher the levels of PTG (Grace et al., 2015). However, PTG is thought to commence relatively early following ABI, with one study reporting a modest degree of change in appreciation for life (as measured by the PTG inventory) as early as 6 months post-injury (Silva et al., 2011). Another study found that stroke survivors showed significantly higher psychological growth 21 months following their injury, and qualitative interviews highlighted key roles for increased appreciation for life and more intense and selective relationships, in particular (Kuenemund et al., 2016).

Research has also examined whether PTG in ABI is influenced by the organic neurological damage and its impact, or whether PTG is associated with having experienced an illness/injury more generally. One study compared ABI and myocardial infarction (MCI, i.e., heart attack) survivors but found no significant differences in levels of PTG between these two groups (Karagiorgou et al., 2017). This suggests that experiences of PTG may be similar across medical groups, reflecting a generalized positive change following illness/injury. However, both MCI and ABI can result in cognitive, physical and psychological problems, and thus a more controlled study with diverse control groups is needed to know if there is something unique about organic ABI damage and PTG.

A recent qualitative study sought to understand the *process* of PTG following ABI (Lyon et al., 2020). The authors described the development of PTG as a four-phase process in which survivors move back and forth. These phases were conceptualized "living with a life-changing injury," "trying to beat it and acceptance," "identifying with a new you and others," and "meaningful positive change". The first phase describes the shock and realization of living with the effects of ABI. The second theme captures the importance of accepting and adjusting to limitations and losses. The third stage involves survivors' comparing themselves to their premorbid identity as well as to other individuals with ABI and reflecting on these comparisons to enable acceptance. Finally, these phases enable survivors to begin to grow in positive ways and appreciate things differently.

Factors Contributing to PTG in ABI

A seminal meta-analysis (Grace et al., 2015) explored a range of demographics and variables correlating with PTG in ABI. While some cannot be manipulated through neurorehabilitation (e.g., gender; age; pre-morbid education history; relationship status or injury severity), others may be specifically targeted in clinical interventions (self-understanding, degree of acceptance, increased positive mindset, level of autonomy, sense of personal meaning and a number of positive social ties). Table 32.1 provides a brief overview of how these factors are associated with PTG in ABI, the ABI barriers associated with each factor and suggested interventions that may support people living with ABI to overcome these barriers.

The aforementioned meta-analysis identified participant characteristics associated with PTG in ABI. These include demographics (gender, age, and pre-injury education), severity of injury, being in a relationship, and psychological factors. Firstly, that being

Table 32.1 Factors Associated with PTG in ABI Barriers and Opportunities for Neurorehabilitation

Factor Associated with PTG in ABI	*Barrier in ABI*	*Suggested Interventions to Facilitate Factor*
Level of self-understanding	Feeling lost and confused. Not knowing what to expect from the outcome of ABI (Karagiorgou et al., 2017).	ABI-specific psycho-education (Seeto et al., 2017), songwriting and storytelling (Baker et al., 2018; D'Cruz et al., 2019; Roddy et al., 2018)
Degree of acceptance	Denial is used by ABI survivors to avoid the negative implications of injury and preserve pre-morbid identity (Fleming et al., 2009).	Acceptance and commitment therapy (Ciarrochi et al., 2010); Compassion-based therapy (Freeman et al., 2014)
Increased positive mindset	Increased negative affect, and reduced capacity for positive emotion (Morton & Wehman, 2009).	Peer mentoring (Kersten et al., 2018); Positive psychology (Andrewes et al., 2014; Tulip et al., 2020).
Level of autonomy	ABI commonly restricts activity levels and independence (Grace et al., 2015). Survivors have reported feeling 'powerless' (Seeto et al., 2017).	Psychoeducational groups (Hart et al., 2018); Adapted activity-based groups in the community (Wilkie et al., 2021).
Sense of personal meaning	Long-term disability prevents return to pre-morbid activity at work, home and community. Become deprived of meaningful activity.	Supporting employment (Sekely & Zakzanis, 2018); Facilitating religious or spiritual needs (Gillespie, 2019); Creating an opportunity to help others through peer support groups (Payne et al., 2020).
Number of positive social ties	Increased loneliness and social withdrawal is common in ABI (Kumar et al., 2020; McClure, 2011).	Peer support groups (Hanks et al., 2012; Struchen et al., 2011); Enhancing community participation (Carbonneau et al., 2011); Creating safety via a 'therapeutic milieu' (Ben-Yishay & Daniels-Zide, 2000)

female is associated with greater levels of PTG following ABI supports wider research, which has found higher levels of PTG in women outside the context of ABI (Vishnevsky et al., 2010). Research suggests that coping behavior may meditate this relationship between gender and PTG, as women are more likely than men to engage in adaptive coping strategies post-trauma, such as seeking social support, engaging in deep and reflective thought and positive re-appraisal (Akbar & Witruk, 2016). *Older* ABI survivors report greater levels of PTG (Grace et al., 2015), in agreement with existing literature on finding meaning after stroke (Thompson, 1991). However, this finding in ABI contradicts the PTG literature on non-ABI samples, which has suggested that younger trauma survivors are more likely to experience PTG, as their expectations and worldviews are more likely to be dramatically shattered. A longer *pre-injury education* is also associated with PTG following an ABI (Grace et al., 2015). Education is considered to act as a cognitive reserve, providing educated survivors with a higher level of cognitive functioning following ABI (Satz, 1993).

Interestingly, a *more severe injury* is associated with higher levels of PTG (Grace et al., 2015) with survivors of moderate to severe traumatic brain injury displaying higher levels of PTG relative to samples with mild injury (Sekely & Zakzanis, 2018). It has been suggested that this is because higher levels of impairment cause higher levels of disruption to the survivor's life and sense of self, and the struggle to accommodate this disruption triggers the cognitive processes leading to PTG (Baseotto et al., 2020).

Being in a relationship, providing a support system and opportunities to foster a new sense of identity and self, is also associated with PTG following ABI (Powell et al., 2012). Many studies have highlighted the importance of social connection in the development of PTG following ABI (Allen et al., 2021; Lefkovits et al., 2020; Lyon et al., 2020; Roundhill et al., 2007), especially partners, who can bolster self-esteem (Roundhill et al., 2007). ABI survivors who are more active in the community are more likely to experience PTG due to an increase in social ties and opportunities to find meaning and purpose through community-based activities (Grace et al., 2015).

Psychological factors associated with PTG in ABI provide opportunities for neurorehabilitation to facilitate the emergence of PTG. Firstly, having a sense of understanding (or self-coherence) can facilitate recovery from ABI (Allen et al., 2021; Lyon et al., 2020; Roundhill et al., 2007; Snell et al., 2016). Survivors also note the importance of self-acceptance, adaptation, and perseverance in the face of disability (Allen et al., 2021; Karagiorgou et al., 2017). A positive mindset toward the injury and the future is important for PTG in ABI (Downing et al., 2020; Karagiorgou et al., 2017) as are gratitude, appreciation (Karagiorgou et al., 2017; Kuenemund et al., 2016) and positive subjective beliefs about change post-injury (Grace et al., 2015). Having a sense of autonomy and agency also facilitates PTG following ABI as is having a sense of meaning (Gillespie, 2019; Lyon et al., 2020). A recent study found that PTG was significantly associated with value-directed living following ABI (Baseotto et al., 2020). They attributed this to ABI survivors' living in alignment with their core personal values, which are meaningful to them and their life. This is consistent with Wong's (2007) meaning-management theory, which emphasizes the role of meaning in psychological well-being despite hardship and suffering. Associations between spirituality and positive outcomes have been reported after ABI, including better psychological coping, mental and physical health, life satisfaction, productivity, functional independence, and posttraumatic growth (Gillespie, 2019; Jones et al., 2018; Mahalik et al., 2007).

Interventions to Promote PTG in ABI

The literature suggests that *self-understanding, acceptance, positive mindset, autonomy, meaning, and social ties* may provide opportunities for promoting PTG via neurorehabilitation services that can utilize interventions targeting the aforementioned factors contributing to PTG in ABI in several ways. For example, to increase self-understanding, brain injury-specific psychoeducational courses may help survivors comprehend that the symptoms and implications of their injury are part of their condition rather than a character flaw (Wilkie et al., 2021). Songwriting and storytelling have been found to promote PTG in ABI by focusing on re-conceptualizing changes to the self (Baker et al., 2018; D'Cruz et al., 2019; Roddy et al., 2018). To facilitate survivors' acceptance, neurorehabilitation services may utilize Acceptance and Commitment Therapy (ACT), a key component of which is acknowledging and embracing one's experiences (Ciarrochi et al., 2010). Compassion-based therapies (CFT) encourage compassion towards oneself and increased acceptance of one's own imperfections (Wang et al., 2017). While initial data suggests that CFT might be beneficial for ABI survivors, relevant research is limited (Freeman et al., 2014).

Evidence suggests that an 8-week Positive psychology (PP) group program, aimed to increase a positive mindset, can promote growth in adults with ABI (Tulip et al., 2020). Preliminary qualitative data indicate that adapted surf and cycling groups can increase personal growth, purpose, and environmental mastery to enhance survivors' level of autonomy (Wilkie et al., 2021). Community-based occupational therapy facilitates functional independence in daily activities such as housework, community participation, shopping, and socializing (Sloan et al., 2009).

Several interventions could be used to increase survivors' positive social relationships. One way to increase meaning-finding in ABI survivors is through the use of peer support groups, which enable survivors to share their experiences and feel value in helping others (Ben-Yishay & Daniels-Zide, 2000; Wilkie et al., 2021). Recent qualitative explorations indicate that delivering ABI interventions in a group can aid social relationships as some ABI survivors report feeling more comfortable forming friendships with fellow survivors who understand their experience and limitations (Tulip et al., 2020; Wilkie et al., 2021). Peer-mentoring programs are beneficial for facilitating PTG in ABI survivors, as mentors can share their stories whilst mentees receive support, guidance, and hope (Kersten et al., 2018). Social support groups enable survivors to feel understood rather than judged or embarrassed, helping to positively redefine themselves (Lyon et al., 2020). Meeting fellow survivors of ABI also facilitates a sense of belongingness, contributing to psychosocial well-being (Bay et al., 2002). Feeling safe and supported by neurorehabilitation professionals may facilitate PTG (Downing et al., 2020) as it creates a therapeutic milieu that provides a sense of safety, trust, and cooperation, which promotes adjustment processes and facilitates social participation (Cattelani et al., 2010).

Implications for Models of Neurorehabilitation

In the Western world, healthcare settings are predominantly underpinned by the medical model, which typically aims to reduce impairment by returning the patient to the pre-injury state (Wade & Halligan, 2017). When Tedeschi and Calhoun began their work on PTG in the 1990s, psychology focused on how to 'fix' dysfunction caused by trauma, as opposed to facilitating potential positive and adaptive outcomes (Rendon, 2015). This was also reflected in neurorehabilitation settings, which were historically concerned with the "reduction of disabilities and handicaps" (Wilson, 2002, p. 209). These pathology-focused approaches assume that reducing impairment improves well-being; yet evidence shows that the absence of impairment is not equivalent to well-being (Anderson, 1995). Because ABI is a chronic condition, and its effects are seldom reversed, survivors must learn to adapt and live with at least some degree of impairment. Accordingly, there is a need for neurorehabilitation to create a context for well-being and PTG in addition to reducing impairment.

In the last decade, ABI neurorehabilitation has seen a shift from principles of the traditional medical model of 'fixing what's wrong' towards principles of positive psychology and 'building what's strong' (Evans, 2011). Neurorehabilitation now favors the holistic model, which considers the dynamic relationship between a person and their environment and the psychological, social, cognitive, and physical impact of the injury and associated bi-directional relationships (Ben-Yishay & Daniels-Zide, 2000; Prigatano, 2000; Tate & Pledger, 2003). The holistic model focuses on six key aspects: a therapeutic milieu, a shared understanding, meaningful, functional, goal-directed activities, compensatory and retraining skills, psychological interventions, and working with carers and families (Wilson, 2002).

While the Holistic Model of Neurorehabilitation is more effective than traditional approaches (Cicerone et al., 2008) it may be enhanced further by considering advances in well-being science (Fisher et al., 2020), and reflecting on how facilitation of well-being might support opportunities for PTG. Our GENIAL model of wellbeing (Kemp et al., 2017; Mead et al., 2019, 2021) proposes that the core domains of wellbeing involve the individual (including a balanced mind and a healthy body), community (social connection), the natural environment (connection with nature), behavior change and socio-structural factors (Fisher et al., 2020). Whilst models of well-being commonly focus on individuals (Fredrickson, 2004; Seligman, 2011), there is a lack of emphasis on promoting connection to nature, health behaviors, long-term community integration, and socio-structural factors. For example, reducing behavioral and psychological barriers to social integration through social skills and communication training is common in neurorehabilitation (Struchen et al., 2011), but this does not in itself facilitate new social connections or social cohesion. Survivors need to actively gain opportunities to meet new people, create friendships, get involved in the community and make lasting bonds which are sustained beyond discharge.

Recently a qualitative service evaluation was conducted on a series of neurorehabilitation interventions designed to integrate components of the holistic model with advances in well-being science, using the core components of the GENIAL well-being model (Wilkie et al., 2021). These included community partnerships with third-sector organizations such as 'Bike-ability' and 'Surf-ability' whereby service users attended adapted cycling and surfing lessons with clinicians from the neurorehabilitation service. Also included were group-based psychotherapy, psychoeducational, and a social 'fun' group. ABI participants reported experiencing safety and trust, purpose and achievement, increased social ties including friendships connections, a sense of community, positive emotions and hopefulness, increased sense of meaning and connection to nature. These interventions were unique in that they were able to facilitate many of the aforementioned manipulable factors associated with PTG and well-being. Moreover, partnerships with local community projects meant that survivors had a stepping stone to bridge the gap between rehabilitation in the health service and community integration.

A core feature of this model implemented by the neurorehabilitation service is the dedication to actively secure funding via collaborative efforts between clinical and community staff, making these opportunities available as part of the 'free at the point of entry' National Health

Service (NHS) treatment. Thus, there was no economic barrier preventing ABI patients from accessing the intervention. This illustrates how socio-structural barriers may be overcome by partnering with community providers and highlights the potential utility of designing holistic interventions to facilitate PTG in ABI using advances in well-being science and partnerships across healthcare settings and third-sector, community projects (Wilkie et al., 2021).

Several theoretical questions on the relationship between well-being and PTG require further consideration. Firstly, might interventions designed to build well-being in ABI populations (Tulip et al., 2020; Wilkie et al., 2021) support efforts to facilitate PTG over the longer term (Jayawickreme et al., 2021; Vazquez et al., 2021)? Is PTG a pathway in itself to experiencing well-being following major life adversity or do the constructs of PTG and wellbeing, particularly eudaimonia, refer to the same construct following trauma (Wong, 2011)? Finally, is the relationship between well-being and PTG more complex, perhaps building well-being may promote PTG, which may subsequently sustain this positive change following trauma, consistent with an upward spiral model (Kok et al., 2012; Kok & Fredrickson, 2010). While a detailed discussion of the relationship between well-being and PTG is beyond the scope of the present chapter, further work is needed to clarify the relationship between these related and overlapping constructs.

Overall, it is apparent that PTG can arise in the ABI population, and that there are a range of demographics that increase the likelihood of it occurring (gender; age; pre-morbid education history; relationship status or injury severity). There are a range of manipulable factors associated with PTG in ABI that can be targeted by neurorehabilitation services to facilitate growth (self-coherence; self-acceptance; positive mindset; autonomy and sense of meaning). We propose that there is a relationship between PTG and wellbeing, whereby the factors which promote PTG overlap considerably with those that promote wellbeing. We further suggest that strategies to improve well-being in people living with ABI may facilitate PTG, laying strong foundations for further improvements in well-being in an upward spiral relationship (Kok et al., 2012; Kok & Fredrickson, 2010).

Future research needs to explore the relationship between PTG and well-being in longitudinal, prospective studies that track the process and changes in both well-being and PTG across time, overcoming the limitations of published research, which often relies on retrospective interviews. Future research might also consider cross-cultural comparisons given the difference in value placed on individual versus social connection in individualistic versus collectivist cultures. Finally, given the large amount of emerging evidence on the benefits of nature on wellbeing, connection to nature has the potential to promote experiences of PTG in the ABI population, and should be a priority for future research in this population. We propose that factors associated with PTG in ABI may potentially be categorized according to 'self-connectedness', 'social-connectedness' and 'nature-connectedness', consistent with our recently developed theoretical models (Mead et al., 2021).

References

Akbar, Z., & Witruk, E. (2016). Coping mediates the relationship between gender and posttraumatic growth. *Procedia - Social and Behavioral Sciences*, *217*, 1036–1043. 10.1016/j.sbspro.2016.02.102

Allen, N., Hevey, D., Carton, S., & O'Keeffe, F. (2021). Life is about "constant evolution": The experience of living with an acquired brain injury in individuals who report higher or lower posttraumatic growth. *Disability and Rehabilitation*, 1–14. 10.1080/09638288.2020.1867654

Anderson, R. M. (1995). Patient empowerment and the traditional medical model: A case of irreconcilable differences? *Diabetes Care*, *18*(3), 412–415. 10.2337/diacare.18.3.412

Andrewes, H. E., Walker, V., & O'Neill, B. (2014). Exploring the use of positive psychology interventions in brain injury survivors with challenging behaviour. *Brain Injury*, *28*(7), 965–971. 10.3109/02699052.2014.888764

Baker, F. A., Tamplin, J., Rickard, N., New, P., Ponsford, J., Roddy, C., & Lee, Y.-E. C. (2018). Meaning making process and recovery journeys explored through songwriting in early neurorehabilitation: Exploring the perspectives of participants of their self-composed songs through the interpretative phenomenological analysis. *Frontiers in Psychology*, *9*, 1422. 10.3389/fpsyg.2018.01422

Baseotto, M. C., Morris, P. G., Gillespie, D. C., & Trevethan, C. T. (2020). Post-traumatic growth and value-directed living after acquired brain injury. *Neuropsychological Rehabilitation*, 1–20. 10.1080/09602011.2020.1798254

Bay, E., Hagerty, B. M., Williams, R. A., Kirsch, N., & Gillespie, B. (2002). Chronic stress, sense of belonging, and depression among survivors of traumatic brain injury. *Journal of Nursing Scholarship*, *34*(3), 221–226. 10.1111/j.1547-5069.2002.00221.x

Ben-Yishay, Y., & Daniels-Zide, E. (2000). Examined lives: Outcomes after holistic rehabilitation. *Rehabilitation Psychology*, *45*(2), 112–129. 10.1037/0090-5550.45.2.112

Berman, S. L., Montgomery, M. J., & Ratner, K. (2020). Trauma and identity: A reciprocal relationship? *Journal of Adolescence*, *79*, 275–278. 10.1016/j.adolescence.2020.01.018

Berntsen, D., & Rubin, D. C. (2006). The centrality of event scale: A measure of integrating a trauma into one's identity and its relation to post-traumatic stress disorder symptoms. *Behaviour Research and Therapy*, *44*(2), 219–231. 10.1016/j.brat.2005.01.009

Calhoun, L., & Tedeschi, R. (1999). *Facilitating posttraumatic growth: A clinician's guide*. Routledge.

Carbonneau, H., Martineau, É., Andre, M., & Dawson, D. (2011). Enhancing leisure experiences post traumatic brain injury: A pilot study. *Brain Impairment*, *12*(2), 140–151. 10.1375/brim.12.2.140

Cattelani, R., Zettin, M., & Zoccolotti, P. (2010). Rehabilitation treatments for adults with behavioral and psychosocial disorders following acquired brain injury: A systematic review. *Neuropsychology Review*, *20*(1), 52–85.

Ciarrochi, J., Bilich, L., & Godsell, C. (2010). Psychological flexibility as a mechanism of change in acceptance and commitment therapy. In R. A. Baer (Ed.), *Assessing mindfulness and acceptance processes in clients: Illuminating the theory and practice of change* (pp. 51–75). Context Press/New Harbinger Publications.

Cicerone, K. D., Mott, T., Azulay, J., Sharlow-Galella, M. A., Ellmo, W. J., Paradise, S., & Friel, J. C. (2008). A randomized controlled trial of holistic neuropsychologic rehabilitation after traumatic brain injury. *Archives of Physical Medicine and Rehabilitation*, *89*(12), 2239–2249. 10.1016/j.apmr.2008.06.017

Corrigan, J. D., Selassie, A. W., & Orman, J. A. (Langlois). (2010). The epidemiology of traumatic brain injury. *Journal of Head Trauma Rehabilitation*, *25*(2), 72–80. 10.1097/htr.0b013e3181ccc8b4

D'Cruz, K., Douglas, J., & Serry, T. (2019). Narrative storytelling as both an advocacy tool and a therapeutic process: Perspectives of adult storytellers with acquired brain injury. *Neuropsychological Rehabilitation*, *30*(8), 1409–1429. 10.1080/09602011.2019.1586733

Downing, M., Hicks, A., Braaf, S., Myles, D., Gabbe, B., Cameron, P., Ameratunga, S., & Ponsford, J. (2020). Factors facilitating recovery following severe traumatic brain injury: A qualitative study. *Neuropsychological Rehabilitation*, 1–25. 10.1080/09602011.2020.1744453

Evans, J. J. (2011). Positive psychology and brain injury rehabilitation. *Brain Impairment*, *12*(2), 117–127. 10.1375/brim.12.2.117

Fisher, Z., Galloghly, E., Boglo, E., Gracey, F., & Kemp, A. (2020). Emotion, wellbeing and the neurological disorders. In *Reference module in neuroscience and biobehavioral psychology*. Amsterdam: Elsevier. 10.1016/b978-0-12-819641-0.00013-x

Fisher, Z., Galloghly, E., Boglo, E., & Kemp, A. H. (2020). Emotion, wellbeing and the neurological disorders. In *Reference module in neuroscience and biobehavioral psychology*. Amsterdam: Elsevier. 10.1016/b978-0-12-819641-0.00013-x

Fitzgerald, J. M., Berntsen, D., & Broadbridge, C. L. (2016). The influences of event centrality in memory models of PTSD. *Applied Cognitive Psychology*, *30*(1), 10–21. 10.1002/acp.3160

Fleming, J. M., Strong, J., & Ashton, R. (2009). Self-awareness of deficits in adults with traumatic brain injury: How best to measure? *Brain Injury*, *10*(1), 1–16. 10.1080/026990596124674
Fredrickson, B. L. (2004). The broaden-and-build theory of positive emotions. *Philosophical Transactions of the Royal Society of London. Series B: Biological Sciences*, *359*(1449), 1367–1377. 10.1098/rstb.2004.1512
Freeman, A., Adams, M., & Ashworth, F. (2014). An exploration of the experience of self in the social world for men following traumatic brain injury. *Neuropsychological Rehabilitation*, *25*(2), 189–215. 10.1080/09602011.2014.917686
Gillespie, E. (2019). A qualitative pilot study of spirituality in long-term recovery in acquired brain injury. *Journal of Pastoral Care & Counseling*, *73*(2), 96–105. 10.1177/1542305019853588
Glenn, M. B., O'Neil-Pirozzi, T., Goldstein, R., Burke, D., & Jacob, L. (2009). Depression amongst outpatients with traumatic brain injury. *Brain Injury*, *15*(9), 811–818. 10.1080/02699050120330
Goldberg, L. D., McDonald, S. D., & Perrin, P. B. (2019). Predicting trajectories of posttraumatic growth following acquired physical disability. *Rehabilitation Psychology*, *64*(1), 37–49. 10.1037/rep0000247
Gould, K. R., & Ponsford, J. L. (2014). A longitudinal examination of positive changes in quality-of-life after traumatic brain injury. *Brain Injury*, *29*(3), 283–290. 10.3109/02699052.2014.974671
Grace, J. J., Kinsella, E. L., Muldoon, O. T., & Fortune, D. G. (2015). Post-traumatic growth following acquired brain injury: A systematic review and meta-analysis. *Frontiers in Psychology*, *6*, 1162. 10.3389/fpsyg.2015.01162
Gracey, F., Evans, J. J., & Malley, D. (2009). Capturing process and outcome in complex rehabilitation interventions: A "Y-shaped" model. *Neuropsychological Rehabilitation*, *19*(6), 867–890. 10.1080/09602010903027763
Hanks, R. A., Rapport, L. J., Wertheimer, J., & Koviak, C. (2012). Randomized controlled trial of peer mentoring for individuals with traumatic brain injury and their significant others. *Archives of Physical Medicine and Rehabilitation*, *93*(8), 1297–1304. 10.1016/j.apmr.2012.04.027
Hart, T., Driver, S., Sander, A., Pappadis, M., Dams-O'Connor, K., Bocage, C., Hinkens, E., Dahdah, M. N., & Cai, X. (2018). Traumatic brain injury education for adult patients and families: A scoping review. *Brain Injury*, *32*(11), 1–12. 10.1080/02699052.2018.1493226
Hawley, C. A., & Joseph, S. (2008). Predictors of positive growth after traumatic brain injury: A longitudinal study. *Brain Injury*, *22*(5), 427–435. 10.1080/02699050802064607
James, S. L., Theadom, A., Ellenbogen, R. G., Bannick, M. S., Montjoy-Venning, W., Lucchesi, L. R., Abbasi, N., Abdulkader, R., Abraha, H. N., Adsuar, J. C., Afarideh, M., Agrawal, S., Ahmadi, A., Ahmed, M. B., Aichour, A. N., Aichour, I., Aichour, M. T. E., Akinyemi, R. O., Akseer, N., ... Murray, C. J. L. (2019). Global, regional, and national burden of traumatic brain injury and spinal cord injury, 1990–2016: A systematic analysis for the Global Burden of Disease Study 2016. *The Lancet Neurology*, *18*(1), 56–87. 10.1016/s1474-4422(18)30415-0
Jayawickreme, E., Infurna, F. J., Alajak, K., Blackie, L. E. R., Chopik, W. J., Chung, J. M., Dorfman, A., Fleeson, W., Forgeard, M. J. C., Frazier, P., Furr, R. M., Grossmann, I., Heller, A. S., Laceulle, O. M., Lucas, R. E., Luhmann, M., Luong, G., Meijer, L., McLean, K. C., Park, C. L., Roepke, A. M., al Sawaf, Z., Tennen, H., White, R. M. B., & Zonneveld, R. (2021). Post-traumatic growth as positive personality change: Challenges, opportunities, and recommendations. *Journal of Personality*, *89*(1), 145–165. 10.1111/jopy.12591
Jones, K. F., Pryor, J., Care-Unger, C., & Simpson, G. K. (2018). Spirituality and its relationship with positive adjustment following traumatic brain injury: A scoping review. *Brain Injury*, *32*(13–14), 1–11. 10.1080/02699052.2018.1511066
Jorge, R. E., Robinson, R. G., Moser, D., Tateno, A., Crespo-Facorro, B., & Arndt, S. (2004). Major depression following traumatic brain injury. *Archives of General Psychiatry*, *61*(1), 42–50. 10.1001/archpsyc.61.1.42
Karagiorgou, O., Evans, J. J., & Cullen, B. (2017). Post-traumatic growth in adult survivors of brain injury: A qualitative study of participants completing a pilot trial of brief positive psychotherapy. *Disability and Rehabilitation*, *40*(6), 1–8. 10.1080/09638288.2016.1274337
Kemp A. H., Arias J. A., & Fisher Z. (2017) Social ties, health and wellbeing: A literature review and model. In A. Ibáñez, L. Sedeño, & A. García (Eds.), *Neuroscience and social science* (pp. 397–427). Cham: Springer. https://doi-org.libproxy.adelphi.edu/10.1007/978-3-319-68421-5_17

Kersten, P., Cummins, C., Kayes, N., Babbage, D., Elder, H., Foster, A., Weatherall, M., Siegert, R. J., Smith, G., & McPherson, K. (2018). Making sense of recovery after traumatic brain injury through a peer mentoring intervention: A qualitative exploration. *BMJ Open*, *8*(10), e020672. 10.1136/bmjopen-2017-020672

Kok, B. E., Coffey, K. A., Cohn, M. A., Catalino, L. I., Vacharkulksemsuk, T., Algoe, S. B., Brantley, M., & Fredrickson, B. L. (2012). How positive emotions build physical health. *Psychological Science*, *24*(7), 1123–1132. 10.1177/0956797612470827

Kok, B. E., & Fredrickson, B. L. (2010). Upward spirals of the heart: Autonomic flexibility, as indexed by vagal tone, reciprocally and prospectively predicts positive emotions and social connectedness. *Biological Psychology*, *85*(3), 432–436. 10.1016/j.biopsycho.2010.09.005

Kuenemund, A., Zwick, S., Rief, W., & Exner, C. (2016). (Re-)defining the self – Enhanced posttraumatic growth and event centrality in stroke survivors: A mixed-method approach and control comparison study. *Journal of Health Psychology*, *21*(5), 679–689. 10.1177/1359105314535457

Kumar, R. G., Ornstein, K. A., Bollens-Lund, E., Watson, E. M., Ankuda, C. K., Kelley, A. S., & Dams-O'Connor, K. (2020). Lifetime history of traumatic brain injury is associated with increased loneliness in adults: A US nationally representative study. *International Journal of Geriatric Psychiatry*, *35*(5), 553–563. 10.1002/gps.5271

Lefkovits, A. M., Hicks, A. J., Downing, M., & Ponsford, J. (2020). Surviving the "silent epidemic": A qualitative exploration of the long-term journey after traumatic brain injury. *Neuropsychological Rehabilitation*, 1–25. 10.1080/09602011.2020.1787849

Lyon, I., Fisher, P., & Gracey, F. (2020). "Putting a new perspective on life": A qualitative grounded theory of posttraumatic growth following acquired brain injury. *Disability and Rehabilitation*, 1–9. 10.1080/09638288.2020.1741699

Mahalik, J. L., Johnstone, B., Glass, B., & Yoon, D. P. (2007). Spirituality, psychological coping, and community integration for persons with traumatic brain injury. *Journal of Religion, Disability & Health*, *11*(3), 65–77. 10.1300/j095v11n03_06

McClure, J. (2011). The role of causal attributions in public misconceptions about brain injury. *Rehabilitation Psychology*, *56*(2), 85–93. 10.1037/a0023354

McLellan, T., Bishop, A., & McKinlay, A. (2010). Community attitudes toward individuals with traumatic brain injury. *Journal of the International Neuropsychological Society*, *16*(4), 705–710. 10.1017/s1355617710000524

Mead, J., Fisher, Z., Tree, J., Wong, P. J., & Kemp, A. H. (2021). Protectors of wellbeing during the COVID-19 pandemic: Key roles for gratitude and tragic optimism in a UK-based cohort. *Frontiers in Psychology*. 10.3389/fpsyg.2021.647951

Mead, J., Fisher, Z., Wilkie, L., Gibbs, K., Pridmore, J., Tree, J., & Kemp, A. (2019). Rethinking wellbeing: Toward a more ethical science of wellbeing that considers current and future generations. *Authorea*. 10.22541/au.156649190.08734276

Morton, M. V., & Wehman, P. (2009). Psychosocial and emotional sequelae of individuals with traumatic brain injury: a literature review and recommendations. *Brain Injury*, *9*(1), 81–92. 10.3109/02699059509004574

NICE (2019). *National institute for health and care excellence (UK) clinical guidelines* (Vol. 176). NICE.

Nochi, M. (1998). "Loss of self" in the narratives of people with traumatic brain injuries: A qualitative analysis. *Social Science & Medicine*, *46*(7), 869–878. 10.1016/s0277-9536(97)00211-6

Osborn, A. J., Mathias, J. L., & Fairweather-Schmidt, A. K. (2014). Depression following adult, non-penetrating traumatic brain injury: A meta-analysis examining methodological variables and sample characteristics. *Neuroscience & Biobehavioral Reviews*, *47*, 1–15. 10.1016/j.neubiorev.2014.07.007

Ownsworth, T., & Haslam, C. (2014). Impact of rehabilitation on self-concept following traumatic brain injury: An exploratory systematic review of intervention methodology and efficacy. *Neuropsychological Rehabilitation*, *26*(1), 1–35. 10.1080/09602011.2014.977924

Payne, L., Hawley, L., Morey, C., Ketchum, J. M., Philippus, A., Sevigny, M., Harrison-Felix, C., & Diener, E. (2020). Improving well-being after traumatic brain injury through volunteering: A randomized controlled trial. *Brain Injury*, *34*(6), 697–707. 10.1080/02699052.2020.1752937

Powell, T., Ekin-Wood, A., & Collin, C. (2007). Post-traumatic growth after head injury: A long-term follow-up. *Brain Injury*, *21*(1), 31–38. 10.1080/02699050601106245

Powell, T., Gilson, R., & Collin, C. (2012). TBI 13 years on: Factors associated with post-traumatic growth. *Disability and Rehabilitation*, *34*(17), 1461–1467. 10.3109/09638288.2011.644384
Prigatano, G. P. (2000). A brief overview of four principles of neuropsychological rehabilitation. In A. L. Christensen, & B. P. Uzzell (Eds.), *International handbook of neuropsychological rehabilitation. Critical Issues in Neuropsychology* (pp. 115–125). Boston, MA: Springer. 10.1007/978-1-4757-5569-5_7
Rendon, J. (2015). *Upside: The new science of post-traumatic growth*. NY: Simon and Schuster.
Roddy, C., Rickard, N., Tamplin, J., Lee, Y.-E. C., & Baker, F. A. (2018). Exploring self-concept, wellbeing and distress in therapeutic songwriting participants following acquired brain injury: A case series analysis. *Neuropsychological Rehabilitation*, *30*(2), 1–21. 10.1080/09602011.2018.1448288
Roundhill, S. J., Williams, W. H., & Hughes, J. M. (2007). The experience of loss following traumatic brain injury: Applying a bereavement model to the process of adjustment. *Qualitative Research in Psychology*, *4*(3), 241–257. 10.1080/14780880701473540
Satz, P. (1993). Brain reserve capacity on symptom onset after brain injury: A formulation and review of evidence for threshold theory. *Neuropsychology*, *7*(3), 273–295. 10.1037/0894-4105.7.3.273
Seeto, E., Scruby, K., & Greenhill, T. (2017). 'Your whole life becomes a recovery': Experiences of young adults following acquired brain injury. *Counselling Psychology Review*, *4*(32), 39–48.
Sekely, A., & Zakzanis, K. K. (2018). The relationship between post-traumatic growth and return to work following mild traumatic brain injury. *Disability and Rehabilitation*, *41*(22), 1–7. 10.1080/09638288.2018.1476598
Seligman, M. (2011). *Flourish: A visionary new understanding of happiness and well-being*. Free Press.
Silva, J., Ownsworth, T., Shields, C., & Fleming, J. (2011). Enhanced appreciation of life following acquired brain injury: Posttraumatic growth at 6 months post discharge. *Brain Impairment*, *12*(2), 93–104. 10.1375/brim.12.2.93
Sloan, S., Callaway, L., Winkler, D., McKinley, K., Ziino, C., & Anson, K. (2009). Changes in care and support needs following community-based intervention for individuals with acquired brain injury. *Brain Impairment*, *10*(3), 295–306.
Snell, D. L., Martin, R., Surgenor, L. J., Siegert, R. J., & Hay-Smith, E. J. C. (2016). What's wrong with me? Seeking a coherent understanding of recovery after mild traumatic brain injury. *Disability and Rehabilitation*, *39*(19), 1–8. 10.1080/09638288.2016.1213895
Struchen, M. A., Davis, L. C., Bogaards, J. A., Hudler-Hull, T., Clark, A. N., Mazzei, D. M., Sander, A. M., & Caroselli, J. S. (2011). Making connections after brain injury. *Journal of Head Trauma Rehabilitation*, *26*(1), 4–19. 10.1097/htr.0b013e3182048e98
Tate, D. G., & Pledger, C. (2003). An integrative conceptual framework of disability. *American Psychologist*, *58*(4), 289–295. 10.1037/0003-066x.58.4.289
Teasdale, T. W., & Engberg, A. W. (2001). Suicide after traumatic brain injury: A population study. *Journal of Neurology, Neurosurgery & Psychiatry*, *71*(4), 436. 10.1136/jnnp.71.4.436
Thompson, S. C. (1991). The search for meaning following a stroke. *Basic and Applied Social Psychology*, *12*(1), 81–96. 10.1207/s15324834basp1201_6
Tulip, C., Fisher, Z., Bankhead, H., Wilkie, L., Pridmore, J., Gracey, F., Tree, J., & Kemp, A. H. (2020). Building wellbeing in people with chronic conditions: A qualitative evaluation of an 8-week positive psychotherapy intervention for people living with an acquired brain injury. *Frontiers in Psychology*, *11*, 66. 10.3389/fpsyg.2020.00066
Vazquez, C., Valiente, C., García, F. E., Contreras, A., Peinado, V., Trucharte, A., & Bentall, R. P. (2021). Post-traumatic growth and stress-related responses during the COVID-19 pandemic in a national representative sample: The role of positive core beliefs about the world and others. *Journal of Happiness Studies*, 1–21. 10.1007/s10902-020-00352-3
Vishnevsky, T., Cann, A., Calhoun, L. G., Tedeschi, R. G., & Demakis, G. J. (2010). Gender differences in self-reported posttraumatic growth: A meta-analysis. *Psychology of Women Quarterly*, *34*(1), 110–120. 10.1111/j.1471-6402.2009.01546.x
Wade, D. T., & Halligan, P. W. (2017). The biopsychosocial model of illness: A model whose time has come. *Clinical Rehabilitation*, *31*(8), 995–1004. 10.1177/0269215517709890
Wang, X., Chen, Z., Poon, K.-T., Teng, F., & Jin, S. (2017). Self-compassion decreases acceptance of own immoral behaviors. *Personality and Individual Differences*, *106*, 329–333. 10.1016/j.paid.2016.10.030

Wilkie, L., Arroyo, P., Conibeer, H., Kemp, A. H., & Fisher, Z. (2021). The impact of psycho-social interventions on the wellbeing of individuals with acquired brain injury during the COVID-19 pandemic. *Frontiers in Psychology*, *12*, 648286. 10.3389/fpsyg.2021.648286

Wilson, B. A. (2002). Cognitive rehabilitation in the 21st century. *Neurorehabilitation and Neural Repair*, *16*(2), 207–210. 10.1177/088843900201600203

Wong, P. (2011). Positive psychology 2.0: Towards a balanced interactive model of the good life. *Canadian Psychology/Psychologie Canadienne*, *52*(2), 69–81. 10.1037/a0022511

Wong, P. T. P. (2007). Meaning management theory and death acceptance. In A. Tomer, E. Grafton, & P. T. P. Wong (Eds.), *Existential and spiritual issues in death attitudes* (pp. 65–87). Erlbaum.

Yeates, G. N., Gracey, F., & Mcgrath, J. C. (2008). A biopsychosocial deconstruction of "personality change" following acquired brain injury. *Neuropsychological Rehabilitation*, *18*(5–6), 566–589. 10.1080/09602010802151532

33
ADVERSARIAL GROWTH IN PERSONS WITH VISION IMPAIRMENT

Bozena Maria Sztonyk

The Nature, Prevalence, and Impact of Vision Loss

Visual Impairment (VI) is the substantial and often irreversible loss of one or more functions of the visual system. VI is a multifaceted and highly heterogeneous condition in terms of the visual function affected, onset age, severity, cause, and prognosis of vision loss. It can be congenital or acquired (Brunes & Heir, 2020b; Colenbrander, 2010). The International Classification of Diseases (ICD-11) indicates that VI results when an eye condition affects the visual system and one or more of its vision functions. Hence, it is measured by visual acuity, and severity is categorized as mild, moderate or severe distance vision impairment or blindness, and near vision impairment (World Health Organization, 1992).

Prevalence

It is estimated that at least 2.2 billion people around the world have a VI of whom at least 1 billion have a VI that could have been prevented (World Health Organization, 2019). Recent statistics show that in 2020, an estimated 43.3 million people were blind, of whom 23.9 were female. About 295 million people had moderate and severe VI, of whom 163 million were female; 258 million had a mild VI, of whom 142 million were female; and 510 million had VI from uncorrected presbyopia (the gradual loss of the eyes' ability to focus on nearby objects), of whom 280 million were female (Bourne et al., 2021). It is predicted that by 2050 about 61 million people will be blind, 472 million will have moderate and severe VI, 360 million will have mild VI and 866 million will be with presbyopia (Bourne et al., 2021). Further, for many the prospect is for their vision to progressively worsen over time (Boerner et al., 2006).

Impact

The loss of vision results in a physical disability that can occur at any point across the lifespan and often dramatically alter a person's life. The experience of vision loss is potentially traumatic and can have major implications for people coping with it as well as

 DOI: 10.4324/9781032208688-42

for people close to them. Moreover, the condition entails a higher risk of experiencing additional types of potentially traumatic events (PTEs) than the general population, especially threats in everyday life that may impact mental health. The increased exposure to PTE is said to be related to vision being a key sensory modality in obtaining rapid and precise information and VI could affect one's ability to predict, prepare for, and flee from dangerous and life-threatening situations (Brunes et al., 2019a, 2019b).

While vision loss itself does not meet the diagnostic criteria for a traumatic experience, PTSD in people with VI is likely to be a result of traumatic events related to it. As VI may increase vulnerability and aggravate posttraumatic stress reactions, a systematic review revealed a prevalence of PTSD in those with VI from 4% to 50% (van der Ham et al., 2021). Loss of vision in adulthood may have a negative impact on well-being and quality of life. For example, adults with VI are generally less physically active due to lower self-efficacy (Haegele et al., 2018). VI increases the risk of mental health problems and affects social participation. However, within the VI population, there is considerable variation in well-being, physical, and mental health, and the relationship between the severity of impairment and the impact on well-being is complex. When individuals are informed about their sight loss, they first experience emotional distress. Negative emotions ensue such as shock, anxiety, fear, anger, denial or disbelief, depression, self-pity, loss of self-esteem, withdrawal, and eventually, after considerable time, a realistic acceptance (Hernandez Trillo & Dickinson, 2012; Senra et al., 2015). The implications of VI are manifold, especially in relation to daily tasks, which are based on visual stimuli. The perception of vision loss is usually a challenging process that requires making sense of the diagnosis and includes major changes in one's life. These changes are often emotionally distressing, as people experience additional losses such as increased dependence on others and limited ability to work, read, walk, cook and drive leading to identity changes.

A developmental perspective emphasizes that to understand adaptation to functional loss due to a physical impairment such as the loss of vision, it is important to consider the stage in life and the context in which a challenge occurs, which internal and external conditions are involved and whether the event is non-normative, all of which shape the experience and its outcomes (Boerner & Wang, 2010). The risk of developing mental health problems for those who lose vision as adults tend to be higher for younger and middle-aged individuals because ultimately the loss of vision interferes with the pursuit of life goals (e.g., career goals, supporting a family), which may lead to significant interruptions of daily routine and emotional distress (Boerner & Wang, 2010; Elsman et al., 2017).

Empirical evidence shows that VI interferes the most with functional and relationship goals and the least with life philosophy-religion goals (Boerner, 2004; Boerner & Cimarolli, 2005; Boerner & Wang, 2010). A study of the views of young and middle-aged persons with VI on life changes due to vision loss, specifically relative to goals, self-views, worldview, and relationships with others found that middle-aged adults reported experiencing more positive changes than their older counterparts (Boerner & Wang, 2010). For some, these life changes were gradual, whereas for others the nature of the change was far more drastic (Popivker et al., 2010).

Psychological adjustment to VI can have a significant impact on individuals' rehabilitation outcomes and quality of life (QoL). Most of the studies on QoL conducted on middle-aged and older populations with VI emphasize that these populations have a higher risk of depression and report less satisfaction than their sighted counterparts (Brown & Barrett, 2011; Brunes & Heir, 2020a, 2020b; Demmin & Silverstein, 2020). Depression in the populations with VI is often unrecognized and untreated and many VI persons do not seek professional help due to inaccessible environments and the stigma attached to being blind (Brunes & Heir, 2020a, 2020b). A meta-analysis of studies reported an estimated prevalence varying between 5% and 57% (mean of 25%) of depression or depressive symptoms in people with vision-related conditions (Zheng et al., 2017).

Social isolation, lower perceived social support, lower feelings of self-efficacy, and experiences of adverse events (particularly bullying and abuse) are independently associated with depressive symptoms in VI (Brunes & Heir, 2020a, 2020b; Horowitz et al., 2005). This population is at risk of social exclusion and experiences a higher probability of bullying than the general population (Brunes et al., 2018). Bullying is predominant among individuals with low vision and blindness and especially among those who are young, in early onset age of VI and experiencing additional impairments. Brunes et al. (2018) also pointed to strong associations between lifetime bullying and lower self-efficacy and life satisfaction.

While loneliness is a higher risk for individuals with VI across all age groups, it is strongly associated with young age, severe degree of impairment, unemployment and past exposure to bullying or abuse and a lower level of life satisfaction (Brunes et al., 2019a, 2019b). Therefore, depressed young adults have considerably lower life satisfaction due to their experiences of discrimination and handling stigma, loneliness and isolation (Brunes & Heir, 2020b).

Psychosocial Resources in the Aftermath of Vision Loss

A range of psychosocial resources, specifically those related to control, play a significant role in stress resistance and growth (Hobfoll, 2002). They include self-efficacy, adopting positive attitudes and outlooks, greater acceptance of the condition, effective coping strategies including developing problem-solving strategies, use of assistive aids (Senra et al., 2015), and social support.

Self-efficacy tends to be found in individuals who are stress-resistant and more likely to exercise successful influence over their environment and the accomplishment of their goals. Studies of adults with VI found that they had higher levels of self-efficacy than the general population (Brunes et al., 2021) and that self-efficacy accounted for about 35% of the effect of VI on depressive symptoms and over 60% of the effect on life satisfaction in older adults (Brown & Barrett, 2011). This higher self-efficacy in VI may arise from extensive mastery experience in managing life with reduced vision (Brunes et al., 2021). Reinhardt et al. (2009) confirmed that focusing on the reality of the condition of one's vision, and on personal strength can facilitate adjustment. Having additional impairments and a previous history of physical and sexual assault were associated with lower self-efficacy whereas higher education and living in an urban municipality were associated with higher self-efficacy (Brunes et al., 2021).

Coping strategies identified as effective in adaptation to sight loss are *assimilative*, i.e., efforts to change one's situation in the face of obstacles in order to pursue goals, and *accommodative*, i.e., re-evaluation of goals, and disengagement from goals that are no longer feasible (Boerner & Wang, 2012). While these coping strategies are not mutually exclusive, they generally represent somewhat antagonistic thought processes (Brandtstädter & Rothermund, 2002). Studies that focused on examining whether accommodative or assimilative coping strategies serve best in dealing with vision loss have shown that accommodative coping facilitated positive adjustment to losses. Accommodative coping involved re-evaluation of goals, and disengagement from goals that are no longer feasible (Boerner & Wang, 2012). A study on middle-aged adults with VI found that an effective rehabilitation process depends on assimilation in goal-specific coping, while general coping tendencies were higher when accommodative modes were used (Boerner & Wang, 2012).

Social support plays an important role in helping individuals with VI to optimize their resources to effectively cope with troubling conditions (Ogińska-Bulik, 2013). Studies of the role of social support at the initial time of vision loss stressed the importance of affective friends and support in adaptation to vision loss (Reinhardt et al., 2009). The most valuable support is motivating people to take responsibility for their lives (Joseph, 2013). Cimarolli and Boerner (2005) who explored both positive and negative aspects of social support and their links to the well-being of working-age adults with VI, found that instrumental help from family members was the most frequent type of positive support received while underestimating the VI persons' capabilities was the most frequent type of negative experience. Less-optimal well-being was linked with experiencing a lack of support and with receiving only negative social exchanges that may have a negative impact on recipients' mental health. For example, overprotective attitudes may affect negatively age-related adjustment to vision loss. McIlvane and Reinhardt (2001) who explored the interactive effects of social support showed that women with high support from both friends and family had better psychological well-being. This confirms prior findings that it is the quality of social relationships, rather than the quantity of network members that enhances psychological functioning (Newsom & Schulz, 1996). Wang and Boerner (2008) reported that adults who lost their vision had difficulties in staying socially connected due to other people's lack of understanding and/or their own lack of visual cues. Responses to these challenges included readjusting own behavior to maintain relationships (e.g., explaining themselves more and being more assertive, relying on other senses for information) or letting relationships turn sour (withdrawing and making fewer initiatives to socialize or getting angry and telling people off).

Understanding Growth through the Lens of the Organismic Valuing Theory of Growth

The Organismic Valuing Theory of Growth through Adversity (OV) was conceptualized by Joseph and Linley (2005, 2008) as a comprehensive perspective aligned with a wider view of positive psychology, giving equal importance to potential positive and negative changes in integrating human experience (Joseph et al., 2012; Linley & Joseph, 2004). Consistent with this wider perception, they posit that the relationship between stress, PTSD and PTG is curvilinear (Joseph et al., 2012), i.e., stress is viewed as the catalyst of growth which does not eliminate one's feeling of sadness, while potentially contributing to greater personal wisdom (Linley, 2003). They view growth as being about personality development, i.e., how people develop an understanding of their place and significance in the world and engage with the existential challenges of life, such as trauma (Joseph & Linley, 2008).

According to OV theory, characteristics of growth related to psychological well-being (PWB) are closer relationships, greater self-acceptance, and deeper spirituality (Joseph & Linley, 2008; Ryff & Singer, 1996). Ryff (1989) explained that PWB comprises self-acceptance, environmental mastery, personal growth, autonomy, positive relations with others, and having a purpose in life. Thus, PWB's dimensions can be associated with three domains of PTG, i.e., changes in life philosophy, changes in a perception of self that indicates recognition of new possibilities in one's life or taking a new and different path in life (Tedeschi & Calhoun, 2004), and changes in relationships with others (Joseph & Linley, 2008). OV theory proposes observing growth following traumatic events as moving toward greater authenticity in living that leads to greater PWB (Joseph & Linley, 2005).

Joseph and Linley (2005, 2008) posit that while people are intrinsically motivated toward positive accommodation, some circumstances and environments may restrict, impede, or distort these intrinsic processes. New trauma-related information can either be assimilated within existing models of the world (e.g., self-blame for misfortune or the disengagement with the significance of the event), or existing models of the world may accommodate the new trauma-related information. Individuals who seek to accommodate their traumatic experience in a new way, modify their existing models and change their worldviews, whether that change is in a positive or a negative direction. When the experiences are accommodated in a negative direction, they lead to problems such as depression and helplessness. When the experiences are accommodated in a positive direction, they lead to growth (i.e., valuing relationships, and appreciating life).

The process of "assimilation or accommodation is influenced by the extent to which people have a supportive social environment and a malleable personality schema that is open to revision" (Joseph & Linley, 2008, p. 14). Assimilation or accommodation can be seen as the outcome and as the direction of processing, which takes time to develop and continue across the lifespan. Thus, a person cannot reach an endpoint at which processing ceases. Furthermore, these processes are multifaceted as a person may emotionally process experiences in one direction, and some facets of self-structure can be accommodated, while other experiences may be assimilated. Joseph and Linley (2008) claim that these directions of processing are not mutually exclusive. Accommodating may be challenging and requires a supportive social environment that facilitates the satisfaction of basic psychological needs for autonomy, competence, and relatedness. Figure 33.1 presents the theory schematically.

Posttraumatic Growth Following Vision Impairment

Limited research exists regarding transformational growth following vision loss in adulthood. Tedeschi and Calhoun (2004) formulated PTG as an experience in which growth and distress can coexist and positive changes predominate over negative changes. This notion was questioned by Wortman (2004) who emphasized the need to consider the impact of negative changes alongside positive changes and argued that most people are diminished, rather than enhanced, by tragedy. The aforementioned study by Boerner and colleagues (2006) on people with VI supported the notion that both positive and negative changes may occur following loss of vision. However, they found that the majority of changes were in-between changes, as opposed to no changes at all, and more negative than positive changes. They explained that their finding may differ as the nature of diseases and subsequent implications are different than other adversities; for example, while cancer patients face mortality, people who experience vision loss face this ongoing adversity throughout their life. Moreover, they face the prospect of their vision loss getting progressively worse over time, which differs from the situation of those who deal with one-time traumas and losses.

Boerner and colleagues (2006) concluded that the most common positive change following the experience of vision loss is that individuals were more likely to discover new aspects of the world that they did not know existed. Positive changes required a proper

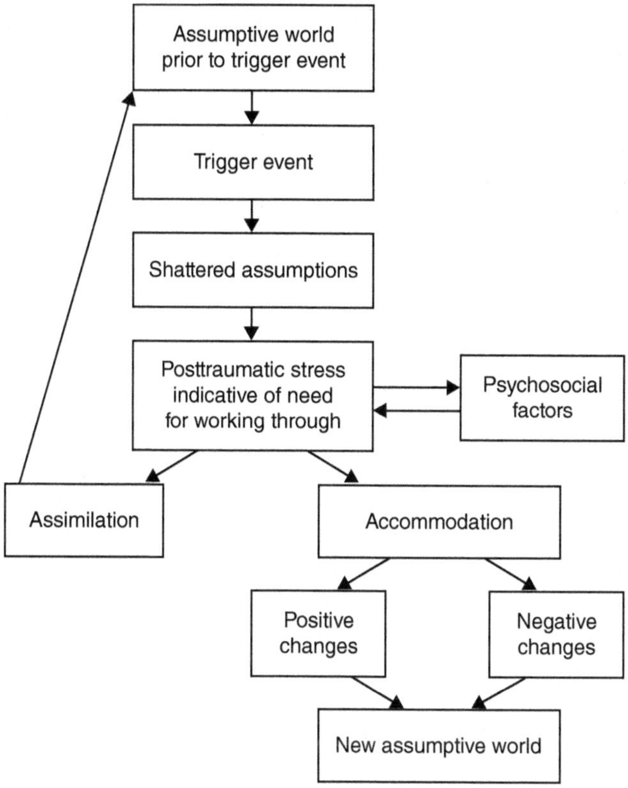

Figure 33.1 Organismic Valuing Theory of Growth through Adversity (Joseph & Linley, 2008, p. 13).

understanding of the situation and implications of vision loss for people at different ages during adulthood can be unique in some regards and similar in others.

Findings from studies on populations with vision loss support the notion that both positive and negative changes occur; however negative changes may prevail in the VI population. A qualitative study of 10 participants with a visual impairment from chronic illness or serious injury yielded a four stages model of trauma and recovery: apprehension, diagnosis and devastation, choosing to go, building a way to live, and integration of the trauma and expansion of the self (Salick & Auerbach, 2006). In the last stage, participants reported integration of their pre-and post-trauma lives via processes of moving forward by coming to terms with the disability in the context of rebuilding life (commitment to life), being involved in giving back in response to feeling empowered to contribute to a social or world community, finding based on their own suffering and experience new empathy, sense of compassion for others, increased sense of purpose, and meaningful goals. Interviewees recognized benefits in their adversity and an increased sense of self and emotional experiences. Nevertheless, for most participants, this final stage of growth integrated both positive and negative aspects of their becoming disabled.

Research on the experience of the population with VI demonstrates that reported growth after vision loss shares some similarities with the existing model of PTG. Tanner and colleagues (2020) conducted a mixed-method study of the experience of VI population with severe related macular degeneration (AMD) and found that in addition to negative outcomes, participants also reported an increased sense of personal strength, spirituality, and empathy for others, all of which are domains of PTG. The findings of this study pointed to the importance of supporting others and deliberate cognitive processing in experiencing PTG. In a study of bullying as a potential precursor to PTG in adults and children with VI, Ratcliff et al. (2017) found that both adults and children spontaneously reported PTG in response to their bullying experiences, suggesting that bullying experiences may engender growth in personal strength or the sense of personal capacity to flourish.

A Case Study

This section focuses on one' woman's story of losing her vision and gaining benefits from the struggle with this loss. Joanna, 57 years old, is a professor at a university in Poland. She was born with a cataract that was corrected when she was one year old. The surgery gave her an opportunity to function with low vision and attend a regular school rather than being sent to one of the few boarding schools for blind children. A year after graduating from the university at the age of 25, she had to undergo an operation because of glaucoma. The operation was unsuccessful due to an infection and Joanna lost her vision. Joanna scored 90 out of a total possible score of 105 on the Posttraumatic Growth Inventory (Tedeschi & Calhoun, 1996). In an in-depth interview she shared the process of transformational change she experienced (Sztonyk & Formella, 2020). Joanna's story is examined to explore the impact of vision loss and experiences upon her life with a focus on the transformational aspects of these experiences. The aforementioned Organismic Valuing Theory of Growth through Adversity (OV) serves as a lens to guide the analysis of the interview. Joanna's story illustrates many of the empirical findings reported above. The direct quotes from the interview are brought with no editing to maintain the authentic tone of her account.

Joanna's growth in the aftermath of vision loss demonstrated a sequential process, from a negative traumatic experience to the gradual discovery of positive changes in different dimensions of life, but most of all a sense of gained personal strength reflected in her sharing of her life paradox: *Despite the loss of independence, I am stronger and more courageous now.* Joanna's life story illustrates the theoretical and empirical knowledge as to how the struggle that leads to adversarial growth is first a struggle to survive and cope and that growth tends to be unplanned and unexpected.

Joanna's view of positive changes in the aftermath of her vision loss was related to three areas that correspond to domains of PTG, i.e., personal strength, heightened appreciation for life and people, and improved quality of relationships. She described these transformational changes:

> I am weaker in a sense that I am dependent on others when it comes to some aspects of my functioning. It is difficult to assess [if I am stronger] because in some situations I feel weaker, in others definitely much stronger than I was, before I lost vision. I think I am a more courageous person now. I am a more tolerant person towards others. I have greater understanding of other people's shortcomings or imperfections.

Joanna related changes relative to her goals as linked to her personality resources such as control and self-efficacy:

> I cannot say that the loss of vision had a significant influence on my life goals. When it comes to doctoral program, I was thinking of that option before I lost my vision. After I lost vision, I returned to that idea but in different circumstances. I think the loss of vision did not change radically my goals in life. I was formerly going to work on my PhD as a sighted person and was going to write on history of the book. After I lost vision my work on history of the book seemed impossible to pursue because required to work on archive resources. I changed the theme and supervisor; these were radical changes, but the idea of pursuing the doctor's degree remained. Then, I started working on the book in the Braille system in Poland.

Joanna's feeling of a strong inner drive serves to integrate new trauma-related information. Janoff-Bulman (1992) explained that over time, people develop assumptions, which provide expectations about their own selves and the world, to allow functioning effectively. The experience of vision loss may uncover fragility, uncertainty about the future, and the fact that what happens can be random. Joanna shared some of her shattered beliefs and how she attempted to re-examine these previous assumptions to comprehend the situation or seek the personal significance of what had happened:

> I never had anger against anyone or God for what happened to me. I accepted that with humility. I took a rational approach. It happened, and I decided to accept that not passively, but actively. I did not feel regret and pretensions to anyone that I lost my vision. I could have blamed doctors, as the infection at the hospital was a result of negligence regarding hygiene. I could have been angry and go to the court with that but what that would change especially at the time in a communistic system? I was dependent on that clinic also regarding my future. It was only one such specialist clinic in Poland that could effectively assist me. It would have turned against me, if I had decided to go to the court. At that time to win with the clinic wouldn't be possible and it would close my future eventual medical assistance. It was rational way of thinking.

Her sudden loss of vision was a strong motive for seeking answers to these existential questions. That an operation expected to be successful led to the loss of vision and raised for Joanna questions of what is worth living, the meaning in life, and what is less important. In searching for meaning in life and finding it, reading a book by Roman [a writer who lost his vision and hands after World War II; his name was changed to protect his privacy] played a significant role:

> My first great loss was a lack of possibility to read printed books. I had loved reading books, was fascinated with books despite I had a low vision but with correction glasses I could read. I loved reading books (devoured books). So, the first loss was that I had realized that I won't ever read printed books with my eyes.
>
> It had a very significant beginning. When I was released from the clinic, we were returning home, my father at the train station in a kiosk spotted a book with the

significant title *When my eyes* and bought it. It was a novelty at that time, the book was published in 1985 and I lost my vision the same year. When my father saw the title, he thought there may be something important in it. He even did not recognize the author of that book. The title was catching, and he bought it. He was reading that book on the train on our way back home. Sometimes he had to leave me for a moment and walk in the corridor, but as we found later he went out to cope and dry his eyes wet ... Everything was fresh for him and this book with such story ...

When we returned home we started to read that book ... It was a first book I did not read myself but it was read to me. Parents read at evenings, and we together were reading it.

Having someone who can be a model, especially if they experienced a similar event can be helpful as they can provide constructive support that may assist in the development of new schemes (Tedeschi et al., 2018). Joanna described the supportive significant persons and other trauma survivors who accompanied her in the aftermath of her trauma. Specifically:

I think it was Roman's personality, his attitude toward life. Meeting him and knowing him, was significant for me in a sense that I was able to find answers to my situation. I was thinking, if Roman without sight and his hands achieved that much, then for me it would be easier. It served a bit as a self-consolation, but also as an objective evaluation of reality for me. It helped me find a new meaning in life and change the life priorities, re-evaluate them.

In agreement with Wang and Boerner's (2008) finding that the nature of social relationships following vision loss is multifaceted and requires re-establishing by both parties in order to stay connected, Joanna shared her perception of social changes she experienced after vision loss that made her decide with whom to be connected:

I do not remember if there were persons that made me feel difficult to handle the trauma, but there were persons with whom was difficult to talk to and find understanding. Some of my good friends did not pass that difficult test (being with me in relation after I lost vision) due to their emotions and they withdrew from being in touch with me. Others decided to stay in touch and these relations got stronger, closer. Most of all, I received the greatest support from my parents with everything.

A person's ability to develop a positive accommodation and growth depends on the extent that basic needs of autonomy, competence and relatedness have been met in the past and can function as factors of resilience (Joseph & Linley, 2005). Indeed, Joanna shared how much experiences from her childhood contributed to her resilience:

I had to deal with many challenges and with my emotions from my childhood ... I was enrolled in the mainstream school on a condition: if I managed and coped, I would be able to continue. I passed successfully probation because my parents supported and helped me a lot in study. But also, thanks to my class teacher, who was a courageous person and decided to work with special needs student, the teacher with real vocation ... From childhood I was confronted with many challenges and these experiences toughen me ... Yes, it was rather a fact that I had a bit different childhood that made me tougher person.

In agreement with the aforementioned empirical knowledge that self-efficacy can support a process of growth, Joanna attributed the realistic attitude that she learned from her parents to help her face life's challenges and execute her goals:

It is my realism as my attitude towards life as I never was easy to resort to dreams or idealism in life. I was able to assess realistically my situation. In general, I think this realism and a bit of cold (pragmatic) approach helps me to go ahead in life. My parents were very realistic persons, walking on the ground. I had these models to follow. I like to have control over the situation, and I also control myself. I do not allow myself to manifest strong emotions in public spaces. I do not try to improvise in life by saying it is going to be somehow, no, it is going to be the way I am planning to be.

Joanna's attitude further illustrates the finding in studies of populations with VI that a strong association exists between self-esteem and psychological adjustment (Augestad, 2017).

In some way, I felt the need to defend my own dignity because after I lost my vision, I evidently became disabled person. Certainly, as a person with low vision my self-esteem was low, and after when I lost vision, I also had that lower self-esteem of not being fully independent person. Knowing that this low self-esteem would not help me but lead to some problems I decided to challenge myself. In some ways this engagement in scientific work, pursuing doctor's degree was meant to rise my self-esteem. I had a need to find the solution for life to avoid as much as it was possible the classical approach to disabled person – feeling of pity.

That the impact of visual loss depends on its timing (Boerner, 2004) is illustrated in Joanna's experience when at the age of 25, a time in life related to establishing goals for adulthood, she lost her vision. Though as per the OV theory, a person may accommodate traumatic material positively, Joseph and Linley (2008) posit that even well-intentioned others may intervene in a way that distorts the natural direction of recovery of those who lost their vision. After Joanna lost her sight, she did not learn mobility orientation as the doctors advised her to stop it and her parents were always there for her to provide guidance for mobility. However, reflecting now on whether she would change something in dealing with trauma at the initial stage, she shares:

I now realise that we missed the opportunity when I could have learned the orientation and using the stick. It was a result of the decision that doctors made. Theoretically there was a danger that I could cause greater damage to my retina if I bumped at something while learning orientation. To protect me from this risk I was stopped from learning mobility orientation. It is characteristic for the blind persons that the most sensitive time to learn orientation is straight after loss of vision. With the time lapse the sensibility to learn that can be missed. Also, at that time when I lost my vision I had always someone to walk with me, to be with me and I think I did not have motivation to do so. Nowadays, I unfortunately pay for that earlier decision as today I have a need to walk independently and also have some problems with availability of a permanent person that could accompany me. Now, it is too late to learn orientation, the opportunity was missed.

References

Augestad, L. B. (2017). Self-concept and self-esteem among children and young adults with visual impairment: A systematic review. *Cogent Psychology*, *4*(1), 1319652. 10.1080/23311908.2017.1319652

Boerner, K. (2004). Adaptation to disability among middle-aged and older adults: The role of assimilative and accommodative coping. *The Journals of Gerontology Series B: Psychological Sciences and Social Sciences*, *59*(1), 35–42. 10.1093/geronb/59.1.P35

Boerner, K., & Cimarolli, V. R. (2005). Optimizing rehabilitation for adults with visual impairment: Attention to life goals and their links to well-being. *Clinical Rehabilitation*, *19*(7), 790–798. 10.1191/0269215505cr893oa

Boerner, K., & Wang, S. (2012). Targets for rehabilitation: An evidence base for adaptive coping with visual disability. *Rehabilitation Psychology*, *57*(4), 320–327. 10.1037/a0030787

Boerner, K., & Wang, S.-W. (2010). How it matters when it happens: Life changes related to functional loss in younger and older Adults. *The International Journal of Aging and Human Development*, *70*(2), 163–179. 10.2190/AG.70.2.d

Boerner, K., Wang, S.-W., & Cimarolli, V. R. (2006). The impact of functional loss: Nature and implications of life changes. *Journal of Loss and Trauma*, *11*(4), 265–287. 10.1080/15325020600662625

Bourne, R., Steinmetz, J. D., Flaxman, S., Briant, P. S., Taylor, H. R., Resnikoff, S., Casson, R. J., Abdoli, A., Abu-Gharbieh, E., Afshin, A., Ahmadieh, H., Akalu, Y., Alamneh, A. A., Alemayehu, W., Alfaar, A. S., Alipour, V., Anbesu, E. W., Androudi, S., Arabloo, J., … , & Vos, T. (2021). Trends in prevalence of blindness and distance and near vision impairment over 30 years: An analysis for the global burden of disease study. *The Lancet Global Health*, *9*(2), e130–e143. 10.1016/S2214-109X(20)30425-3

Brandtstädter, J., & Rothermund, K. (2002). The life-course dynamics of goal pursuit and goal adjustment: A two-process framework. *Developmental Review*, *22*(1), 117–150. 10.1006/drev.2001.0539

Brown, R. L., & Barrett, A. E. (2011). Visual impairment and quality of life among older adults: An examination of explanations for the relationship. *The Journals of Gerontology Series B: Psychological Sciences and Social Sciences*, *66B*(3), 364–373. 10.1093/geronb/gbr015

Brunes, A., Hansen, M. B., & Heir, T. (2019a). Loneliness among adults with visual impairment: Prevalence, associated factors, and relationship to life satisfaction. *Health and Quality of Life Outcomes*, *17*(1), 24. 10.1186/s12955-019-1096-y

Brunes, A., Hansen, M. B., & Heir, T. (2019b). Post-traumatic stress reactions among individuals with visual impairments: A systematic review. *Disability and Rehabilitation*, *41*(18), 2111–2118. 10.1080/09638288.2018.1459884

Brunes, A., Hansen, M. B., & Heir, T. (2021). General self-efficacy in individuals with visual impairment compared with the general population. *PLoS One*, *16*(7), e0254043. 10.1371/journal.pone.0254043

Brunes, A., & Heir, T. (2020a). Social interactions, experiences with adverse life events and depressive symptoms in individuals with visual impairment: A cross-sectional study. *BMC Psychiatry*, *20*(1), 224. 10.1186/s12888-020-02652-7

Brunes, A., & Heir, T. (2020b). Visual impairment and depression: Age-specific prevalence, associations with vision loss, and relation to life satisfaction. *World Journal of Psychiatry*, *10*(6), 139–149. 10.5498/wjp.v10.i6.139

Brunes, A., Nielsen, M. B., & Heir, T. (2018). Bullying among people with visual impairment: Prevalence, associated factors and relationship to self-efficacy and life satisfaction. *World Journal of Psychiatry*, *8*(1), 43–50. 10.5498/wjp.v8.i1.43

Cimarolli, V. R., & Boerner, K. (2005). Social support and well-being in adults who are visually impaired. *Journal of Visual Impairment & Blindness*, *99*(9), 521–534. 10.1177/0145482X0509900904
Colenbrander, A. (2010). Assessment of functional vision and its rehabilitation. *Acta Ophthalmologica*, *88*(2), 163–173. 10.1111/j.1755-3768.2009.01670.x
Demmin, D. L., & Silverstein, S. M. (2020). Visual impairment and mental health: Unmet needs and treatment options. *Clinical Ophthalmology*, *14*, 4229–4251. 10.2147/OPTH.S258783
Elsman, E. B. M., van Rens, G. H. M. B., & van Nispen, R. M. A. (2017). Impact of visual impairment on the lives of young adults in the Netherlands: A concept-mapping approach. *Disability and Rehabilitation*, *39*(26), 2607–2618. 10.1080/09638288.2016.1236408
Haegele, J. A., Kirk, T. N., & Zhu, X. (2018). Self-efficacy and physical activity among adults with visual impairments. *Disability and Health Journal*, *11*(2), 324–329. 10.1016/j.dhjo.2017.10.012
Hernandez Trillo, A., & Dickinson, C. M. (2012). The impact of visual and nonvisual factors on quality of life and adaptation in adults with visual impairment. *Investigative Opthalmology & Visual Science*, *53*(7), 4234. 10.1167/iovs.12-9580
Hobfoll, S. E. (2002). Social and psychological resources and adaptation. *Review of General Psychology*, *6*(4), 307–324. 10.1037/1089-2680.6.4.307
Horowitz, A., Reinhardt, J. P., & Kennedy, G. J. (2005). Major and subthreshold depression among older adults seeking vision rehabilitation services. *The American Journal of Geriatric Psychiatry*, *13*(3), 180–187. 10.1097/00019442-200503000-00002
Janoff-Bulman, R. (1992). *Shattered assumptions: Towards a new psychology of trauma*. Free Press; Maxwell Macmillan Canada; Maxwell Macmillan International.
Joseph, S. (2013). *What doesn't kill us: The new psychology of posttraumatic growth*. Basic Books Perseus Books Group. http://public.ebookcentral.proquest.com/choice/publicfullrecord.aspx?p=796098
Joseph, S., & Linley, P. A. (2005). Positive adjustment to threatening events: An organismic valuing theory of growth through adversity. *Review of General Psychology*, *9*(3), 262–280. 10.1037/1089-2680.9.3.262
Joseph, S., & Linley, P. A. (Eds.). (2008). *Trauma, recovery, and growth: Positive psychological perspectives on posttraumatic stress*. John Wiley & Sons.
Joseph, S., Murphy, D., & Regel, S. (2012). An affective-cognitive processing model of post-traumatic growth. *Clinical Psychology & Psychotherapy*, *19*(4), 316–325. 10.1002/cpp.1798
Linley, P. A. (2003). Positive adaptation to trauma: Wisdom as both process and outcome. *Journal of Traumatic Stress*, *16*(6), 601–610. 10.1023/B:JOTS.0000004086.64509.09
Linley, P. A., & Joseph, S. (2004). Positive change following trauma and adversity: A review. *Journal of Traumatic Stress*, *17*(1), 11–21. 10.1023/B:JOTS.0000014671.27856.7e
McIlvane, J. M., & Reinhardt, J. P. (2001). Interactive effect of support from family and friends in visually impaired elders. *The Journals of Gerontology Series B: Psychological Sciences and Social Sciences*, *56*(6), 374–382. 10.1093/geronb/56.6.P374
Newsom, J. T., & Schulz, R. (1996). Social support as a mediator in the relation between functional status and quality of life in older adults. *Psychology and Aging*, *11*(1), 34–44. 10.1037/0882-7974.11.1.34
Ogińska-Bulik, N. (2013). The role social support in posttraumatic growth in people struggling with cancer. *Health Psychology Report*, *1*, 1–8. 10.5114/hpr.2013.40464
Popivker, L., Wang, S., & Boerner, K. (2010). Eyes on the prize: Life goals in the context of visual disability in midlife. *Clinical Rehabilitation*, *24*(12), 1127–1135. 10.1177/0269215510371421
Ratcliff, J. J., Lieberman, L., Miller, A. K., & Pace, B. (2017). Bullying as a source of posttraumatic growth in individuals with visual impairments. *Journal of Developmental and Physical Disabilities*, *29*(2), 265–278.
Reinhardt, J. P., Boerner, K., & Horowitz, A. (2009). Personal and social resources and adaptation to chronic vision impairment over time. *Aging & Mental Health*, *13*(3), 367–375. 10.1080/13607860902860912
Ryff, C. D. (1989). Happiness is everything, or is it? Explorations on the meaning of psychological well-being. *Journal of Personality and Social Psychology*, *57*(6), 1069–1081. 10.1037/0022-3514.57.6.1069

Ryff, C. D., & Singer, B. (1996). Psychological well-being: Meaning, measurement, and implications for psychotherapy research. *Psychotherapy and Psychosomatics*, *65*(1), 14–23. 10.1159/000289026

Salick, E. C., & Auerbach, C. F. (2006). From devastation to integration: Adjusting to and growing from medical trauma. *Qualitative Health Research*, *16*(8), 1021–1037. 10.1177/1049732306292166

Senra, H., Barbosa, F., Ferreira, P., Vieira, C. R., Perrin, P. B., Rogers, H., Rivera, D., & Leal, I. (2015). Psychologic adjustment to irreversible vision loss in adults. *Ophthalmology*, *122*(4), 851–861. 10.1016/j.ophtha.2014.10.022

Sztonyk, B. M., & Formella, Z. S. (2020). The role of social support in contributing to posttraumatic growth in persons with vision impairment. *Health Psychology Report*, *8*(3), 238–247.

Tanner, C., Caserta, M., Guo, J.-W., Clayton, M., Bernstein, P., & Kleinschmidt, J. (2020). The positive legacy of vision loss: Pathways to posttraumatic growth. *Innovation in Aging*, *4*(Suppl 1), 616–617. 10.1093/geroni/igaa057.2094

Tedeschi, R. G., & Calhoun, L. G. (1996). The posttraumatic growth inventory: Measuring the positive legacy of trauma. *Journal of Traumatic Stress*, *9*(3), 455–471. 10.1002/jts.2490090305

Tedeschi, R. G., & Calhoun, L. G. (2004). TARGET ARTICLE: 'Posttraumatic growth: conceptual foundations and empirical evidence'. *Psychological Inquiry*, *15*(1), 1–18. 10.1207/s15327965pli1501_01

Tedeschi, R. G., Shakespeare-Finch, J., Taku, K. K., & Calhoun, L. G. (2018). *Posttraumatic growth: Theory, research and applications*. Routledge.

van der Ham, A. J., van der Aa, H. P. A., Brunes, A., Heir, T., de Vries, R., van Rens, GHMB, & van Nispen, R. M. A. (2021). The development of posttraumatic stress disorder in individuals with visual impairment: A systematic search and review. *Ophthalmology and Physiology Optics*, *41*(2), 331–334. 10.1111/opo.12784

Wang, S.-W., & Boerner, K. (2008). Staying connected: Re-establishing social relationships following vision loss. *Clinical Rehabilitation*, *22*(9), 816–824. 10.1177/0269215508091435

Wortman, C. B. (2004). Posttraumatic growth: Progress and problems. *Psychological Inquiry*, *15*(1), 81–90.

World Health Organization (1992). *The ICD-10 classification of mental and behavioural disorders: Clinical descriptions and diagnostic guidelines*. World Health Organization.

World Health Organization (2019). *World report on vision*. World Health Organization. https://apps.who.int/iris/handle/10665/328717

Zheng, Y., Wu, X., Lin, X., & Lin, H. (2017). The prevalence of depression and depressive symptoms among eye disease patients: A systematic review and meta-analysis. *Scientific Reports*, *7*(1), 46453. 10.1038/srep46453

34
THE PAINS AND GAINS OF IMPRISONMENT
Posttraumatic Growth among Incarcerated Individuals

Esther F.J.C. van Ginneken

At present, roughly eleven million people are incarcerated worldwide (Fair & Walmsley, 2021). The United States has the highest incarceration rate at 629 per 100,000 inhabitants, while the world prison population rate is 140 per 100,000 people (Fair & Walmsley, 2021). Imprisonment affects both the people who are incarcerated and their families, friends, and communities. The harmful effects of incarceration have been extensively researched, and include psychological distress (Crewe et al., 2017; Haney, 2012), decreased opportunities in the labor market after release (Decker et al., 2015; Ramakers et al., 2014), ruptured relationships, and intergenerational problems, such as a heightened risk of criminal behavior among children of (formerly) incarcerated individuals (Besemer et al., 2011; Mears & Siennick, 2015). It is also well-established that incarcerated people are more vulnerable than their non-incarcerated counterparts in terms of physical health, mortality after release, and mental health (Butler et al., 2006; Fazel & Baillargeon, 2011; Zlodre & Fazel, 2012). Many incarcerated people have histories of traumatic experiences and these are associated with various negative outcomes, including posttraumatic stress disorder (Bowen et al., 2018; Liu et al., 2021). Incarceration may exacerbate these traumatic experiences, especially when people are victimized in prison (Wolff et al., 2007). More surprising – and not nearly as well researched and documented – is the manifestation of posttraumatic growth (PTG) among (formerly) incarcerated people. In the context of imprisonment, PTG can be understood as self-reported positive changes attributed to the experience of incarceration. These changes can occur in a variety of domains, including personal development, relationships, and opportunities for the future (Tedeschi & Calhoun, 2004). This chapter starts with a description of psychologically stressful aspects of imprisonment, followed by descriptions of growth, and the mechanisms that may contribute to such experiences.

Pains of Imprisonment

Imprisonment is a potentially psychologically traumatic event, because it forcefully disrupts the life course, strips people of their autonomy and liberty, and incarcerates them in a possibly hostile environment. As a result, people are separated from family and friends, and

DOI: 10.4324/9781032208688-43

may face irreparable consequences such as the loss of custody over children, and the loss of employment and housing. The first period of imprisonment demands adjustment to the new and stressful circumstances and is often also associated with uncertainty related to trial outcomes. Studies have consistently found that entry into prison and pre-trial detention are associated with high levels of psychological distress and an increased risk of suicide and self-harm (Fazel et al., 2008; Hawton et al., 2014; Marzano et al., 2016). Thus, imprisonment is both existentially threatening and a real peril to a person's physical well-being. Yet, the traumatic nature of imprisonment may be 'frontloaded' leading to possible PTG during, rather than following, imprisonment (and arguably, while the trauma is still ongoing), after a period of entry shock and adjustment.

The pains of imprisonment are extensively described in the criminological literature and are universal (Crewe, 2011; Haggerty & Bucerius, 2020; McKendy & Ricciardelli, 2021; Sykes, 1958), although the effects can vary depending on prison conditions and individual vulnerabilities. Relative to *prison conditions*, even in places where prisons have been characterized as exceptionally humane, in countries such as Norway, the experience of imprisonment inevitably causes distress (Crewe et al., 2022; Shammas, 2014). Many negative consequences following imprisonment do not depend on prison conditions (e.g., loss of employment or housing), although some can be ameliorated (e.g., contact with loved ones). Thus, it is appropriate to apply the psychological framework of PTG to understand why some individuals attribute a positive transformation to the experience of imprisonment. Importantly, this does not diminish the negative consequences that these individuals and others may face, because similar to other potentially psychologically traumatic events, growth, and trauma can co-exist in relation to imprisonment (Shakespeare-Finch & Lurie-Beck, 2014). Regarding *individual vulnerabilities*, it is necessary to recognize the complex interplay between the potential trauma of imprisonment and possible traumatic events prior to imprisonment. Incarcerated individuals are likely to have histories of multiple traumatic experiences, including sexual and violent victimization, combat exposure, and adverse childhood experiences (Ford et al., 2020; Henry, 2020; Skarupski et al., 2016). Imprisonment may aggravate previous experiences of trauma as well as sometimes offer opportunities for support in dealing with trauma; in fact, higher levels of PTG are associated with more (post)traumatic stress (Hearn et al., 2021; Schubert et al., 2016).

Gains of Imprisonment

Imprisonment can constitute a 'turning point' in people's life stories; it may be simultaneously the apex of despair and an opportunity for positive change, despite its well-known harmful effects. People may literally describe their imprisonment as a turning point; for example, participants in Van Ginneken's study (2016) stated "It sounds bad, but I am kind of glad I've come to prison because it's just turned my life around really" and "Coming to prison was the best thing to happen to me. Because it turned my life around" (p. 217). The key element in these narratives is that people perceive the transformation from a bad pre-incarceration situation to a better situation during incarceration, accompanied by the hope and conviction that life will improve after release. Such positive interpretations of the prison experience can be seen as indications of PTG. However, because such experiences have received scant research attention, it is difficult to estimate how prevalent they are.

PTG among incarcerated individuals is not widely recognized or discussed in the literature. Only recently have more scholars started paying attention to positive experiences and interpretations of imprisonment, next to its better-known painful experiences (Crewe & Ievins, 2020; Frois, 2017; Liebling et al., 2019; Maier & Ricciardelli, 2021; Ugelvik, 2022). Even in the literature on extreme experiences of incarceration, specifically prolonged solitary confinement, some individuals demonstrate an extraordinary capacity to cultivate meaning in the experience and emerge stronger (O'Donnell, 2014). Studies of PTG among incarcerated individuals conducted in Belgium by Vanhooren and colleagues (2016, 2017, 2018) used different methods to gauge levels of PTG and their relation to the search for meaning and coping strategies. The average score on the Posttraumatic Growth-Inventory (PTG-I) in a sample of 365 incarcerated men and women was 2.52, on a 6-point scale (Vanhooren et al., 2018). There was no significant difference in scores between men and women, but levels of PTG were higher among participants who received therapy. Emotional support (e.g., "I have been getting comfort and understanding from someone"), religious coping (e.g., "I have been praying or meditating"), and search for meaning (e.g., "I am looking for something that makes my life feel meaningful") predicted PTG. Behavioral disengagement (e.g., "I have been giving up trying to deal with it"), on the other hand, was negatively associated with PTG (Vanhooren et al., 2018).

A qualitative study of 30 therapy-involved individuals convicted of sexual offenses revealed that the difficult experience of incarceration was related to experiences of growth. In the words of a participant in Vanhooren et al.'s study (2017): "It is weird. Prison was one of the worst episodes in my life, but at the same time, it gave me the opportunity to change for the better." (p. 183). Participants in this study reported that therapy helped them find meaning in their incarceration experience, and contributed to personal growth.

A study conducted in England by Hearn et al. (2021) found that 48% of 160 surveyed men in prison experienced at least moderate levels of PTG (average scores of 3 or higher on the 6-point Posttraumatic Growth-Inventory scale). This was correlated with perceptions of the quality of relationships with staff, and with the trauma of imprisonment such that if relationships were rated more positively and imprisonment was experienced as more traumatic, levels of PTG were higher.

Other accounts of positive narratives of imprisonment resemble PTG in the sense that they attribute growth in various domains to the (simultaneously stressful) experience of incarceration. For example, Crewe and Ievins (2020) described narratives of positive transformation expressed by a minority of incarcerated men and women in different research projects in England, Wales, and Norway. The analysis of these narratives within a theoretical framework that considers the interaction between the institutional impact of the prison and the individual's biographical experiences showed that together, these individual and institutional factors explain "discourses of reinvention' among incarcerated individuals" (p. 572). The researchers identify three sub-groups among incarcerated individuals whose biographies could help account for their positive experiences. First, women who narrated positive transformation felt protected from abusive relationships, drug addictions, and damaging and degrading forms of sex work. Second, men with histories of serious drug abuse welcomed the constraints imposed by imprisonment on the use of drugs and engagement with damaging social relationships, and saw it as an opportunity to improve their health, moral identity, and prosocial relationships. Finally, men convicted of sexual offenses expressed a desire to be punished, so that they could stop offending and demonstrate a reformed identity (Crewe & Ievins, 2020). Such reinvention narratives can be understood as expressions of PTG.

Criminological scholars are critical of the idea of positive prison experiences and there is still a debate about whether PTG constitutes a real and lasting change rather than merely an illusion of change. There is a strand of research that supports the idea that cognitive change and positive expectations are associated with successful desistance, i.e., the cessation of criminal behavior (Burnett & Maruna, 2004; Doekhie et al., 2017; Giordano et al., 2002; Kazemian, 2020; Paternoster & Bushway, 2009; Ugelvik, 2022). Narratives of PTG and positive transformation have been identified among people who have successfully desisted (Comfort, 2008; Mapham & Hefferon, 2012), although Comfort (2008) argues that these individuals adopt the rhetoric of reform in the absence of true correctional support.

Conversely, experiences of PTG during imprisonment may be of a temporary nature when they are a strategy for coping with the stress and inescapability of imprisonment. Narratives of transformation and an expressed motivation to cease committing a crime may be driven by an instrumental motive to demonstrate change in order to be able to progress in the system. For example, Crewe (2009) discusses how 'pragmatists' in prison complied with institutional rules and sought to gain rewards through good behavior to make their time easier. Others have argued that prison sentences fail to support narratives of reform with proper rehabilitation support and thus positive intentions are unlikely to translate into a sustained change after release (Hart, 2017; Liebling et al., 2019; Schinkel, 2014; Soyer, 2014). Cognitive change is different from behavioral change, and even those who express a strong intention to live a conventional life may face such substantial hardship that they fall back on crime. Future research on PTG in relation to imprisonment should seek to further examine the interplay between previous traumatic experiences and imprisonment in relation to growth, the influence of prison conditions on growth, how different theoretical frameworks on positive narratives can be understood, and to what extent PTG is durable beyond release.

Mechanisms of PTG

Various mechanisms can explain why the experience of imprisonment can (eventually) contribute to PTG. These mechanisms fall into two broad categories: cognitive processes leading to a re-evaluation of one's life, and socio-supportive aspects of imprisonment that trigger and facilitate personal growth.

Cognitive Processes

These processes may include reflection and searching for meaning. A recurrent theme in different studies is that a prison sentence offers space and time for reflection (Crewe & Ievins, 2020; Kazemian, 2020; Maier & Ricciardelli, 2021; O'Donnell, 2014). It confronts people with the precarious state of their lives, and the image of what life will be like if they do not change their ways. This image of an undesirable future has been termed the 'feared self' in the Identity Theory of Criminal Desistance (Paternoster & Bushway, 2009), and can trigger a deliberate process of change towards a more desirable future ('the positive possible self'). This is illustrated by Maier and Ricciardelli's (2021) discussion of narratives of change by 56 men who were formerly incarcerated in a Canadian federal prison. Imprisonment "pushed them to reflect on their past lives ... and consider how they envisioned their future selves" (p. 779). Since their past was often characterized by poor choices, substance abuse, low self-worth, and hurting loved ones, they wanted to achieve a future different from their pre-incarceration lifestyle. In the Maier and Ricciardelli (2021) study this future entailed being calmer, drug-free, and having a greater appreciation by loved ones. Positive identities and future goals in other studies similarly involved romantic relationships, fulfilling work, family life, and religion in both men and women (Hoskins & Cobbina, 2019; Kazemian, 2020).

The aforementioned attempts to construct a positive identity are closely tied to a presumed existential need for meaning. The attribution to imprisonment of positive changes can fulfill this need for meaning because it gives the prison sentence a place in a person's life story. This framing is not easy because imprisonment challenges one's assumptions about the world and about oneself, such as the supposition of the self as a good person. The strict regulation of expressions of the self (e.g., in terms of clothing and possessions), activities, and contact with the outside world can be regarded as assaults on individuals' identities and their sense of self-worth (Cohen & Taylor, 1972; Goffman, 1961). Indeed, even narratives of PTG are characterized by descriptions of the initial period of imprisonment as extremely difficult (Van Ginneken, 2016), 'shocking', and 'brutal' (Kazemian, 2020, p. 106). Vanhooren et al. (2015) who studied 365 incarcerated people in Belgium found that imprisonment was associated with a loss of meaning, which, in turn, was related to higher levels of distress, whereas searching for meaning was associated with higher levels of PTG (Vanhooren et al., 2018). There is also evidence that religion can give meaning to the experience of incarceration, for example by interpreting it as part of God's plan (Ellis, 2021). Furthermore, religion can help rebuild a person's sense of identity and self-worth, through a narrative of forgiveness and agency (Maruna et al., 2006), the need for which can be acute when people question if they are good persons and have to come to terms with their offenses and their (sometimes very long) sentences. A participant in Maruna et al., 2006, p. 171) stated:

> So what happened to me was, I was desperate. I was charged with murder, first time ever in prison, my whole life had kind of exploded really. It was lying in pieces all around me, I didn't know whether I wanted to live or die … . I contemplated suicide, couldn't do that … . I was praying, praying more than I … had ever prayed before in my life you know, because I really needed some help, and nothing seemed to be happening you know in a really kind of, in a desperate situation you want an answer and you want it now, no answer.

This quote illustrates that the need for meaning may be attached to the need for survival. Religious and non-religious narratives of growth and purpose can help make sense of the difficult and potentially psychologically traumatic situation of incarcerated individuals. A further benefit of religion is that it provides individuals with a community, which can also support and help sustain positive change after release from prison. The impact of prosocial relationships on growth should not be underestimated.

Socio-Supportive Mechanisms

Three mechanisms that potentially contribute to PTG are contact with loved ones, protection from harm, and meaningful activities.

Contact with Loved Ones

Imprisonment can have both a positive and a negative impact on relationships. Despite the fact that imprisonment disrupts relationships with loved ones, some people may rekindle relationships with family while in prison, which can offer them support during imprisonment and assist with reintegration (Kazemian, 2020; Van Ginneken, 2015). The disruption of relationships may strengthen the appreciation of their importance as "being held away from their families appeared to increase feelings of identifying with and belonging to their loved ones on the outside" (Maier & Ricciardelli, 2021, p. 6). Another source of social support can be relationships with staff when officers are accessible, understanding, attentive to individual strengths, and willing to listen and give counsel (Frois, 2017; Hearn et al., 2021; Liebling et al., 2019).

Protection from Harm

Another explanation for experiences of growth is that paradoxically imprisonment can sometimes protect individuals from further harm. This protection narrative is found particularly among women with histories of abuse who report that prison helped them escape from a destructive situation (Bucerius et al., 2021; Crewe & Ievins, 2020; Van Ginneken, 2016). While entering prison is often experienced as highly stressful, women may come to see it as a respite from their difficult lives, and an opportunity to set out on a new path. This can only be understood with the knowledge that imprisonment is often one of many potentially psychological traumatic episodes in women's lives (Carlton & Segrave, 2011). Narratives of imprisonment as protection from further harm often speak to the broader abysmal context in which they arise, and can also be interpreted as evidence of the failure of the social welfare system to intervene well before criminal justice agencies became involved (Bucerius et al., 2021). While many women may have lost trust in people and institutions, positive interactions with staff and other incarcerated women in prison can help them rebuild their self-worth and trust in others while they are protected from harm from the outside world. Additionally, prison may present a lower threshold than the outside environment for access to counseling services regarding prior experiences. For example, prison may often be the first place that acknowledges and addresses women's histories of victimization (Van Ginneken, 2016). Similarly, practical support may be more easily accessible, such as finding accommodation away from the previously harmful situation. These reports of positive experiences do not preclude the possibility that imprisonment itself is harmful and it can compound negative experiences and extend patterns of abuse and control (Carlton & Segrave, 2011; Hoskins & Cobbina, 2019).

Meaningful Activities

Growth may also result from the availability of substance abuse treatment and purposeful activities, such as helping others, training, and education. Individuals with severe substance abuse problems have been documented to report growth following imprisonment and treatment in residential settings (Crewe & Ievins, 2020; Frois, 2017; Hoskins & Cobbina, 2019; Sufrin, 2017; Van Ginneken, 2016). Prison is often seen as the last resort because it forcibly removes people from environments where drugs and alcohol are easily available. For example, participants in Crewe and Ievins' (2020) study reported that "[they] wouldn't have got off the drugs if [they were] outside" (p. 576). Hoskins and Cobbina (2019) found that positive changes were more commonly reported by women in a residential substance abuse treatment setting than in jail or prison. Recovery from substance abuse can then lead to new prosocial roles like becoming peer support workers, in which recovered individuals help others who have problems with substance addiction, contributing to a sense of purpose and self-worth (Hoskins & Cobbina, 2019). Helping others can be described as a generative narrative or redemption script, both of which are reported in multiple studies (Maruna et al., 2006; Van Ginneken, 2016), and help reestablish a person's sense of moral worth.

A sense of moral worth, purpose, and positive identity can also be derived from education and training in prison. These activities can give individuals the opportunity to use their time in a meaningful way and reveal possible pathways for life after release, although the availability of programs is limited (Kazemian, 2020; Van Ginneken, 2015). In Kazemian's (2020) study, 70% of the participants reported that they developed useful skills during incarceration, which could vary from specific vocational skills to passions, such as writing, art, and working with computers. In their description of a high-achieving prison, Liebling et al. (2019) ascribe importance to the availability of a range of diverse meaningful and creative activities, and the opportunity and support for individual projects as these activities can contribute to a greater sense of self-worth, a sense of meaning, and a positive possible self. Indeed, a large majority of individuals incarcerated in this particular prison reported that they perceived their prison time as an opportunity to change, as illustrated by the statement of one participant:

> From cooking meals for those with no cooking skills, bee keeping, taking care of an aquarium, or working with birds of prey, to becoming a barista or a gardener – prisoners were able to find their niche, and along with it, purpose and some gratification. (p. 118).

Conclusion and Implications

This chapter has documented emerging insights on PTG (or otherwise labeled positive interpretations) attributed to imprisonment. These experiences are not as prevalent and visible as the harms of imprisonment, which can explain why they have not received as much scholarly attention. Nonetheless, the evidence suggests that positive transformations can be observed among incarcerated individuals in different countries including Portugal (Frois, 2017), France (Kazemian, 2020), England and Wales (Crewe & Ievins, 2020; Hearn et al., 2021; Van Ginneken, 2016), Belgium (Vanhooren et al., 2018), Israel (Vignansky et al., 2018), Canada (Maier & Ricciardelli, 2021), and the United States (Hoskins & Cobbina, 2019). The descriptions of growth against a backdrop of despair are a testament to the extraordinary capacity of human beings to overcome difficulty and find meaning in even the bleakest of places.

In summary, experiences of PTG among incarcerated individuals may derive from internal cognitive processes on the one hand and socio-supportive aspects of imprisonment on the other hand. The cognitive processes can entail reflection and a search for meaning that lead to the identification of new purposes, increased self-worth, and a sense of imprisonment as a meaningful turning point. The socio-supportive aspects are related to practical support, substance abuse treatment, protection from harmful life circumstances, and emotionally supportive relationships with staff, peers, and people outside prison. Both processes likely interact with a person's individual characteristics and circumstances, their history, and the prison's climate and resources; for example, individuals with more chaotic life circumstances may be more likely to perceive imprisonment as a respite (Bucerius et al., 2021), and prisons with a greater variety of meaningful activities may encourage more experiences of growth (Liebling et al., 2019). This offers important practical implications for supporting PTG among incarcerated and formerly incarcerated people.

Akin to the dual nature of the mechanisms that contribute to growth, support should also target these two pathways. Importantly, support to sustain positive changes should aim to buffer the stressors associated with re-entry, so that material (e.g., housing and income), health, and emotional needs are met as much as possible. Another important area of support is the recovery from substance addiction, which is more difficult to maintain outside the prison in the face of greater temptation (Frois, 2017). Positive identity changes can be supported by the provision of meaningful activities and contact with other people who recognize and reinforce this positive change (Maruna et al., 2004; Nugent & Schinkel, 2016). It would be helpful to connect incarcerated individuals with organizations and volunteers who can fulfill the role of a prosocial and supportive community after imprisonment (e.g., religious organizations). Positive identities can also be reaffirmed by formerly incarcerated individuals' fulfilling a meaningful role as peer support workers, drawing on their own experiences of incarceration, transformation, or recovery from substance abuse to help others (Heidemann et al., 2016; Scannell, 2021). Finally, interventions informed by positive psychology and strengths-based approaches may facilitate growth while simultaneously supporting desistance among (formerly) incarcerated individuals (Mapham & Hefferon, 2012). Overall, it is likely that effective interventions and support need to address both a person's life circumstances and mindset in order to achieve durable positive growth.

References

Besemer, S., van der Geest, V., Murray, J., Bijleveld, C. C. J. H., & Farrington, D. P. (2011). The relationship between parental imprisonment and offspring offending in England and The Netherlands. *The British Journal of Criminology*, *51*(2), 413–437. 10.1093/bjc/azq072

Bowen, K., Jarrett, M., Stahl, D., Forrester, A., & Valmaggia, L. (2018). The relationship between exposure to adverse life events in childhood and adolescent years and subsequent adult psychopathology in 49,163 adult prisoners: A systematic review. *Personality and Individual Differences*, *131*, 74–92. 10.1016/j.paid.2018.04.023

Bucerius, S., Haggerty, K. D., & Dunford, D. T. (2021). Prison as temporary refuge: Amplifying the voices of women detained in prison. *The British Journal of Criminology*, *61*(2), 519–537. 10.1093/bjc/azaa073

Burnett, R., & Maruna, S. (2004). So 'Prison Works', does it? The criminal careers of 130 men released from prison under Home Secretary, Michael Howard. *The Howard Journal of Criminal Justice*, *43*(4), 390–404. 10.1111/j.1468-2311.2004.00337.x

Butler, T., Andrews, G., Allnutt, S., Sakashita, C., Smith, N. E., & Basson, J. (2006). Mental disorders in Australian prisoners: A comparison with a community sample. *Australian & New Zealand Journal of Psychiatry*, *40*(3), 272–276. 10.1080/j.1440-1614.2006.01785.x

Carlton, B., & Segrave, M. (2011). Women's survival post-imprisonment: Connecting imprisonment with pains past and present. *Punishment & Society*, *13*(5), 551–570. 10.1177/1462474511422174

Cohen, S., & Taylor, L. (1972). *Psychological survival: The experience of long-term imprisonment.* Penguin.

Comfort, M. (2008). The best seven years I could'a done: The reconstruction of imprisonment as rehabilitation. In P. Carlen (Ed.), *Imaginary penalties* (pp. 252–274). Willan Publishing.

Crewe, B. (2009). *The prisoner society: Power, adaptation, and social life in an English prison.* Oxford University Press.

Crewe, B. (2011). Depth, weight, tightness: Revisiting the pains of imprisonment. *Punishment & Society, 13*(5), 509–529. 10.1177/1462474511422172

Crewe, B., Hulley, S., & Wright, S. (2017). Swimming with the tide: Adapting to long-term imprisonment. *Justice Quarterly, 34*(3), 517–541. 10.1080/07418825.2016.1190394

Crewe, B., & Ievins, A. (2020). The prison as a reinventive institution. *Theoretical Criminology, 24*(4), 568–589. 10.1177/1362480619841900

Crewe, B., Ievins, A., Larmour, S., Laursen, J., Mjåland, K., & Schliehe, A. (2022). Nordic penal exceptionalism: A comparative, empirical analysis. *The British Journal of Criminology*, azac013. 10.1093/bjc/azac013

Decker, S. H., Ortiz, N., Spohn, C., & Hedberg, E. (2015). Criminal stigma, race, and ethnicity: The consequences of imprisonment for employment. *Journal of Criminal Justice, 43*(2), 108–121. 10.1016/j.jcrimjus.2015.02.002

Doekhie, J., Dirkzwager, A., & Nieuwbeerta, P. (2017). Early attempts at desistance from crime: Prisoners' prerelease expectations and their postrelease criminal behavior. *Journal of Offender Rehabilitation, 56*(7), 473–493. 10.1080/10509674.2017.1359223

Ellis, R. (2021). 'You're not serving time, you're serving Christ': Protestant religion and discourses of responsibilization in a women's prison. *The British Journal of Criminology, 61*(6), 1647–1664. 10.1093/bjc/azab022

Fair, H., & Walmsley, R. (2021). *World prison population list* (13th edition). Institute for Crime & Justice Policy Research. https://www.prisonstudies.org/sites/default/files/resources/downloads/world_prison_population_list_13th_edition.pdf

Fazel, S., & Baillargeon, J. (2011). The health of prisoners. *The Lancet, 377*(9769), 956–965. 10.1016/S0140-6736(10)61053-7

Fazel, S., Cartwright, J., Norman-Nott, A., & Hawton, K. (2008). Suicide in prisoners: A systematic eeview of risk factors. *The Journal of Clinical Psychiatry, 69*(11), 1721–1731.

Ford, K., Bellis, M. A., Hughes, K., Barton, E. R., & Newbury, A. (2020). Adverse childhood experiences: A retrospective study to understand their associations with lifetime mental health diagnosis, self-harm or suicide attempt, and current low mental wellbeing in a male Welsh prison population. *Health & Justice, 8*(1), 13. 10.1186/s40352-020-00115-5

Frois, C. (2017). *Female imprisonment: An ethnography of everyday life in confinement.* Palgrave Macmillan.

Giordano, P. C., Cernkovich, S. A., & Rudolph, J. L. (2002). Gender, crime, and desistance: Toward a theory of cognitive transformation. *American Journal of Sociology, 107*(4), 990–1064. 10.1086/343191

Goffman, E. (1961). *Asylums: Essays on the social situation of mental patients and other inmates.* Doubleday.

Haggerty, K. D., & Bucerius, S. (2020). The proliferating pains of imprisonment. *Incarceration, 1*(1), 2632666320936432. 10.1177/2632666320936432

Haney, C. (2012). Prison effects in the era of mass incarceration. *The Prison Journal*, 0032885512448604. 10.1177/0032885512448604

Hart, E. L. (2017). Women prisoners and the drive for desistance: Capital and responsibilization as a barrier to change. *Women & Criminal Justice, 27*(3), 151–169. 10.1080/08974454.2016.1217814

Hawton, K., Linsell, L., Adeniji, T., Sariaslan, A., & Fazel, S. (2014). Self-harm in prisons in England and Wales: An epidemiological study of prevalence, risk factors, clustering, and subsequent suicide. *The Lancet, 383*(9923), 1147–1154. 10.1016/S0140-6736(13)62118-2

Hearn, N., Joseph, S., & Fitzpatrick, S. (2021). Post-traumatic growth in prisoners and its association with the quality of staff–prisoner relationships. *Criminal Behaviour and Mental Health, 31*(1), 49–59. 10.1002/cbm.2173

Heidemann, G., Cederbaum, J. A., Martinez, S., & LeBel, T. P. (2016). Wounded healers: How formerly incarcerated women help themselves by helping others. *Punishment & Society, 18*(1), 3–26. 10.1177/1462474515623101

Henry, B. F. (2020). Typologies of adversity in childhood & adulthood as determinants of mental health & substance use disorders of adults incarcerated in US prisons. *Child Abuse & Neglect*, *99*, 104251. 10.1016/j.chiabu.2019.104251

Hoskins, K. M., & Cobbina, J. E. (2019). It depends on the situation: Women's identity transformation in prison, jail, and substance abuse treatment settings. *Feminist Criminology*, *15*(3), 340–358. 10.1177/1557085119878268

Kazemian, L. (2020). *Positive growth and redemption in prison: Finding light behind bars and beyond*. Routledge.

Liebling, A., Laws, B., Lieber, E., Auty, K., Schmidt, B. E., Crewe, B., Gardom, J., Kant, D., & Morey, M. (2019). Are hope and possibility achievable in prison? *The Howard Journal of Crime and Justice*, *58*(1), 104–126. 10.1111/hojo.12303

Liu, H., Li, T. W., Liang, L., & Hou, W. K. (2021). Trauma exposure and mental health of prisoners and ex-prisoners: A systematic review and meta-analysis. *Clinical Psychology Review*, *89*, 102069. 10.1016/j.cpr.2021.102069

Maier, K., & Ricciardelli, R. (2021). "Prison didn't change me, I have changed": Narratives of change, self, and prison time. *Criminology & Criminal Justice*, *22*(5), 774–789. 10.1177/1748895 8211031336

Mapham, A., & Hefferon, K. (2012). "I used to be an offender—now I'm a defender": Positive psychology approaches in the facilitation of posttraumatic growth in ofenders. *Journal of Offender Rehabilitation*, *51*(6), 389–413. 10.1080/10509674.2012.683239

Maruna, S., Lebel, T. P., Mitchell, N., & Naples, M. (2004). Pygmalion in the reintegration process: Desistance from crime through the looking glass. *Psychology, Crime & Law*, *10*(3), 271–281. 10.1080/10683160410001662762

Maruna, S., Wilson, L., & Curran, K. (2006). Why God is often found behind bars: Prison conversions and the crisis of self-narrative. *Research in Human Development*, *3*(2–3), 161–184. 10.1 080/15427609.2006.9683367

Marzano, L., Hawton, K., Rivlin, A., Smith, E. N., Piper, M., & Fazel, S. (2016). Prevention of suicidal behavior in prisons: An overview of initiatives based on a systematic review of research on near-lethal suicide attempts. *Crisis: The Journal of Crisis Intervention and Suicide Prevention*, *37*(5), 323–334. 10.1027/0227-5910/a000394

McKendy, L., & Ricciardelli, R. (2021). The pains of imprisonment and contemporary prisoner culture in Canada. *The Prison Journal*, *101*(5), 528–552. 10.1177/00328855211048166

Mears, D. P., & Siennick, S. E. (2015). Young adult outcomes and the life-course penalties of parental incarceration. *Journal of Research in Crime and Delinquency*, *53*(1), 3–35. 10.1177/002242 7815592452

Nugent, B., & Schinkel, M. (2016). The pains of desistance. *Criminology & Criminal Justice*, *16*(5), 568–584. 10.1177/1748895816634812

O'Donnell, I. (2014). *Prisoners, solitude, and time*. Oxford University Press.

Paternoster, R., & Bushway, S. (2009). Desistance and the 'feared self': Toward an identity theory of criminal desistance. *The Journal of Criminal Law and Criminology*, *99*(4), 1103–1156. http://www.jstor.org/stable/20685067

Ramakers, A., Apel, R., Nieuwbeerta, P., Dirkzwager, A., & Van Wilsem, J. (2014). Imprisonment length and post-prison employment prospects. *Criminology*, *52*(3), 399–427. 10.1111/1745-9125. 12042

Scannell, C. (2021). By helping others we help ourselves: Insights from peer support workers in substance use recovery. *Advances in Mental Health*, *20*(3), 232–241. 10.1080/18387357.2021. 1995452

Schinkel, M. (2014). *Being imprisoned: Punishment, adaptation and desistance*. Palgrave Macmillan.

Schubert, C. F., Schmidt, U., & Rosner, R. (2016). Posttraumatic growth in populations with posttraumatic stress disorder—A systematic review on growth-related psychological constructs and biological variables. *Clinical Psychology & Psychotherapy*, *23*(6), 469–486. 10.1002/ cpp.1985

Shakespeare-Finch, J., & Lurie-Beck, J. (2014). A meta-analytic clarification of the relationship between posttraumatic growth and symptoms of posttraumatic distress disorder. *Journal of Anxiety Disorders*, *28*(2), 223–229. 10.1016/j.janxdis.2013.10.005

Shammas, V. L. (2014). The pains of freedom: Assessing the ambiguity of Scandinavian penal exceptionalism on Norway's Prison Island. *Punishment & Society*, *16*(1), 104–123. 10.1177/1462474513504799

Skarupski, K. A., Parisi, J. M., Thorpe, R., Tanner, E., & Gross, D. (2016). The association of adverse childhood experiences with mid-life depressive symptoms and quality of life among incarcerated males: Exploring multiple mediation. *Aging & Mental Health*, *20*(6), 655–666. 10.1080/13607863.2015.1033681

Soyer, M. (2014). The imagination of desistance: A juxtaposition of the construction of incarceration as a turning point and the reality of recidivism. *The British Journal of Criminology*, *54*(1), 91–108. 10.1093/bjc/azt059

Sufrin, C. (2017). *Jailcare: Finding the safety net for women behind bars*. University of California Press.

Sykes, G. (1958). *The society of captives: A study of a maximum security prison*. Princeton: Princeton University Press.

Tedeschi, R. G., & Calhoun, L. G. (2004). Posttraumatic growth: Conceptual foundations and empirical evidence. *Psychological Inquiry*, *15*(1), 1–18. 10.1207/s15327965pli1501_01

Ugelvik, T. (2022). The transformative power of trust: Exploring tertiary desistance in reinventive prisons. *The British Journal of Criminology*, *62*(3), 623–638. 10.1093/bjc/azab076

Van Ginneken, E. F. J. C. (2015). Doing well or just doing time? A qualitative study of patterns of psychological adjustment in prison. *Howard Journal of Criminal Justice*, *54*(4), 352–370. 10.1111/hojo.12137

Van Ginneken, E. F. J. C. (2016). Making sense of imprisonment: Narratives of posttraumatic growth among female prisoners. *International Journal of Offender Therapy and Comparative Criminology*, *60*(2), 208–227. 10.1177/0306624X14548531

Vanhooren, S., Leijssen, M., & Dezutter, J. (2015). Loss of meaning as a predictor of distress in prison. *International Journal of Offender Therapy and Comparative Criminology*, *61*(13), 1411–1432. 10.1177/0306624X15621984

Vanhooren, S., Leijssen, M., & Dezutter, J. (2016). Profiles of meaning and search for meaning among prisoners. *The Journal of Positive Psychology*, *11*(6), 622–633. 10.1080/17439760.2015.1137625

Vanhooren, S., Leijssen, M., & Dezutter, J. (2017). Posttraumatic growth in sex offenders: A pilot study with a mixed-method design. *International Journal of Offender Therapy and Comparative Criminology*, *61*(2), 171–190. 10.1177/0306624X15590834

Vanhooren, S., Leijssen, M., & Dezutter, J. (2018). Coping strategies and posttraumatic growth in prison. *The Prison Journal*, *98*(2), 123–142. 10.1177/0032885517753151

Vignansky, E., Addad, M., & Himi, H. (2018). Despair will hold you prisoner, hope will set you free: Hope and meaning among released prisoners. *The Prison Journal*, *98*(3), 334–358. 10.1177/0032885518764920

Wolff, N., Blitz, C. L., Shi, J., Siegel, J., & Bachman, R. (2007). Physical violence inside prisons: Rates of victimization. *Criminal Justice and Behavior*, *34*(5), 588–599. 10.1177/0093854806296830

Zlodre, J., & Fazel, S. (2012). All-cause and external mortality in released prisoners: Systematic review and meta-analysis. *American Journal of Public Health*, *102*(12), e67–e75. 10.2105/AJPH.2012.300764

35

POSTTRAUMATIC GROWTH AMONG MILITARY VETERANS

Michael A. LaRocca

Military service is a transformative human experience, presenting both a unique set of stressors as well as opportunities for personal development and growth. In addition to the major stressors associated with combat deployment, service members face separation from family, long hours of physically-exhausting training, and frequent changes of duty station and work environment; this sequence of challenging experiences concludes in the cultural readjustment to civilian life. Among veterans, coping with the aftermath of these stressors can impose some of the greatest challenges in their lives. Moreover, it is well established that veterans suffer from elevated rates of PTSD and depression, with veterans of the recent wars in Afghanistan and Iraq having rates of PTSD as high as 11 to 20% (National Center for PTSD, 2018; Tanielian & Jaycox, 2008). Regardless of whether military stressors lead to problems in mental health, recovering from these stressors may provide an avenue for PTG (Tedeschi & McNally, 2011). This chapter explores the military experience, with a focus on combat and being a prisoner of war as a precursor to PTG. In addition to summarizing research on the link between combat and PTG, it discusses how PTSD and depression – possible outcomes of military stressors – may also give rise to personal growth. The chapter concludes with implications for clinicians as well as military leaders.

The Military Experience of PTG

Literature regarding PTG related to military service includes knowledge about PTG in the aftermath of combat, PTG following being a prisoner of war, and knowledge about war-related PTG in general beyond these two specific experiences. The following sections summarize this literature.

Combat and PTG

Overview

The experience of combat may involve a prolonged major stressor or reoccurrences of traumatic experiences, often within a closely-knit military unit (Tedeschi & McNally,

 DOI: 10.4324/9781032208688-44

2011). Research on the psychological effects of a range of military conflicts suggests that, in addition to negative effects, veterans may experience a positive personal change in the aftermath of combat. Much of the early research on this topic involved studies of Vietnam War veterans. For example, Fontana and Rosenheck (1998) examined data from the National Vietnam Veterans Readjustment Study and found dual effects of combat exposure. While combat in Vietnam was positively associated with self-impoverishment and alienation from others (i.e., "psychological liabilities"), it was also associated with self-improvement and solidarity with others (i.e., "psychological benefits"). Fontana and Rosenheck (1998) found that intermediate levels of traumatic exposure were linked with the greatest feelings of solidarity. Their study also revealed that war zone exposure in the form of participation in atrocities was not associated with psychological benefits. Based on the positive and negative effects of trauma on their sample of veterans, Fontana and Rosenheck (1998) endeavored to prevent "interpreting logical opposites as psychological opposites" (p. 501), meaning that positive and negative effects may occur together.

Similar findings of PTG have occurred among veterans of conflicts after the Vietnam War. Based on a heterogeneous sample of combat veterans of the wars in Vietnam, Afghanistan, and Iraq, and other conflicts, LaRocca and Avery (2020) found overall combat experiences to be positively associated with total PTG, as well as with the PTG-specific aspects of personal strength, new possibilities, and appreciation of life. The link between combat experiences and PTG was most evident among veterans reporting low-to-moderate depression symptom severity. Similarly, based on data from the National Health and Resilience in Veterans Study, Greenberg et al. (2021) found that combat severity and number of deployments predicted the level of PTG. Their study also revealed that PTG was reported more by those who were deployed two or more times.

Social Support and Combat-Related PTG

Social support has been found to play an important role in PTG among combat veterans. For example, Maguen and colleagues (2006) explored deployment-related predictors of PTG among Gulf War I veterans. In this study, while overall exposure to warfare was not associated with PTG, the perceived threat was associated with the appreciation of life, which is a dimension of PTG. Moreover, post-deployment social support was associated with PTG overall as well as with its dimensions of relating to others and personal strength. Maguen and colleagues (2006) concluded that subjective perceptions of danger in combat may deepen one's appreciation of the value of life, as well as that supportive social networks after deployment may facilitate individual perceptions of personal growth.

Researchers have also explored how certain types of social support may relate to PTG among combat veterans. Specifically, in a study of over 3,000 Norwegian veterans of the War in Afghanistan, Nordstrand et al. (2020) found that perceptions of quality and quantity of social support contributed to PTG, while barriers to the discussion of combat experiences were associated with posttraumatic deprecation. Studies of combat veteran social support and its effects on PTG have also included the veteran-sibling dyad. For example, Zerach (2020a) found that among Israeli combat veterans, warm sibling relationships were linked with higher veteran PTG. Similarly, combat veterans' immediate family members may also benefit from veterans' PTG. In a separate but related study, Zerach (2020b) found that Israeli combat veterans' PTG was positively associated with sibling secondary PTG. As a whole, these studies suggest that trusted social networks and supportive conversations are essential to recovering and thriving after a military stressor.

In addition to exploring how types of social support may relate to PTG among combat veterans, some researchers have explored how social support within a veteran's developmental trajectory may associate with PTG. For example, in a study of treatment-seeking veterans of Operation Enduring Freedom and Operation Iraqi Freedom, Marotta-Walters et al. (2015) found that psychosocial development mediated the association between PTSD symptoms and PTG, although no direct link between combat experiences and PTG was found.

Cohesion and Combat-Related PTG

Similar to social support, feelings of cohesion while deployed may also foster PTG among combat veterans. In a large study of Operation Enduring Freedom and Operation Iraqi Freedom soldiers, Mitchell et al. (2013) found greater combat intensity to be associated with PTG. Their study also revealed that strong unit cohesion, being married, minority status, and being a junior enlisted soldier predicted PTG. To explain the link between combat and PTG, the researchers applied Schnurr et al.'s (1993) idea that the repeated stressors of combat lead to stress inoculation among soldiers, allowing them to tolerate increasing levels of adversity, while also building coping skills through greater confidence in their ability to tolerate stress. Based on their findings, Mitchell et al. (2013) recommended that bolstering unit cohesion before, during, and after combat may maximize PTG.

Specific Wartime Events and PTG

Research on PTG among combat veterans also suggests that personal growth may originate from specific events during combat or from combat-related stress in general. For example, Staugaard et al. (2015) explored how the memory of significant combat-related events, either positive or negative, may relate to PTG among Danish veterans of the War in Afghanistan. Their study found that perceptions of significant positive and negative combat events were associated with PTG, as was openness to experience, social support, and combat exposure itself. Staugaard and colleagues (2015) suggested that balanced processing of positive and negative memories may be most effective in producing PTG among combat veterans. In another study of specific events predicting PTG, Evans et al. (2018) explored PTG among veterans, the majority of whom had experienced combat, and all of whom were experiencing religious and spiritual struggles. Veterans who specifically reported violating their own morals (i.e., experiencing moral injury) and those with higher life satisfaction were more likely to report PTG. To describe the mechanism of PTG, Evans, and colleagues used Hayes et al.'s (2012) idea of the desire to revise life priorities around the moral or personal value that was violated.

PTG Among POWs

An important body of PTG research comes from studies of former prisoners of war (POWs). Among earlier studies in this area, Sledge et al. (1980) investigated self-concept changes among U.S. Air Force personnel who were repatriated Vietnam War POWs. Reported POW experiences included solitary confinement, torture, and disease, as well as enduring long periods of monotony that were punctuated by physical and psychological abuse, threats, and extreme distress. Remarkably, 61.1% of former POWs reported positive psychological change, whereas only 32.0% of control participants (i.e., pilots and navigators who had served combat tours in Southeast Asia but were not POWs) reported such changes. Psychological benefits included optimism, discerning important matters from the trivial, interpersonal effectiveness, patience, and understanding of others.

More recent studies have also found a link between war captivity and PTG. For example, Erbes et al. (2005) used the Posttraumatic Growth Inventory (Tedeschi & Calhoun, 1996) to assess PTG among former POWs from World War II and the Korean War. Predictors of PTG included the personality component of positive activity, while POW trauma exposure was positively related to perceived strength. According to Erbes and colleagues (2005), experiences of starvation, abuse, and torture taught these former POWs that they were stronger than they had initially believed. A study by Solomon and Dekel (2007) compared PTG levels of former POWs of the 1973 Yom Kippur War with non-POW veterans of the war. While the former POWs reported higher PTG, they also had higher levels of PTSD symptoms. These researchers also found that the POW coping strategy of detachment was positively associated with PTG. Given the powerlessness of being in captivity, some POWs appeared to adapt by compartmentalizing their suffering and mentally withdrawing from their environment (Sledge et al., 1980; Solomon & Dekel, 2007; Solomon et al., 1999). In another study, Feder et al. (2008) explored PTG among 30 former POWs in the Vietnam War, most of whom were aviators who had been shot down. Using the Posttraumatic Growth Inventory, the authors found that most study participants reported moderate or greater PTG, with the greatest growth occurring in the dimensions of personal strength and appreciation of life. PTG was also associated with optimism and duration of captivity, supporting the idea that significant hardships confront individuals with a need to find meaning, which may lead to a revision of life goals (Feder et al., 2008; Tedeschi & Calhoun, 1996).

PTG Related to General Wartime Experiences

Alternative to reflection on specific combat-related events, a more general assessment of wartime events may also lead to PTG. For example, Rosner and Powell (2006) found that the total traumatic events experienced by veterans of the war in Bosnia and Herzegovina were positively associated with the PTG aspect of relating to others. Their study also revealed that total PTG was positively associated with task-oriented, emotion-oriented, and avoidance-oriented coping. In interpreting these findings, the researchers noted that the war in Bosnia and Herzegovina often involved former friends and acquaintances fighting on opposite sides. As such, surviving the war required the cultivation of trust and mutual support with others while enduring shared hardships.

In sum, the body of research linking combat experiences to PTG spans many decades, conflicts, and service member experiences. Although the horrors of combat are a notable risk factor for mental health problems such as PTSD (e.g., National Center for PTSD, 2018), the research described here suggests that PTG may result when military stressors are framed as opportunities for personal growth and development. As illustrated in PTG studies involving social support (e.g., Nordstrand et al., 2020), growth may be fully realized when military trauma survivors are embedded in trusted support systems. The role of these support systems is further discussed in this chapter's section on clinical implications.

PTSD and Depression as Impetus for Veterans' PTG

A large body of research suggests that veterans suffer from high rates of PTSD and depression (e.g., National Center for PTSD, 2018; Tanielian & Jaycox, 2008), both of which may provide the impetus for PTG. Overall, the research on both PTSD and depression as they relate to PTG among veterans presents a mixed set of findings. Perhaps what is most clear from the review of relevant studies is that both PTSD and depression present important opportunities for PTG among veterans.

Veterans' PTSD and PTG

Consistent with the notion that adversarial experiences are often necessary to give rise to personal growth, some research has found a positive association between PTSD symptoms and PTG among veterans of the wars in Afghanistan and Iraq (e.g., Pietrzak et al., 2010), as well as among mixed veteran samples (e.g., Martz et al., 2018; Morgan et al., 2017). However, research on the relationship between PTSD symptom severity and PTG among veterans presents inconsistent findings. In an early study, Fontana and Rosenheck (1998) explored psychological benefits and liabilities among veterans of the Vietnam War. Although they did not examine PTG as we now know it, the authors found psychological benefits (i.e., affirmation, self-improvement, and feelings of solidarity with others) to negatively associate with PTSD, while psychological liabilities (i.e., disillusionment, self-impoverishment, and alienation) were positively associated with it. They noted that the sense of self-improvement was the greatest protective factor against PTSD among these veterans. Other studies, however, have not found a meaningful relationship between PTSD and PTG. For example, Feder et al. (2008) found no relation between current psychopathology and PTG in a sample of former POWs of the Vietnam War. They proposed that while trauma may give rise to a search for personal meaning, the specific relationship between PTSD and PTG is complex. Similarly, Hijazi et al. (2015) explored potential predictors of PTG among a clinical sample of veterans of the Korean War, Vietnam War, first Persian Gulf War, and the recent wars in Afghanistan and Iraq. Although they found that minority ethnicity, cognitive flexibility, and perception of moral wrongdoing were associated with greater PTG, PTSD symptoms were not associated with growth. These findings provided further support for a potentially complex relationship between PTSD and PTG, and the researchers suggested a need to explore mediators and moderators of the relationship.

A considerable body of research suggests that the relationship between PTSD and PTG is not linear. For example, Solomon and Dekel (2007) found a curvilinear (inverted-U) relationship between PTSD symptom severity and PTG among Israeli former POWs, in which medium symptom severity was associated with the most growth. These findings have been replicated among a variety of samples. McCaslin et al. (2009) found a similar inverted-U relationship between posttraumatic stress symptoms and PTG among Sri Lankan medical students. This unique sample, which had experienced civil war and political uprising, also yielded a curvilinear relationship between peritraumatic dissociation (i.e., dissociation occurring during or immediately after the trauma) and PTG. Similarly, studies by Tsai et al. (2015), Whealin and colleagues (2020), and Greenberg et al. (2021) of large, nationally representative cohorts of U.S. veterans found curvilinear relationships between PTSD and PTG, where moderate PTSD was most associated with PTG, providing further support for a nonlinear relationship between PTSD and PTG. The results suggested that in addition to PTSD having an inverted-U relationship with PTG, it also appears to drive PTG across time. Adding greater specificity to the link between PTSD and PTG, Greenberg et al. (2021), who examined the relationship between PTSD symptom clusters and PTG among veterans participating in the National Health and Resilience in Veterans Study, found that re-experiencing symptoms were independently associated with PTG among other symptom clusters, suggesting that intrusive thoughts set the stage for attempts to understand and make meaning of trauma (Greenberg et al., 2021; Tedeschi & Calhoun, 2004). On the whole, these studies suggest that PTSD symptoms and PTG are not mutually exclusive and that an optimal distress level appears to give rise to personal growth. While very low and very high levels of PTSD present challenges to PTG, moderate PTSD levels appear to provide a strong impetus for recovery and growth.

Veterans' Depression and PTG

While intuitively depression symptoms limit the ability to derive meaning and personal growth following a trauma, compared to the amount of studies on PTSD and PTG, research on depression as it relates to PTG is limited, especially in the context of veterans. Studies of the relation of depression to PTG are both preliminary and inconsistent, although overall findings suggest that negative thinking accompanying depression may be a barrier to the meaning-making necessary for PTG. One notable study by Bush et al. (2011) explored whether PTG was a protective factor against suicidal ideation among combat veterans. Based on a sample of over 5,000 predominantly Army-veteran participants, depression was negatively associated with PTG, as was suicidal ideation, even after adjusting for depression, emotional lability, substance abuse, and PTSD. While these findings are promising, more research should further test whether PTG is a protective factor against suicide among combat veterans. More recently, Palmer et al. (2016) found that among a sample of veterans receiving treatment for PTSD, there was a significant negative linear relationship between depression and PTG in general as well as with its individual dimensions. Thus, it is unclear if the relationship between depression and PTG takes on an inverted-U shape (as with PTSD and PTG), although such a relationship appears possible based on preliminary research (e.g., Kleim & Ehlers, 2009).

While some studies have not directly investigated the link between PTG and depression, they have arguably shed light on the relationship. For example, Feder et al. (2008) explored the role of optimism on PTG among former POWs of the Vietnam War. Although not measuring depression directly, the study found a positive association between optimism (which is arguably incompatible with depression) and PTG, even after adjusting for length of captivity, religious coping, and purpose in life. Similarly, Currier et al. (2013) found no association between PTG and depression among a clinical sample of veterans within six months of returning from service in the wars in Afghanistan and Iraq but reported a connection between PTG and feeling a need to disclose a trauma. Such disclosure may be an important first step to explore and challenge self-blame, feelings of worthlessness, or other depression symptoms relating to the trauma. Moreover, studying a mixed sample of veterans, Morgan et al. (2017) found a positive association between PTG and satisfaction with life as well as with deliberate rumination, a form of cognitive processing that may provide the underpinnings for recovering from depression. Finally, LaRocca and Avery (2020) found that combat experiences were positively associated with PTG, and that this association was strongest among those with low-to-moderate depression levels. Although depression was not directly related to PTG, results suggested that restructuring of depression-related cognitions may provide the foundation for PTG after combat.

Clinical Implications for PTG among Veterans

Clinicians working with veterans are in an important position to highlight personal meaning and growth in the context of military stressors. However, research on clinical interventions to enhance PTG is extremely limited. Among the few studies in this area, Hagenaars and van Minnen (2010) found that the therapeutic technique of prolonged exposure to PTSD increased PTG. In addition, Roepke (2015) found in a meta-analysis that cognitive-behavioral therapy, cognitive-based stress management, and emotional disclosure led to increases in PTG. Moreover, based on their robust findings of the positive association between PTSD and PTG, Greenberg et al. (2021) suggested that assessment, monitoring, and clinical emphasis on PTG may bolster the quality of life of combat veterans, including their mental health. Finally, a recent study evaluating a PTG training program found that growth increased by the 18-month follow-up (Moore et al., 2021). This study also found that by the end of the program, PTG was associated with psychological well-being, including lower PTSD, depression, and insomnia, as well as higher psychological flexibility and self-compassion.

Although research is limited on whether established clinical approaches increase PTG, the literature suggests that the experience of combat and its aftermath provides an opportunity for positive personal change. Accordingly, in addition to using evidence-based treatments of PTSD and depression, clinicians working with veterans may facilitate the exploration of how trauma recovery provides a pathway to personal growth and life meaning (Tedeschi & Calhoun, 2006). According to Tedeschi and McNally (2011), clinical approaches to promoting PTG focus on cognitive, existential, humanistic, and storytelling techniques. In line with these approaches, factors of the Posttraumatic Growth Inventory (Tedeschi & Calhoun, 1996) provide guideposts to explore areas of potential clinical value. These factors, which consist of new possibilities, relating to others, personal strength, spiritual change, and appreciation of life, have had broad clinical applications in the U.S. and other Western cultures.

Through therapy, a clinician may serve as an "expert companion" (Tedeschi & Calhoun, 2006) by showing humility and respect toward the veteran's experience, while also pointing out areas of strength and personal growth. In a recent elaboration of expert companionship, as it applies to interventions to increase PTG, Moore and colleagues (2021) noted that expert companions facilitate growth through five elements. These are psychoeducation on trauma response and personal growth, training in meditation and mindfulness to regulate emotions, constructive disclosure about trauma and its aftermath using natural conversation, narrative perspectives, and helping others who have not been exposed to PTG perspectives. In addition, Tedeschi and Calhoun (2006) noted that in treating combat veterans with negative interpretations of their experiences, clinicians may emphasize that PTG often consists of a co-occurrence of positive and negative cognitions about a traumatic experience and its aftermath. Clinicians may also encourage reflective rumination, in which the veteran identifies cognitive distortions or other errors in thinking that perpetuate distress and impose a barrier to growth (Tedeschi & Moore, 2016). These negative thoughts may then be replaced with more objective, realistic, and helpful thoughts.

According to Janoff-Bulman (2006), trauma recovery may also build hardiness to negotiate future stressors with greater self-efficacy and wisdom. As other researchers have documented (e.g., Hawker & Nino, 2017), veterans may find it both refreshing and salutary to go beyond a symptoms focus to one that includes newfound personal growth and meaning. Moreover, in a culturally-informed model of PTG, Calhoun et al. (2010) proposed several coping mechanisms for facilitating PTG. These include reflective rumination, expressing concerns about the traumatic event, seeking responses from others to one's personal disclosures, and the distal and proximate sociocultural context.

Military Leadership and PTG

Although PTG may arise through clinical interventions, military leaders are also in an important position early on to set the stage for growth. Because PTG may be maximized when supportive structures for personal growth are present, service members may benefit from supportive military leadership before, during, and immediately after combat or other major military stressors. A developing body of research suggests that psychologically-informed leaders may support follower well-being by serving as a buffer against major stressors. For example, supportive military leadership has been found to associate with fewer symptoms of PTSD (e.g., LaRocca et al., 2018; Wood et al., 2012). In a similar vein, positive, supportive leadership styles may influence PTG among followers. For example, the approaches that Tedeschi and McNally (2011) proposed for fostering PTG among veterans arguably apply to military leadership during a combat trauma or its aftermath. They note that the psychoeducational training on PTG incorporated in the U.S. Army's Comprehensive Soldier Fitness Program may be implemented prior to deployment. They also suggest that leaders or other supportive people reassure service members that distress is a normal reaction to combat, as well as that leader's model and encourage healthy responses to stressors. For example, while their units face major stressors, military leaders may emphasize help-seeking behavior, supportive conversations with leaders and peers, as well as the use of mental health services and other resources available from the military and the greater community. Military leaders may discuss with followers how to combat stress or other major stressors that may lay the groundwork for PTG, resilience, and post-deployment readjustment (Tedeschi & McNally). Tedeschi (2013) called on military leaders to educate soldiers about PTG prior to deployment, as well as serve as an expert companion after deployment to help service members achieve their potential for PTG. However, Tedeschi recommended that military leaders discuss PTG only when the timing is right, such as when service members are more open to it. In addition to the suggestions put forth by Tedeschi and McNally (2011) and Tedeschi (2013), it is noted here that military leaders may further support PTG by discouraging risky behaviors such as substance use, aggression, and isolation.

In line with research on how leaders may influence PTG, Bartone (2006) proposed that military leaders may set an example for adaptive interpretations of military stressors, which in turn may promote follower resilience. He noted that stress-hardy individuals interpret major stressors as interesting and worthwhile challenges that serve as opportunities for learning and personal growth. Given the structure and cohesion of military units, stress-hardy military leaders may transmit these interpretations to followers. According to Bartone, resilience-promoting leaders may use advice and counsel, positive storytelling and reconstruction of shared stressful events, and sharing of examples of resilience, all of which may help followers make sense of and find meaning in stressful experiences. Bartone further suggested that military after-action reviews, which have long been a standard method of post-event debriefing to improve future operations, present an opportunity for military leaders to communicate positive interpretations of stressors to promote resilience and growth.

Transformational leadership, which decades of research have established as a style that is both supportive of followers and effective for organizations, is an example of a leadership approach that may foster personal growth among followers. Transformational leaders create positive change by communicating an inspiring vision and raising the motivation and enthusiasm of followers to achieve this vision (Avolio & Bass, 1995; Burns, 1978). Transformational leaders inspire change through four behavioral dimensions: (1) *idealized influence*, in which leaders exemplify positive characteristics and behaviors; (2) *inspirational motivation*, in which leaders encourage followers to achieve a shared vision; (3) *individualized consideration*, in which leaders recognize the uniqueness of each follower while providing coaching and mentorship; and (4) *intellectual stimulation*, in which leaders encourage diverse feedback and innovation (Avolio & Bass, 1995; Bass & Riggio, 2006). Although transformational leadership is well-established in its association with follower performance and organizational effectiveness (e.g., Judge & Piccolo, 2004; Wang & Howell, 2012), follower well-being (e.g., LaRocca et al., 2018; Perko et al., 2014), and organizational, team, and subordinate resilience (Dimas et al., 2018; Harland et al., 2005; Witmer & Mellinger, 2016), very little research has explored transformational leadership's role in follower PTG among service members or veterans. More research in this area may provide support for theoretical models of transformational leadership (e.g., MacIntyre et al., 2013), authentic leadership, and other supportive leadership approach nurturing followers' ability to recover from major stressors. In a preliminary study in this area among combat veterans, LaRocca and Groves (2021) found that perceived transformational leadership in combat was positively associated with PTG, particularly among longer deployments. They concluded that while longer deployments present more opportunities for stressors, there is also more time for leaders to cultivate psychologically-supportive relationships with followers and lay the groundwork for follower PTG. Despite these promising findings, more research is needed to verify the association between transformational leadership and follower PTG across contexts, as well as whether other supportive leadership approaches (e.g., servant leadership, authentic leadership, and other positive, encompassing leadership styles) similarly associate with personal growth.

Conclusion

The experience of combat imposes significant and repeated military-related stressors, often over a lengthy deployment. Although combat may be one of the most difficult human experiences, conditions such as PTSD and depression are not inevitable outcomes, and combat may provide the groundwork for PTG. When PTSD does result, research suggests that moderate levels of symptoms provide the greatest opportunity for positive rumination and other bases for PTG. Accordingly, PTG may be an important adjunct to manualized PTSD treatment approaches. Similarly, the cognitive underpinnings of depression treatment are also the basis for finding meaning and growth after a life stressor. Treatment programs involving PTG show promise in their efficacy, and clinicians would do well to emphasize avenues for personal growth in addition to attending to symptom reduction. Finally, military leaders may foster a PTG mindset among followers before, during, and after combat and other military stressors. Proactive approaches to growth modeled by leaders provide coping tools to service members early on, serving to maximize recovery and growth among service members and veterans.

References

Avolio, B. J., & Bass, B. M. (1995). Individual consideration viewed at multiple levels of analysis: A multi-level framework for examining the diffusion of transformational leadership. *The Leadership Quarterly*, *6*(2), 199–218. 10.1016/1048-9843(95)90035-7

Bartone, P. T. (2006). Resilience under military operational stress: Can leaders influence hardiness? *Military Psychology*, *18*(Suppl.), S131–S148. 10.1207/s15327876mp1803s_10

Bass, B. M., & Riggio, R. E. (2006). *Transformational leadership* (2nd ed.). Mahwah, NJ: Erlbaum.

Burns, J. M. (1978). *Leadership*. New York: Harper & Row.

Bush, N. E., Skopp, N. A., McCann, R., & Luxton, D. D. (2011). Posttraumatic growth as protection against suicidal ideation after deployment and combat exposure. *Military Medicine*, *176*(11), 1215–1222. 10.7205/milmed-d-11-00018

Calhoun, L. G., Cann, A., & Tedeschi, R. G. (2010). The posttraumatic growth model: Sociocultural considerations. In T. Weiss, & R. Berger (Eds.), *Posttraumatic growth and culturally competent practice: Lessons learned from around the globe* (pp. 1–14). Hoboken NJ: Wiley.

Currier, J. M., Lisman, R., Harris, J. I., Tait, R., & Erbes, C. R. (2013). Cognitive processing of trauma and attitudes toward disclosure in the first six months after military deployment. *Journal of Clinical Psychology*, *69*(3), 209–221. 10.1002/jclp.21930

Dimas, I. D., Rebelo, T., Lourenço, P. R., & Pessoa, C. I. P. (2018). Bouncing back from setbacks: On the mediating role of team resilience in the relationship between transformational leadership and team effectiveness. *The Journal of Psychology: Interdisciplinary and Applied*, *152*(6), 358–372. 10.1080/00223980.2018.1465022

Erbes, C., Eberly, R., Dikel, T., Johnsen, E., Harris, I., & Engdahl, B. (2005). Posttraumatic Growth among American former prisoners of War. *Traumatology* *11*(4), 285–295. 10.1177/1534765605 01100407

Evans, W. R., Szabo, Y. Z., Stanley, M. A., Barrera, T. L., Exline, J. J., Pargament, K. I., & Teng, E. J. (2018). Life satisfaction among veterans: Unique associations with morally injurious events and posttraumatic growth. *Traumatology*, *24*(4), 263–270. 10.1037/trm0000157

Feder, A., Southwick, S. M., Goetz, R. R., Wang, Y., Alonso, A., Smith, B. W., Buchholz, K. R., Waldeck, T., Ameli, R., Moore, J., Hain, R., Charney, D. S., & Vythilingam, M. (2008). Posttraumatic growth in former Vietnam prisoners of war. *Psychiatry*, *71*(4), 359–370.

Fontana, A., & Rosenheck, R. (1998). Psychological benefits and liabilities of traumatic exposure in the war zone. *Journal of Trauma Stress*, *11*(3), 485–503.

Greenberg, J., Tsai, J., Southwick, S. M., & Pietrzak, R. H. (2021). Can military trauma promote psychological growth in combat veterans? Results from the national health and resilience in veterans study. *Journal of Affective Disorders*, *282*(8), 732–739. 10.1016/j.jad.2020.12.077

Hagenaars, M. A., & van Minnen, A. (2010). Posttraumatic growth in exposure therapy for PTSD. *Journal of Traumatic Stress*, *23*(4), 504–508. 10.1002/jts.20551

Harland, L., Harrison, W., Jones, J. R., & Reiter-Palmon, R. (2005). Leadership behaviors and subordinate resilience. *Journal of Leadership and Organizational Studies*, *11*(2), 2–14. 10.1177/1 07179190501100202

Hawker, M. E., & Nino, A. (2017). Factors contributing to posttraumatic growth in Iraq and Afghanistan combat veterans. *Journal of Aggression, Maltreatment & Trauma*, *26*(10), 1104–1116. 10.1080/10926771.2017.1341442

Hayes, S. C., Strosahl, K. D. & Wilson, K. G. (2012). *Acceptance and commitment therapy: The process and practice of mindful change* (2nd ed.). Guilford Press.

Hijazi, A. M., Keith, J. A., & O'Brien, C. (2015). Predictors of posttraumatic growth in a multiwar sample of U.S. combat veterans. *Peace and Conflict: Journal of Peace Psychology*, *21*(3), 395–408. 10.1037/pac0000077

Janoff-Bulman, R. (2006). Schema-change perspectives on posttraumatic growth. In L. G. Calhoun, & R. G. Tedeschi (Eds.), *Handbook of posttraumatic growth: Research and practice* (pp. 81–99). Mahwah, NJ: Erlbaum.

Judge, T. A., & Piccolo, R. F. (2004). Transformational and transactional leadership: A meta-analytic test of their relative validity. *Journal of Applied Psychology*, *89*(5), 755–768. 10.1037/0021-9010. 89.5.755

Kleim, B., & Ehlers, A. (2009). Evidence for a curvilinear relationship between posttraumatic growth and posttrauma depression and PTSD in assault survivors. *Journal of Traumatic Stress*, *22*(1), 45–52. 10.1002/jts.20378

LaRocca, M. A., & Avery, T. J. (2020). Combat experiences link with posttraumatic growth among veterans across conflicts: The influence of PTSD and depression. *Journal of Nervous and Mental Disease*, *208*(6), 445–451. 10.1097/NMD.0000000000001147

LaRocca, M. A., & Groves, K. S. (2022). Transformational leadership in extreme contexts: Associations with posttraumatic growth and self-efficacy among combat veterans. *Armed Forces & Society*, *48*(4), 849–871. 10.1177/0095327X211030610

LaRocca, M. A., Scogin, F. R., Hilgeman, M. M., Smith, A. J., & Chaplin, W. F. (2018). The impact of posttraumatic growth, transformational leadership, and self-efficacy on PTSD and depression symptom severity among combat veterans. *Military Psychology*, *30*(2), 162–173. 10.1080/08995605.2018.1425073

MacIntyre, A., Charbonneau, D., & O'Keefe, D. (2013). The role of transformational and ethical leadership in building and maintaining resilience. In R. R. Sinclair, & T. W. Britt (Eds.), *Building psychological resilience in military personnel: Theory and practice* (pp. 85–111). American Psychological Association. 10.1037/14190-005

Maguen, S., Vogt, D. S., King, L. A., King, D. W., & Litz, B. T. (2006). Posttraumatic growth among Gulf War I veterans: The predictive role of deployment-related experiences and background characteristics. *Journal of Loss and Trauma*, *11*(5), 373–388. 10.1080/15325020600672004

Marotta-Walters, S., Choi, J., & Shaine, M. D. (2015). Posttraumatic growth among combat veterans: A proposed developmental pathway. *Psychological Trauma: Theory, Research, Practice, and Policy*, 7(4), 356–363. 10.1037/tra0000030

Martz, E., Livneh, H., Southwick, S. M., & Pietrzak, R. H. (2018). Posttraumatic growth moderates the effect of posttraumatic stress on quality of life in U.S. military veterans with life-threatening illness or injury. *Journal of Psychosomatic Research*, *109*, 1–8. 10.1016/j.jpsychores.2018.03.004

McCaslin, S. E., De Zoysa, P., Butler, L. D., Hart, S., Marmar, C. R., Metzler, T. J., & Koopman, C. (2009). The relationship of posttraumatic growth to peritraumatic reactions and posttraumatic stress symptoms among Sri Lankan university students. *Journal of Traumatic Stress*, *22*(4), 334–339. 10.1002/jts.20426

Mitchell, M. M., Gallaway, M. S., Millikan, A. M., & Bell, M. R. (2013). Combat exposure, unit cohesion, and demographic characteristics of soldiers reporting posttraumatic growth. *Journal of Loss and Trauma*, *18*(5), 383–395. 10.1080/15325024.2013.768847

Moore, B. A., Tedeschi, R. G., & Greene, T. C. (2021). A preliminary examination of a posttraumatic growth-based program for veteran mental health. *Practice Innovations*, *6*(1), 42–54. 10.1037/pri0000136

Morgan, J. K., Desmarais, S. L., Mitchell, R. E. & Simons-Rudolph, J. M. (2017). Posttraumatic stress, posttraumatic growth, and satisfaction with life in military veterans. *Military Psychology*, *29*(5), 434–447. 10.1037/mil0000182

National Center for PTSD. (2018). How common is PTSD in veterans? Retrieved September 30, 2021, from https://www.ptsd.va.gov/understand/common/common_veterans.asp#:~:text=The%20number%20of%20Veterans%20with,PTSD%20in%20a%20given%20year.

Nordstrand, A. E., Bøe, H. J., Holen, A., Reichelt, J. G., Gjerstad, C. L., & Hjemdal, O. (2020). Social support and disclosure of war-zone experiences after deployment to Afghanistan – Implications for posttraumatic deprecation or growth. *Traumatology*, *26*(4), 351–360. 10.1037/trm0000254

Palmer, G. A., Graca, J. J., & Occhietti, K. E. (2016). Posttraumatic growth and its relationship to depressive symptomatology in veterans with PTSD. *Traumatology*, *22*(4), 299–306. 10.1037/trm0000101

Perko, K., Kinnunen, U., & Feldt, T. (2014). Transformational leadership and depressive symptoms among employees: Mediating factors. *Leadership & Organization Development Journal*, *35*(4), 286–304. 10.1108/LODJ-07-2012-0082

Pietrzak, R. H., Goldstein, M. B., Malley, J. C., Rivers, A. J., Johnson, D. C., Morgan, C. A. III, & Southwick, S. M. (2010). Posttraumatic growth in veterans of operations enduring freedom and Iraqi freedom. *Journal of Affective Disorders*, *126*(1-2), 230–235. 10.1016/j.jad.2010.03.021

Roepke, A. M. (2015). Psychosocial interventions and posttraumatic growth: A meta-analysis. *Journal of Consulting and Clinical Psychology*, *83*(1), 129–142. 10.1037/a0036872

Rosner, R., & Powell, S. (2006). Posttraumatic growth after war. In L. G. Calhoun, & R. G. Tedeschi (Eds.), *Handbook of posttraumatic growth: Research and practice* (pp. 197–213). Mahwah, NJ: Erlbaum.

Schnurr, P. P., Rosenberg, S. D., & Friedman, M. J. (1993). Change in MMPI scores from college to adulthood as a function of military service. *Journal of Abnormal Psychology*, *102*(2), 288–296. 10.1037/0021-843X.102.2.288

Sledge, W. H., Boydstun, J. A., & Rabe, A. J. (1980). Self-concept changes related to war captivity. *Archives of General Psychiatry*, *37*(4), 430–443. 10.1001/archpsyc.1980.01780170072008

Solomon, Z., & Dekel, R. (2007). Posttraumatic stress disorder and posttraumatic growth among Israeli ex-POWs. *Journal of Trauma Stress*, *20*(3), 303–312. 10.1002/jts.20216

Solomon, Z., Waysman, M. A., Neria, Y., Ohry, A., Schwarzwald, J. & Wiener, M. (1999). Positive and negative changes in the lives of Israeli former prisoners of war. *Journal of Social and Clinical Psychology*, *18*(4), 419–435. 10.1521/jscp.1999.18.4.419

Staugaard, S. R., Johannessen, K. B., Thomsen, Y. D., Bertelsen, M., & Berntsen, D. (2015). Centrality of positive and negative deployment memories predicts posttraumatic growth in Danish veterans. *Journal of Clinical Psychology*, *71*(4), 362–377. 10.1002/jclp.22142

Tanielian, T., & Jaycox, L. H. (2008). *Invisible wounds of war: Psychological and cognitive injuries, their consequences, and services to assist recovery*. Santa Monica, CA: The RAND Center for Military Health Policy Research.

Tedeschi, R. G. (2013). Posttraumatic growth. In G. B. Graen, & J. A. Graen (Eds.), *Management of team leadership in extreme context: Defending our homeland, protecting our first responders* (pp. 101–111). Information Age Publishing.

Tedeschi, R. G., & Calhoun, L. G. (1996). The posttraumatic growth inventory: Measuring the positive legacy of trauma. *Journal of Traumatic Stress*, *9*(3), 455–471. 10.1007/BF02103658.

Tedeschi, R. G., & Calhoun, L. G. (2004). Posttraumatic growth: Conceptual foundations and empirical evidence. *Psychological Inquiry*, *15*(1), 1–18. 10.1207/s15327965pli1501_01

Tedeschi, R. G., & Calhoun, L. G. (2006). Expert companions: Posttraumatic growth in clinical practice. In L. G. Calhoun, & R. G. Tedeschi (Eds.), *Handbook of posttraumatic growth: Research and practice* (pp. 291–310). Mahwah, NJ: Erlbaum.

Tedeschi, R. G., & McNally, R. J. (2011). Can we facilitate posttraumatic growth in combat veterans? *American Psychologist*, *66*(1), 19–24. 10.1037/a0021896

Tedeschi, R. G., & Moore, B. A. (2016). *The posttraumatic growth workbook: Coming through trauma wiser, stronger, and more resilient*. New Harbinger Publications, Inc.

Tsai, J., El-Gabalawy, R., Sledge, W. H., Southwick, S. M., & Pietrzak, R. H. (2015). Posttraumatic growth among veterans in the USA: Results from the National Health and Resilience in Veterans Study. *Psychological Medicine*, *45*(1), 165–179. 10.1017/S0033291714001202

Wang, X., & Howell, J. M. (2012). A multilevel study of transformational leadership, identification, and follower outcomes. *The Leadership Quarterly*, *23*(5), 775–790. 10.1016/j.leaqua.2012.02.001

Whealin, J. M., Pitts, B., Tsai, J., Rivera, C., Fogle, B. M., Southwick, S. M., & Pietrzak, R. H. (2020). Dynamic interplay between PTSD symptoms and posttraumatic growth in older military veterans. *Journal of Affective Disorders*, *269*(6), 185–191. 10.1016/j.jad.2020.03.020

Witmer, H., & Mellinger, M. S. (2016). Organizational resilience: Nonprofit organizations' response to change. *Work*, *54*(2), 255–265. 10.3233/WOR-162303

Wood, M. D., Foran, H. M., Britt, T. W., & Wright, K. M. (2012). The impact of benefit finding and leadership on combat-related PTSD symptoms. *Military Psychology*, *24*(6), 529–541. 10.1080/08995605.2012.736321

Zerach G. (2020a). Posttraumatic growth among combat veterans and their siblings: A dyadic approach. *Journal of Clinical Psychology*, *76*(9), 1719–1735. 10.1002/jclp.22949

Zerach, G. (2020b). "He ain't heavy, he's my brother": Distress tolerance moderates the association between secondary posttraumatic symptoms and secondary posttraumatic growth among siblings of combat veterans. *Psychological Trauma: Theory, Research, Practice, and Policy*, *12*(7), 687–697. 10.1037/tra0000582

36

POSTTRAUMATIC GROWTH IN THE CONTEXT OF TRAUMATIC LOSS

Leia Y. Saltzman, Sophie Brickman, and Michal Toporek

The documentation of instances of posttraumatic growth (PTG) has spanned multiple populations (e.g., Bellet et al., 2018; Palgi, 2016; Saltzman et al., 2018; Tian & Solomon, 2020), different geographical regions (e.g., Lee et al., 2019; Lumb et al., 2017; Ogińska-Bulik, 2015; Pat-Horenczyk et al., 2015; Sattler et al., 2018; Xu et al., 2015) and different types of trauma (e.g., Feder et al., 2008; Kleim & Ehlers, 2009; Pat-Horenczyk et al., 2015; Saltzman et al., 2018; Solomon & Dekel, 2007; Spain et al., 2019; Sumalla et al., 2008). This chapter focuses specifically on bereavement. While bereavement can be understood as a universal reality, a subset of individuals experience traumatic loss, and subsequently may experience PTG.

Outcomes of Traumatic Loss

Traumatic loss is a bereavement experience in which the loss is sudden, violent, unexpected, or "off time" (Green, 2000). Examples of traumatic loss may include homicide, suicide, or the loss of a child. The criteria for trauma exposure (Criterion A for posttraumatic stress disorder) in the Diagnostic and Statistical Manual (DSM-V) include exposure to death or threatened death as a form of trauma (American Psychiatric Association, 2013), confirming the potential psychological ramifications of traumatic loss.

The experience of traumatic loss may be associated with posttraumatic stress disorder (Green, 2000; Krosch & Shakespeare-Finch, 2017). For example, several large studies suggest that the rates of PTSD diagnosis in homicide survivors were approximately 20-30% (Green, 2000; Rheingold & Williams, 2015). Beyond PTSD, survivors of traumatic loss may experience disruptions in sleep (Bonanno et al., 2007), eating disorders (Kersting et al., 2007), disintegration of important or intimate relationships (Bonanno et al., 2007), substance use disorders (Zinzow et al., 2009), anxiety (Kersting et al., 2007), depression (McDevitt-Murphy et al., 2012) and suicidal ideation (Latham & Prigerson, 2004).

While traumatic loss overlaps with other forms of trauma exposure, it has unique features in that survivors may experience *both* grief and posttraumatic stress. For example, a survivor of a school shooting may grieve the loss of their peers (bereavement symptoms) and simultaneously experience trauma symptoms including a persistent sense of threat, a desire to

 DOI: 10.4324/9781032208688-45

avoid reminders of the shooting, or intrusive memories about the shooting (Green, 2000). As a result of this combination, a traumatic loss may also result in a diagnosis of persistent complex bereavement disorder (American Psychiatric Association, 2013; Green, 2000).

Mourning is the external expression of grief resulting from bereavement (Kubler Ross & Kessler, 2005). Kubler-Ross (1969; Kubler Ross & Kessler, 2005) provided the seminal theoretical perspective outlining the process of mourning by identifying five stages of grief: (1) denial; (2) anger; (3) bargaining; (4) depression; and (5) acceptance. Over time, her theoretical perspective has been refined to shift from a sequential stage model to a cyclical process highly interconnected to the experience of time (Saltzman, 2019). Yet the inclusion of PTG in formal models of grief and mourning remains lackluster.

Growth Following Traumatic Loss

Theories of human adaptation have long focused on how individuals, families, and communities cope with and grow from challenging circumstances. Distinct among these theories is the notion of benefit finding following traumatic events. Over decades of research, the picture of how individuals find benefits in the face of trauma has refined (Kobasa, 1979; Linley & Joseph, 2004; McMillen et al., 1997; Park et al., 1996; Ryff & Singer, 1998) and is now commonly referred to as PTG (Tedeschi & Calhoun, 1996). As a concept, PTG extends the expectations of survivors' adaptability from 'bouncing back' (i.e., resilience) to 'bouncing forward' in the wake of trauma (Walsh, 2002). Once PTG was established as a potential outcome following traumatic events, attention turned to identifying the factors that predict PTG and developing clinical approaches to maximize the possibility of experiencing growth after trauma. The development of literature regarding PTG has led to four important realizations, which are outlined focusing on their application to contexts of traumatic loss.

There Is Something Unique in the Experience of Traumatic Loss

Compatible with Janoff-Bulman's (1992) idea that humans have basic assumptions that the world is predictable, controllable, meaningful, just, fair, safe, secure, and trusting, a traumatic loss can shatter these basic assumptions and trigger a process by which survivors attempt to reduce the gap between these foundational worldviews and the new realities of their world following a loss (Davis et al., 2000). Traumatic loss engages survivors in a psychological struggle to modify their beliefs about the world, which is an important catalyst for PTG (Bellet et al., 2018; Calhoun et al., 2010; Davis et al., 2007; Green, 2000; Krosch & Shakespeare-Finch, 2017; Tedeschi & Calhoun, 2004). PTG can occur as survivors struggle with challenges associated with the loss and subsequently, modify their beliefs and views to account for, and explain, the traumatic experience (Tedeschi & Calhoun, 2004). The domains of PTG (appreciation of life, relating to others, spirituality, new possibilities, and personal strength) describe some of the specific ways in which individuals report growth as they adapt their worldviews to accommodate the experience of trauma and loss (Tedeschi & Calhoun, 1996).

In their conceptual model of PTG within the context of grief, Calhoun and colleagues (2010) posit that the degree to which the experience of loss challenges pre-trauma world beliefs is predictive of adaptation trajectories, and specifically of the potential for PTG to occur. In addition to universal aspects relative to PTG, the uniqueness of traumatic loss that allows for the possibility of PTG includes also the degree of grief symptoms (Engelkemeyer & Marwit, 2008; Hirooka et al., 2017; Krosch & Shakespeare-Finch, 2017) or the nature of the relationship of the survivor with the decedent (Hirooka et al., 2017; Ningning et al., 2018; Ogińska-Bulik, 2015; Sawyer & Brewster, 2019).

A few PTG studies focus exclusively on violent or sudden loss and only a handful included a large number of respondents with sudden and/or violent bereavement experiences. In a study of 374 college students impacted by sudden and /or violent death, Captari and colleagues (2021) found that positive world assumptions were related to PTG in the context of traumatic loss. Michael and Cooper (2013) conducted a systematic review of 70 articles focusing on PTG specifically as it related to bereavement and concluded that PTG is a documented outcome associated with bereavement and that key factors such as age, time since the loss, social support, active cognitive coping strategies, and religiosity may mediate the relationship between loss and PTG. A meta-analysis of PTG among suicide loss survivors found similar factors associated with PTG including time since loss, adaptative coping, help-seeking, and social support (Levi-Belz et al., 2021).

Factors that Increase the Potential to Experience PTG Following a Traumatic Loss

While profiles of risk and protective factors associated with PTG continue to be identified, two broad categories have emerged in the literature thus far i.e., internal characteristics and contextual factors.

Internal Characteristics

Levels of distress, psychological well-being, autonomous motivation, coping strategies, and meaning-making are associated with PTG following a traumatic loss. A study by Lumb and colleagues (2017) used Self Determination Theory to identify factors that predict PTG in the context of bereavement and presented two studies. The first study included 98 University students and found that current levels of distress, psychological well-being, and autonomous motivation were predictors of PTG. The second study was a mediation analysis with 133 university students and indicated an indirect effect of autonomous motivation on PTG via task-oriented coping.

Additionally, coping strategies are thought to influence the occurrence of PTG. Specifically, emotion regulation (Tedeschi & Calhoun, 2004), flexibility in coping (Cohen & Katz, 2015) as well as specific kinds of coping including problem-focused coping, religious coping (Yilmaz & Zara, 2016), and positive reframing (Lafarge et al., 2017) have been found to increase PTG. An offshoot of coping strategies is the notion of meaning-making (Davis et al., 2007; Larner & Blow, 2011; Milman et al., 2018), which is an important cognitive process associated with PTG (Tian & Solomon, 2020) as individuals contextualize their loss and create a narrative that integrates the experience. In a study of individuals who experienced a violent loss, those who reported more experiences of meaning-making also reported fewer symptoms of prolonged grief disorder, compared to those who experience less meaning-making (Milman et al., 2018). Specifically, violent loss was indirectly related to prolonged grief disorder symptoms when meaning-making focused on cultivating a sense of peace and a continuing bond with the deceased, suggesting that these particular themes may be helpful for traumatic loss survivors engaged in meaning-making (Milman et al., 2018). Davis et al. (2007) examined profiles of PTG following a traumatic loss and identified meaning-making as a unique indicator that characterized profiles of growth and adaptation after a traumatic loss. The profile of individuals that appeared to represent the conceptual model of PTG was characterized by meaning-making whereas the profile of individuals who did not report growth was characterized by the inability to find meaning.

Contextual Factors

Religion and spirituality, sex, and social support were found to predict PTG in the context of traumatic loss. *Religion and spirituality* offer a context for survivors to find meaning. Issues of religiosity are particularly important to the assessment of PTG in the context of bereavement as religious doctrine frames the experience of the "afterlife" or what happens to a loved one after death. Thus, religion can offer "meaning" in death or provide comfort regarding the current situation of the deceased (e.g., in heaven) and the potential for a continued relationship (Yilmaz & Zara, 2016). Additionally, spiritual changes are an area where PTG may emerge and is measured by the Post Traumatic Growth Inventory ([PTGI]; Tedeschi & Calhoun, 1996), which is the most commonly used tool to assess PTG. Sawyer and Brewster (2019) evaluated differences in PTG, complicated grief, and psychological distress among 299 individuals and compared those who self-identified as atheists with those with strong religious belief systems. They found that belief in God, search for and sense of meaning, and the interaction of search for meaning and belief, all positively influence PTG, suggesting differences between survivors who utilize religious beliefs in their coping process and those that do not.

Sex differences exist in bereavement (Doka & Martin, 2011) and in related PTG (Sawyer & Brewster, 2019; Vishnevsky et al., 2010). Patrick and Henrie (2016) surveyed 414 adults regarding their bereavement experiences and noted sex differences for two subscales of the PTGI – spiritual change and relationships with others, with females reporting higher levels on both subscales when compared to males. Sex also moderated the relationship between current grief symptoms and PTG and was reported regarding help-seeking behaviors (Nam et al., 2010), engagement in social support (Day & Livingstone, 2003), and attachment style (Schmidt et al., 2012; Xu et al., 2015) all factors influential in PTG development (Levi-Belz et al., 2021; Nelson et al., 2019). A systematic review of studies on bereaved parents found that mothers reported higher levels of PTG than fathers (Waugh et al., 2018).

Social support has been identified as related to PTG in the context of traumatic loss. In a study of 76 adults following the loss of a child, emotional and instrumental supports were found to mediate the relationship between trauma intensity and PTG suggesting an important role for social support in the process of developing PTG among those with traumatic loss (Ogińska-Bulik & Kobylarczyk, 2019). While these factors may influence the trajectory of adaptation and promote PTG, doing so does not eliminate the potential for psychological distress.

Growth and Suffering Are Not Mutually Exclusive

The relationship between psychological distress and PTG has received attention in the literature (Maercker & Zoellner, 2004; Pat-Horenczyk et al., 2015; Saltzman et al., 2018; Wortman, 2004). Some scholars suggest that growth is a mechanism to reduce psychological distress (Maercker & Zoellner, 2004; Wortman, 2004) predicting later PTG (Hall et al., 2015), a few found that grief intensity was inversely correlated with reported PTG (Engelkemeyer & Marwit, 2008; Krosch & Shakespeare-Finch, 2017), while others found that psychological distress was not related to PTG at all (Eisma et al., 2019). For example, in a study of 412 bereaved adults, Eisma et al., (2019) found that symptoms of anxiety, depression, PTSD, or prolonged grief did not predict PTG, suggesting that PTG may occur independently of psychological distress.

A more nuanced approach suggests a curvilinear model in which a threshold of PTSD symptoms can facilitate PTG, but the effect of PTSD symptoms, when above the threshold, can reduce PTG (Captari et al., 2021; Shakespeare-Finch & Lurie-Beck, 2014). In their aforementioned study, Eisma and colleagues (2019) found that the highest levels of PTG were experienced by survivors with moderate levels of depression, anxiety, PTSD, and symptoms of prolonged grief whereas those with lower and higher levels of psychological distress endorsed lower levels of PTG (an inverted U pattern).

We propose that PTSD and PTG co-occur simultaneously in the same survivor – a concept we refer to as struggling growth (Pat-Horenczyk et al., 2015; Saltzman et al., 2018). A pattern of co-occurring distress and growth was found in a study of 273 bereaved Chinese adults (Ningning et al., 2018) that used latent class analysis and identified three latent classes (1) a resilient class (2) a growth class, and (3) a grief *and* growth class, characterized by high levels of functional impairment. Membership in the grief and growth class was predicted by a younger age of the deceased loved one and the deceased loved one being a parent, child, or spouse of the participant. While they account for traumatic loss (i.e., non-natural death), the vast majority (92.3%) of their sample died from illness, which the authors did not classify under traumatic loss; thus the lack of results specific to traumatic loss may be related to statistical power.

Similarly, in another recent study of 422 Chinese adults bereaved as a result of COVID-19, Chen and Tang (2021) identified four latent classes that indicate interconnectivity between PTSD and PTG: (1) resilience; (3) growth; (3) moderate combined; and (4) high combined –highlighting that PTG may characterize adaptation in and of itself but may also be present even with high levels of psychological distress. They also found that a close relationship with the deceased increased the chances of membership in the high combined latent class while a conflictual relationship with the deceased decreased the chances of belonging to the growth latent class.

The aforementioned contradictory findings regarding the relationship between PTG and PTSD speak to a longstanding debate regarding the utility of the concept of PTG and its relationship to other indicators of posttraumatic adaptation. These inconsistent findings, as they pertain to traumatic loss, may reflect the failure to account for time, which is an important element of PTG adaptation.

Growth Unfolds over Time

Adaptation to trauma is recognized as a process that unfolds over time (Bonanno, 2004). Trajectories of trauma adaptation, including PTG, have been identified and tracked as far as 24 months posttrauma (Bonanno, 2004; Layne et al., 2007) suggesting that changes in adaptation are malleable and can be influenced over time (Pat-Horenczyk et al., 2015). Trajectories of PTG can change over time both when accounting for the amount of PTG and when considering the quality of growth over time (Pat-Horenczyk et al., 2015;

Saltzman et al., 2018). In their Janus Face Model, Maercker and Zoellner (Maercker & Zoellner, 2004; Zoellner & Maercker, 2006) propose two components of PTG that are differentially associated with psychological distress over time. The first component is referred to as illusory growth and is expected to emerge in the immediate aftermath of trauma to reduce distress symptomology. Over time, illusory growth may give way to the second component of growth, i.e., constructive growth that is inversely related to psychological distress and positively associated with other indicators of well-being. Similarly, scholars have focused on the utility of PTG in facilitating and predicting other forms of well-being (Hobfoll et al., 2002; Wortman, 2004). To our knowledge, no empirical studies have confirmed illusory and constructive growth patterns in the context of bereavement.

Saltzman (2019) focused on the process of adaptation over time, suggested that the relationship between PTG and psychological distress may be influenced by subjective experiences of time, and proposed understanding grief and bereavement from the new perspective of meaningful time. This approach suggests that the process of mourning interacts with a system of meaningful time treating time as a cyclical experience, in which temporal triggers can re-initiate the process of coping with loss rather than as a linear construct with equal intervals. In this conceptualization, coping "looks different" at different moments in time. A meaningful-time approach considers the possibility that the relationship between PTSD and PTG may be inverse, positive, or curvilinear at different moments in time in one survivor's trajectory depending on the subjective meaning attributed to the moment in time or the passage of time more broadly. As of yet, studies to empirically test this approach are unavailable.

Clinical Applications

While PTG has been established in the context of traumatic loss theoretically and empirically, it is also important to transfer this knowledge to the practice realm. How does PTG present in clinicians' environments when working with diverse groups of individuals experiencing traumatic loss? What techniques can mental health practitioners harness to enhance the possibility of achieving growth among those with bereavement experiences? This section introduces intervention modalities that can be used by mental health practitioners to facilitate growth among their bereaved clients.

First, it is important to relinquish the view of PTG as the optimal outcome of bereavement. While seeking to enhance well-being and reduce symptoms, it is important to remember that not all clients will, or desire to, achieve PTG. The pressure to achieve growth may create for clients new challenges such as the feeling of "not grieving correctly" or feeling shame or guilt for not experiencing PTG, all of which may inadvertently create barriers to adaptation and to the clinical process. As such, introducing PTG to clients (if at all) should occur organically and be framed to align with the value and language used by the client to describe their bereavement process.

Interventions for PTG

While research on PTG has grown immensely since the late 1990s, the development of interventions designed specifically to promote it is less prolific. One of the few interventions that specifically aims to facilitate PTG is a component of the Comprehensive Soldier Fitness Program, which is designed to teach skills to foster resilience to trauma, and may promote

PTG in U.S. Army Service Members prior to deployment (Tedeschi & McNally, 2011). The program provides psychoeducation about trauma responses, emotion regulation, constructive self-disclosure, creating a trauma narrative with PTG domains, and using PTG to improve functioning and influence values. A sample of 49 combat veterans who participated in the 7-day program prior to deployment demonstrated significant reductions in PTSD symptoms, insomnia, and negative affect 18 months after program completion; of most relevance, participants also exhibited significant increases in PTG and psychological flexibility (Moore et al., 2021). While this intervention may not focus specifically on bereavement it may be applicable to populations that have experienced traumatic loss as well.

While early data from smaller-scale studies suggest that PTG can be fostered via psychological intervention, research on individuals with traumatic loss is significantly underdeveloped. We identified one randomized controlled trial that tested an intervention specifically targeting PTG as an outcome in bereaved adults (Roepke et al., 2018). This study tested a psychosocial group intervention model called "SecondStory" in a sample of 112 bereaved adults and did not find differences in PTG gains between the intervention and control group, suggesting that improvements in PTG may be due to other factors, or the natural passage of time, rather than the intervention. Roepke (2015) conducted a meta-analysis in search of knowledge about psychosocial interventions designed to facilitate PTG more generally and identified 12 randomized controlled trials in trauma-affected populations, but none specifically targeted PTG as an outcome. Similarly, Li and colleagues (2020) identified 15 randomized controlled trials of interventions designed to facilitate PTG in cancer patients and found that mindfulness-based approaches were the most common and most effective in improving PTG, followed by cognitive-behavioral interventions. Despite the lack of interventions specifically designed to foster PTG among bereaved individuals, there are a handful of interventions that have enhanced PTG among other trauma-affected populations. In the section below we outline the evidence for and provide examples of mindfulness approaches, meaning reconstruction, and cognitive behavioral interventions.

Mindfulness Approaches

Eleven studies using mindfulness approaches to facilitate PTG among survivors of medical trauma were evaluated by Shiyko and colleagues (2017) finding a small positive effect of these interventions on PTG. Intervention models included mindfulness-based stress reduction and mindfulness-based cancer recovery with components of group sessions, meditation, and yoga. Mindfulness-based stress reduction often included physical components (e.g., yoga), which aligns with a new application of mindfulness approaches focused on physical activity as an intervention (e.g., yoga, snowboarding, and health coaching). Zhang and colleagues (2022) reviewed 12 such intervention models and found posttests a modest effect on PTG with positive effects remaining significant over six months.

Attunement, trust, therapeutic touch, egalitarianism, nuance, and death education (ATTEND), is an example of a mindfulness-based intervention, developed by Cacciatore and Flint. This mindfulness-based bereavement care model focuses on self-care and compassion (Cacciatore & Flint, 2012; Cacciatore et al., 2014). The intervention relies heavily on the clinician modeling the use of mindfulness to engage and have a deep connection with the suffering clients. At the same time, the clients practice mindfulness techniques to help them increase their tolerance to pain following a traumatic loss. This allows for reflection and self-compassion among providers and enhances the provider's ability to help the bereaved individual. The attunement of the bereaved individual prevents the avoidance of pain and grief and enhances a meaning-making process among the bereaved. These processes interact with each other and can foster PTG for clients who have had a traumatic loss. This model can offer the bereaved an opportunity to fully experience grief while allowing a process of meaning-making and experiencing a higher likelihood of PTG.

Meaning Reconstruction

Meaning reconstruction approaches bereavement with the goal of developing a narrative that details the meaning of the loss or the events surrounding it; which can facilitate PTG among those with traumatic loss (Neimeyer, 2004; 2016; Neimeyer & Thompson, 2014). In their conceptual model of the process of PTG within the context of grief, Calhoun and colleagues (2010) posit that prior to the traumatic loss, individuals form assumptive world beliefs that help them make sense of their experiences. The experience of traumatic loss leads to emotional distress, which can be either heightened or mitigated by pre-existing beliefs. When an individual's worldviews and beliefs mitigate their emotional distress (e.g., *I believe everything happens for a reason, so I know there must be a reason for this tragedy*), this individual is likely to follow a resilient trajectory of adaptation as their emotional distress subsides. However, when an individual's worldviews and beliefs are challenged, (e.g., *I believed that bad things don't happen to good people, so why did an innocent infant suffer such a horrible death*), that individual begins a process of psychological struggle, emotion regulation, and rumination that can lead them to modify their narrative of the traumatic experience or their worldviews and beliefs, and this struggle may also result in PTG. The degree to which core beliefs are disrupted or challenged by the experience of traumatic loss is proportional to the potential for PTG to occur, such that the greater the disruption, the more potential for the occurrence of PTG (Calhoun et al., 2010).

Meaning reconstruction approaches use techniques such as the development of oral narratives called "Restorative Retelling" and writing in therapeutic journals called "Directed Journaling" (Neimeyer, 2004; 2016). The aim is to facilitate meaning-making by encouraging clients to reflect on how they have made sense of their loss, the philosophical and personal resources that built their resilience, and the positive parts of grief they experience. This process is linked with the cognitive challenges posed by grief that are outlined in the Calhoun (2010) model.

Cognitive Behavioral Interventions

More traditional approaches to trauma intervention focus on cognitive-behavioral approaches. Trauma-focused cognitive behavioral therapy, which goes further than meaning reconstruction to modify core beliefs, has been associated with significantly higher reports of PTG, in comparison to control groups (Farnia et al., 2018; Knaevelsrud et al., 2010; Zoellner et al., 2011). Cognitive behavioral interventions may also focus on: (1) psychoeducation; (2) facilitating emotional disclosure; (3) practicing communication skills; (4) cognitive processing and rumination; (5) mindfulness and reflection; and (6) problem-solving techniques (Shakiba et al., 2020). In their evaluation of a cognitive-emotional intervention, Shakiba and colleagues (2020) found that PTG increased significantly among participants in the intervention group as compared to the control, suggesting that cognitive approaches to foster growth may be beneficial.

As the COVID-19 pandemic has demonstrated, the ability to transfer trauma and bereavement treatments to the virtual space is becoming increasingly important, allowing for a greater reach in providing care to clients who previously had difficulty accessing mental health treatment. Bereavement is also a critical outcome of the COVID-19 pandemic impacting millions of people worldwide creating a rapid influx of bereaved individuals from diverse backgrounds. Knaevelsrud and colleagues (2007; 2010) proposed a cognitive-behavioral online intervention to promote PTG and found significant changes in PTG among those who took part in the intervention, including a group of bereaved respondents. Their primarily online writing-based intervention protocol included three treatment components, i.e., self-confrontation, cognitive reconstruction, and social sharing (Knaevelsrud et al., 2010; Lange et al., 2002). These tasks focus on the cognitive processes outlined by Calhoun and colleagues (2010) in their model of PTG. Similarly, Wagner et al. (2007) examined the effects of internet-based cognitive behavioral therapy specifically for individuals experiencing complicated grief. Targeting exposure to bereavement cues, cognitive reappraisal, and integration of loss into life, they found that bereaved individuals who participated in the intervention demonstrated significant increases in PTG compared to a control group. The virtual nature of these interventions offers hope that online interventions may effectively foster PTG while providing opportunities to reach traditionally underserved populations.

Summary

While we outline a handful of interventions focused on facilitating PTG, it is important to note that few interventions have been designed and evaluated specifically to promote PTG among individuals experiencing traumatic loss. Despite the limitations of the research, PTG remains a possible outcome for individuals who experience traumatic loss (Michael & Cooper, 2013) and there are several factors that influence individual trajectories of adaptation, some of which may promote PTG. Further, achieving PTG is a process that unfolds over time. While the larger body of literature on PTG continues to navigate criticisms of the construct and challenges regarding its utility, we propose that PTG and psychological distress in the context of traumatic loss should not be considered mutually exclusive; rather, survivors may experience changes in the quality of growth that differentially interacts with psychological distress and other indicators of well-being based on their unique and subjective experience of time.

There are several limitations to the material presented in this chapter. Firstly, the experiences of loss, trauma, and PTG are subjective and highly influenced by context and culture. As a result, what defines a traumatic loss may vary from person to person as may their meaning-making process and subsequent experiences of PTG. Further, there are many forms of traumatic loss not addressed in this chapter; for example, experiencing disenfranchised loss and ambiguous loss may have unique risk and protective profiles potentially generating a different experience of PTG than the experience of survivors of other kinds of loss. We similarly underscore that loss and PTG look different across the lifespan. While some attention has been paid to adolescents (e.g., Hirooka et al., 2017; Stein et al., 2018) and children (Howell et al., 2015; Layne et al., 2017) experiencing loss, the primary focus in this chapter is adult populations. Despite these limitations, this chapter has provided an overview of the experience of PTG within the context of traumatic loss and calls on clinicians and researchers to develop, implement, and evaluate interventions that specifically target PTG as a primary outcome among survivors of traumatic loss.

References

American Psychiatric Association. (2013). *Diagnostic and statistical manual of mental disorders* (5th ed.). Washington, DC: American Psychiatric Publishing.

Bellet, B. W., Jones, P. J., Neimeyer, R. A., & McNally, R. J. (2018). Bereavement outcomes as causal systems: A network analysis of the co-occurrence of complication grief and posttraumatic growth. *Clinical Psychological Services*, *6*(6), 797–809. 10.1177/2167702618777454.

Bonanno, G. A. (2004). Loss, trauma, and human resilience: Have we underestimated the human capacity to thrive after extremely aversive events? *American Psychologist*, *59*(1), 20–28. 10.1037/0003-066X.59.1.20.

Bonanno, G. A., Neria, Y., Mancini, K. G., Coifman, B., Litz, B., & Insel, B. (2007). Is there more to complicated grief than depression and posttraumatic stress disorder? A test of incremental validity. *Journal of Abnormal Psychology*, *116*(2), 342–351. 10.1037/0021-843X.116.2.342.

Cacciatore, J., & Flint, M. (2012). Attend: Toward a mindfulness-based bereavement care model. *Death Studies*, *36*(1), 61–82. 10.1080/07481187.2011.591275.

Cacciatore, J., Thieleman, K., Osborn, J., & Orlowski, K. (2014). Of the soul and suffering: Mindfulness-based interventions and bereavement. *Clinical Social Work Journal*, *42*(3), 269–281. 10.1007/s10615-013-0465-y.

Calhoun, L. G., Tedeschi, R. G., Cann, A., & Hanks, E. A. (2010). Positive outcomes following bereavement: Paths to posttraumatic growth. *Psychological Belgica*, *50*(1/2), 125–143.

Captari, L. E., Riggs, S. A., & Stephen, K. (2021). Attachment processes following traumatic loss: A mediation model examining identity distress, shattered assumptions, prolonged grief, and posttraumatic growth. *Psychological Trauma: Theory, Research, Practice, and Policy*, *13*(1), 94–103. 10.1037/tra0000555.

Chen, C., & Tang, S. (2021). Profiles of grief, posttraumatic stress, and post-traumatic growth among people bereaved due to COVID-19. *European Journal of Psychotraumatology*, *12*(1), 1947563. 10.1080/20008198.2021.1947563.

Cohen, O., & Katz, M. (2015). Grief and growth of bereaved siblings as related to attachment style and flexibility. *Death Studies*, *39*(3), 158–164. 10.1080/07481187.2014.923069.

Davis, C. G., Wohl, M. J., & Verberg, N. (2007). Profiles of posttraumatic growth following an unjust loss. *Death Studies*, *31*(8), 693–712.

Davis, C. G., Wortman, C. B., Lehman, D. R., & Silver, R. C. (2000). Searching for meaning in loss: Are clinical assumptions correct. *Death Studies*, *24*(6), 497–540. 10.1080/07481180050121471.

Day, A. L., & Livingstone, H. A. (2003). Gender differences in perceptions of stressors and utilization of social support among university students. *Canadian Journal of Behavioural Science / Revue Canadienne des Sciences du Comportement*, *35*(2), 73–83. 10.1037/h0087190.

Doka, K. J., & Martin, T. L. (2011). *Grieving beyond gender: Understanding the ways men and women mourn*. London, UK: Routledge.

Eisma, M. C., Lenferink, L. I. M., Stroebe, M. S., Boelen, P. A., & Chut, H. A. W. (2019). No pain no gain: Cross lagged analysis of posttraumatic growth and anxiety, depression, posttraumatic stress, and prolonged grief symptoms after loss. *Anxiety, Stress, and Coping*, *32*(3), 231–243. 10.1080/10615806.2019.1584293.

Engelkemeyer, S. M., & Marwit, S. J. (2008). Posttraumatic growth in bereaved parents. *Journal of Traumatic Stress*, *21*(3), 344–346. 10.1002/jts.20338.

Farnia, V., Naami, A., Zargar, Y., Davoodi, I., Salemi, S., Tatari, F., Kazemi, A., Basanj, B., Jouybari, T. A., & Alikhani, M. (2018). Comparison of trauma-focused cognitive behavioral therapy and theory of mind: Improvement of posttraumatic growth and emotion regulation strategies. *Journal of Education and Health Promotion*, *7*(1), 58–64. 10.4103/jehp.jehp_140_17.

Feder, A., Southwick, S. M., Goetz, R. R., Wang, Y., Alonso, A., Smith, B. W., Buchholz, K. R., Waldeck, T., Ameli, R., Moore, J., Hain, R., Charney, D. S., & Vythilingam, M. (2008). Posttraumatic growth in former Vietnam prisoners of war. *Psychiatry*, *71*(4), 359–370. 10.1521/psyc.2008.71.4.359.

Green, B. L. (2000). Traumatic loss: Conceptual and empirical links between trauma and bereavement. *Journal of Personal & Interpersonal Loss*, *5*(1), 1–17. 10.1080/10811440008407845.

Hall, B. J., Saltzman, L. Y., Canetti, D., & Hobfoll, S. E. (2015). A longitudinal investigation of the relationship between posttraumatic stress symptoms and posttraumatic growth in a cohort of

Israeli Jews and Palestinians during ongoing violence. *PloS one*, *10*(4), e0124782. 10.1371/journal.pone.0124782.
Hirooka, K., Fukahori, H., Ozawa, M., & Akita, Y. (2017). Differences in posttraumatic growth and grief reactions among adolescents by relationships with the deceased. *Journal of Advanced Nursing*, *73*(4), 955–965. 10.1111/jan.13196.
Hobfoll, S. E. (2002). Social and Psychological Resources and Adaptation. *Review of General Psychology*, *6*(4), 307–324. 10.1037/1089-2680.6.4.307.
Howell, K. H., Shapiro, D. N., Layne, C. M., & Kaplow, J. B. (2015). Individual and psychosocial mechanisms of adaptive functioning in parentally bereaved children. *Death Studies*, *39*(5), 296–306.
Janoff-Bulman, R. (1992). *Shattered assumptions: Towards a new psychology of trauma*. New York, NY, US: Free Press.
Kersting, A., Kroker, K., Steinhard, J., Lüdorff, K., Wesselmann, U., Ohrmann, P., Arolt, V., & Suslow, T. (2007). Complicated grief after traumatic loss: A 14-month follow up study. *European Archives of Psychiatry and Clinical Neuroscience*, *257*(8), 437–443. 10.1007/s00406-007-0743-1.
Kleim, B., & Ehlers, A. (2009). Evidence for a curvilinear relationship between posttraumatic growth and posttrauma depression and PTSD in assault survivors. *Journal of Traumatic Stress*, *22*(1), 45–52. 10.1002/jts.20378.
Knaevelsrud, C., & Maercker, A. (2007). Internet-based treatment for PTSD reduces distress and facilitates the development of a strong therapeutic alliance: A randomized controlled trial. *BMC Psychiatry*, *7*(13). 10.1186/1471-244X-7-13.
Knaevelsrud, C., Liedl, A., & Maercker, A. (2010). Posttraumatic growth, optimism, and openness as outcomes of a cognitive behavioral intervention for posttraumatic stress reactions. *Journal of Health Psychology*, *15*(7), 1030–1038. 10.1177/1359105309360073.
Kobasa, S. (1979). Stressful life events, personality, and health: An inquiry into hardiness. *Journal of Personality and Social Psychology*, *37*(1), 1–11.
Krosch, D. J., & Shakespeare-Finch, J. (2017). Grief, traumatic stress, and posttraumatic growth in women who have experienced pregnancy loss. *Psychological Trauma: Theory, Research, Practice, and Policy*, *9*(4), 425–433. 10.1037/tra0000183.
Kubler-Ross, E. (1969). *On death and dying*. New York: The Macmillan Company.
Kübler-Ross, E., & Kessler, D. (2005). *On grief and grieving: Finding the meaning of grief through the five stages of loss*. NY: Simon and Schuster.
Lafarge, C., Mitchell, K., & Fox, P. (2017). Posttraumatic growth following pregnancy termination for fetal abnormality: The predictive role of coping strategies and perinatal grief. *Anxiety, Stress, & Coping*, *30*(5), 536–550. 10.1080/10615806.2016.1278433.
Lange, A., Schoutrop, M., Schrieken, B., & Ven, J.-P. v. d. (2002). Interapy: A model for therapeutic writing through the Internet. In S. J. Lepore, & J. M. Smyth (Eds.), *The writing cure: How expressive writing promotes health and emotional well-being* (pp. 215–238). American Psychological Association. 10.1037/10451-011.
Larner, B., & Blow, A. (2011). A model of meaning-making coping and growth in combat veterans. *Review of General Psychology*, *15*(3), 187–197. 10.1037/a0024810.
Latham, A. E., & Prigerson, H. G. (2004). Suicidality and bereavement: Complicated grief as psychiatric disorder presenting greatest risk for suicidality. *Suicide and Life-Threatening Behaviors*, *34*(4), 350–362. 10.1521/suli.34.4.350.53737.
Layne, C. M., Kaplow, J. B., & Youngstrom, E. A. (2017). Applying evidence-based assessment to childhood trauma and bereavement: Concepts, principles, and practices. In *Evidence-based treatments for trauma related disorders in children and adolescents* (pp. 67–96). NY: Springer.
Layne, C. M., Warren, J. S., Watson, P. J., & Shalev, A. Y. (2007). Risk, vulnerability, resistance, and resilience: Toward an integrative conceptualization of posttraumatic adaptation. In M. J. Friedman, T. M. Keane, & P. A. Resick (Eds.), *Handbook of PTSD: Science and practice* (pp. 497–520). NY: The Guilford Press.
Lee, E., won Kim, S., & Enright, R. D. (2019). Beyond grief and survival: Posttraumatic growth through immediate family suicide loss in South Korea. *OMEGA- Journal of Death and Dying*, *79*(4), 414–435. 10.1177/0030222817724700.
Levi-Belz, Y., Krysinska, K., &Andriessen, K. (2021). "Turning personal tragedy into triumph": A systematic review and meta-analysis of studies on posttraumatic growth among suicide-loss

survivors. *Psychological Trauma: Theory, Research, Practice, and Policy, 13*(3), 322–332. ISSN: 1942-9681. 10.1037/tra0000977.

Li, J., Peng, X., Su, Y., He, Y., Zhang, S., & Hu, X. (2020). Effectiveness of psychosocial interventions for posttraumatic growth in patients with cancer: A meta-analysis of randomized controlled trails. *European Journal of Oncology Nursing, 48*, 101798.

Linley, P. A., & Joseph, S. (2004). Positive change following trauma and adversity: A review. *Journal of Traumatic Stress, 17*(1), 11–21. 10.1023/B:JOTS.0000014671.27856.7e.

Lumb, A. B., Beaudry, M., & Blanchard, C. (2017). Posttraumatic growth and bereavement: The contribution of self-determination theory. *OMEGA-Journal of Death and Dying, 75*(4), 311–336. 10.1177/0030222816652971.

Maercker, A., & Zoellner, T. (2004). The Janus face of self-perceived growth: Toward a two-component model of posttraumatic growth. *Psychological Inquiry, 15*(1), 41–48.

McDevitt-Murphy, M. E., Neimeyer, R. A., Burke, L. A., Williams, J. L., & Lawson, K. (2012). The toll of traumatic loss in African Americans bereaved by homicide. *Psychological Trauma: Theory, Research, Practice, and Policy, 4*(3), 303–311. 10.1037/a0024911.

McMillen, J. C., Smith, E. M., & Fisher, R. H. (1997). Perceived benefit and mental health after three types of disaster. *Journal of Consulting and Clinical Psychology, 65*(5), 733–739. 10.1037/0022-006X.65.5.733.

Michael, C., & Cooper, M. (2013). Post-traumatic growth following bereavement: A systematic review of the literature. *Counselling Psychology Review, 28*(4), 18–33.

Milman, E., Neimeyer, R. A., Fitzpatrick, M., MacKinnon, C. J., Muis, K. R., & Cohen, S. R. (2018). Prolonged grief symptomatology following violent loss: The mediating role of meaning. *European Journal of Psychotraumatology, 8*(Suppl 6), 1503522. 10.1080/20008198.2018.150352.

Moore, B. A., Tedeschi, R. G., & Greene, T. C. (2021). A preliminary examination of a posttraumatic growth-based program for veteran mental health. *Practice Innovations, 6*(1), 42–54. 10.1037/pri0000136.

Nam, S. K., Chu, H. J., Lee, M. K., Lee, J. H., Kim, N., & Lee, S. M. (2010). A meta-analysis of gender differences in attitudes toward seeking professional psychological help. *Journal of American College Health, 59*(2), 110–116. 10.1080/07448481.2010.483714.

Neimeyer, R. A. (2004). Fostering posttraumatic growth: A narrative elaboration. *Psychological Inquiry, 15*(1), 53–59.

Neimeyer, R. A. (2016). Meaning reconstruction in the wake of loss: Evolution of a research program. *Behaviour Change, 33*(2), 65–79. 10.1017/bec.2016.4.

Neimeyer, R. A., & Thompson, B. E. (2014). Meaning making and the art of grief therapy. In B. E. Thompson, & R. A. Neimeyer (Eds.), *Grief and the expressive arts: Practices for creating meaning* (pp. 3–13). Routledge/Taylor & Francis Group.

Nelson, K. M., Hagedorn, W. B., & Lambie, G. W. (2019). Influence of attachment style on sexual abuse survivors' posttraumatic growth. *Journal of Counseling & Development, 97*(3), 227–237. 10.1002/jcad.12263.

Ningning, Z., Wei, Y., Suqin, T., Jianping, W., & Killikelly, C. (2018). Prolonged grief and posttraumatic growth after loss: Latent class analysis. *Psychiatry Research, 267*, 221–227. 10.1016/j.psychres.2018.06.006.

Ogińska-Bulik, N. (2015). The relationship between resiliency and posttraumatic growth following the death of someone close. *OMEGA Journal of Death and Dying, 71*(3), 233–244. 10.1177/0030222815575502.

Ogińska-Bulik, N., & Kobylarczyk, M. (2019). The experience of trauma resulting from the loss of a child and posttraumatic growth- the mediating role of coping strategies (loss of a child, PTG, and coping). *OMEGA- Journal of Death and Dying, 80*(1), 104–119. 10.1177/0030222817724699.

Palgi, Y. (2016). Subjective age and perceived distance to death moderating the association between posttraumatic stress symptoms and posttraumatic growth among older adults. *Aging and Mental Health, 20*(9), 948–954. 10.1080/13607863.2015.1047320.

Pat-Horenczyk, R., Saltzman, L. Y., Hamama-Raz, Y., Perry, S., Ziv, Y., Ginat-Frolich, R., & Stemmer, S. M. (2015). Stability and transitions in posttraumatic growth trajectories among cancer patients: LCA and LTA analyses. *Psychological trauma: Theory, research, practice and policy, 8*(5), 541–549. 10.1037/tra0000094.

Park, C. L., Cohen, L. H., & Murch, R. L. (1996). Assessment and prediction of stress-related growth. *Journal of Personality*, *64*(1), 71–105. 10.1111/j.1467-6494.1996.tb00815.x.
Patrick, J. H., & Henrie, J. (2016). Up from the ashes: Age and gender effects on post-traumatic growth in bereavement. *Women & Therapy*, *39*(3–4), 296–314. 10.1080/02703149.2016.1116863.
Rheingold, A. A., & Williams, J. L. (2015). Survivors of homicide: Mental health outcomes, social support, and service use among a community-based sample. *Violence and Victims*, *30*(5), 870–883. 10.1891/0886-6708.VV-D-14-00026.
Roepke, A. M. (2015). Psychosocial interventions and posttraumatic growth: A meta-analysis. *Journal of Consulting and Clinical Psychology*, *83*(1), 129–142. 10.1037/a0036872.
Roepke, A. M., Tsukayama, E., Forgeard, M., & Blackie, L. (2018). Randomized controlled trial of SecondStory, an intervention targeting posttraumatic growth with bereaved adults. *Journal of Consulting and Clinical Psychology*, *86*(6), 518–532. 10.1037/ccp0000307.
Ryff, C. D., & Singer, B. (1998). The contours of positive human health. *Psychological Inquiry*, *9*(1), 1–28. 10.1207/s15327965pli0901_1.
Saltzman, L. Y. (2019). It's about time: Reconceptualizing the role of time in loss and trauma. *Psychological Trauma: Theory, Research, Practice, and Policy*, *11*(6), 663–670. 10.1037/tra0000435.
Saltzman, L. Y., Pat-Horenczyk, R., Lombe, M., Weltman, A., Ziv, Y., McNamara, T., Takeuchi, D., & Brom, D. (2018). Post-combat adaptation: Improving social support and reaching constructive growth. *Anxiety, Stress, and Coping*, *31*(4), 418–430. 10.1080/10615806.2018.1454740.
Sattler, D. N., Claramita, M., & Muskavage, B. (2018). Natural disasters in Indonesia: Relationships among posttraumatic stress, resource loss, depression, social support, and posttraumatic growth. *Journal of Loss and Trauma*, *23*(5), 351–365. 10.1080/15325024.2017.1415740.
Sawyer, J. S., & Brewster, M. (2019). Assessing posttraumatic growth, complicated grief, and psychological distress in bereaved atheists and believers. *Death Studies*, *43*(4), 224–234. 10.1080/07481187.2018.1446061.
Shakespeare-Finch, J., & Lurie-Beck, J. (2014). A meta-analytic clarification of the relationship between posttraumatic growth and symptoms of posttraumatic distress disorder. *Journal of Anxiety Disorders*, *28*(2), 223–229. 10.1016/j.janxdis.2013.10.005.
Shakiba, M., Latifi, A., & Navidian, A. (2020). The effect of cognitive-emotional intervention on growth and posttraumatic stress in mothers of children with cancer: A randomized clinical trial. *Journal of Pediatric Hematology and Oncology*, *42*(2), 118–125. 10.1097/MPH.0000000000001558.
Shiyko, M. P., Hallinan, S., & Naito, T. (2017). Effects of mindfulness training on posttraumatic growth: A systematic review and meta-analysis. *Mindfulness*, *8*, 848–858. 10.1007/s12671-017-0684-3.
Schmidt, S. D., Blank, T. O., Bellizzi, K. M., & Park, C. L. (2012). The relationship of coping strategies, social support, and attachment style with posttraumatic growth in cancer survivors. *Journal of Health Psychology*, *17*(7), 1033–1040. 10.1177/1359105311429203.
Solomon, Z., & Dekel, R. (2007). Posttraumatic stress disorder and posttraumatic growth among Israeli ex-pows. *Journal of Traumatic Stress*, *20*(3), 303–312. 10.1002/jts.20216.
Spain, B., O'Dwyer, L., & Moston, S. (2019). Pet loss: Understanding disenfranchised grief, memorial use, and posttraumatic growth. *Anthrozoös*, *32*(4), 555–568. 10.1080/08927936.2019.1621545.
Stein, C. H., Petrowski, C. E., Gonzales, S. M., Mattei, G. M., Hartl Majcher, J., Froemming, M. W., Greenberg, S. C., Dulek, E. B., & Benoit, M. F. (2018). A matter of life and death: Understanding continuing bonds and post-traumatic growth when young adults experience the loss of a close friend. *Journal of Child and Family Studies*, *27*(3), 725–738. 10.1007/s10826-017-0943-x.
Sumalla, E. C., Ochoa, C., & Blanco, I. (2008). Posttraumatic growth in cancer: Reality or illusion? *Clinical Psychology Review*, *29*(1), 24–33. 10.1016/j.cpr.2008.09.006.
Tedeschi, R. G., & Calhoun, L. G. (1996). The Posttraumatic Growth Inventory: Measuring the positive legacy of trauma. *Journal of Traumatic Stress*, *9*(3), 455–471. 10.1007/BF02103658.
Tedeschi, R. G., & Calhoun, L. G. (2004). Target article: Posttraumatic growth: Conceptual foundations and empirical evidence. *Psychological Inquiry*, *15*(1), 1–18. 10.1207/s15327965pli1501_01.
Tedeschi, R. G., & McNally, R. J. (2011). Can we facilitate posttraumatic growth in combat veterans? *American Psychologist*, *66*(1), 19–24. 10.1037/a0021896.

Tian, X., & Solomon, D.H. (2020). Grief and posttraumatic growth following miscarriage: The role of meaning reconstruction and partner supportive communication. *Death Studies*, *44*(4), 237–247. 10.1080/07481187.2018.1539051.

Vishnevsky, T., Cann, A., Calhoun, L. G., Tedeschi, R. G., & Demakis, G. J. (2010). Gender differences in self-reported posttraumatic growth: A meta-analysis. *Psychology of Women Quarterly*, *34*(1), 110–120. 10.1111/j.1471-6402.2009.01546.x.

Wagner, B., Knaevelsrud, C., & Maercker, A. (2007). Post-traumatic growth and optimism as outcomes of an internet-based intervention for complicated grief. *Cognitive Behaviour Therapy*, *36*(3), 156–161. 10.1080/16506070701339713.

Walsh, F. (2002). Bounding forward: Resilience in the aftermath of September 11. *Family Process*, *41*(1), 34–36. 10.1111/j.1545-5300.2002.40102000034.x.

Waugh, A., Kiemle, G., & Slade, P. (2018). What aspects of post-traumatic growth are experienced by bereaved parents? A systematic review. *European Journal of Psychotraumatology*, *9*(1), 1506230. 10.1080/200008198.2018.1506230.

Wortman, C. B. (2004). Posttraumatic growth: Progress and problems. *Psychological Inquiry*, *15*(1), 81–90.

Xu, W., Fu, Z., He, L., Schoebi, D., & Wang, J. (2015). Growing in times of grief: Attachment modulates bereaved adults' posttraumatic growth after losing a family member to cancer. *Psychiatry Research*, *230*(1), 108–115. 10.1016/j.psychres.2015.08.035.

Yilmaz, M., & Zara, A. (2016). Traumatic loss and posttraumatic growth: The effect of traumatic loss related factors on posttraumatic growth. *Anatolian Journal of Psychiatry*, *17*(1), 5–11. 10.5455/apd.188311.

Zhang, N., Xiang, X., Zhou, S., Liu, H., He, Y., & Chen, J. (2022). Physical activity intervention and posttraumatic growth: A systematic review and meta-analysis. *Journal of Psychosomatic Research*, *152*. 10.1016/j.jpsychores.2021.110675.

Zinzow, H. M., Rheingold, A. A., Hawkins, A. O., Saunders, B. E., & Kilpatrick, D. G. (2009). Losing a loved one to homicide: Prevalence and mental health correlates in a national sample of young adults. *Journal of traumatic stress*, *22*(1), 20–27. 10.1002/jts.20377.

Zoellner, T., & Maercker, A. (2006). Posttraumatic growth in clinical psychology- A critical review and introduction of a two-component model. *Clinical Psychology Review*, *26*(5), 626–653. 10.1016/j.cpr.2006.01.008.

Zoellner, T., Rabe, S., Karl, A., & Maercker, A. (2011). Post-traumatic growth as outcome of a cognitive-behavioural therapy trial for motor vehicle accident survivors with PTSD. *Psychology and Psychotherapy: Theory, Research and Practice*, *84*(2), 201–213. 10.1348/147608310X520157.

37

BLOOMING IN UNLIKELY PLACES

Posttraumatic Growth in Survivors of Sex Trafficking

Heather Evans

Understanding Trafficking and Its Traumatic Impact

Human trafficking is a global human rights violation, enslaving men, women, and children. Trafficking is the commodification of a human being, made possible by a demand for the sex industry and a supply of human beings, particularly those who are vulnerable and isolated. The Justice for Victims of Trafficking Act (2015) defines human trafficking as the recruitment, harboring, transportation, provision, obtaining, patronizing, or soliciting of a person for the purpose of labor or a commercial sex act, in which the labor or commercial sex act is induced by force, fraud, or coercion, or in which the person induced to perform such act has not obtained 18 years of age (Department of State, 2022).

Human trafficking occurs in every nation of the world. Sex trafficking is the most prevalent form of trafficking, and remains a hidden, misunderstood, and largely underreported crime worldwide (Department of State, 2022). Because of its nature, there are no reliable estimates of the scope and scale of the problem. The U.N. Office of Drugs and Crime (UNODC) estimates that in 2016, 72% of all detected trafficking victims were women and girls and that 94% of detected sex trafficking victims globally were women and girls, making human trafficking primarily a crime of gender (Bender et al., 2019). Though we have limited data, boys and men are also trafficked for sexual exploitation, and in 2018, 50% of boy trafficking victims were victims of sexual exploitation (Counter Trafficking Data Collaborative, 2019).

The prevalence of sex trafficking is far-reaching, spanning multiple demographic characteristics such as age, socioeconomic status, nationality, education level, and gender. Risk factors for being trafficked include poverty, young age, limited education, lack of support system (e.g., being orphaned or in the child welfare system), family instability/abuse, runaway/throwaway, homelessness, history of previous sexual abuse, health or mental health challenges, living in vulnerable areas (e.g., areas with high crime, or economic/political instability), gender, or sexual identity (Clawson et al., 2009; Evans, 2019; 2020; 2022; Orme & Ross-Sheriff, 2015) and ethnicity (FBI, 2019; Ferguson, 2016). Additionally, globalization, demographic disparities between the developing and developed world, and the worldwide feminization of poverty are also contributors (Shelley, 2010).

DOI: 10.4324/9781032208688-46

A trafficker most often begins with a romantic relationship, using seduction, promises, and relationships as his or her greatest weapon to create a complex dynamic with the victim. This often results in a "trauma bond," a phenomenon in which trafficking victims have strong feelings of attachment to their abusers. In situations of captivity like human trafficking, the perpetrator becomes the most powerful person in the life of the victim, and the psychology of the victim is shaped by the actions and beliefs of the perpetrator (Evans, 2022).

The impact on a victim of human sex trafficking is layered and complex. The physical violence, sexual violence, and psychological control of a trafficker and the events during the time of sexual exploitation often compound early childhood trauma (Evans, 2019; 2022; Hardy et al., 2013). The effects of these experiences continue after the exploitation ends. Upon identification as a victim and separation from the trafficker, a victim faces complicating factors and needs, including issues of poverty, homelessness, and the absence of a safe social support network. They may have much capacity and potential, but lack education and job experience, or have a criminal record from their time in exploitation. This can generate a cycle of exploitation that requires immense social and health interventions to pause and reverse (Clawson et al., 2009; Evans, 2019; 2022; Farley, 2003).

Issues observed in and described by victims of human sex trafficking can be explained as complex trauma. Terminology formulated to capture trauma that is extreme, chronic or repetitious, interpersonal, and premeditated includes Complex Trauma (Courtois & Ford, 2009) or Disorders of Extreme Stress Not Otherwise Specified (DESNOS) (Spinazzola et al., 2001). Complex trauma is "resulting from exposure to severe stressors that are repetitive or prolonged, involves harm or abandonment by caregivers or other adults, and occurs at developmentally vulnerable times in the victim's life" (Courtois & Ford, 2009, p.13). While not an official diagnosis listed in the *Diagnostic and Statistical Manual of Mental Disorders*, 5th edition, this diagnosis accurately describes the trauma seen in victimization within human sex trafficking (Choi et al., 2009).

Complex trauma emphasizes alterations in six areas: regulation of affect and impulses, attention or consciousness, self-perception, relations with others, somatization, and systems of meaning (Spinazzola et al., 2001). To cope with it, victims who present with complex trauma often resort to substance abuse, self-injury, disordered eating, suicidal ideation, or other forms of self-destructive behaviors, which can in turn create additional barriers to trauma recovery. These outcomes are commonly observed in human sex trafficking victims, along with the effects of the captivity which contribute to trauma bonds, confusion, fear, and guilt (Clawson et al., 2009; Evans, 2019; 2022; Hardy et al., 2013; Herman, 1992).

PTG in Survivors of Sex Trafficking

PTG in trafficking survivors has been addressed to a very limited degree. Perry and de Castro Pecanha (2017) conducted a quantitative study to explore if there is a relationship between PTG and quality of life and found small positive levels of PTG, as some survivors experienced psychological growth that manifested through behavioral changes in particular life domains responsible for enhancing the quality of life. In another quantitative study, Schultz et al. (2020) investigated links between posttraumatic stress, PTG, and religious coping and discovered moderately high levels of PTG as well as high connections between religious coping and PTG. Evans (2019; 2022) conducted a qualitative study to capture the voices of survivors of human sex trafficking, especially women, in the United States who have been separated from their traffickers for more than one year. Using the theoretical lenses of ecological systems, complex trauma, and PTG, in-depth interviews were conducted to explore survivors experience of services, support systems, and barriers, and identify factors that seem to be most helpful and pertinent. Incorporated into the interview process as an additional means for survivors to express their experiences was the Photovoice methodology (i.e., a research methodology where research participants are empowered to express their lived experiences through photography) including individual expression, participatory group reflection, and awareness-raising about important community issues through the display and discussion of the photography (Wang & Burris, 1997). The study was designed to create an opportunity for survivors to share their experiences in a way that promotes the nuanced impact of their experiences and highlights their voices and wisdom to further define, recommend, and test effective interventions and support systems.

The study provided salient findings on all aspects of complex trauma and all five domains of PTG. These findings are discussed below. Participants' stories and photos reflected long-term ongoing challenges related to mental and physical stabilization as well as a significant struggle with identity and relationships. Yet, these expressions of continual need and challenges are accompanied by stories and photos that remarkably express the domains of PTG. Participants are identified in the following description by name or number as per their preference. Quotes are unedited to maintain authenticity.

PTG Domain 1: Personal Strength

This domain refers to an individual identifying and being surprised by his/her power or strength. Phrases illustrating this domain are "vulnerable, yet stronger" or "I am more vulnerable than I thought but much stronger than I ever imagined" (Calhoun & Tedeschi, 2006 p.5). Traffickers abuse power as a tool to strip survivors of their own sense of agency and exploit trust to create psychological captivity, which are core aspects of humanity (Herman, 1992). Yet, it is survivors' strength that enables them to endure, escape, and heal. Survivors reported how they found personal strength to exit the trafficking situation, testify against their trafficker, seek services, and become an advocate for others. Personal strength was described as a form of coping during or after the trafficking experience. For example, Cat grew up in and out of foster homes and was sexually abused at a young age. She was first trafficked by her mother but later was recruited by two different traffickers. Out of this life for four years at the time of the interview, she describes her own personal strength and how it has helped her survive:

> I just keep trying to stay positive. I think that … I'm really stubborn and really hard-headed and I'm the kind of person that, if you tell me I can't do something, I'm gonna do it anyway. And I think that, that's helped me a lot because through all this – even when times have been hard, and I have to admit, that even now, I've been out of the life for a couple years, it's still hard. It's still really hard.

Some survivors described personal strength as a characteristic that developed as a *result* of the trafficking experience. Cat further stated:

> … it's impacted my life in the way that I don't trust people. It's impacted me that I felt that I'm not worth anything, used up. But, I've also grown very strong because of it … I could say this 100 times and I really know that it's true. I hate what's happened to

> me. I hate that I've been a victim. I hate that I have to identify as a victim. It's very uncomfortable because I've been so strong and fearless but I would not take it back because I feel that I am ferocious, and that I know that because of what has happened to me, it's made me who I am and it's made me to be so strong now. My mind is much stronger than it used to be ...

PTG Domain 2: New Possibilities

New possibilities include the development of new interests or opportunities, sometimes related to the experienced trauma (Calhoun & Tedeschi, 2006). Survivors of trafficking described their ways of finding purpose, opportunities for learning, and goals and dreams they have for the future. Much of this was focused on helping others illustrating Herman's (1992) observation "But we do know that the women who recover most successfully are those who discover some meaning in their experience that transcends the limits of personal tragedy. Most commonly, women find this meaning by joining with others in social action" (p.73). Two main aspects of new possibilities were seeking purpose and developing goals and dreams.

Seeking Purpose

Almost all the participants made references to things that give them purpose, meaning, and value that these things provide. Particularly, almost every participant made reference to finding purpose in the post-trafficking phase through helping others, or joining the anti-trafficking movement as a survivor leader who seeks justice, provides advocacy, and trains others about human trafficking. For example, Megan, trafficked as a young adult for five years, and out of it for five years at the time of the interview said: "It's very fulfilling and my wish is to be that person and to have that organization that wasn't there." Grace was trafficked as a young adult. With a history of childhood abuse, family instability, and an abusive relationship, she became involved with drugs, making her vulnerable to sexual exploitation. Out of the trafficking for three years, she commented:

> It's not what you're trying to gather up for yourself. It has nothing to do with that. It's how can you serve in this world to make it better? How can you help somebody not be so broken? How can you breathe life back into somebody is what keeps me going every day. I want to give back in every way that I can and I want to leave my mark here, however I can.

Approximately half of those interviewed described coming to this sense of purpose as part of their healing process. Victoria was trafficked by two women she met through a local organization. Out of that life for three years, she reflected:

> It was definitely just like this hell that I have been living in for so long and I spent a good year-and-a-half in therapy and then, it's been the past year where I've really started to bloom and move past ... I'm healing, I'm doing good. Now I want to bring justice. I want to help stop what's happening.

Developing Goals and Dreams

When participants were asked about their goals and dreams, the majority talked about having a career, with most of them wanting jobs or wanting to start programs where they can help other women. Grace stated: "Hopefully, open up my own practice of some sort or open up my own housing situation for women ... I want to give back in every way that I can and I want to leave my mark here, however I can." One participant stated:

> I would like to write books, continue to speak, continue to educate, train, and I really want to use my degree in clinical psychology to give me credibility as a trainer, as a speaker, and as an author. I want to help non-profits and organizations working with survivors – really be able to do it well. So, what does complex trauma look like within your organization and how can you respond to needs in a way that really meets just the unique and specific needs of a victim of human trafficking.

Their goals and dreams are related to giving back, contributing to services, and providing what they wish they would have received or what they have identified as a need from their own experience. Two-thirds mentioned the goal of education; for example, Grace said: "I do want to finish this Bachelor's Degree. I want to eventually get my Masters"; One participant was trafficked all of her life; starting with her family at a young age, she was sexually abused, exploited for pornography, and then sold to other traffickers. At the time she was out of the trafficking experience for eight years, she concurred:

> So, I went to school and got my degree in counseling in undergrad in counseling, a B.A. and left there with a dream to eventually get my doctorate in clinical psychology ... It's given me this huge dream to like continue in these academic pursuits and it's like, oh, my goodness, I now do not have to believe the stupid shit I was told growing up but, I can come and create my own way of thinking and being able to come to conclusions.

PTG Domain 3: Relating to Others

This domain refers to a greater connection to other people and increased compassion for those who suffer. Calhoun and Tedeschi (2006) report that this increased experience of compassion translates into a greater degree of frequency of altruistic acts. The exploitation of sex trafficking occurs within a relationship and trust in a relationship is one of the greatest tools of the trafficker. Therefore, the profound damage to trust, safety, and intimacy in friendships, family, and intimate-partner relationships have long-reaching implications. Indeed, for a trafficking survivor, the relationship was the greatest need and primary source of healing. It is in relationships that some were able to exit the trafficking experience, form and strengthen their identity, and be encouraged to flourish (Evans, 2019; 2020; 2022). One research participant eloquently described how relationships may provide the opposite of the abuse in the trafficking experience:

> I really believe that just as the trauma takes place in relationships – I believe that healing takes place in relationships as well and just as I have seen the pure sickness of individuals, I believe now that there is a lot of good individuals in this world and, so, those people are very much a part of my life on a daily basis and I know I can call them at any moment.

Some survivors described how they were able to find their personal power to make choices and set boundaries: " ... developing that in relationships and learning I can say no to things and what consent means and all of those things" (Participant 14). Of special importance were key support persons or service providers who had confidence in the survivors, verbalized what they saw, and were with them on a journey of naming and helping them to discover their beliefs, values, skills, interests, and preferences. This provided a mirror for participants to begin to see and further develop themselves. For example, Grace explained how she found relationships that were exceptions to her past experiences and perceptions, and how these relationships impacted her, particularly when expressing understanding and confidence in her.

> The smallest things, are the people that I've come in contact with ... it's just the way that people were put – and I can't deny it and I know that, that was for me and that I'm walking the right way. And, if it wasn't for those signs, I think I'd probably have given up because, when you're surrounded by people that don't understand or don't know what you're thinking, feeling, or what it's even like, it's hard to see that there's a path and that you can kind of come out of it ... Just people that kind of surrounded me and said that I could do this. And, I'm like, if you say so, and I just kept walking and here I am.

Participants also described the role of unconditional love and having someone who would not give up, would provide acceptance of where they were at, and who provided presence, tangible support, accountability, and the opportunity to practice healthy attachment.

> I'm currently in a mentor program and that has been absolutely incredible having a community, being able to build relationships with a person who I've been able to create attachments with that are healthy attachments. But, knowing that they have accountability, knowing that it's not an isolation which is an isolation which absolutely terrifies me because my trauma happened in isolation ... So, she has been through a lot of life with me, sat in a lot of doctor's appointments with me and stuff ... People that are safe have really changed my life (Participant 14)

PTG Domain 4: Appreciation for Life

An increased appreciation for life or a changed sense of what is of most importance may occur for those who have experienced threat or danger in their suffering is applicable to trafficking survivors (Calhoun & Tedeschi, 2006). Most participants referenced changes in their perceptions of themselves and of their life (Evans, 2019; 2022).

Perception of Self

More than two-thirds described how the experience made them stronger or how they saw that something good came from the experience, particularly their being able to help others or the strength they gained from the experience. "Some of the ways it shaped my life have been positive. I wouldn't be doing this work if I hadn't been through that, and I wouldn't live where I live and I wouldn't have the job that I have that I love and it's not that I think it's all bad" (Participant 15). Audrey shared:

> As far as my identity and my recovery, how I look at my life now is that good, bad, or indifferent what I've done what a lot of other people have not done, was that I lived two different lives in one lifetime. And, so, I'm very fortunate because I also work in the field-what was meant for bad, turned out to be good.

Perception of Life

A repetitious theme was the description that their eyes were open to see and appreciate life and beauty to a greater or different degree as a result of the trafficking experience. Participant 10 stated, "it caused me to open my eyes to the world." Grace shared this experience after being released from sexual exploitation as well as incarceration:

> It was a totally different world. Everything looked big. I saw trees and I was just isolated for months. It seemed like years. Because, technically, it was years. I didn't pay attention to trees for years. I didn't pay attention to any of that and, for once, my eyes were just opened.

Some participants specifically mentioned photography being something they learned or that was helpful for them in their recovery, as a result of their ability to see and appreciate beauty. Participant 14 said:

> It was like this really cool life came alive to me because I was seeing these little intricate details – things outside for the first time with my human eye and, so, here I was going on my hands and knees, crawling all over fields and all of that getting pictures of bugs and leaves and just twigs and fun stuff. And I was seeing all this fun – in an hour I would get one picture of a butterfly ... So, it's been part of my healing to realize that, I can create my own healing through a camera ... I think for most of my life I felt so invisible to people that I love taking pictures of, like – macro photography – taking pictures of things that nobody sees and making them visible to the seeing eye because it makes me feel like I'm seen in some way.

Grace concurred:

> I'll go outside and some bird will fly by and I will be reminded that I am still in the present and where I'm at. I just went to park, took a little hike, sat by this waterfall, prayed and then I ended up sending a picture to the two girls on my cell phone and I was like, this is how I've learned to walk it off.

This repeated description of an increased capacity to *see* reflects their perspective, intuition, and depth. Kristine explained, "I think you feel like you're an old person in a young person's body. I think you've already lived a life and appreciate life a lot more and see things that people don't see ... " Participant 14 also described how she can find beauty because of the perspective she now has:

> It just makes me so excited because that's the reason why I had to go through so much crap then, maybe there's a little bit of beauty. And, I will always see things differently than most people ... I see little things and it's not like I don't see a big picture. It's not like I don't have dreams and like I dream and see big pictures but I also see little things and they just bring me a lot of smiles and happiness and I'll always probably be like that.

Grace explained that she is more in touch with emotions and has a greater appreciation for relationships:

> ... I'm more emotional than some people, but I'm also more in tune with that. And, honestly, that's something I wouldn't change because I don't want to ever walk around this world again not being in touch with that – not being in touch with my senses and not understanding how I'm feeling or being in the moment. I don't want to ever lose that again. So, that's kind of been a blessing ... I think I value relationships a lot more. I have also learned that not everybody is like me. Not everybody is as deep as I go. Not everybody thinks or feels the way I feel.
>
> I have a new perspective on a lot of things. I have gratitude that I never had. I have a humility that I never had. I have a passion that I have never had. I have an eye for beauty in the little things that I never had. And, I just have a really good way about making any situation positive. There's times that I don't, but most times I can always turn it around somehow. Yeah, and just my whole idea about what life is, it's not about the big car and all that, it's about how you feel about yourself and what you're doing to help somebody else. It's not what you're trying to gather up for yourself. It has nothing to do with that. It's how can you serve in this world to make it better? How can you help somebody not be so broken? How can you breathe life back into somebody is what keeps me going every day? And, I think a lot of people that I come in contact with see that about me.

PTG Domain 5: Spiritual Change

Some individuals who have experienced trauma report increased spiritual or existential meaning in their lives (Little et al., 2011). Tedeschi and Calhoun (2006) report that they observe the most significant PTG in this domain, which reflects greater satisfaction, and greater clarity with answers to fundamental existential questions. Almost all of the survivors mentioned experiences of faith or religion. Half of them credit spirituality as a form of coping or means of survival during the time of being trafficked. For example, Kristine said: "I had some really supernatural experiences out there and I know that I was being watched over – stuff that just doesn't happen. And, so, I do feel like that God was watching me, no doubt." The same feeling resonates in Cat's statement:

> When I was in the life I prayed a lot actually. I prayed for my protection. Every time I would have a date I would always pray, God bless me and please keep me safe and even though I know I'm sinning right now ... I really started to feel God's love and,

> now, I constantly – I battle with God sometimes, because I can be disobedient and I tend to want to do things on my own because I always have so I don't want him to take the wheel and it's affected me because I get myself in some sticky situations and, it just makes me realize how much more I need Him to depend on.

More than half of the participants in the study described how spiritual beliefs as a part of their healing process helped after the trafficking experience. Kristine shared:

> I went back to church ... I think I felt like I didn't have anybody in the world that I could trust – even my parents – anyone. I felt like God was my father and if I really get into that message ... just tried to learn a different way of living, whatever that was like to practice the lessons. So, I think that it has healed me. I mean, you know, those things of guilt and shame that many survivors carry, I think that has, you know, definitely subsided because of it.

Cat explained:

> I pray. I pray a lot. And, I really do a lot of self-talk. I – it's been something – I never really realized that I did but it's actually a coping mechanism and it's been really good for me because I think when I vocally hear myself and I look at myself and I talk to myself and I look at myself in my eyes, I can see – I started to see myself as God sees me. And, when I started to look at myself as God sees me, I started to kind of see like a sparkle in my eye, like a light in my eye.

Approximately one-third of participants described additional spiritual growth *because* of the trafficking experience. Participant 14 stated:

> I have found a lot of healing in spirituality in practicing my own faith. I use the term spiritual resiliency because I have experienced so much spiritual abuse and so much horrific stuff on a spiritual level, whether that's supposed to be from well-intentioned people or from my experiences with my biological people ... I really have found a lot of peace and being able to practice my faith, my religion. And, also, learning to define it my way instead of letting people define it for me. I am religious and I don't go to church every week because I don't like going to church and, so, yeah, I would say that I have a faith and I do have a belief system.

Supporting PTG in Survivors of Sex Trafficking

PTG blooms in unlikely places, including survivors of sex trafficking. What is our role in supporting survivors that may water the seeds of PTG? PTG is not inevitable, yet it is a universal phenomenon. Therefore, any helper should remain attentive to emerging signs of growth, and may sensitively introduce the topic, meeting the person where they are, while also recognizing the potential for growth and facilitating spaces for that growth to occur (Weiss & Berger, 2010). Offering and honoring choice promotes finding and nurturing personal strength. Support persons have the role of maintaining a balance between coping with posttraumatic distress, while also encouraging the development of goals, dreams and exercise of new possibilities. Clinical work can be conducted within a client's existential or spiritual framework, thus encouraging them to find meaning and perspective from their stated spiritual beliefs (Weiss & Berger, 2010).

Creative and expressive means can be used to foster a survivors' seeing and appreciating beauty. Similar therapeutic means have been used with populations in treatment for PTSD, including veterans (Ezparza, 2015; Sornborger et al., 2017), and survivors of sexual abuse and other forms of trauma (Hass-Cohen et al., 2018; Meston et al., 2013). Creative and expressive arts reduced symptoms of depression and PTSD (Ezparza, 2015; Meston C. et al., 2013; Sornborger et al., 2017) and increased indicators of PTG (Hass-Cohen et al., 2018).

Strategies for helping to promote PTG in survivors may include activities that incorporate art, music, cooking, photography, nature, fashion, and interior design. For example, participants in photovoice communicated its impact, showing the value of finding other ways to expose survivors to expressions of beauty. Grace stated:

> It reminds me that I am not alone with the experience of trying to fit back into society after you have been so branded and broken. Everyone finds their way differently but we are also searching for the same thing. Survivors take different avenues, but everyone can still see beauty. Out of all that darkness you can still see something that's beautiful. That to me just shows a spirit of complete power and such strength ... Pictures are a lot more powerful than words sometimes and it comes from such a creative ... it makes people think.

Participant 14 shared:

> I hope others see the power of Photovoice and the ways that it can be utilized to give expression to an individual, and as a survivor, the ways that I have found healing in the midst of it and the ways that it can really share that narrative and not just share the narrative but also share the future as well. It doesn't just tell the past narrative, it can also share the creation of a future narrative. This is what I am leaving this experience with, which has been so powerful for me

Finally, practitioners must not underestimate the role of relationships. Interventions should occur on multiple levels (individual, family, peer group, community). The relationship includes bearing witness, which happens in the context of a relationship and is crucial for supporting survivors of sex trafficking. To bear witness means to testify to, give or afford evidence of something that has happened, which is usually unfair, unjust, or problematic. To bear witness is to enter in, listen, seek to understand, and be a student of the one whom we are witnessing. Bloom (1997) states that in this century of genocide, totalitarian control, mass oppression, and torture, bearing witness has become one of the most potent and nonviolent methods for transforming experienced and witnessed traumatic experiences. Bearing witness changes both the one who is bearing witness and the one who is being witnessed.

Relationships are also the context where voice, choice, and dignity are revived and honored. When an individual can be seen and heard, it serves as a mirror to the discovery of identity. Relationships provide models for safety, trust, and health, and have the capacity to serve as the exception, the reversal of trauma, exploitation, and betrayal by giving hope and meaning. It is essential that any intervention provides opportunities for survivors to connect with other survivors, mentors, and support persons that will provide lifelong acceptance and model mutuality and shared power. This may require exploring nontraditional service models or creating resources to connect survivors to support persons who are committed to a long-term, empowering, trauma-informed relationship.

Additionally, survivors point to the importance of training families, faith communities, and organizations about the needs of trafficking survivors, and the importance of providing supportive relationships for them. When working with survivors, providers should address aspects of healthy relationships such as communication, boundaries, and intimacy. It is the hope borrowed from someone else's confidence that becomes the soil and fertilizer for PTG.

References

Bender, R., Bien-Aime', Feifer, K., Foster, R., Hatcher, M., Hersh, L., Meyers, A., Ream, A., Rhodes, S., & Zipkin, R. (November 2019). *Equality not exploitation: An overview of the global sex trade and trafficking crisis, and the case for the Equality Model.* New York: World Without Exploitation.

Bloom, S. (1997). By the crowd they have been broken, by the crowd they shall be healed: The social transformation of trauma. In C. P. Tedeschi, & L. Calhoun (Eds.), *Post-traumatic growth: Theory and research on change in the aftermath of crises* (pp. 173–208). Mahwah, NJ: Lawrence Erlbaum Associates.

Calhoun, L., & Tedeschi, R. (2006). The foundations of posttraumatic growth: An expanded framework. In *Handbook of Posttraumatic Growth Research and Practice* (pp. 1–23). Mahwah, NJ: Lawrence Erlbaum.

Choi, H., Klein, C., Shin, M., & Lee, H. (2009). Posttraumatic stress disorder and disorders of extreme stress (desnos) symptoms following prostitution and childhood abuse. *Violence Against Women*, *15*(8), 933–951. 10.1177/1077801209335493

Clawson, H., Dutch, N., Salomon, A., & Grace, L. G. (2009). *Study of HHS programs serving human trafficking final report.* US Department of Health and Human Services, Office of the Assistant Secretary for Planning and Evaluation.

Counter Trafficking Data Collaborative. (2019). *Global data hub on human trafficking.* https://www.ctdatacollaborative.org/global-dataset-0

Courtois, C., & Ford, J. (2009). Defining and understanding ocmplex trauma and complex traumatic stress disorders. In F. Courtois (Ed.), *Treating complex traumatic stress disorders* (pp. 13–30). New York: Guilford Press.

Department of State, U. S. (2022). *Trafficking in Persons Report.* Washington, D.C.: Department of State.

Evans, H. (2019). *From the voices of domestic sex trafficking survivors: Experiences of complex trauma and posttraumatic growth. Doctorate in Social Work Dissertations*, 126. https://repository.upenn.edu/edissertations_sp2/126

Evans, H. (2020). The integral role of relationships in experiences of complex trauma in sex trafficking survivors. *International Journal of Human Rights in Healthcare*, *13*(2), 109–123. 10.1108/ijhrh-07-2019-0054

Evans, H. (2022). *Understanding complex trauma and post-traumatic growth in survviors of sex trafficking: Foregroudning women's voices for effective care and prevention.* New York: Routledge.

Ezparza, J. (2015). Using person-centered expressive arts group therapy with combat-related PTSD veterans. Doctoral dissertation, Saybrook University. ProQuest 1732168278.

Farley, M. (2003). *Prostitution, trafficking, and traumatic stress.* Binghamton: Haworth Press.

FBI. (2019). *Uniform crime reports, arrests by race and ethnicity.* https://ucr.fbi.gov/crime-in-the-u.s/2019/crime-in-the-u.s.-2019/tables/table-43.

Ferguson, D. (27 August 2016). *Native communities focus on sex trafficking prevention training.* Retrieved from Argus Leader: www.argusleader.com

Hardy, V. L., Compton, K. D., & McPhatter, V. S. (2013). Domestic minor sex trafficking: Practice implications for mental health professionals. *Affilia*, *28*(1), 8–18. 10.1177/088610991247
Hass-Cohen, N., Bokoch, R., Clyde Findlay, J., & Banford Witting, A. (2018). A four-drawing art therapy trauma and resiliency protocol study. *The Arts in Psychotherapy*, *61*, 44–56. 10.1016/j.aip.2018.02.003
Herman, J. (1992). *Trauma and recovery*. New York: Harpercollins.
Little, S. G., Akin-Little, A., & Somerville, M. P. (2011). Response to trauma in children: An examination of effective intervention in response to post-traumatic growth. *School Psychology International*, *32*(5), 448–463. 10.1177/0143034311402916
Meston, C., Lorenz, T., & Stephenson, K. (2013). Effects of expressive writing on sexual dysfunction, depression, and PTSD in women with a history of childhood sexual abuse: Results from a randomized clinical trial. *Journal of Sexual Medicine*, *10*(9), 2177–2189. 10.1111/jsm.12247
Orme, J., & Ross-Sheriff, F. (2015). Sex trafficking: Policies, programs and services. *Social Work*, *60*(4), 287–294. 10.1093/sw/swv031
Perry, C. L., & de Castro Pecanha, V. (2017). Sex-trafficked survivors: The relation between post-traumatic growth and quality of life. *Journal of Human Trafficking*, *3*(4), 271–284. 10.1080/23322705.2016.1224761
Schultz, T., Canning, S. S., & Eveleigh, E. (2020). Posttraumatic stress, posttraumatic growth, and religious coping in individuals exiting sex trafficking. *Journal of human trafficking*, *6*(3), 358–374. 10.1080/23322705.2018.1522924
Shelley, L. (2010). *Human trafficking: A global perspective*. New York: Cambridge University Press.
Sornborger, J., Fann, A., Serpa, G., Ventrelle, J., Sornborger, J., Fann, A., Serpa, J.G., Ventrelle, J., Ming Foynes, M., Carleton, M., Sherrill, A., Kao, L., Jakubovic, R., Bui, E., & Normand, P. (2017). Integrative therapy approaches for posttraumatic stress disorder: a special focus on treating veterans. *Focus: The Journal of Lifelong Learning in Psychiatry*, *15*(4), 390–398. 10.1176/appi.focus.20170026
Spinazzola, J., Blaustein, M., Kisiel, C., & Van der Kolk, B. (2001). *Beyond PTSD: Further evidence for a complex adaptational response to traumatic life events*. New Orleans: Paper presented at American Psychiatric Association Annual Meeting.
Wang, C., & Burris, M. A. (1997). Photovoice: Concept, methodology, and use for participatory needs assessment. *Affilia*, *24*(3), 87–100.
Weiss, T., & Berger, R. (2010). *Posttraumatic growth and culturally competent practice: Lessons learned from around the globe*. Hoboken: John Wiley & Sons.

PART 6

Vicarious PTG: Growth of "Others" by Affiliation

38

VICARIOUS POSTTRAUMATIC GROWTH

The Benefits of Indirect Exposure to Trauma

Nina Ogińska-Bulik and Zygfryd Juczyński

Studies conducted over the last twenty-five years have provided a wealth of evidence indicating that surviving a traumatic event not only leads to negative consequences but can also be a source of positive posttraumatic changes, which are commonly described as *Posttraumatic Growth* (PTG). PTG includes changes in self-perception, relationships with others, and philosophy of life (Berger, 2015; Calhoun et al., 2010; Calhoun & Tedeschi, 2013; Tedeschi & Calhoun, 1996; 2004). Although both the negative and positive consequences of experienced trauma have been the subject of numerous studies, much less is known about the effects of indirect exposure to trauma, especially positive ones.

While the greatest indirect exposure to trauma has been attributed to those who provide assistance to trauma victims as part of their professional duties, particularly therapists, social workers, probation officers, and medical staff, people who care for the seriously ill or disabled are also frequently exposed. Following frequent contact with traumatized clients and listening to their reports about their experiences, the helpers may begin looking at the world through the eyes of their charges, and experience similar emotions and behaviors. As a consequence, the helpers may also indirectly become victims of trauma, i.e., the trauma of others becomes their own.

Apart from *Secondary Posttraumatic Stress Disorder* (STSD), indirect exposure to trauma can also generate positive posttraumatic changes, known as *Vicarious/Secondary Posttraumatic Growth* (VPTG/SPTG). As this phenomenon mainly affects representatives of certain professions, the term Professional Posttraumatic Growth is also used. This issue has received little research attention to date.

Before the posttraumatic growth construct was popularized, Pearlman and Mac Ian (1995) drew attention to the possibility of positive changes resulting from secondary exposure to trauma. People who empathically engage in helping trauma victims open themselves up to deep personal transformation entailing personal growth, deeper relationships with others experiencing adversity events, and a greater awareness of various aspects of life.

It is assumed that vicarious growth after trauma consists of a set of positive changes related to the psychosocial functioning of those who have been exposed to indirect trauma (Arnold et al., 2005; Brockhouse et al., 2011; Manning-Jones et al., 2016; 2017). As with

DOI: 10.4324/9781032208688-48

posttraumatic growth, these positive changes following vicarious traumatization include changes in self-perception, relationships with others, and philosophy of life.

It is worth noting that the positive consequences of secondary exposure to trauma are also described in other terms. One such example is the concept of *secondary resilience* (SR), referring to the transformation of the inner experience of helpers associated with demonstrating empathy towards trauma victims (Engstrom et al., 2008). This is a unique positive effect that occurs in helpers in response to the development of secondary resilience. The components of this are faith in the ability of the client to recover, looking at their problems from a different perspective, incorporating spirituality into the healing process, developing hope and engagement, and recognizing the strength of the community. Another term that refers to the possible positive consequences of secondary exposure to trauma is *compassion satisfaction*, understood as the pleasure that can be experienced when providing effective help (Stamm, 2002). Compassion satisfaction manifests as a state of fulfillment, balance, and well-being, and can be regarded as the opposite of compassion fatigue.

In the following sections, we present models explaining the occurrence of VPTG, measurements of VPTG, empirical findings regarding VPTG, its occurrence and determinants, and finally suggestions for promoting VPTG.

Models Explaining the Occurrence of VPTG

Vicarious growth after trauma is often explained by models developed for posttraumatic growth. Two leading such models are the functional-descriptive model by Tedeschi and Calhoun (1996; 2004) and the VPTG in Trauma Workers model by Cohen and Collens (2013).

The Functional-Descriptive Model by Tedeschi and Calhoun (Calhoun et al., 2010; Tedeschi & Calhoun, 1996; 2004) draws on cognitive psychology and the existential approach. This model assumes that PTG occurs when a traumatized person experiences changes in their perception of themselves and the world, resulting in a deeper understanding of experienced traumatic events and the ability to give them meaning. Consequently, the loss experienced through suffering is transformed into a deeper understanding of oneself and the surrounding reality, an essential value for a human being and allows the individual to deal more effectively with adversity in the future. The authors emphasize that this is a complex and extended process, which includes stages of stagnation or even regression, indirectly indicating that the experienced trauma can yield both positive and negative consequences.

The VPTG in Trauma Workers model was developed by Cohen and Collens (2013) based on a meta-analysis of 20 studies. In emphasizing the importance of the cognitive activity of the helper, the authors take the position that secondary trauma and VPTG are independent processes and lead to different effects. The trauma experienced by the directly injured person may challenge the cognitive schemas of the helper leading to their questioning their own basic assumptions about the world, and to attempts to understand the experience of the victim and their meaning. The first reaction is typically negative and usually results in the emergence of new negative beliefs about the world and oneself or the consolidation of already existing ones. The second type of reaction, which is positive in nature, leads to positive posttraumatic changes, especially if the helper witnessed growth in the trauma victim.

According to Cohen and Collens (2013), the starting point for the positive effects of indirect exposure to trauma on professionals involved in helping traumatized persons is empathic engagement in victims' problems. Such engagement may lead to stress, negative emotions, and somatic reactions in the professionals, which in turn, are associated with their taking remedial activity, primarily in the form of seeking social support and using personal resources, particularly optimism and spirituality. Over the passage of time, these coping strategies contribute to the reduction in stress and can lead to growth. Optimism and spirituality can be treated both as coping strategies and as the results of resolving the client's situation, thus constituting an element of vicarious growth following the trauma. With regard to remedial activity, the authors point to the importance of strategies for self-care and separating oneself from the victim, i.e., separating work from personal life. Positive changes observed in the helpers concern their beliefs about the world and self, personal values, and everyday life; thus, helpers can express beliefs that they have high resistance to traumatic events and value life to a greater extent. They may display an increase in compassion, wisdom, self-awareness, self-esteem, and self-confidence, and assign greater importance to family and friends.

While both models aim to explain the occurrence of vicarious growth after trauma, they differ primarily in the understanding of the processes that determine posttraumatic changes. Tedeschi and Calhoun (1996; 2004) assume that PTG is based on the same psychological processes as the negative effects of a traumatic experience. They emphasize the interrelationships between the consequences of trauma and indicate that the initial negative changes gradually transform into positive ones. They also emphasize the dynamic of changes in cognitive functioning while helping trauma victims. Cohen and Collens (2013) propose that negative and positive posttraumatic changes should be treated as separate processes, although they may be interrelated. They also suggest that the development of negative or positive changes in helpers depends on the nature of the work performed, and particularly on the type of traumatic situations experienced by their clients.

Measurement of Vicarious Posttraumatic Growth

Multiple tools for measuring PTG have been used in studies assessing VPTG. The *Posttraumatic Growth Inventory (PTGI)*, developed by Tedeschi and Calhoun (1996), is the most popular among them and has been used in 87% of studies aimed at assessing the occurrence of vicarious positive posttraumatic changes (Bybee, 2018). The PTGI is a 21-item Likert-type self-report scale measuring positive changes after struggling with adversity. It includes five dimensions: New possibilities, Personal strengths, Relating to Others, Appreciating of Life and Spiritual Change. The PTGI-SF was developed as a short form of PTG (Cann et al., 2009). While it measures the same five dimensions of posttraumatic growth, it only includes 10 items, i.e., two from each of the five subscales of the original PTGI.

The *Shared Trauma and Professional Posttraumatic Growth Inventory* (STPPGI) has been developed to understand the dual nature of trauma exposure (Tosone et al., 2012). The scale examines the experiences of dual trauma among mental health professionals exposed to both human-made and natural disasters. It is a 14-item, Likert-type scale composed of three subscales: Technique-specific shared trauma, Personal trauma, and Professional PTG. The STPPG accommodates the reciprocal nature of shared trauma and correlates well with existing measures for posttraumatic stress, secondary trauma, shared trauma, and PTG.

The *Vicarious Resilience Scale* (VRS) may also be used to assess the perceived benefits of secondary exposure to trauma (Killian et al., 2017). It consists of 27 items and measures seven aspects of secondary resilience: changes in life goals and perspectives, client-inspired hope, increased recognition of clients' spirituality as a therapeutic resource, increased self-awareness and self-care practices, consciousness about power and privilege relative to the social location of the client, increased capacity for resourcefulness, and increased capacity for remaining present while listening to trauma narratives. The seven subscales have demonstrated adequate to very good reliability. Although it was developed to assess vicarious resilience, rather than vicarious growth, the scale has been found to moderately and positively correlate with PTG and compassion satisfaction, indicating convergent validity.

In addition to questionnaires, inventories, and scales, VPTG may also be evaluated using qualitative methods such as narrative techniques, structured interviews and open-ended questions. McCormack et al. (2011) emphasize the advantages of this type of research when evaluating VPTG because it may reveal unique aspects that questionnaire-based research cannot capture such as humility, love, gratitude, and empathy. However, these methods have rarely been used in VPTG research.

The scarcity of tools for measuring VPTG necessitates the development of a specific tool for its assessment, particularly since differences exist between positive posttraumatic changes deriving from direct and indirect trauma. In order to meet this task, *the Secondary Posttraumatic Growth Inventory* (SPTGI) was developed for professionals working with trauma victims including therapists, medical rescuers, nurses in palliative care, social workers, and probation officers (Ogińska-Bulik & Juczyński, 2020).

An initial set of items was obtained from various tools for measuring PTG, such as the PTGI, as well as developing some new items. The original version of 40 items was narrowed down to a final list of 12 items (e.g., "I have learned to accept others more"); the participant indicates the frequency of their experience on a scale of 0 ("I have not experienced this change at all") to 5 ("I experienced this change to a very great degree). The scale was administered to a sample of 500 respondents (Ogińska-Bulik & Juczyński, in press). A factor analysis of the SPTGI yielded a four-factor solution comprising: 1. New challenges and an increase in professional competences; 2. Increase in spiritual experiences and a greater sense of responsibility for others; 3. Greater confidence in oneself and appreciating life; 4. Increased acceptance and actions for others. The four factors (dimensions) together accounted for 76.43% of the total variance. The Cronbach's alpha of the SPTGI was .90. The test demonstrated high stability in a two-month test-retest value (.78). Its scoring positively correlate with those of the PTGI-SF, two positive cognitive strategies, *viz.* cognitive restructuring and resolution/acceptance from *the Cognitive Processing of Trauma Scale* (CPOTS), and two aspects of empathy, *viz.* perspective taking and empathetic concern, and with secondary traumatic stress symptoms. Thus, the SPTGI appears to be a reliable and valid instrument for measuring positive posttraumatic changes among professionals exposed to secondary trauma and can be useful in scientific research and in clinical practice.

As the SPTGI confirms the concept of PTG (Tedeschi & Calhoun, 1996; 2004), and its dimensions accurately reflect possible positive posttraumatic changes among professionals exposed to secondary trauma, it can be a good alternative to the PTGI, which is commonly used in research on VPTG. Both tools share common elements such as new challenges/ possibilities, appreciation of life or spiritual changes, which seem to be universal in nature, regardless of whether they relate to posttraumatic changes following direct trauma, or those associated with indirect trauma. However, the SPTGI draws on a broader and slightly different spectrum of positive posttraumatic changes, which mainly concern an increase in professional competences, a greater sense of responsibility for others, or increased acceptance and actions for others. Thus, it can help therapists, psychiatrists, social workers, and medical personnel in providing crisis intervention to trauma victims at high risk for adverse outcomes (Ogińska-Bulik & Juczyński, 2020).

Empirical Findings Regarding VPTG

Studies have found VPTG to confirm the general assumptions of the PTG model in regard to diverse groups of human service providers. For example, professionals serving victims of violence-related trauma have shown beneficial personality changes (Arnold et al., 2005; Hyatt-Burkhart, 2013). These changes are manifested in greater sensitivity, compassion, and self-confidence, increased tolerance and empathy, all of which were found to promote a better understanding of trauma victims, greater acceptance of their reactions and behaviors, and a more accurate recognition of their ability to cope effectively. Some therapists in the Hyatt-Burkhart (2013) study emphasized that they began to appreciate their own lives and learn from them more as a result of working with traumatized clients. While some noted an increased awareness of the negative consequences of this type of work, this awareness also appeared to lead to a deeper understanding of the complexity of the entire spectrum of human functioning. Most of the respondents also noticed spiritual changes, manifested mainly in deepened faith and emphasized their belief that the spiritual changes contributed most to the expansion and deepening of their own spirituality and religiosity. These types of observations indicate that positive changes may be transmitted from trauma victims to professionals and that helpers may also "become infected with" the positive posttraumatic changes observed among their charges.

Similarly, research on mental health professionals serving victims following additional types of trauma showed positive changes, which included increased compassion, a deepened understanding of others, an increased sense of self-efficacy, and the presence of positive emotions in situations of providing effective help (Froman, 2014). The helpers also demonstrated greater resilience, especially in situations where their charges also displayed highly effective coping skills, and increased gratitude and appreciation for what they have. Professionals further reported better relationships with others, a greater ability to assign meaning to traumatic situations, increased spirituality, and the need to develop their own personality. Professionally, they noted a greater sense of belonging to the therapeutic community and increased motivation to undertake practices aimed at self-protection.

Studies report the potential for increased self-esteem, increased life wisdom, greater acceptance of others and faith in the effectiveness of their actions, as well as a broader appreciation of their own work with trauma victims (Cohen & Collens, 2013). The positive changes constituting VPTG do not appear suddenly; rather, they occur gradually, suggesting that they result from long-term work with traumatized clients.

Despite the clear similarity between VPTG and PTG, some differences also exist. Arnold et al. (2005) showed that those experiencing VPTG exhibit slightly greater human resilience than trauma survivors; however, they also display slightly fewer changes in their sense of personal strength. In the spiritual realm, those who experience traumatic events directly tend to indicate a personal increase in spirituality, while those who help trauma victims report their spirituals broadening. In other words, the acceptance of spiritual beliefs was viewed as a factor conducive to the process of posttraumatic adaptation without experiencing changes in personal beliefs (Arnold et al., 2005). There are also some aspects unique to VPTG such as increasing awareness of work as a value and the need to increase professional capabilities and competences (Barrington & Shakespeare-Finch, 2013; Guhan & Leibling-Kalifani, 2011; Splevins et al., 2010). Helpers tend to demonstrate a lower intensity of positive posttraumatic changes compared to direct trauma survivors, as indicated in a comparative study by Lambert and Lawson (2013) who found that hurricane victims showed significantly higher levels of posttraumatic growth than those who helped them.

VPTG in Diverse Groups

VPTG can occur in professionals of various specialities working with trauma victims. Despite the paucity of research, previous studies indicate that VPTG appears to be fairly common among medical personnel (Ogińska-Bulik, 2018; Shiri et al., 2008), members of public services (Linley et al., 2003), those helping refugees (Barrington & Shakespeare-Finch, 2013), psychotherapists (Arnold et al., 2005), social workers (Shamai & Ron, 2009), probation officers (Ogińska-Bulik & Juczyński, 2020), people helping addicts (Cosden et al., 2016), professionals working in the social and mental health services sector (Cieslak et al., 2016), as well as translators working with refugees (Splevins et al., 2010).

However, it is difficult to determine the degree of the prevalence of VPTG in diverse occupational groups. This is mainly due to the small number of studies, especially those of a comparative nature, as well as the ambiguity of the results. One study of five professional groups serving trauma victims (Manning-Jones et al., 2017) identified the highest intensity of VPTG in social workers, who also displayed the highest intensity of symptoms of secondary traumatic stress, followed by nurses, counselors, and doctors. The lowest rates were recorded among psychologists. However, a similar study by Ogińska-Bulik and Juczyński (2020) did not confirm such a high intensity of VPTG among social workers; in fact, the findings indicate a lower severity of VPTG in this professional group compared to therapists, paramedics, and nurses.

Studies of VPTG among medical personnel are also inconclusive. Lev-Wiesel et al. (2009) report that nurses show a greater intensity of VPTG than social workers, while Beck et al. (2017) indicate a rather low degree of positive posttraumatic changes among nurses. An Israeli study identified low VPTG among medical staff and found that nurses in the pediatric ward revealed a slightly higher intensity of VPTG than doctors (Taubman-Ben-Ari & Weintroub, 2008). In contrast, Zerach and Shalev (2015) report a moderate intensity of VPTG in psychiatric and community nurses, with the former showing a slightly lower intensity of vicarious positive posttraumatic change.

Findings regarding therapists are also indeterminate. Arnold et al. (2005) found that all surveyed therapists reported at least one positive change as a result of working with trauma victims. Ogińska-Bulik and Juczyński (2020) report that out of five groups of professionals working with trauma victims, therapists obtained the highest level of VPTG; however, Juczyński et al. (in press) note higher levels of VPTG among clergymen providing pastoral care in hospitals, hospices, health care centers, prisons, resocialization centers and penitentiary institutions in Poland. In contrast, Linley et al., (2005), indicate a low level of VPTG among therapists and Manning-Jones et al. (2017) report a low intensity of VPTG among psychologists.

One possible explanation for the high variation in findings may be the type of traumatic events experienced by clients. Indeed, Ben-Porat and Itzhaky (2009) indicate that therapists working with victims of domestic violence display a milder severity of VPTG than those working with clients who experienced other types of traumatic events. Additionally, the comparative studies of Ogińska-Bulik and Juczyński (2020) indicated that among five groups of professionals working with trauma victims, the intensity of STS in therapists was the lowest and they demonstrate greater competence in helping trauma victims than in other groups of professionals. A possible explanation is that therapists tend to be both highly knowledgeable about the dangers involved in helping others and have the appropriate skills to deal with traumatic situations experienced by others. Due to their knowledge and competences, their cognitive schemas are more resistant to interference than those possessed by other support professions. Thus, the traumatic events experienced by clients do not necessarily pose a significant challenge to the therapist's cognitive schemas, which may reduce the occurrence of VPTG.

The phenomenon of VPTG applies also to those who informally offer support to trauma victims such as relatives and family members of individuals who have suffered trauma, for example, wives of war veterans. One of the first studies showing the occurrence of PTG in wives of PTSD-afflicted war veterans was conducted by Dekel and Solomon (2007) who found that positive posttraumatic changes in veterans coexisted with VPTG in their wives. Later, an interview-based study by McCormack et al. (2011) found that wives of Vietnam veterans who suffered from PTSD noticed positive changes in themselves following the problems experienced by their husbands. The women indicated *inter alia* an improvement in the quality of their marital relationship and a change in their relationship with their husbands, which became more valuable and more meaningful for them. The women felt stronger and more determined and showed a greater understanding of the problems faced by their husbands. They also reported having greater self-esteem and changes in their self-perception from being a victim and suffering person focused on the past, to being more confident and oriented towards the present and the future.

A longitudinal study by Bachem et al. (2018) employed three measurements over a 30-year period to examine both war veterans who experienced primary trauma and their spouses who suffered secondary trauma. They found that the severity of PTG in veterans and VPTG in their wives decreased over time. Veterans reported a decline in positive change in more areas of growth than their secondary traumatized spouses. The greatest degree of stability was shown in appreciating life among the veterans and in personal strength among their wives. The presence of VPTG has also been confirmed in caregivers of people struggling with life-threatening somatic diseases, especially cancer (Arnedo & Casellas-Grau, 2015).

Factors Determining the Occurrence of Vicarious Posttraumatic Growth

Not every person exposed to secondary trauma will experience vicarious growth after trauma; it depends on external/environmental and subjective factors.

Environmental factors are primarily related to work. They pertain generally to workload, comprising such factors as the number of hours of work with traumatized persons, the number of clients, and the severity of cases. These elements are often treated as indicators of secondary exposure to trauma. While studies have noted the existence of a positive association between workload and VPTG (Abel et al., 2014; Arnold et al., 2005; Brockhouse et al.,

2011; Cohen & Collens, 2013; Froman, 2014; Linley & Joseph, 2007), other studies do not confirm such relationship (Fedele, 2018; Ogińska-Bulik & Juczyński, 2020). Another organizational/environmental factor that may favor the occurrence of VPTG is social support, especially in the workplace. The received support helps regulate the experienced emotions, fosters the use of more effective coping strategies, and enables the correction of cognitive schemas distorted by the trauma experienced by the client. Most available studies confirm that social support plays an important role in the occurrence of VPTG, with support from colleagues or associates being a positive predictor of VPTG among groups of professionals dealing with the health of people after traumatic experiences (Manning-Jones et al., 2017; Ogińska-Bulik & Juczyński, 2020; Ogińska-Bulik et al., 2021). Social support, expressed in the form of subjective support, objective support, and seeking support, demonstrated a positive relationship with VPTG among the employees of ambulance teams from six emergency centers in Jinan, China (Kang et al., 2018). Similarly, positive links between social support and VPTG were reported among therapists working with trauma victims (Linley & Joseph, 2007). These findings suggest that the provision of supportive professional or peer supervision may increase the reflectivity and meaningfulness of the undertaken professional activity, and promote cognitive processing of trauma, thus fostering the occurrence of personal growth. However, no such relationship was observed between social support and VPTG in groups of therapists (Brockhouse et al., 2011).

Preferred therapeutic orientation and therapeutic bond may also contribute to the occurrence of secondary positive posttraumatic changes. A humanistic and transpersonal orientation, as indicated by Linley and Joseph (2007), turned out to be positively related to VPTG, while the use of cognitive-behavioral therapy was negatively related. The relationship with the client turned out to be the main predictor of observed positive posttraumatic changes among therapists (Linley & Joseph, 2005). A similar role may be played by job satisfaction and attributing high value to work, as shown in studies conducted among social workers (Gibbons et al., 2011).

Personal factors that determine the occurrence of VPTG include gender, age, own history of trauma, personality characteristics of the helpers, as well as the remedial activity undertaken by them. However, the available data do not give a clear picture of the relationship between these variables and the intensity of vicarious positive posttraumatic change. For example, in a group of therapists, women obtained higher levels of VPTG than men (Froman, 2014; Linley & Joseph, 2007). However, no differences in the intensity of VPTG were found between women and men in a study of five professional groups of people working with trauma victims (doctors, psychologists, nurses, social workers, and counselors), (Manning-Jones et al., 2017). In a group of therapists (Brockhouse et al., 2011), older age was found to be associated with higher severity of VPTG and, most significantly, with positive changes in personal strength and appreciation of life. Positive, albeit weak, relationships between age and VPTG were also observed among midwives who participated in complicated births (Beck et al., 2017).

The occurrence of VPTG may be fostered by the personal traumatic experiences of the helper (Linley & Joseph, 2007; Lev-Wiesel et al., 2009). Such a history of trauma seems to result in greater empathetic involvement in the problems experienced by the client, as well as a better ability to address such situations.

An important factor in the development of VPTG is the helper's empathetic engagement in helping the client. This is indicated by studies conducted among therapists (Brockhouse et al. 2011; Linley & Joseph, 2007; Ogińska-Bulik et al., 2021). In a study by Brockhouse et al. (2011) vicarious exposure to trauma and empathy positively predicted VPTG levels in therapists. Additionally, empathy was a moderator in the relationship between secondary exposure to trauma and the relating to others aspect of VPTG. The findings suggest that therapists with highly emphatic abilities are more likely to accommodate their relating to others' schema, even if vicarious exposure is poor. In Ogińska-Bulik and Juczyński study (2020) VPTG was positively related to two aspects of empathy (measured by Interpersonal Reactivity Index), i.e., empathic concern and perspective taking (it was not related to the third aspect of empathy, i.e., personal suffering).

Additionally, self-compassion in the face of trauma combined with self-care has also been found to promote the occurrence of VPTG. Resilience was found to be positively related to VPTG among groups of therapists (Ogińska-Bulik & Juczyński, 2020), doctors (Taku, 2014), nurses working in palliative care (Ogińska-Bulik, 2018), and among the staff of ambulance teams (Kang et al., 2018).

Another resource conducive to the occurrence of positive changes resulting from vicarious exposure to trauma is life optimism, which is associated with positive affect. Cohen and Collens (2013) emphasize the importance of a positive view of the world and a sense of humor as factors influencing the occurrence of VPTG. Optimism turned out to be positively related to VPTG in a group of nurses and rehabilitators (Shiri et al., 2010) and in those involved in the burial of the deceased (Linley & Joseph, 2005).

The occurrence of secondary positive posttraumatic changes may also be fostered by spirituality and religiosity. As such, is not surprising to find a high level of positive changes in clergymen helping trauma victims; Juczyński et al. (in press) report the occurrence of VPTG in 61.4% of studied clergy. Religious beliefs were also positively associated with VPTG among child protection social workers (Rhee et al., 2013).

A significant role in the development of VPTG is played by the cognitive activity undertaken by the individual, including the change of beliefs about the world and oneself, and the coping strategies used. Cohen and Collens (2013) indicate the importance of both behavioral and cognitive remedial efforts. Studies of midwives who have participated in complicated births have shown positive associations between changes in key beliefs and the VPTG (Beck et al., 2017). This suggests that some kind of flexibility in cognitive schemas, expressed in readiness to change, favors the positive consequences of secondary exposure to trauma.

Studies involving five different groups of professionals working with trauma victims showed positive associations between VPTG and ruminations, especially deliberate ones, as well as using cognitive restructuring and resolution/acceptance (measured by CBI) for coping with trauma. It suggests that the greater the challenge to one's core beliefs, the higher the posttraumatic growth (Ogińska-Bulik & Juczyński, 2020). These two strategies also acted as VPTG predictors in studies of medical personnel exposed to secondary trauma (Ogińska-Bulik et al., 2021). However, cognitive activity appears to have a weaker influence on VPTG than on PTG. This may mean that experiencing trauma indirectly involves cognitive processes to a lesser extent than in the case of directly experienced trauma. It may also result from the specificity of the work of professionals helping trauma victims, who usually have little time to significantly engage cognitively in processing the trauma experienced by their charges. Moreover, helping people who have experienced a variety of traumatic events may hinder cognitive processing, especially when the helper works with a large number of such people.

It is also noted that the occurrence of vicarious positive posttraumatic changes is favored by behavioral coping strategies, and above all, various types of self-care activities. Several studies have shown that exercise, healthy eating, and hobbies are positively associated with VPTG (Arnold et al., 2005; Barrington & Shakespeare-Finch, 2013; Splevins et al., 2010).

Promoting Vicarious Posttraumatic Growth

VPTG can be promoted by increasing knowledge and awareness of the phenomenon of secondary trauma among helpers, as well as of various types of interventions designed to foster it. Interventions, especially those of a cognitive nature, may contribute to a revision of the existing cognitive schemas and enable the creation of new ones better adapted to the new reality. Particular attention should be paid to the development of the ability to reformulate basic beliefs about oneself and the world and shape reflectivity to support active information processing and cognitive involvement in the search for new points of view.

Because the importance of group interventions is emphasized in the process of shaping positive posttraumatic changes, special attention should be attributed to the support of colleagues and supervision, mainly from work colleagues. The possibility of expressing painful experiences and emotions related to traumatic events of others in a group may increase the helpers' belief in their own ability to cope and their sense of security. Members of support groups can provide examples of new perspectives and goals in life, and professionals who have experienced vicarious posttraumatic growth can serve as models for others who find it more difficult to deal with the trauma experienced by their clients (Froman, 2014; Kang et al., 2018).

Interventions intended to foster VPTG should take into account the development of personal resources and personality traits conducive to the occurrence of positive changes, including empathy. This is particularly true for cognitive processing, resilience, life optimism, self-efficacy, and extraversion. Shaping and developing empathy seems to be particularly important as it can contribute to greater reflection and acceptance of the inevitable in addition to allowing the helper to understand better the suffering of trauma victims. The aforementioned resources are associated with positive affect, which can reduce negative emotions resulting from the experience of secondary trauma. These properties are also important factors contributing to greater well-being. To promote VPTG, it is important to mobilize and multiply resources for those exposed to secondary trauma.

The significance of such multiplication and mobilization of resources that favor the adoption of an active attitude to adversities is emphasized by Conservation of Resources theory (COR; Hobfoll, 1989). COR theory provides a medium for understanding how loss of resources impacts both individuals and the larger community and offers a framework to enhance coping with daily stressors and crises. Research to date has often concluded that posttraumatic growth was positive by virtue of the fact that people report more meaning, spirituality, or intimacy with others, rather than whether these changes resulted in improved functioning, decreased psychopathology, or rebuilding their lives (Hall et al., 2006). Perceived gains that are bound to traumatic events may not offset losses but be specious insofar as they reflect attempts at coping and mastery that are maintained at a cognitive level of beliefs rather than actual real gains of tangible resources.

VPTG is a similar but not identical construct to PTG, as the areas of growth include specific aspects such as becoming a better professional (Cohen & Collens, 2013). The existence of similar dependencies can be assumed with regard to the phenomenon of vicarious posttraumatic growth; however, further studies of the consequences of posttraumatic growth are advisable, both in people directly affected by trauma and in people who are secondarily traumatized.

References

Abel, L., Walker, C., Samios, C., & Morozow, L. (2014). Vicarious posttraumatic growth: Predictors of growth and relationships with adjustment. *Traumatology*, *20*(1), 9–18. 10.1037/h0099375

Arnedo, C. O., & Casellas-Grau, A. (2015). Vicarious or secondary posttraumatic growth: How are positive changes transmitted to significant others after experiencing a traumatic event? In C. Martin, V. Predey, & V. Patel (Eds.), *Comprehensive Guide to Post-Traumatic Stress Disorder* (1767–1782). Springer Publishing.

Arnold, D., Calhoun, L. G., Tedeschi, R., & Cann, A. (2005). Vicarious posttraumatic growth in psychotherapy. *Journal of Humanistic Psychology*, *45*(2), 239–263. 10.1177/0022167805274729

Bachem, R., Mitreuter, S., Levin, Y., Stein, J. Y., Xiao, Z., & Solomon, Z. (2018). Longitudinal development of primary and secondary posttraumatic growth in aging veterans and their wives: Domain-specific trajectories. *Journal of Traumatic Stress*, *31*(5), 730–741. 10.1002/jts.22331

Barrington, A. G., & Shakespeare-Finch, J. (2013). Working with refugee survivors of torture and trauma: An opportunity for vicarious post-traumatic growth. *Counselling Psychology Quarterly*, *26*(1), 89–105. 10.1080/09515070.2012.727553

Beck, C., Rivera, J., & Gable, R. (2017). A mixed-methods study of vicarious posttraumatic growth in certified nurse-midwives. *Journal of Midwifery and Women's Health*, *62*(1), 80–87. 10.1111/jmwh.12523

Ben-Porat, A., & Itzhaky, H. (2009). Implications of treating family violence for the therapist: Secondary traumatization, vicarious traumatization, and growth. *Journal of Family Violence*, *24*(7), 507–515. 10.1007/s10896-009-9249-0

Berger, R. (2015). *Stress, Trauma, and Posttraumatic Growth. Social Context, Environment, and Identities*. Routledge.

Brockhouse, R., Msetfi, R. M., Cohen, K., & Joseph, S. (2011). Vicarious exposure to trauma and growth in therapists: The moderating effects of sense of coherence, organizational support, and empathy. *Journal of Traumatic Stress*, *24*(6), 735–742. 10.1002/jts.20704

Bybee, S. (2018). Vicarious posttraumatic growth in end-of-life care: How filling gaps in knowledge can foster clinicians' growth. *Journal of Social Work in End-of-Life & Palliative Care*, *14*(4), 257–273. 10.1080/15524256.2018.1498820

Calhoun, L. G., Cann, A., & Tedeschi, R. G. (2010). The posttraumatic growth model: Sociocultural considerations. In T. Weiss, & R. Berger (Eds.), *Posttraumatic growth and culturally competent practice: Lessons learned from around the globe* (pp. 1–14). John Wiley & Sons.

Calhoun, L. G., & Tedeschi, R. G. (2013). *Posttraumatic growth in clinical practice*. Routledge.

Cann, A., Tedeschi, R. G., Calhoun, L. G., & Taku, K. (2009). A short form of the posttraumatic growth inventory. *Anxiety, Stress, and Coping*, *23*(2), 127–137. 10.1080/10615800903094273

Cieslak, R., Benight, Ch., Rogala, A., Smoktunowicz, E., Kowalska, M., Zukowska, K., Yeager, C., & Luszczynska, A. (2016). Effects on internet-based self-efficacy on secondary traumatic stress and secondary posttraumatic growth among health and human service professionals exposed to indirect trauma. *Frontiers in Psychology*, *4*(7), 1009. 10.3389/fpsyg.2016.01009

Cohen, K., & Collens, P. (2013). The impact of trauma work on trauma workers: A metasynthesis on vicarious trauma and vicarious posttraumatic growth. *Psychological trauma: Theory, research, practice, and policy*, *5*(6), 570–580. 10.1037/a0030388

Cosden, M., Sanford, A., Koch, L. M., & Lepore, C. E. (2016). Vicarious trauma and vicarious posttraumatic growth among substance abuse treatment providers. *Substance Abuse*, *37*(4), 619–624. 10.1080/08897077.2016.1181695

Dekel, R., & Solomon, Z. (2007). Secondary traumatization among wives of war veterans with PTSD. In C. Figley, & W. Nash (Eds.), *Combat stress injury: Theory, research, and management* (pp. 137–157). Routledge.

Engstrom, D., Hernandez, P., & Gangsei, D. (2008). Vicarious resilience: A qualitative investigation into its description. *Traumatology*, 14(3), 13–21. 10.1177/1534765608319323

Fedele, K. M. (2018). *An investigation of factors impacting vicarious traumatization and vicarious posttraumatic growth in crisis workers: Vicarious exposure to trauma, feminist beliefs, and feminist self-labeling* [Doctoral dissertation, University of Akron]. http://rave.ohiolink.edu/etdc/view?acc_num=akron1519564198322496

Froman, M. (2014). *A mixed methods study of the impact of providing therapy to traumatized clients: Vicarious trauma, compassion fatigue, and vicarious posttraumatic growth in mental health therapists* [Doctoral dissertation, the University of Minnesota]. https://conservancy.umn.edu/handle/11299/165355

Gibbons, S., Murphy, D., & Joseph, S. (2011). Countertransference and positive growth in social workers. *Journal of Social Work Practice*, *25*(1), 17–30. 10.1080/02650530903579246

Guhan, R., & Leibling-Kalifani, H. (2011). The experiences of staff working with refugees and asylum seekers in the United Kingdom: A grounded theory exploration. *Journal of Immigrant and Refugee Studies*, *9*(3), 205–228. 10.1080/15562948.2011.592804

Hall, B. J., Rattigan, S., Walter, K. H., & Hobfoll, S. E. (2006). Conservation of resources theory and trauma: An evaluation of new and existing principles. In P. Buchwald (Ed.), *Stress and Anxiety – Application to Health, Community, Work Place, and Education* (pp. 230–250). Cambridge Scholar Press Ltd. https://www.researchgate.net/publication/269711011_Conservation_of_resources_theory_and_trauma_An_evaluation_of_new_and_existing_principles

Hobfoll, S. E. (1989). Conservation of resources: A new attempt at conceptualizing stress. *American Psychologist*, *44*(3), 513–524. 10.1037/0003-066X.44.3.513

Hyatt-Burkhart, D. (2013). The Experience of Vicarious Posttraumatic Growth in mental health workers. *Journal of Loss and Trauma*, *19*(5), 452–461. 10.1080/15325024.2013.797268

Juczyński, Z., Ogińska-Bulik, N., & Binnenbesel, J. (in press). Empathy and cognitive processing as factors determining the consequences of secondary exposure to trauma among Roman Catholic clergymen. *Journal of Religion and Health*.

Kang, X., Fang, Y., Li, S., Liu, Y., Zhao, D., Feng, X., Wang, Y., & Li, P. (2018). The benefits of indirect exposure to trauma: The relationship among vicarious posttraumatic growth, social support, and resilience in ambulance personnel in China. *Psychiatry Investigation*, *15*(5), 452–459. 10.30773/pi.2017.11.08.1

Killian, K., Hernandez-Wolfe, P., Engstrom, D., & Gangsei, D. (2017). Development of the Vicarious Resilience Scale (VRS): A measure of positive effects of working with trauma survivors. *Psychological Trauma: Theory, Research, Practice, and Policy*, *9*(1), 23–31. 10.1037/tra0000199

Lambert, F., & Lawson, G. (2013). Resilience of professional counselors following hurricanes Katrina and Rita. *Journal of Counseling & Development*, *91*(3), 261–268. 10.1002/j.1556-6676.2013.00094.x

Lev-Wiesel, R., Goldblatt, H., Eiskovits, Z., & Admi, H. (2009). Growth in the shadow of war: the case of social workers and nurses working in a shared war reality. *British Journal of Social Work*, *39*(6), 1154–1174. 10.1093/bjsw/bcn021

Linley, P. A., & Joseph, S. (2005). Positive and negative changes following occupational death exposure. *Journal of Traumatic Stress*, *18*(6), 751–758. 10.1002/jts.20083

Linley, P. A., & Joseph, S. (2007). Therapy work and therapists' positive and negative well-being. *Journal of Social and Clinical Psychology*, *26*(3), 385–403. 10.1521/jscp.2007.26.3.385

Linley, P. A., Joseph, S., Cooper, R., Harris, S., & Meyer, C. (2003). Positive and negative changes following vicarious exposure to the September 11 terrorists attack. *Journal of Traumatic Stress*, *16*(5), 481–485. 10.1023/A:1025710528209

Linley, P. A., Joseph, S., & Loumidis, K. (2005). Trauma work, sense of coherence, and positive and negative changes in therapists. *Psychotherapy and Psychosomatics*, *75*(3), 185–188. 10.1159/000084004

Manning-Jones, S., de Terte, I., & Stephens, C. (2016). Secondary traumatic stress, vicarious posttraumatic growth, and coping among health professionals: A comparison study. *New Zealand Journal of Psychology*, *45*(1), 20–29. https://www.semanticscholar.org/paper/Secondary-Traumatic-Stress%2C-Vicarious-Posttraumatic-Manning-Jones-Terte/aacc6ce93e64725c50e25943b470a76a11fd05f4

Manning-Jones, S., de Terte, I., & Stephens, C. (2017). The relationship between vicarious posttraumatic growth and secondary traumatic stress among health professionals. *Journal of Loss and Trauma*, *22*(3), 256–270. 10.1080/15325024.2017.1284516

McCormack, L., Hagger, M. S., & Joseph, S. (2011). Vicarious growth in wives of Vietnam veterans: A phenomenological investigation into decades of "Lived" Experience. *Journal of Humanistic Psychology*, *51*(3), 273–290. 10.1177/0022167810377506

Ogińska-Bulik, N. (2018). Secondary traumatic stress and vicarious posttraumatic growth in nurses working in palliative care – the role of psychological resiliency. *Advances in Psychiatry and Neurology*, *27*(3), 196–210. 10.5114/ppn.2018.78713

Ogińska-Bulik, N. Gurowiec, P., Michalska, P., & Kędra, E. (2021). Prevalence and determinants of secondary posttraumatic growth following trauma work among medical personnel: A cross-sectional study. *European Journal of Psychotraumatology*, *12*(1). 10.1080/20008198.2021.1876382

Ogińska-Bulik, N., & Juczyński, Z. (2020). *Kiedy trauma innych staje się własną. Negatywne i pozytywne konsekwencje pomagania osobom po doświadczeniach traumatycznych*. [When the trauma of others becomes one's own. Negative and positive consequence of helping people after traumatic experiences]. Wydawnictwo Naukowe PWN.

Ogińska-Bulik, N., & Juczyński, Z. (in press). Assessing positive posttraumatic changes among professionals working with trauma victims: The Secondary Posttraumatic Growth Inventory. *Annals of Psychology*.

Pearlman, L. A., & Mac Ian, P. S. (1995). Vicarious traumatization: An empirical study on the effects of trauma work on trauma therapists. *Professional Psychology Research and Practice*, *26*(6), 558–565. 10.1037/0735-7028.26.6.558

Rhee, Y. S., Ko, Y. B., & Han, I. Y. (2013). Posttraumatic growth and relating factors of child protective service workers. *Annals of Occupational and Environmental Medicine*, *25*(1). 10.1186/2052-4374-25-6

Shamai, M., & Ron, P. (2009). Helping direct and indirect victims of national terror: Experiences of Israeli social workers. *Qualitative Health Research*, *19*(1), 42–54. 10.1177/1049732308327350

Shiri, S., Wexler, I. D., Alkalay, Y., Meiner, Z., & Kreitler, S. (2008). Positive psychological impact of treating victims of politically motivated violence among hospital-based health care providers. *Psychotherapy and Psychosomatics*, *77*(5), 315–318. 10.1159/000142524

Shiri, S., Wexler, I. D., & Kreitler, S. (2010). Cognitive orientation is predictive of posttraumatic growth after secondary exposure to trauma. *Traumatology*, *16*(1), 42–48. 10.1177/1534765609348243

Splevins, K. A., Cohen, K., Joseph, S. Murray, C., & Bowley, J. (2010). Vicarious posttraumatic growth among interpreters. *Qualitative Health Research*, *20*(12), 1705–1716. 10.1177/1049732310377457

Stamm, B. H. (2002). Measuring compassion satisfaction as well as fatigue: Developmental history of the Compassion Satisfaction and Fatigue Test. In C. R. Figley (Ed.), *Treating compassion fatigue* (pp. 107–119). Brunner-Routledge.

Taku, K. (2014). Relationship among perceived psychological growth, resilience and burnout in physicians. *Personality and Individual Differences*, *59*, 120–123. 10.1016/j.paid.2013.11.003

Taubman-Ben-Ari, O., & Weintroub, A. (2008). Meaning in life and personal growth among pediatric physicians and nurses. *Death Studies*, *32*(7), 621–645. 10.1080/07481180802215627

Tedeschi, R. G., & Calhoun, L. G. (1996). The Post-Traumatic Growth Inventory: Measuring the positive legacy of trauma. *Journal of Traumatic Stress*, *9*(3), 455–471. 10.1007/BF02103658

Tedeschi, R. G., & Calhoun, L. G. (2004). Posttraumatic growth: Conceptual foundations and empirical evidence. *Psychological Inquiry*, *15*(1), 1–8. 10.1207/s15327965pli1501_01

Tosone, C., Nuttman-Shwartz, O., & Stephens, T. (2012). Shared trauma: When the professional is personal. *Clinical Social Work Journal*, *40*(2), 231–239. 10.1007/s10615-012-0395-0

Zerach, G., & Shalev, T. (2015). The relations between violence exposure, posttraumatic stress symptoms, secondary traumatization, vicarious posttraumatic growth and illness attribution among psychiatric nurses. *Archives of Psychiatric Nursing*, *29*(3), 135–142, 10.1016/j.apnu.2015.01.002

39

SECONDARY POSTTRAUMATIC GROWTH AND RESILIENCE IN SHARED TRAUMATIC SITUATIONS

Orit Nuttman-Shwartz

Large-scale life-threatening events such as war, terror attacks, natural disasters, and global collective stressors like the COVID-19 pandemic, affect clients as well as trauma workers, who may experience primary and secondary trauma as well as growth. Trauma workers may undergo these experiences both as members of the exposed society and as mental health professionals serving the community (Ali et al., 2021; Baum, 2010; Nuttman-Shwartz & Shaul, 2021; Saakvitne, 2002). Such situations are conceptualized as a shared reality, a phenomenon whereby helping professionals, their communities, and their clients are exposed to the same traumatic, life-threatening circumstances.

Although a review of the literature shows an increase in the number of studies that have addressed the consequences of shared realities, far less attention has been given to the salutogenic dynamics that take place in these situations, such as shared resilience in a traumatic reality (Nuttman-Shwartz, 2015b; Tosone, 2021); shared growth; compassion satisfaction (Ali et al., 2021); and shared and secondary/vicarious posttraumatic growth (Bauwens & Tosone, 2014; Day et al., 2017). Various terms, including trauma worker, worker, professional, social worker, therapist, and mental health care provider will be used interchangeably for professionals who work in these situations.

Shared Traumatic Reality

In recent years, professional literature has begun to acknowledge that when the whole community is exposed to a traumatic event, helping professionals who live and work in the same community as the people they serve, are threatened by the same circumstances and must help their clients cope with the trauma while simultaneously coping with these same traumatic experiences themselves. Thus, trauma workers are exposed to trauma on two levels in most of these instances. First, they are vicariously/indirectly exposed via interactions with clients (e.g., hearing clients' traumatic stories), and second, they are directly exposed, as they belong to and live in the affected community (Baum, 2010; 2012). This experience has typically been referred to in the professional literature from a negative perspective, as reflected in the terms shared traumatic reality (Nuttman-Shwartz & Dekel,

 DOI: 10.4324/9781032208688-49

2008), shared trauma (Saakvitne, 2002), shared tragedy (Eidelson et al., 2003), and shared traumatic stress, all of which have been increasingly used to reflect the distinct impact of trauma that is simultaneously personal and professional (Tosone, 2012).

An early reference to the concept "shared trauma", can be found in a study by the psychoanalyst Schmideberg (1942) who described the impact of the London Blitz shared traumatic reality on her relationships with her patients during their psychotherapy when the author and her patients were exposed to the same ongoing threat of injury and death. Since then, the concept has been commonly used specifically in the U.S. and Israel, relative to recurrent terror events, natural disasters, and the global collective stressor of the COVID-19 pandemic (Nuttman-Shwartz, 2021).

Most existing theoretical and clinical literature on trauma has examined shared traumatic reality situations from a pathological perspective, emphasizing the individual, mainly the helping professional, and the therapeutic relationship between therapist and client (Bauwens & Naturale, 2017; Nuttman-Shwartz & Shaul, 2021; Nuttman-Shwartz & Sterenberg, 2017). For example, scholars have claimed that direct experience of shared trauma may cause trauma workers to become potentially more susceptible to posttraumatic stress, the blurring of professional and personal boundaries, and increased self-disclosure. Such shared trauma responses are attributed to the dual (direct/indirect) nature of the exposure, and findings have indicated that trauma workers feel their ability to help under these circumstances is impaired. They experience heightened work-related stress as a result of greater demands on their professional time and feel professionally unprepared for the situation, and a loss of boundaries between their personal and professional selves (Cronin et al., 2007; Dekel & Baum, 2010; Nuttman-Shwartz, 2015a; Tosone et al., 2012).

Baum (2014) termed the unique characteristics of professional double exposure in the context of shared traumatic realities as intrusive anxiety, lapses of empathy, lack of immersion in the professional role, role expansion, and changes in the place and time of work. The first three characteristics refer to trauma workers' emotional and behavioral responses to the dangers their family members face during times when they are working whereas the latter two reflect expanded or changing professional demands on them. Despite these reactions, a low level of secondary traumatization was found among workers who provided emergency treatment to victims or their families in the wake of shared traumatic situations in Israel as well as following the 9/11 attacks in the U.S. (Adams et al., 2008; Baum & Ramon, 2010; Dekel et al., 2007; Lev-Wiesel et al., 2009; Shamai & Ron, 2009). Further, findings have revealed that working in a shared traumatic reality can have also positive effects on professional performance, and that posttraumatic growth (PTG) can coexist with symptoms of distress for these workers (Bauwens & Tosone, 2010; Dekel & Baum, 2010; Lev-Wiesel et al., 2009; Shamai & Ron, 2009).

Attempts to shed light on the positive consequences of working in a shared traumatic reality have sought to identify and create new measurement tools to evaluate professional growth following working with trauma clients and in traumatic situations (Baum, 2014; Bauwens & Tosone, 2010). Baum (2014) highlighted the unique contribution of professionals' lapses of empathy to their distress and, by contrast, the contribution of immersion in their professional role to their growth. Bauwens and Tosone (2010) explored the long-term impact of the 9/11 terrorist attack on the professional lives of 201 Manhattan clinicians and found that together with adverse effects, increased compassion and connectedness with clients characterized their professional growth. Participants reported that 9/11 was the impetus for enhancing self-care, changing their clinical modality, and forging new skills. A study using the shared traumatic and professional PTG (STPPG) inventory scale (Tosone et al., 2016) showed that professional growth and having the skills to work in a shared reality impact trauma workers' perceptions of the shared reality as well as its effects (Nuttman-Shwartz & Shaul, 2021).

Notwithstanding, to date, the positive effects of shared traumatic realities have not been referred to as a unique or distinct phenomenon. Such positive effects include the reciprocity that typifies the client-therapist relationship in these situations (Nuttman-Shwartz, 2015b); however, they have been overshadowed by the negative consequences of working in a shared traumatic reality. This chapter describes opportunities for positive personal and professional responses among trauma workers who work in a shared traumatic reality. These responses derive from workers' "double exposure" and from the experiences they undergo together with their clients.

Positive Perceptions of Trauma Work in Shared Traumatic Realities

The ecological perspective on trauma includes a conceptualization of positive responses following direct or indirect exposure to trauma work, mainly following exposure to clients who have undergone traumas. These responses are in line with the growing recognition that many people show positive outcomes, including PTG, resilience, and recovery, following direct exposure to traumatic events such as violence (Bonanno et al., 2015; Rosshandler et al., 2016; Tol et al., 2013). Regarding trauma workers, and in line with PTG and resilience processes, scholars have offered three main concepts to capture this phenomenon: vicarious resilience (Hernandez et al., 2007); secondary PTG, which has also been coined vicarious PTG (Arnold et al., 2005); and compassion satisfaction (Figley, 2002). These concepts provide a basis for viewing trauma workers as possibly empowered, experiencing growth or resilience via someone else's trauma and story, and offering a counterbalance to the perception that trauma work is only harmful to trauma workers (Manning-Jones et al., 2015). Further, these concepts suggest that if trauma workers are open to and aware of the possibility and utility of vicarious resilience, vicarious PTG, and/or compassion satisfaction, their ability to reframe negative events, as well as their coping skills, may be enhanced through working with trauma survivors.

A review of the literature reveals that positive responses to working in a shared traumatic reality include professionals' being in better contact with their clients' emotions and learning to respond in session more empathically and effectively (Batten & Orsillo, 2002; Tosone et al., 2003); experiencing vicarious resilience as a result of witnessing clients' overcoming adversity, thereby changing professionals' attitudes and emotions regarding people's capacity to heal and to view their problems differently (Hernandez et al., 2007); experiencing a renewed commitment to their profession and their clients (Seeley, 2003); and increasing positive feelings about their work (Eidelson et al., 2003). These positive responses have been found to contribute to trauma workers' own personal and professional growth (Shamai & Ron, 2009), compassion satisfaction (Racanelli, 2005), and PTG (Lev-Wiesel et al., 2009), as well as to their feelings of professional competence (Dekel et al., 2016). It has been suggested that these effects go beyond the therapeutic relationship with clients and significantly shape workers' perceptions, relations, and environment, serving as protective factors for trauma workers in shared traumatic realities (Bell & Robinson, 2013).

Based on Ungar's (2013) concept of resilience, it was suggested that the process and manifestations of resilience could be affected by the client-trauma worker and the ability of both to function successfully in a shared traumatic reality (Nuttman-Shwartz, 2015b). Specifically, when either worker or client feels resilient and can function well in a traumatic reality, such resilience/functionality can affect the other party. The "shared resilience in a traumatic reality" concept describes the mutual growth process that takes place between worker and client as a result of joint learning and a shared experience and even an exchange of roles in the relationship. This reciprocal learning, which is undertaken to find a creative solution to the shared threat, may accelerate the therapeutic alliance and process (Nuttman-Shwartz, 2015b) making the term shared resilience useful in referring to this phenomenon.

Shared resilience and shared growth refer to a mental health care provider's endurance, coping skills, and ability to adjust despite the adverse circumstances that characterize a shared collective stressor. Shared PTG (abbreviated to "shared growth", for the sake of simplicity and because for some communities, the "post" in posttraumatic is non-applicable, given the ongoing and continuous nature of the trauma) refers to positive effects that go beyond shared resilience (i.e., return-to-baseline) of the trauma worker following a shared traumatic reality. Such positive effects may include improved abilities, greater awareness of new possibilities, increased compassion, and changed life philosophies and priorities; Going a step further than previous conceptualizations of reactions of trauma workers exposed to collective stressor environments (e.g., vicarious posttraumatic growth, vicarious resilience, and compassion satisfaction), Ali et al. (2021) recently proposed a uniquely but appropriately inclusive shared resilience and growth model. This model reflects trauma workers' twofold potential for direct and indirect forms of resilience and growth, and the acute, chronic, collective, or transgenerational effects of these positive effects, all of which are influenced by cultural context. This model is also informed by social identity processes, stressor appraisals, consequent meaning-making systems, and the contextual nature of therapists' cultures, on a spectrum ranging from individualism to collectivism. The direct, indirect, and cultural components of these positive psychological factors influence each other and culminate in the individual nature and degree of resilience and growth of the therapist/trauma worker. Diagram 39.1 presents a variation of Ali et al.'s (2021) abovementioned shared resilience and growth model.

In sum, the literature review suggests that positive responses and the ability to articulate shared growth and resilience under stress may result from the shared reality experienced together by trauma workers and clients. Moreover, the shared reality may help trauma workers understand that empathic bonding, which results from these mutual, symmetric relationships, provides the basis for positive responses to the traumatic reality and may help workers become aware of the dual and shared growth and resilience taking place. In this way, positive consequences of a shared traumatic reality may go beyond the micro-level client-therapist relationship and also affect relationships at the meso level, such as with colleagues, managers, and family members (Ungar, 2013) as well as extend even more widely to the community, society as a whole, and to the next generation (Ali et al., 2021; Nuttman-Shwartz, 2021).

Shared Traumatic Reality Assessment Instruments

Several tools have been developed to capture the negative and positive dynamics of working in a shared traumatic reality.

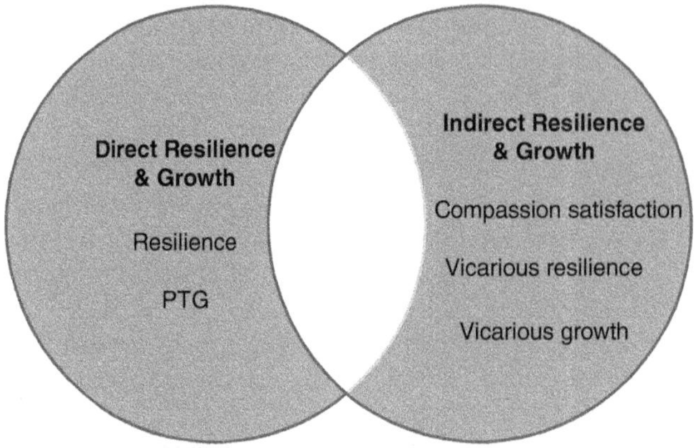

Diagram 39.1 Shared resilience and growth model.

The ***Working in a Shared Traumatic Reality*** measure (Baum, 2014) includes five factors: (1) intrusive anxiety, which consists of statements referring to professionals' anxiety regarding their own and their family's safety when they are working; (2) lapses in empathy, which consists of statements indicating that the professionals' anxiety impairs their ability to empathize with their clients' fears; (3) changes in place and time of work, which consists of statements regarding the need for professionals to meet clients in ever-changing locations or to report for work outside their usual hours; (4) immersion in the professional role, which consists of statements regarding how focusing on helping others helps to alleviate the professionals' anxiety; and (5) role expansion, which consists of statements indicating that professionals must perform out-of-role tasks for clients or extend professional assistance to non-clients. Baum's (2014) findings, based on her research of 63 Israeli social workers who lived and worked in communities exposed to missile attacks during the 2014 Gaza War, showed that intrusive anxiety and changes in place and time of work correlated significantly with the professionals' personal growth, lapses of empathy uniquely contributed to professionals' distress, whereas immersion in own role uniquely contributed to the professionals' professional growth.

The ***STPPG* scale** mentioned above (Tosone et al., 2016) consists of three subscales: (1). the therapist's personal trauma; (2). the therapist's professional PTG; and (3). the therapist's own technique-specific way of dealing with shared trauma. The total combined score for all of the subscales and the individual scores for each subscale indicate the therapists' perceptions regarding whether their level of growth resulted from their working in a shared traumatic reality. This is the only existing scale that specifically allows evaluating trauma workers' positive responses and trauma outcomes by asking them to assess their professional PTG as a result of working in a shared traumatic reality and to address their own technique-specific way of dealing with shared trauma. Using the STPPG, one study showed that after Hurricane Katrina, U.S. trauma workers who experienced this particular shared traumatic reality perceived themselves as having high levels of professional PTG (Tosone et al., 2016). By contrast, Israeli trauma workers during the shared traumatic reality of the novel coronavirus pandemic (Nuttman-Shwartz & Shaul, 2021) revealed lower levels of professional PTG although they reported experiencing the pandemic as a stressful event, particularly regarding the aspect of personal trauma on the STPPG scale. They seemed to believe that the skills at their disposal were not valuable or relevant at this particular time and, thus, reported a low level of professional PTG.

The ***Shared Concerns Index*** developed by Nuttman-Shwartz and Shaul (2021) to measure the shared concerns aspect of the shared traumatic reality was used to examine similarities and differences in trauma workers' and clients' concerns. This measure was constructed on the basis of trauma workers' perceived symmetry between themselves and their clients in situations of a shared reality (Boulanger, 2013). The index includes five main areas of concern: (1) security concerns (related to the fact that Israel is typified by an ongoing and continuous traumatic security situation), (2) economic concerns, (3) emotional problems, (4) problems with family relationships, and (5) health concerns. The domains were based on an accepted assessment questionnaire that maps clients' problem areas (i.e., reason/reasons for seeking treatment to assess the suitability of the type of service and therapist). The shared concerns index examines the difference between trauma workers' evaluations of their own distress and of their clients' distress in the designated area. The closer the score, the smaller the gap between therapist and client concerns.

While the Working in a Shared Traumatic Reality measure and the STPPG scale relate only to the effects of the therapeutic dynamic on the therapist and were developed to pertain to war and terror events, with the former relating to ongoing/continuous traumatic situations and the later to one-time war/terror events (the 9/11 terror attack), the Shared Concerns measure was developed in light of the COVID-19 pandemic. A study of 150 trauma workers using the STPPG scale (Tosone et al., 2016) showed that professional growth and having the appropriate skills to work in a shared traumatic reality seemed to determine trauma workers' perceptions of COVID-19 as a shared reality, as well as its effects (Nuttman-Shwartz & Shaul, 2021). Specifically, the more experience trauma workers had, the less they perceived the situation (i.e., the pandemic) as a shared traumatic reality, reducing their perceived skills and sense of professional growth.

The three tools combined may help to better identify (1) trauma workers' personal and professional negative and positive responses, and the specific techniques they use to address shared trauma; (2) trauma workers' lack of awareness regarding their responses within the therapeutic relationship (such as intrusive anxiety, lapses in empathy, role expansion, and professional immersion); and (3) areas of concern they share with their clients. Although using all three measures together can help professionals in the field arrive at a better understanding of the shared traumatic reality phenomenon on multiple levels (therapist, client, dyadic relations), both separately and as a whole, more attention must be given to positive outcomes. To date, the tools at our disposal mainly measure therapists' negative perceptions of the therapist/patient relationship in light of the shared reality, their own negative responses, and their own concerns. More room must be given to the multitude of responses, learning more about the reciprocal therapist and client dynamic, and expanding the tools to measure professional and personal, direct and indirect, growth by hearing therapists' and clients' voices on these matters.

Trauma Workers Sharing and Assessing Positive Changes Following Working in a Shared Traumatic Reality

This section illustrates and discusses themes of positive perceptions of working in a shared traumatic reality. The themes emerged from a thematic analysis of interviews conducted in a mixed-methods study of the cumulative and coexisting shared traumatic reality of living and working near Israel's border with Gaza amidst the COVID-19 pandemic. Residents of Israel's area boarding with Gaza, who are trauma and resilience workers in the area, have been interviewed. All were exposed to missile attacks, and about half of them experienced a missile hit close to their home. They were experienced social workers (60%), educators (20%), and paraprofessional personnel affiliated with an emergency team (20%).

My Client Taught Me Something

During a period of escalation in our area, I entered a shelter, could barely breathe, and sat down next to my client. He encouraged me, showed me how to do breathing exercises, and calmed me down. As I did the breathing exercises, he continued talking to me. He said: "It will take about five minutes and then you'll be able to return to routine." At that moment, I admired him and thought about how this was the first time I had been able to see his strength. To be honest, he helped me feel I had enough strength of my own to overcome my sense of fear. During the [regularly scheduled] team meeting we had afterward, I became aware of my client's contribution to my own abilities and was glad I allowed myself to rely on him and his ability to take care of me.

Working in a Shared Reality Is a Mission

I've worked in the Resilience Center for the last five years and have met many people with acute stress responses and other traumatic reactions. But one day I realized when talking with my family that I actually benefit from working with trauma clients, and even convinced them that this was true. I think this is so because I see this work as a mission, and I get a lot of satisfaction from the compassion I feel toward my clients. A shared reality allows you to see that you as a therapist have lots of personal and professional resources and even new skills despite the difficulties you go through while you're helping others.

I Am Better than I Thought I Was – I Have Lots of Professional Skills

I feel competent. After so many years, I finally realize that I have a great many skills in my toolbox. I have a sense of satisfaction, perhaps in part from knowing how to go back and forth between my personal role and my professional role, and after having received so much training. I can honestly say that I'm an expert, and I've received excellent feedback from my clients. I know what to do. Recently I was invited to give a talk in front of students, and it was great. I can share, I know how to conceptualize my skills, and I have something to offer young professionals. It was a great experience. I feel growth, I feel proud, I feel good. Yes, I have learned a lot. I can say that part of my resilience is a result of my good relationships with my clients. And I have also learned from them how to cope, how to deal. I have the feeling that my clients and I make good teams. And this is in addition to my colleagues and my supervisor and my manager. All of them are essential resources.

I'm More Attuned to My Clients

When COVID-19 coincided with the "regular" shared traumatic reality, I felt troubled by my anxieties, and perhaps as a result of that, and knowing that I had experience working in shared traumatic realities, my meetings with my clients became more effective and organized. I felt that my thoughts had become more precise, and I made an effort to achieve the therapeutic outcomes that were previously planned and to follow them with my activities. I focused on the here and now rather than on reflective thinking. That is, less involvement but more listening, guiding, and supervising my clients. And I think maybe I was more verbal, more active, gave more concrete advice in the sessions, and perhaps I was a little more emotionally detached. More than anything else, I was flexible. I succeeded in moving and changing my therapeutic plan and offering something more suitable to my clients ... I was even more aware of using the theories I subscribe to during the session.

I'm Just Like My Clients – Shared Concerns and Shared Growth

Yesterday I met with a client of mine. It has been a long time since we met, and he asked me to meet again now as the pandemic had reawakened some of his fears. During our meeting, he shared his concerns, and at first I found the things he said to be similar to the way my wife talks. After several minutes I felt he was saying the kinds of things that I myself could have been saying. He said, "Again I'm having difficulties sleeping, I over-control my children" and then immediately he changed course, and said, "To be honest I can handle it. While talking to you I'm realizing that I have previous experiences that I can rely on, and I know what to do. I have enough tools to help me. I know how to reduce stress; I belong to a running group, and I even like to cook." So I found myself saying to myself: I'm just like my clients, I too go back and forth between feelings of worry and feelings of strength. And I feel he helped me carry out an inner process, after which I was able to return to help him.

Via several vignettes that illustrate the experience of working in a shared reality, this chapter provides a theoretical understanding that had previously been conceptualized as shared resilience in a traumatic reality.

These vignettes manifest shared growth and resilience as well as reflect direct and indirect positive outcomes resulting from personal and reciprocal therapeutic encounters between trauma workers and their clients. The themes also reflect the fact that the positive processes highlight the importance of empathic and mutually beneficial relationships, and trauma workers' motivations for doing their work, all of which have been found to be essential components for promoting resilience in a shared traumatic reality (Nuttman-Shwartz, 2015b) and may also be considered PTG components of meaning-making, growth, and change (Calhoun & Tedeschi, 2014). Moreover, the vignettes offered above reveal how trauma workers' appreciation and awareness of their client's strengths, resilience, and capacity to grow extended to their own internalizing of and benefiting from their clients' positive experiences (Puvimanasinghe et al., 2015). Establishing a more reciprocal therapist/client relationship, increased empathic bonding, greater therapeutic flexibility, and exchanging of therapist and client roles may be seen as positive shared reality outcomes on both the emotional and behavioral levels.

The positive dimension of working in a shared reality is also reflected in aspects of the assessment tools described above, such as the subscale that assesses professional growth (Tosone et al., 2016). In fact, the vignettes provide empirical support for the STPPG scale, which measures therapists' perceptions of their professional growth and skills. The vignettes also support Baum's (2014) Working in a Shared Traumatic Reality measure, as they show that working in a shared traumatic reality strengthens trauma workers' ability to be empathic and attuned to their clients within sessions. Such findings may be the result of the workers' continuous exposure to traumatic events, being well-trained, and perhaps even of having become accustomed to living and working "under fire." Overall, it seems that working in a shared traumatic reality enhances growth, a sense of competence, and even resilience among workers.

The vignettes also illustrate the notion of continuous traumatic stress, as coined by Nuttman-Shwartz and Shuval-Zukerman (2016), in the context of a shared reality. In line with the idea that trauma workers must be able to oscillate, and have the flexibility to do so when needed, and in line with Stein et al. (2018), the vignettes suggest a habituation effect to continuous traumatic stress. This habituation effect characterized participants in the Nuttman-Shwartz and Shuval-Zukerman study (2016), and seemed to contribute to their ability to develop a sense of shared professional growth. The vignettes also demonstrate that these direct and indirect positive responses might coincide during a shared traumatic reality, and trauma workers must be keenly aware of the dual nature of the situation – their clients, themselves, and both counter-responses, which may alter the nature of their relationships with their clients (Tosone et al., 2012).

Although this chapter has highlighted the potentially positive outcomes of shared traumatic realities, including shared resilience and professional growth resulting from the heightened reciprocity in the client-therapist relationship, negative aspects must be taken into account as well. Reciprocity allows for the dyad members reach the desired outcome jointly and can promote the mental health of both parties (Nuttman-Shwartz, 2015b; Tosone, 2021), but there are potentially negative effects as well, including burden resulting from working in a shared traumatic reality and a decrease in feelings of professional competence within the therapeutic process (Baum, 2014; Nuttman-Shwartz & Shaul, 2021).

Other unique aspects of shared reality are the ability to move between different domains, the flexibility that trauma workers show in these situations, and the extent to which they have a holding environment (Dekel & Nuttman-Shwartz, 2014). As such, it is essential to adopt a broader ecological perspective of shared traumatic realities, given that trauma workers' responses, including the positive ones, may also affect their families and be transmitted intergenerationally, and vice versa (Nuttman-Shwartz, 2021).

Based on the positive perspective, the vignettes support the idea that trauma workers may undergo positive personal and professional changes in response to coping with both direct and indirect trauma, i.e., PTG (Tedeschi & Moore, 2016). As seen in the vignettes and aligning with previous findings, PTG outcomes seem to include discovering new personal strengths, gaining wisdom regarding professional practices, resilience, and sense of purpose (Tedeschi et al., 2018), as well as increased self-confidence, emotional expressiveness, sensitivity, and compassion satisfaction, (Arnold et al., 2005; Figley, 1995; Hernández et al., 2007; Stamm, 2002).

In the same vein, the vignettes support the idea that for vicarious PTG to occur, trauma workers must be exposed to clients' growth and vice versa. Such an understanding implies a non-binary view of the impact of trauma work (Barrington & Shakespeare-Finch, 2013; Cohen & Collens, 2013; Hernandez-Wolfe, 2018).

Summary and Conclusions

The current chapter marks a step forward in expanding our understanding of the positive dynamics that develop following client-therapist encounters in a shared traumatic reality. This understanding is in keeping with current research-based positive psychology and salutogenic approaches (Ali et al., 2021; Nuttman-Shwartz, 2016; Nuttman-Shwartz & Sagy, in press). This chapter sheds light on the importance of mutual client/therapist learning in the therapeutic encounter as well as "practice wisdom," and highlights the transition to a perspective of positivity in trauma research in general and social work research in particular (Joseph & Murphy, 2014).

This view is a unique and appropriately inclusive approach toward shared resilience and growth, highlighting positive responses to double exposure and the twofold potential of trauma workers for direct and indirect forms of resilience and growth, in a variety of collective adversities resulting both from acute events and continuous cumulative shared traumatic situations (Nuttman-Shwartz & Green, 2021; Nuttman-Shwartz & Shaul, 2021). As shared trauma and shared resilience coexist during times of war, terror, natural disasters, and global pandemics, it is necessary to think about protective factors for trauma workers in such situations. It should also be recognized that just like trauma workers are affected both directly and indirectly by their own and their clients' traumas, so too are their clients multiply affected (e.g., directly via their own exposure, as well as indirectly by the exposure of their neighbors, friends, and community members). All these factors must be taken into consideration to provide proper training for those working in a shared traumatic reality.

References

Adams, R. E., Figley, C. R., & Boscarino, J. A. (2008). The Compassion Fatigue Scale: Its use with social workers following urban disaster. *Research on Social Work Practice*, *18*(3), 238–250. 10.1177/1049731507310190

Ali, D. A., Figley, C. R., Tedeschi, R. G., Galarneau, D., & Amara, S. (2021). Shared trauma, resilience, and growth: A roadmap toward transcultural conceptualization. *Psychological Trauma: Theory, Research, Practice, and Policy*. Advance online publication. 10.1037/tra0001044

Arnold, D., Calhoun, L. G., Tedeschi, R., & Cann, A. (2005). Vicarious posttraumatic growth in psychotherapy. *Journal of Humanistic Psychology*, *45*(2), 239–263.

Barrington, A. J., & Shakespeare-Finch, J. (2013). Working with refugee survivors of torture and trauma: An opportunity for vicarious post-traumatic growth. *Counselling Psychology Quarterly*, *26*(1), 89–105. 10.1080/09515070.2012.727553

Batten, S. V., & Orsillo, S. M. (2002). Therapist reactions in the context of collective trauma. *The Behavior Therapist*, *25*(2), 36–40.

Baum, N. (2010). Shared traumatic reality in communal disasters: Toward a conceptualization. *Psychotherapy (Chicago, Ill.)*, *47*(2), 249–259. 10.1037/a0019784

Baum, N. (2012). 'Emergency routine': The experience of professionals in a shared traumatic reality of war. *British Journal of Social Work*, *42*(3), 424–442. 10.1093/bjsw/bcr032

Baum, N. (2014). Professionals' double exposure in the shared traumatic reality of wartime: Contributions to professional growth and stress. *The British Journal of Social Work*, *44*(8), 2113–2134. 10.1093/bjsw/bct085

Baum, N., & Ramon, S. (2010). Professional growth in turbulent times: An impact of political violence on social work practice in Israel. *Journal of Social Work*, *10*(2), 139–156. 10.1177/1468017310363636

Bauwens, J., & Naturale, A. (2017). The role of social work in the aftermath of disasters and traumatic events. *Clinical Social Work Journal*, *45*(2), 99–101. 10.1007/s10615-017-0623-8

Bauwens, J., & Tosone, C. (2010). Professional posttraumatic growth after a shared traumatic experience: Manhattan clinicians' perspectives on post-9/11 practice. *Journal of Loss and Trauma*, *15*(6), 498–517.

Bauwens, J., & Tosone, C. (2014). Posttraumatic growth following Hurricane Katrina: The influence of clinicians' trauma histories and primary and secondary traumatic stress. *Traumatology*, *20*(3), 209–218. 10.1037/h0099851

Bell, C. H., & Robinson, W. H. (2013). Shared trauma in counseling: Information and implications for counselors. *Journal of Mental Health Counseling*, *35*(4), 310–323. 10.17744/mehc.35.4.7v33258020948502

Bonanno, G. A., Romero, S. A., & Klein, S. I. (2015). The temporal elements of psychological resilience: An integrative framework for the study of individuals, families, and communities. *Psychological Inquiry*, *26*(2), 139–169. 10.1080/1047840X.2015.992677

Boulanger, G. (2013). Fearful symmetry: Shared trauma in New Orleans after Hurricane Katrina. *Psychoanalytic Dialogues*, *23*(1), 31–44. 10.1080/10481885.2013.752700

Calhoun, L. G., & Tedeschi, R. G. (2014). The foundations of posttraumatic growth: An expanded framework. In L. G. Calhoun, & R. G. Tedeschi (Eds.), *Handbook of posttraumatic growth* (pp. 17–37). Routledge.

Cohen, K., & Collens, P. (2013). The impact of trauma work on trauma workers: A metasynthesis on vicarious trauma and vicarious posttraumatic growth. *Psychological Trauma: Theory, Research, Practice, and Policy*, *5*(6), 570–580. 10.1037/a0030388

Cronin, M. S., Ryan, D. M., & Brier, D. (2007). Support for staff working in disaster situations: A social work perspective. *International Social Work*, *50*(3), 370–382. 10.1177/0020872807076050

Dekel, R., & Baum, N. (2010). Intervention in a shared traumatic reality: A new challenge for social workers. *British Journal of Social Work*, *40*(6), 1927–1944. 10.1093/bjsw/bcp137

Dekel, R., Hantman, S., Ginzburg, K., & Solomon, Z. (2007). The cost of caring? Social workers in hospitals confront ongoing terrorism. *British Journal of Social Work*, *37*(7), 1247–1261. 10.1093/bjsw/bcl081

Dekel, R., & Nuttman-Shwartz, O. (2014). Being a parent and a helping professional in the ongoing shared traumatic reality in southern Israel. In R. Pat-Horenczyk, D. Brom, & J. M. Vogel (Eds.), *Helping children cope with trauma: Individual, family and community perspectives* (pp. 224–240). Routledge.

Dekel, R., Nuttman–Shwartz, O., & Lavi, T. (2016). Shared traumatic reality and boundary theory: How mental health professionals cope with the home/work conflict during continuous security threats. *Journal of Couple & Relationship Therapy*, *15*(2), 121–134. 10.1080/15332691.2015.1068251

Eidelson, R. J., D'Alessio, G. R., & Eidelson, J. I. (2003). The impact of September 11 on psychologists. *Professional Psychology: Research and Practice*, *34*(2), 144–150. 10.1037/0735-7028.34.2.144

Figley, C. R. (Ed.). (1995). *Compassion fatigue: Coping with secondary traumatic stress disorder in those who treat the traumatized*. Brunner/Mazel.

Figley, C. R. (2002). Compassion fatigue: Psychotherapists' chronic lack of self-care. *Journal of Clinical Psychology*, *58*(11), 1433–1441. 10.1002/jclp.10090

Joseph, S., & Murphy, D. (2014). Trauma: A unifying concept for social work. *British Journal of Social Work*, *44*(5), 1094–1109. 10.1093/bjsw/bcs207

Hernández, P., Gangsei, D., & Engstrom, D. (2007). Vicarious resilience: A new concept in work with those who survive trauma. *Family Process*, *46*(2), 229–241. 10.1111/j.1545-5300.2007.00206.x

Hernandez-Wolfe, P. (2018). Vicarious resilience: A comprehensive review. *Revista de Estudios Sociales*, *66*, 9–17. 10.7440/res66.2018.02

Lev-Wiesel, R., Goldblatt, H., Eisikovits, Z., & Admi, H. (2009). Growth in the shadow of war: The case of social workers and nurses working in a shared war reality. *British Journal of Social Work*, *39*(6), 1154–1174. 10.1093/bjsw/bcn021

Manning-Jones, S., de Terte, I., & Stephens, C. (2015). Vicarious posttraumatic growth: A systematic literature review. *International Journal of Wellbeing*, *5*(2), 125–139. 10.5502/ijw.v5i2.8

Nuttman-Shwartz, O. (2015a). Post-traumatic stress in social work. In J. Wright (Ed.), *The international encyclopedia of social & behavioural sciences* (2nd ed., Vol. 18, pp. 707–713). Elsevier Ltd.

Nuttman–Shwartz, O. (2015b). Shared resilience in a traumatic reality: A new concept for trauma workers exposed personally and professionally to collective disaster. *Trauma, Violence, & Abuse*, *16*(4), 466–475. 10.1177/1524838014557287

Nuttman–Shwartz, O. (2016). Research in a shared traumatic reality: Researchers in a disaster context. *Journal of Loss and Trauma*, *21*(3), 179–191. 10.1080/15325024.2015.1084856

Nuttman-Shwartz, O. (2021). The long-term effects of living in a shared and continuous traumatic reality: The case of Israeli families on the border with Gaza. *Trauma, Violence, & Abuse*. Advance online publication. 10.1177/15248380211063467

Nuttman-Shwartz, O. (in press) Shared reality as a result of war and terror. In A. Goelitz (Ed), *Shared mass trauma in social work: Implications and strategies for resilient practice.* Routledge.

Nuttman-Shwartz, O., & Dekel, R. (2008). Training students for a shared traumatic reality. *Social Work, 53*(3), 279–281. 10.1093/sw/53.3.279

Nuttman-Shwartz, O., & Green, O. (2021). Resilience truths: Trauma resilience workers' points of view toward resilience in continuous traumatic situations. *International Journal of Stress Management, 28*(1), 1–10. 10.1037/str0000223

Nuttman-Shwartz, O. & Sagy, S. A. (in press). Wounded childhood – The case of migration children. In E. Shahar & Z. Valdan (Eds). *The International School of Peace.* Resling. [Hebrew].

Nuttman-Shwartz, O., & Shaul, K. (2021). Online therapy in a shared reality: The coronavirus as a test case. *Traumatology, 27*(4), 365–374. 10.1037/trm0000334

Nuttman-Shwartz, O., & Shuval-Zukerman, Y. (2016). Continuous traumatic situations in the face of ongoing political violence: The relationship between CTS and PTSD. *Trauma, Violence & Abuse, 17*(3), 562–570. 10.1177/1524838015585316

Nuttman–Shwartz, O., & Sterenberg, R. (2017). Social work in the context of an ongoing security threat: Role description, personal experiences, and conceptualization. *British Journal of Social Work, 47*(3), 903–918. 10.1093/bjsw/bcw053

Puvimanasinghe, T., Denson, L. A., Augoustinos, M., & Somasundaram, D. (2015). Vicarious resilience and vicarious traumatisation: Experiences of working with refugees and asylum seekers in South Australia. *Transcultural Psychiatry, 52*(6), 743–765. 10.1177/1363461515577289

Racanelli, C. (2005). Attachment and compassion fatigue among American and Israeli mental health clinicians working with traumatized victims of terrorism. *International Journal of Emergency Mental Health, 7*(2), 115–124.

Rosshandler, Y., Hall, B. J., & Canetti, D. (2016). An application of an ecological framework to understand risk factors of PTSD due to prolonged conflict exposure: Israeli and Palestinian adolescents in the line of fire. *Psychological Trauma: Theory, Research, Practice, and Policy, 8*(5), 641–648. 10.1037/tra0000124

Saakvitne, K. W. (2002). Shared trauma: The therapist's increased vulnerability. *Psychoanalytic Dialogues, 12*(3), 443–449. 10.1080/10481881209348678

Schmideberg, M. (1942). Some observations on individual reactions to air raids. *The International Journal of Psychoanalysis, 23*, 146–176.

Seeley, K. (2003). The psychotherapy of trauma and the trauma of psychotherapy: Talking to therapists about 9–11. *Working Paper Series, Center on Organizational Innovation, Columbia University.* http://www.coi.columbia.edu/pdf/seeley_pot.pdf

Shamai, M., & Ron, P. (2009). Helping direct and indirect victims of national terror: Experiences of Israeli social workers. *Qualitative Health Research, 19*(1), 42–54. 10.1177/1049732308327350

Stamm, B. H. (2002). Measuring compassion satisfaction as well as fatigue: Developmental history of the fatigue and satisfaction test. In C. R. Figley (Ed.), *Treating compassion fatigue* (pp. 107–119). Brunner/Mazel.

Stein, J. Y., Levin, Y., Gelkopf, M., Tangir, G., & Solomon, Z. (2018). Traumatization or habituation? A four-wave investigation of exposure to continuous traumatic stress in Israel. *International Journal of Stress Management, 25*(S1), 137–153. 10.1037/str0000084

Tedeschi, R. G., & Moore, B. A. (2016). *The posttraumatic growth workbook: Coming through trauma wiser, stronger, and more resilient.* New Harbinger Publications.

Tedeschi, R. G., Shakespeare-Finch, J., Taku, K., & Calhoun, L. G. (2018). *Posttraumatic growth: Theory, research, and applications.* Routledge.

Tol, W.A., Song, S., & Jordans, M.J. (2013). Annual Research Review: Resilience and mental health in children and adolescents living in areas of armed conflict-A systematic review of findings in low- and middle-income countries. *Journal of Child Psychology and Psychiatry, and Allied Disciplines, 54*(4), 445–460. 10.1111/jcpp.12053

Tosone, C. (2012). Shared reality. In C. R. Figley (Ed.), *Encyclopedia of trauma: An interdisciplinary guide* (pp. 624–627). Sage.

Tosone, C. (Ed.). (2021). *Shared trauma, shared resilience during a pandemic.* Springer.

Tosone, C., Bauwens, J., & Glassman, M. (2016). The shared traumatic and professional post-traumatic growth inventory. *Research on Social Work Practice*, *26*(3), 286–294. 10.1177/1049731514549814

Tosone, C., Bialkin, L., Campbell, M., Charters, M., Gieri, K., Gross, S., Grounds, C., Johnson, K., Kitson, D., Lanzo, S., Lee, M., Martinez, A., Martinez, M. M., Milich, J., Riofrio, A., Rosenblatt, L., Sandler, J., Scali, M., Spiro, M., & Stefan, A. (2003). Shared trauma: Group reflections on the September 11th disaster. *Psychoanalytical Social Work*, *10*(1), 57–77. 10.1300/J032v10n01_06

Tosone, C., Nuttman–Shwartz, O., & Stephens, T. (2012). Shared trauma: When the professional is personal. *Clinical Journal of Social Work*, *40*(2), 231–239. 10.1007/s10615-012-0395-0

Ungar, M. (2013). Resilience, trauma, context, and culture. *Trauma, Violence & Abuse*, *14*(3), 255–266. 10.1177/1524838013487805

40

VICARIOUS RESILIENCE IN CLINICAL SUPERVISION

Finding Hummingbirds' Nectar

Pilar Hernández-Wolfe, Victoria Acevedo, and Lauren D'Agostino

Like hummingbirds, those who attend to and integrate vicarious resilience (VR) in clinical work find nectar that sustains us as we work to honor the helping relationships we develop with our clients, supervisees, mentees, and consultants. VR refers to the positive impact that clients' resilience has on therapists as a result of witnessing it occurring in the therapeutic relationship (Acevedo & Hernández-Wolfe, 2014; 2017; Hernández et al., 2007; Woodwick, 2021). Therapists who cultivate VR are intentionally attuned to how we vicariously grow as we witness our clients' growth.

Vicariously resilient supervisors attend to the nuances of how social location and larger political and socioeconomic issues impact the relational experience of therapy (Hernández et al., 2007; Hernández-Wolfe et al., 2010). Our work acknowledges that resilience in contexts of exposure to significant adversity involves examining the processes by which people struggle, adapt, and navigate their way to a state of well-being, and how they negotiate, recreate, and affirm their way of life (Ungar, 2015; 2019). Ungar and Theron (2019) posit that research shows that the protective processes at play in a person's life are social, ecological, and individual. We believe that VR must also be grounded in the embodied voices that are a part of the meaning-making process that occurs in therapy. Access to resources and social capital, opportunities for coping, and an outlook open to possibilities are critical as well.

In clinical supervision, VR implies the presence of a stressor or multiple stressors that a client overcomes. The nature of the stressors influences how well a client can navigate and negotiate a situation. Mental health professionals witness and are affected by multiple stressors with multiple and varied outcomes, the cumulative effects of which are not easily sustainable in the long term. We argue that clinical supervision of therapists should address the impact of traumatic stress on therapists and clients alike at a social and personal level, and highlight VR to identify and expand recognition, repair, compassion, wellness, and possibility.

VR in Clinical Supervision

The concept of VR illuminates the reciprocal nature of therapy, inviting clinicians to balance the painful, difficult aspects of trauma work with those that bring hope and

DOI: 10.4324/9781032208688-50

promote growth. VR addresses the positive impact of exposure to someone's positive psychological change resulting from struggling with traumatic experiences.

The supervisory relationship is founded on the intention to influence the therapist's behavior to resemble that of an experienced therapist and in which an experienced therapist safeguards the welfare of clients by monitoring a less experienced therapist's performance with real clients in clinical settings (Bernard & Goodyear, 2019). In the context of trauma work, supervisors may influence supervisees to learn, expand and affirm the ways the client's resilience informs the therapeutic relationship. The primary goals of clinical supervision are to "foster the supervisee's professional development" and to "ensure client welfare" (Bernard & Goodyear, 2019, p. 12).

In a supervisory relationship, both supervisor and supervisee influence each other, albeit not necessarily in equitable ways. A trauma and resilience lens in supervision integrates foundational knowledge of the impact of trauma on clients, awareness of the effects of indirect trauma (Knight, 2018), and social, ecological, and individual protective processes in a person's life (Ungar & Theron, 2019).

Specifically, VR in clinical supervision highlights the idea that a mutual influence exists in the therapist-client relationship and in the supervisor-supervisee relationship. Albeit not equal, the levels of reciprocity in these relationships open up the possibility of appreciating, attending to, and making meaning of the process whereby therapists may heal, learn, and change concurrent with clients. Supervisors, supervisees, therapists, and clients mutually influence each other and construct meaning together. These relationships are framed within organizational, familial, communal, and social layers of contexts and include dimensions of power inherent in the therapeutic relationship and structured by the parties' social locations (Hernández-Wolfe et al., 2014).

Using a trauma and resilience lens to view and conduct supervision involves a supervisor's ability to model an understanding of how a trauma survivor's multiple identities and social contexts lend meaning to the experiences of trauma and resilience. A focus on VR in supervision requires supervisors to attend to the impact of witnessing growth in clients and supervisees considering layers of multiple identities and social contexts.

VR and Vicarious Posttraumatic Growth (VPTG)

Arnold and colleagues (2005) advanced the concept of VPTG based on Tedeschi and Calhoun's work on posttraumatic growth (PTG) who defined PTG as "positive psychological change experienced as a result of the struggle with highly challenging life circumstances" (Tedeschi & Calhoun, 2004, p.1). VPTG captures the personal growth effects of working with traumatized clients and describes positive changes in the therapists' self-perception, their interpersonal relationships, and their philosophy of life (Arnold et al., 2005). Unlike VR, these categories do not include changes in the therapists' practice or view on trauma work.

Like VPTG, VR addresses the observational positive impact of exposure to someone's positive psychological change resulting from struggling with traumatic experiences. However, VR focuses on the unique and positive effects that transform therapists in response to client trauma survivors' resiliency. VR refers to the positive meaning-making, growth, and transformations in the therapist's experience resulting from exposure to clients' resilience in the course of therapeutic processes addressing trauma recovery (Hernández et al., 2007). In addition, it is founded on addressing resilience as "the potential for personal and relational transformation and growth that can be forged out of adversity" (Walsh, 2021, p.130). It exists within evolving systems that encounter transformation and growth from an ecological perspective, which captures how systems evolve, adapt, and cope, both individually and collectively. VR is founded on the assumption that the client and therapist influence each other in the therapeutic relationship. Therapists and clients exist in a relationship in which they mutually influence each other and construct meaning in the therapeutic relationship (Anderson, 2007). Obviously, this relationship is framed within layers of contexts (organizational, familial, communal, social) and includes dimensions of power inherent in the therapeutic relationship and structured by the parties' social locations.

Research on VR in Clinical Supervision

VR has been examined qualitatively in practitioners' work with populations who have survived extreme traumatic experiences, such as torture survivors and asylum seekers (Edelkott et al., 2016; Engstrom et al., 2008; Puvimanasinghe et al., 2015), large-scale natural disaster survivors (Nishi et al., 2016), individuals who work in environments where the threat of trauma is constant (Dekel et al., 2016; Nuttman-Shwartz & Sternberg, 2017), nurses working with children with cancer (Cherven et al., 2020) and law enforcement officials (Pair, 2018). Research has also focused on child protection workers in Argentina, Canada, and Ireland (Hurley et al., 2015) and clinicians who work with at-risk children and youth (Silveira & Boyer, 2015; Tassie, 2015). These studies offer clinicians opportunities to examine how VR may develop in various contexts with different populations. An examination of the diversity and differences in the meaning-making process involving VR is central to helping the supervisee tease out how the therapeutic relationship may be both a burden and a source of learning and nurturance. For example, supervisees may examine the journey of Guatemalan, Mexican or Colombian clients seeking residency in the U.S. to learn how families navigate their members' migration journey using practices wherein exchanges and reciprocities are fundamental. Supervisees may be invited to explore how these journeys have embedded lessons in negotiating and navigating new and challenging social contexts. Similarly, VR might be a focus of attention in working with terminally ill children as these experiences bring to the fore existential questions about the meaning of life and the cycles of death and change embedded in nature.

Quantitative studies have focused on investigating VR in advocates, counselors, and volunteers in agencies that provide services for sexual assault and domestic violence victims. Frey et al. (2017) tested the prevalence of VR, VPTG, compassion satisfaction, and perceived organizational support amongst 222 advocates for survivors of sexual assault and domestic violence. Their analysis revealed that the experience of personal trauma and peer relational quality predicted increased VR. This supports the possibility that clinicians' experiences of adversity might strengthen their ability to handle stressors later in life. Frey et al. (2017) also found that organizational support and peer relationships were positive predictors of VR. Organizational support was the sole predictor of compassion satisfaction, and peer relational quality was the sole predictor of VPTG These findings can be integrated into the supervision process to encourage supervisors to offer supervisory relationships in which supervisees can safely affirm and strengthen their meaning-making of personal trauma and resilience, identify specific ways in which an organization may support supervisees (e.g., participation in decision-making processes, recognition of their work, increased opportunities for professional development), and affirm peer collaborative relationships with opportunities to bond meaningfully and emotionally. Frey et al.'s research (2017) highlights the conditions that allow VR to emerge and flourish. When supervisees work in environments that value them, where attention is paid to the wisdom of their own journeys involving trauma and resilience, and interpersonal relationships offer possibilities for affirmation and bonding, it is easier to pay attention to how clients impact them in positive ways.

In another study, Gallegos (2021) examined the dimensions of VR among volunteers and counselors at a rape crisis center. She explored the relationship between intrapersonal and organizational factors and VR among trauma workers and found that organizational and interpersonal factors identified as coping strategies were associated with high VR. The dimensions of increased capacity for resourcefulness, changes in life goals and perspectives, and increased self-awareness and self-care practices subscales of the VR scale (VRS) (Killian et al., 2017) were the most significant. In the supervision context, counselors and other helpers working with victims of sexual assault may use the VRS didactically to help supervisees assess their own levels of VR, and encourage them to develop specific action plans to examine how their clients increased capacity for resourcefulness informed their own capacity, reassess the impact of a client's journey to healing on their own life goals, and expand their awareness and care for self and others.

Recent findings from quantitative VR studies identified several differences from past studies. For example, Reynolds (2019) and Trivedi (2017) found that clinicians' increase in experience and client contact hours working with trauma survivors were positively correlated with the increased capacity for resourcefulness on the VRS subscale suggesting that possibly VR increases as clinicians' experience grows. This is a key finding for clinical supervision. Novice clinicians may benefit from supervision that helps them track the impact of witnessing trauma and resilience in their clients, strengthen and expand their ability to emotionally hold a therapeutic container that allows for depth and intensity, and expand their ability to co-construct narratives of resilience with their clients.

Reynolds (2019) further found that VR has a stronger negative correlation with burnout than with secondary traumatic stress, which suggests that the pathways for generating positive and negative effects in the therapist might be different depending on the work environment. Reynolds (2019) suggests that "interventions to reduce burnout might be more useful for promoting VR than interventions targeted at preventing secondary traumatic stress in practitioners." (p. 69). This finding signals the importance of establishing fair working conditions for therapists working in organizations with clients needing a high level of care; i.e., it is challenging to focus on VR in supervision when therapists are overwhelmed by paperwork, underpaid, and operate in environments that resemble factory assembly work.

Overall, the aforementioned studies on VR emphasize the core themes of *changes in life goals and perspectives, client-inspired hope, increased recognition of clients' spirituality as a therapeutic resource, increased self-awareness and self-care practices, increased capacity for resourcefulness,* and *increased capacity for remaining present while listening to trauma narratives* (Hernández-Wolfe & Acevedo, 2020; Killian et al., 2017). However, Reynolds (2019) found that the *awareness of power and privilege* subscale of the VRS did not correlate with compassion satisfaction and compassion fatigue measures but showed a positive correlation with burnout and posited:

> In contrast to the other subscales in the VRS, an awareness of inequities in power and privilege—particularly if the practitioner were [*sic*] unable to assist the client in addressing them—could contribute to feelings of burnout and stress on the part of the practitioner. (p. 70)

Theoretically, this finding supports Weingarten's (2003) witnessing model. Her model explains that a witness who has awareness or knowledge regarding the meaning of the events being witnessed but is helpless or unable to act or lacks avenues for doing so is likely to experience burnout, helplessness, and hopelessness. Although therapists may find themselves in any of these positions at different times and in various contexts, Weingarten (2003) speculated that therapists who often find themselves in this position are most vulnerable to burnout. Evidence from a study by Lines et al. (2020) suggests that therapists with moderate exposure to trauma in the workplace have greater VR than their counterparts who are exposed to very high or very low levels of trauma and that therapists with moderate to light workloads are also more likely to experience higher levels of VR.

Awareness of issues of power and privilege in supervision can be a challenging aspect in the context of identifying VR. Oftentimes, supervisors and supervisees find themselves bearing witness to abuses of power in clients' experiences without a way to provide even minimal support, let alone advocacy. In our experience, as supervisors from gendered and racially marginalized locations, we often acknowledge the pain, invite silence to honor the sacrifices people make, and invite rituals of recognition and protection in alignment with the cultural and spiritual beliefs of our supervisees.

How Shared Resilience in a Traumatic Reality Complicates VR

Nuttman-Shwartz (2015) proposed the concept of shared resilience in a traumatic reality (SRTR) to capture the experiences of trauma workers who share a traumatic reality with their clients, and their ability to cope, show resilience, and grow as a result of the relationship with their clients. She highlighted the importance of empathic mutual aid relationships as a basic component for promoting resilience in a shared traumatic reality. This concept emerged in the context of clinical work in the border zone between Israel and Palestine (Dekel et al., 2016; Nuttman-Shwartz, 2015; Nuttman-Shwartz & Sternberg, 2017), post 9/11 New York City (Tosone, 2011; Tosone et al., 2012), and survivors of the Great East Japan Earthquake (Nishi et al., 2016).

Nuttman-Shwartz (2015) examined personal and professional aspects of a traumatic experience shared by clients and therapists and explained that in some situations, trauma is reciprocal, and as such impacts the nature of a clinician's practices. This is the case in the context of the Covid 19 pandemic and its aftermath. In our view, shared resilience in a traumatic reality "complicates" the emergence and identification of VR. In a relationship where there is already an acknowledgment of mutual influence, and where there is a shared traumatic reality, both supervisor and supervisee may have to navigate the complexity of their own trauma responses and circumstances while supporting each other and the supervisees' clients. Nevertheless, therapists and clients may share their resilience and impact each other in positive ways. For example, therapists may show flexibility, hope, and tolerance in shared challenging situations as well as the ability to remain empathic and present in the therapy process. Shared resilience in a shared traumatic reality is proposed as a way of looking at the positive effects that can develop within the therapeutic encounter between the practitioner and the client. Specifically, the empathic bond within a situation of mutual aid can alter the practitioner's emotions, behaviors, and outlook.

Nuttman-Shwartz's (2015) understanding of resilience in a shared traumatic reality sheds light on the complexities that therapists from marginalized social locations must address in clinical practice. Her approach confirms and expands the results that Acevedo and Hernández-Wolfe (2014; 2017) found in working with teachers and community leaders. These studies of two distinct Colombian populations unveiled the commonalities between teachers and students, and leaders and community members, in situations where both teachers and leaders shared a traumatic reality and were able to move to a place in which they could help their communities in various ways.

In her work supervising and training teachers working in marginalized communities in the city of Cali, Colombia, Acevedo (Hernández-Wolfe et al., 2014) shared a traumatic reality with the teachers. This reality involved government-sponsored, guerrilla, and common street violence that impacted people's daily lives generating a high level of hypervigilance. Oppression related to race, class, and gender generated additional layers of potential for the trauma that school teachers and Acevedo, in her capacity as a university professor and supervisor, shared. Within this social context of educational and supervision relationships, they were in a helping position that demanded going beyond traditional expectations to respond to learners with varied and complex needs. For example, the emotional connections that teachers reported with some of their learners, and that Acevedo developed with the teachers she supervised, were emotionally fluid, flexible, and close. These connections helped both learners and teachers beyond their immediate relationship and reverberated into the teachers' personal histories and interpersonal relationships outside the classroom. VR involved witnessing and articulating how supervisors and teachers provided a stable warm relationship, firm boundaries, reliability, and emotional responsiveness to the learners and each other (e.g., in group supervision). This relational attunement with affect regulation occurred amid ongoing and layered levels of violence. From Acevedo's perspective, her ability to attend to VR required having enough time to separate herself from her supervisees, and a support network outside of work or outside of the immediacy of her relationship with the teachers. These conditions allowed her to come back to the relationship with the teachers in supervision with fewer trauma responses of her own and more capacity to be present and to differentiate her reactions from the teachers' reactions.

In clinical contexts, oftentimes, clinicians from marginalized social locations devote their practices to working with their communities, leading the cumulative experience of historical and individual trauma of therapists and clients to converge in a therapeutic situation. This shared traumatic reality has the potential to allow clinicians to achieve the cognitive and emotional levels needed for tapping into their clients' resilience. In clinical supervision, a more experienced therapist from a marginalized social location can help a novice therapist identify and affirm VR based on her own journey of overcoming adversities grounded in similar oppressive circumstances. For example, a Latina supervisor working with a Latina supervisee who works with Latinx clients can assist her in dissecting how her clients make meaning and navigate adversity while attending to legacies of intergenerational trauma. Understanding how to navigate with supervisees the positive cultural aspects of family legacies, access, opportunity, and other aspects of social location is key to affirming both the supervisee and the client.

ccording to Berger and Quiros (2016, p. 145), "the concept trauma-informed refers to a system of care that demonstrates an understanding and recognition of trauma as both interpersonal and sociopolitical and is, therefore, aligned with principles of social justice." Accordingly, working with resilience requires as much sociocultural and political attunement as a trauma lens because studies of resilience show that in contexts with high exposure to adversity, a precondition for resilience, individuals with adequate resources show more resilience than rugged ones. Therefore, the impact of trauma and the potential for navigating and negotiating adversities must be addressed with an understanding of specific social contexts (Acevedo & Hernández-Wolfe, 2017; Hernández-Wolfe, 2013).

Berger and Quiros (2014; 2016) and Varghese et al. (2018) developed a model for trauma-informed care that includes trauma-informed supervision. They assert that the latter is guided by the principles of safety, trustworthiness, choice, collaboration, and empowerment. In this section, we discuss and illustrate how to integrate VR into trauma-informed supervision to assist clinicians in learning from witnessing their clients develop trust, discernment about safety, empowerment, and collaboration.

Safety

Safety is a condition for trauma and resilience-informed supervision; furthermore, it is a condition for exploring the potential of VR in supervisors' and supervisees' relationships. Safety involves sufficient trust, fluidity, and relaxation in the supervision relationship to explore the impact of the client's therapy journey in supervision.

Oftentimes supervisees have experienced abuses and traumatic realities that are similar to those that their clients have experienced, and/or they share a traumatic reality (Acevedo & Hernández-Wolfe, 2017; Nuttman-Shwartz, 2015). Our goal as supervisors is to create the safest environment possible for supervisees within a given context. This may be limited by multiple consistent or temporary constraints. For example, a clinical supervisor who is queer and of a racial minority sometimes must contend with racial microaggressions and homophobia in the workplace that impact her work and the work of her supervisees. In such situations, the supervisor and supervisee may share a reality in which both must navigate safety in their respective environments. Therefore, supervisors should be mindful of relative safety, move away from binary language that allows only two options, e.g., safe or unsafe, and instead discuss safety in terms of what would make it safe enough to be in a supervisory relationship. Unpacking what "enough safety" means and feels like for supervisors and supervisees teaches the latter to discern their boundaries and refine their sense of what is tolerable and what is not at a given moment. It also helps both to remember that we do not intend to harm one another and that we all are participants in a process involving comfort and discomfort.

After having a mutual understanding of what is safe enough for the supervisory relationship and the supervisee, we can invite, when appropriate, a conversation about VR. For instance, we can ask supervisees to pay attention to what and how a client develops a feeling of safety in the therapeutic relationship and in other relationships, and how they navigate safety differently in different relationships. An illustrative example is a supervisee of color who had experienced victimization by the police and shared in supervision that she is triggered by her client's experiences with the police. Supervision allowed space for her to express the impact of such violence and how it awakened her traumatic response; it also helped her discern the difference between her reaction and that of her client. The supervisor observed that the supervisee was challenged by her client's desire to gain more control over his reactions to the police in potential future encounters. The client was not at risk of being involved with the law and knew that many police personnel are respectful and had treated him with consideration. Nevertheless, he experiences a flight-freeze response when stopped for driving over the limit or if he simply sees a police officer across the street. Supervision involved helping the supervisee track experientially what felt safe and unsafe for her client and becoming aware of the negative thinking and rumination triggered by seeing someone in a police uniform. As her work with her client developed, the supervisee was encouraged to observe her client's choices, how his determination to listen and attend to the triggers and trauma response impacted her, and what she learned about "enough safety" given the client's discernment of his emotional limits. Specifically, she was impacted by how he tracked his own thoughts and how he held somatic and emotional connections with other experiences of victimization. As she witnessed and helped him track his chain of negative thoughts in response to the police stimuli, she learned how he became aware of the stories of violence and victimization that he imagined and made him feel sick. As she helped him discern his experiences, the stories, and the images he created, she endeavored to do the same work for herself. In addition, she witnessed how her client sorted out layers of associations between someone in power with a uniform and experiences of severe parental emotional and physical abuse in his childhood. She helped him delve into his childhood trauma experiences and identified the impact of his courage to address these wounds. As a result of this work, she developed a greater capacity to remain present while listening to trauma narratives, shifted her perspective on her trauma responses to police, and pursued somatic experiencing training, which changed her work as a trauma therapist.

Trustworthiness

Knight (2018) notes that trust and feelings of safety are interdependent. Trust involves supervisors' behaviors that allow supervisees to know that they can count on supervisors' honesty, guidance, and understanding. Actions modeling these characteristics must be integrated with those that invite supervisees to develop critical consciousness, empowerment, and accountability. Trust evolves when an experienced therapist shows, guides, invites, and affirms learning about being in a relationship as well as the tasks of clinical work (e.g., assessment, treatment planning, and intervention). Additionally, supervisees need to feel, know, and see, through supervisors' actions, that they can be vulnerable and that there are ways to take care of the impact of witnessing trauma via therapy, balancing work and personal life, spirituality, music, relationships with nature and animals, dance, art, and any other pursuits that uplift us and help us enjoy being emotionally regulated. Supervisees also need to feel, know, and see, through supervisors' actions, the value of coming back to the relationships with humans and other-than-human beings that bring beauty, love, compassion, tolerance, and joy. Supervisors may, and perhaps should, make visible how they tap into their own resilience to do the work they do. This is especially important for supervisors and supervisees from marginalized social locations, as oftentimes novice clinicians of color and those who are Queer benefit from role models that they feel close to. Such clinicians often need more guidance on how to pay attention to resilience and VR and focus on it. Supervisees with histories of enduring trauma need to see what is possible, experience positive and affirming possibilities, and own who they can become.

For example, in guiding a supervisee's work with an interracial, middle-class, cisgender heterosexual couple whose adult child disclosed that one of their siblings molested them, the supervisee learned to discuss questions about safety in a hypothetical way, to offer a conversational space for exploring what is like talking about the potential for sexual abuse in their family, and ultimately to navigate the initial sessions with enough skill to engage this reluctant couple in therapy. Integrating VR into supervision meant inviting the supervisee to reflect on how this couple was able to trust him, specifically, how they moved slowly until they felt reassured that they would not be further traumatized in therapy, and how they got to a place where they could safely release their pain in therapy. Attending VR involved tracking the supervisor's questions and the supervisee's responses and stepping back to learn what it felt like to carefully navigate the clients from distrust to trust. For example, initially, this couple expressed concern about reporting to law enforcement authorities and the impact of reporting on their family. The supervisee role played with the supervisor on how to hypothetically address these concerns and how to attend to the circumstances and requests of the adult child who disclosed incest. Once the couple decided to continue therapy, the supervisee learned in supervision how to help them navigate and set boundaries with the offending child, and with both sets of grandparents to respect the children's request to limit sharing the issue to the immediate nuclear family. Paying such attention to his client's pain and caution, challenged the supervisee to see that the clients' way was resilient and logically responded to their values and concerns. The supervisee's diligent work with these clients led him to reassess his problems and develop more compassion for others in his personal life. As a result of working with this couple, the supervisee became motivated to adopt a more strengths-based approach and began to let his clients take the lead more often during therapy.

Collaboration

Collaboration in supervision requires transparency by both the supervisor and the supervisee, active participation by the supervisee in developing training goals, and disclosure of how they feel in the supervisory relationship. It also involves acknowledgment of their expertise in their own life, and in making decisions about how they want to integrate therapy models into their practice. Active participation should be balanced with embracing guidance and accountability. Group supervision is an excellent space in which to develop a supervisee's voice and collaboration on clinical and workplace-related matters. In our experience, it has been essential to work across social locations with supervisors and supervisees who share the desire to have collaborative group supervision. Such groups serve multiple purposes, including helping members discuss how they have been positively impacted by their clients rather than focusing solely on how to resolve clients' issues (Hernández-Wolfe & Acevedo, 2020). Hernández-Wolfe et al. (2010) suggested questions to invite shared learning and collaboration around VR, e.g., What challenges have you witnessed your clients overcoming in the therapeutic process? What did your client stimulate in you that you want to nurture and expand? Supervisors can outline the following questions and ask supervisees to entertain the ones that resonate with them. In examining how you may have been positively impacted by your clients' ways of coping with adversity, do you: (a) Have any thoughts about how your perception of yourself may have been changed by your clients' resilience? (b) Feel that your general outlook on the world has changed in some way? (c) Identify any impact on your own views about spirituality? (d) Have any thoughts about how your views on trauma work may have been positively impacted by your clients' resilience? (e) Have any thoughts how your taking care of yourself has been impacted by your clients' resilience? Supervisors may also ask social location questions to invite critical consciousness; e.g., What role do your clients; and your own ethnicity, class, sexual orientation, gender, and religion play in shaping your experience and how so?

Group responses can be discussed with an emphasis on identifying and amplifying the learning processes that occur as a result of witnessing clients overcome adversity during trauma work. Because therapists often have not thoroughly articulated these learning experiences, these questions allow them to begin reflecting on these issues.

Empowerment

Empowerment in supervision refers to the co-creation of meaning and the promotion of "power with" supervisees (Hernández-Wolfe, 2013). The supervisee's participation in this process presupposes that social context shapes the lives of both clients and supervisees and acknowledges the contribution of supervisees' own lives to the supervisory relationship. Integrating VR in supervision to foster empowerment involves inviting supervisees to track their growth as a result of their work with their clients. For example, a queer supervisee of color working with a couple in their 60s consisting of an interracial queer and a white cisgender helped them understand and navigate the impact of racism and homophobia that emerged from the white partner's ex-husband and daughter. The partner of color did not have children and was a fairly independent person who had retired from law enforcement; the white partner, who came out in her 50s, had three adult children, of whom two were queer and one was heterosexual. In couple therapy, the supervisee worked experientially to assist them with attachment wounds, letting go of negative patterns of interaction, and building cycles of constructive and reparative interaction. The supervisee became deeply moved by their story and was unexpectedly impacted by the couple. At the time of working with this couple, the supervisee was in their early 50s, after a very difficult divorce eight years prior, and with no hope of finding a partner. The supervisee witnessed how the couple made meaning of their story, navigated difficult relationships, and remained committed to each other in their retirement years. In supervision, we discussed the many gifts that this couple offered to the therapist including overcoming fears about intimate relationships due to ageism, enhancing the ability to take risks to connect with others more deeply, and, the hope to find someone by using the internet as this couple had.

The Coexistence of Vicarious Trauma (VT) and VR: Implications for Clinical Supervision

Historically, literature about the impact of traumatic content on the therapist has been dominated by investigating the toxic effects of trauma work. However, a surge in strength-based approaches to therapy and supervision in the last two decades generated interest and support to investigate how therapists develop growth (Roepke, 2015), satisfaction (Garner & Golijani-Moghaddam, 2021), and resilience (Aafjes-van Doorn et al., 2022) from their work. Clinical supervision must integrate the positive and negative impact of trauma work as it relates to the real lives of supervisees. Clinical work cannot be accomplished by intellectually dissecting and analyzing only segments of experience. Helping supervisees develop maturity in the practice of therapy requires that they attend to and sit with multiple perspectives and connections. Thus, we advocate that clinical supervision assists in naming and expanding supervisees' experiences of overcoming adversity and the positive impact that clients may have as a result of overcoming adversity, in addition to acknowledging traumatic experiences. This explicit examination of both/and has the potential of influencing supervisees' appreciation of the reciprocal nature of therapy and of strengthening the use of self and adopting a lens that balances the painful and difficult aspects of trauma work with those that bring hope and promote growth.

For example, in the context of working with torture survivors, Edelkott et al. (2016) noted that many therapists mentioned that their clients often do not show or develop resilience before they are granted asylum and that viewing resilience in a social context is necessary to appreciate how social location, legal status, language barriers, and social support may influence clients' resilience. These authors further argued that VR and VT probably operate independently, possibly affect one another, and that therapists experience elements of both phenomena.

VT has been defined as "the transformation that occurs within the therapist (or another trauma worker) as a result of empathic engagement with clients' trauma experiences and their sequelae" (Pearlman & Mac Ian, 1995, p. 558). Oftentimes this transformation entails changes in the cognitive schema in which practitioners develop a worldview characterized by suspicion, pessimism, and powerlessness (Pearlman & Saakvitne, 1995). In supervision, supervisees learn with and from their clients about how to address the complexities, variations, and depth of traumatic injuries. In a parallel manner, supervisors can help supervisees identify resilience processes in their clients and the therapeutic relationship. The sophistication of trauma and resilience-informed supervision lies in holding a both/and approach to clinical work.

For example, despite the many risk factors associated with race, class, gender, ability, age, and sexual orientation for Latinx, Chavez-Dueñas et al. (2019) posited that the impact of traumatic experiences and pathways for resilience can coexist. Adversity can unintentionally yield changes in oneself, others, and the world that may result in adaptive and positive experiences. When experiences of adversity are seen in therapy in their social and historical context, it is possible to find interstices in potential positive change over time.

The processes of overcoming adversity are scaffolded as is the process of witnessing it. Such processes evolve over time and in the context of learning to survive, adapt, and thrive (Masten, 2014; 2018). In clinical supervision with a bilingual Spanish/English, white, cisgender, heterosexual female therapist of privileged economic background, working as a mental health counselor at a public school, supervisor and supervisee worked with a high school-aged, Latinx female-identified student who experienced abuse from her oldest sister. It was established that the family environment was not always emotionally safe due to parental preferential treatment, sibling rivalry, and sometimes emotional chaos. The supervisee worked with the student to help her navigate a somewhat emotionally unsafe family environment for two years, threading lightly on how much trauma work the client could emotionally tolerate given that she had to return to her family. The supervisee witnessed how after her high school graduation, the client made choices to increase her autonomy and safety and was encouraged to examine how much the client was helped by the seemingly not impactful work done before she was able to work and attend a trade school. The supervisee was asked to look back at how her client used opportunities at school and elsewhere to protect herself and navigate her way out of her familial home. At a macro level, the supervisee understood the real complexities and challenges of marginalized social locations, identified the impact of a safe relational attachment in therapy, and opportunities and continued support. At a micro-level, the supervisee witnessed momentary self-organization and co-regulation as a result of individual regulation and co-regulation with her in therapy.

Supervisors can invite supervisees to witness the resilience of their clients and help them track how clients coregulate with others and with the therapist. Benjamin's (2004) conceptualization of the ability "to sustain connectedness to the other's mind while accepting his separateness and difference" (p. 8) is useful in clinical supervision as it invites supervisees to seek their own way of establishing attunement to self, others, and the interaction between the two. Supervisees can safely invite clients to explore connections with another person by taking small risks until they can attune to themselves and to others and take responsibility for each person's contribution to the relationship. Supervisees can further be encouraged to notice how exploring deeper connections in a paced and safe manner builds resilience. Witnessing resilience is a key factor leading to the experience of VR and it may occur at different times in therapy.

Relevant to the integration of VT and VR is the consideration of SRTR. In a context involving SRTR, VR, and VT are likely to be present simultaneously for supervisees and their clients. For example, a transmasculine non-binary supervisee with a practice focused on serving the non-binary community worked with children and adolescents who experienced rejection from their families and sometimes abuse from family members and at school. The supervisee was particularly triggered by a transmasculine adolescent boy whose father was emotionally abusive and denied their identity. The supervisee worked with the teenager to find enough space for safety with the mother at home and at the school, assisted the parents in mourning the loss of who they wanted their child to be, and invited them to accept the child as he was becoming. The supervisee tracked how the parents were able to make changes for the benefit of the child over a long period. Supervision focused on inviting the supervisee to take small risks to explore a connection with both parents until sensing enough attunement with them. By noticing how exploring deeper connections in a paced and safe enough manner, the supervisee nurtured resilience in the relationship and witnessed it grow among family members. Over time, this and other experiences helped the supervisee address their distance from their own family, their experiences of rejection, and the fear of coming out to their siblings, who were cisgender and gay. The supervisee reflected on how they helped families learn about and go through transitions, while the reality of their own family relationships felt like limbo lacking real acceptance. The supervisee was able to develop enough hope and courage to open up to their own family, fully come out, and share more of their own life. While the family was not completely ready to see and accept them right away, this decision paved the way for opening the family system and gaining more affirmation and acceptance. From sharing a traumatic reality with the client, the supervisee learned vicariously how to navigate family situations and develop the courage to work with their own families. This example illustrates how SRTR may be at play when working with marginalized social locations.

Finally, this supervisee and supervisor challenged the idea that their intersectional identities could increase their burden. The first author and this supervisee discussed how fluid yet marked by oppression their histories were, unpacked meaningful distinctions and similarities to overcome discrimination, and discussed what all people need to fully enjoy their human rights.

Organizational Support and Peer Relationships as Predictors of VR

Frey et al. (2017) found that organizational support and peer relationships were predictors of VR. This affirms that resilience and VR are likely to occur and flourish in organizational and collegial contexts where mental health providers are valued and respected. While prior research on VR (Edelkott et al., 2016) helped understand how clinicians working with trauma survivors changed their perception of self-care in individual ways, we advocate for addressing the integration of trauma and resilience-informed practices at the organizational level. Organizations must address the complexity of trauma work by embracing multiple perspectives and connections between the micro-level of interpersonal relationships, and the various macro-levels of community and social impacts on supervisees. We highlight the importance of a continued emphasis on integrating the processes by which supervisors and supervisees understand how their identities and social contexts lend meaning to trauma and resilience experiences. For example, Edelkott et al. (2016) found that mental health providers working with survivors of torture examined their ability to set boundaries between their professional and personal lives and to be mindful and detach from work, assessed intentions behind their actions when implementing care for their clients. Such changes resulting from witnessing their clients' resilience should not be underestimated. Edelkott et al. (2016) and Engstrom et al. (2008) showed that torture survivor centers that pioneered trauma-informed practices and interpersonal environments enacted a high level of care among staff and practitioners. Hernández et al. (2007) acknowledged how Survivors of Torture in San Diego was a cradle of practice in which emerging knowledge developed in a context of very caring and mindful staff. Clinical supervision can foster coherence for supervisees when the work occurring in supervision mirrors the work of the organization with the community of supervisors, therapists, staff, and clients as a whole. When there is enough safety in an organizational environment, supervisees can relax and observe how clients impact them in positive ways. When a trauma service organization offers an environment in which supervisors and supervisees can have enough moments of self-regulation and co-regulation, supervisors and supervisees can engage in compassionately witnessing and appreciating how clients grow.

Additionally, trauma and resilience-informed supervision should examine the impact of privilege and marginalization, and enact practices involving both equity and emotional attunement to foster staff efforts to increase empowerment or/and accountability to balance the power in their relationships as well as to learn from each other. Conversations in supervision about how social structures support privileges for some and lack of privileges for others, and issues of relational power embedded in the organizational hierarchy of training shaping the supervisor-clinician-client relationship allow for questioning the frame of reference of supervision and clinical methods, the politics of the profession, and the ethics of clinical service practices in today's society (Hernández-Wolfe & McDowell, 2010). These discussions must occur in a supervisory environment that nurtures relational safety because societal oppression traumatizes clinicians who are from marginalized social locations regularly and in multiple ways (Ngadjui, 2021). Relational safety and attentiveness to professional development and maturity are key in addressing the needs of supervisors in training and novice supervisors who supervise novice clinicians because evidence has shown that the risk of indirect trauma is higher among professionals who have less education, are newer to their jobs and have the most and least experience working with trauma survivors (Harr & Moore, 2011; Molnar et al., 2017).

Implementing Trauma- and Resilience-Informed Supervision

From a supervisory perspective, the interpersonal level of trauma-informed practice involves centering the life experiences of clients and supervisees alongside developing knowledge and supporting trustworthiness, empowerment, choice, collaboration, and safety within the microsystems of therapy and supervision, and within the larger organization. Farkas and Romaniuk (2021) posit that "trauma-informed care practices are no longer only for therapeutic practice with clients. They should be introduced as part of supervisory education for those who will train and guide newly emerging professionals who have the enthusiasm, energy, and courage to push for social change." (p. 35). This orientation to care will benefit everyone.

A trauma and resilience-informed practice challenges the assumption that resilience is a given, or an automatic process that supervisors and clinicians possess. Supervisors and supervisees come to the profession with a range of coping skills that they further develop in supervision and therapy, while also learning new ways of coping as they mature and as they continue to get exposure to new and challenging situations.

Self-care must be situated in a social context and be critically examined to acknowledge that any "self" exists in a relational context and that individual options available to some supervisees are not available to others. For example, there needs to be an explicit and thoughtful acknowledgment of reciprocity in therapeutic and supervisory relationships. Recognizing how we benefit from each other as colleagues, supervisors, therapists, and clients in a manner that honors what we do, encourages us to give back, and allows us to earn what we deserve is a step toward transparency and balance with all our relationships.

Humans' ability to overcome adversity varies over time. A life cycle perspective may help us understand the continuities of life, the beginnings, the endings, and the transformations that all living beings go through. Thus, young supervisees may benefit from vicariously learning through their older clients about the challenges of life cycle transitions. Likewise, older supervisors can vicariously learn from young supervisees the possibilities of resilience for their generation.

Clinical supervision that integrates VR can help therapists find intrinsic sources of learning, recognition, and hope. The therapeutic relationship itself provides this possibility when supervisors pay attention to how clients impact supervisees over time and when we follow the continuities and discontinuities of emerging resilience in clients. For example, in communities with great economic and geographical limitations, families face challenges related to survival, integrity, and dignity; yet, they find ways to build a sense of hope that impacts their capacity to love and care for each other (Acevedo & Hernández-Wolfe, 2017; Hernández-Wolfe et al., 2010). For example, supervisees working with immigrants may focus on learning how transnational families stay connected and how their clients repair ruptures with their loved ones despite physical distance. VR may be the focus of attention as it relates to how clients work out to repair over time within the limitations of financial constraints and lack of physical contact.

VRS can be used to assess and discuss how a supervisee is being impacted by their work (Killian et al., 2017). Discussions about the supervisees' experiences of VR may illuminate the supervisee's parallel processes as learners and therapists. The scale explores seven factors: changes in life goals and perspectives, client-inspired hope, increased recognition of clients' spirituality as a therapeutic resource, increased self-awareness and self-care practices, consciousness about power and privilege relative to clients' social location, increased capacity for resourcefulness, and increased capacity for remaining present while listening to trauma narratives. These areas can be examined in clinical supervision to guide supervisees in looking at potential positive impacts on their clients.

Group supervision offers an ideal setting for community learning as peers can learn from each other using the VRS. It can foster VR in settings with diverse participants in which supervisors and supervisees explore the positive impact of clients' navigation of life cycle transitions. Likewise, when appropriate, supervisors and supervisees can learn vicariously from each other about overcoming adversity professionally and personally.

Laughlin and Rusca (2020) suggested that supervisees reflect on past potential experiences of VR. An assignment that the first author includes in her supervision courses for training master's level couple and family therapists involves asking students to identify and discuss a personal experience of VR. This may steer supervisees' mindset from the outset of training toward a relational growth-oriented perspective.

Supervisors should be encouraged to expand their relational views in supervision. Humans exist in relationships with everyone else on the planet rather than alone. When we open ourselves to relationships with all beings, possibilities for resilience may appear. Working with humans who rehabilitate abused animals has shown that helpers are positively impacted by the bond and the recovery they witness in the animals they help. Supervisors and supervisees can expand their sensorial awareness to the realms of other-than-human beings. Thus, they vicariously learn about taking perspective, expanding sensory awareness to include non-human communication, inspiration and hope, patience and consistency, the sense of contributing to something greater than oneself, and death (Hernández-Wolfe & Acevedo, 2021).

Conclusion

Humans, like hummingbirds, exist within an ecology of relationships with all beings on the planet. Some of these relationships are harmful and some are nurturing. Like hummingbirds, we can seek the nectar that witnessing resilience brings to us, to nurture ourselves and continue serving our communities. VR is a concrete way in which clients can impact growth in therapists. Therapists can learn and change with clients when they attend, identify, and process how the reciprocity of the therapeutic relationship opens the possibility of appreciating and constructing the meaning of the clinical process. Supervisees and supervisors exist in the context of a relationship in which they influence each other and construct meaning. This relationship is framed in organizational, familial, community, and social contexts, and the impact of these contexts influences the supervisor's ability to integrate VR into the supervision process. How larger organizational and social contexts impact supervision and clinical work must be attended to with honesty and humility, knowing that in such a complex and unjust world we will not always succeed in living out the ideals that are so important to us.

References

Aafjes-van Doorn, K., Békés, V., Luo, X., Prout, T. A., & Hoffman, L. (2022). Therapists' resilience and posttraumatic growth during the COVID-19 pandemic. *Psychological Trauma: Theory, Research, Practice, and Policy*, *14*(S1), S165–S173. 10.1037/tra0001097

Acevedo, V., & Hernández-Wolfe, P. (2014). Vicarious resilience: An exploration in work with Colombian educators. *Journal of Trauma, Aggression & Maltreatment*, *23*(5), 473–493. 10.1080/10926771.2014.904468

Acevedo, V., & Hernández-Wolfe, P. (2017). Community mothers and vicarious resilience: An exploration in a Colombian community, *Journal of Humanistic Psychology*, *60*(3), 365–383. 10.1177/0022167817717840

Anderson, H. (2007). Dialogue: People creating meaning with each other and finding ways to go on. In Anderson, H. Gehart, D. (Eds.), *Collaborative therapy: Relationships and conversations that make a difference* (pp. 33–41). Routledge/Taylor & Francis Group.

Arnold, D., Calhoun, L. G., Tedeschi, R., & Cann, A. (2005). Vicarious posttraumatic growth in Psychotherapy. *Journal of Humanistic Psychology*, *45*(2), 239–263. 10.1177/0022167805274729

Benjamin, J. (2004) Beyond doer and done to: An intersubjective view of thirdness. *The Psychoanalytic Quarterly*, *73*(1), 5–46. 10.1002/j.2167-4086.2004.tb00151.x

Berger, R., & Quiros, L. (2014). Supervision for trauma-informed practice. *Traumatology*, *20*(4), 296–301. 10.1037/h0099835

Berger, R., & Quiros, L. (2016). Best practices for training trauma-informed practitioners: Using a qualitative approach to elevate supervisors' voice. *Traumatology*, *22*(2), 145–154. 10.1037/trm0000076

Bernard, J. M., & Goodyear, R. K. (2019). *Fundamentals of clinical supervision* (6th ed.). Boston, MA: Allyn & Bacon.

Chavez-Dueñas, N. Y., Adames, H. Y., Perez-Chavez, J. G., & Salas, S. P. (2019). Healing ethno-racial trauma in Latinx immigrant communities: Cultivating hope, resistance, and action. *American Psychologist*, *74*(1), 49–62.

Cherven, B., Jordan, D., Hale, S., Wetzel, M., Travers, C., & Smith, K. (2020). Nurse-patient connectedness and nurses' professional quality of life: Experiences of volunteering at a pediatric oncology camp. *Journal of Pediatric Oncology Nursing*, *37*(2), 136–147. 10.1177/1043454219887671

Dekel, R., Nuttman-Shwartz, O., & Lavi, T. (2016). Shared traumatic reality and boundary theory: How mental health professionals cope with the home/work conflict during continuous security threats. *Journal of Couple & Relationship Therapy*, *15*(2), 121–134. 10.1080/15332691.2015.1068251

Edelkott, N., Engstrom, D., Hernández-Wolfe, P. & Gangsei, D. (2016). Vicarious resilience: Complexities and variations. *American Journal of Orthopsychiatry*, *86*(6), 713–724. 10.1037/ort0000180

Engstrom, D., Hernández, P., & Gangsei, D. (2008). Vicarious resilience: A qualitative investigation into its description. *Traumatology*, *14*(3), 13–21.

Farkas, K. J., & Romaniuk, J. R. (2021). Supervision for advocacy: Supporting self-care. *Society Register*, *5*(4), 23–40.

Frey, L. L., Beesley, D., Abbott, D., & Kendrick, E. (2017). Vicarious resilience in sexual assault and domestic violence advocates. *Psychological Trauma: Theory, Research, Practice and Policy*, *9*(1), 44–51.

Gallegos, I. (2021). *Vicarious resilience among employees and volunteers at a rape crisis center* (Doctoral Dissertation). Denton, Texas: Texas Woman's University.

Garner, E. V., & Golijani-Moghaddam, N. (2021). Relationship between psychological flexibility and work-related quality of life for healthcare professionals: A systematic review and meta-analysis. *Journal of Contextual Behavioral Science*, *21*, 98–112. 10.1016/j.jcbs.2021.06.007

Harr, C., & Moore, B. (2011). Compassion fatigue among social work students in field placements. *Journal of Teaching in Social Work*, *31*(3), 350–363

Hernández, P., & McDowell, T. (2010). Intersectionality, power and relational safety: Key concepts in clinical supervision. *Training and Education in Professional Psychology*, *4*(1), 29–35. 10.103/a0017064

Hernández, P., Engstrom, D., & Gangsei, D. (2007). Vicarious resilience: A qualitative investigation into a description of a new concept. *Family Process*, *46*(2), 229–241.

Hernández-Wolfe, P. (2013). *Latinos, a borderlands view of Latinos, Latin Americans and decolonization: Rethinking mental health*. Jason Aronson.

Hernández-Wolfe, P., & Acevedo, V. (2020). Towards grounding transnational feminism in borderland spaces, *Women and Therapy*, *44*(1–2), 156–171. 10.1080/02703149.2020.1775994

Hernández-Wolfe, P., & Acevedo, V. (2021). Helping injured animals helps the helper, too: Vicarious resilience and the animal-human bond. *Ecopsychology*, *13*(1), 19–26. 10.1089/eco.2020.0038

Hernández-Wolfe, P., Engstrom, D., & Gangsei, D. (2010). Exploring the impact of trauma on therapists: Vicarious resilience and related concepts in training. *Journal of Systemic Therapies*, *29*(10), 67–83.

Hernández-Wolfe, P., Killian, K., Engstrom, D., & Gangsei, D. (2014). Vicarious resilience, vicarious trauma and awareness of equity in trauma work. *Journal of Humanistic Psychology*, *55*(2), 153–172.

Hurley, D. J., Alvarez, L., & Buckley, H. (2015). From the zone of risk to the zone of resilience: Protecting the resilience of children and practitioners in Argentina, Canada, and Ireland. *International Journal of Child, Youth and Family Studies*, *6*(1), 17–51.

Killian, K., Hernández-Wolfe, P., Engstrom, D., & Gangsei, D. (2017). Development of the Vicarious Resilience Scale (VRS): A measure of positive effects of working with trauma survivors. *Psychological Trauma: Theory, Research, Practice, and Policy*, *9*(1), 23–31. 10.1037/tra0000199

Knight, C. (2018). Trauma-informed supervision: Historical antecedents, current practice, and future directions. *The Clinical Supervisor*, *37*(1), 7–37. 10.1080/07325223.2017.1413607

Laughlin, C. F., & Rusca, K. A. (2020). Strengthening vicarious resilience in adult survivors of childhood sexual abuse: A narrative approach to couples therapy. *The Family Journal*, *28*(1), 15–24. 10.1177/1066480719894938

Lines, R. L. J., Crane, M., Ducker, K. J., Ntoumanis, N., Thøgersen-Ntoumani, C., Fletcher, D., & Gucciardi, D. F. (2020). Profiles of adversity and resilience resources: A latent class analysis of two samples. *British Journal of Psychology*, *111*(2), 174–199. 10.1111/bjop.12397

Masten, A. S. (2014). *Ordinary magic: Resilience in development*. New York: Guilford Press.

Masten, A. S. (2018). Resilience theory and research on children and families: Past, present, and promise. *Journal of Family Theory and Review*, *10*(1), 12–31.

Molnar, B. E., Sprang, G., Killian, K. D., Gottfried, R., Emery, V., & Bride, B. E. (2017). Advancing science and practice for vicarious traumatization/secondary traumatic stress: A research agenda. *Traumatology*, *23*(2), 129–142. 10.1037/trm0000122

Ngadjui, O. T. (2021). Integrating vicarious resilience into counselor education programs. *Journal of Counselor Preparation and Supervision*, *14*(4). Retrieved from https://digitalcommons.sacredheart.edu/jcps/vol14/iss4/10.

Nishi, D., Kawashima, Y., Noguchi, H., Usuki, M., Yamashita, A., Koido, Y., & Matsuoka, Y. J. (2016). Resilience, post-traumatic growth, and work engagement among health care professionals after the Great East Japan Earthquake: A 4-year prospective follow-up study. *Journal of Occupational Health*, *58*(4), 347–353.

Nuttman-Shwartz, O. (2015). Shared resilience in a traumatic reality: A new concept for trauma workers exposed personally and professionally to collective disaster. *Trauma, Violence, & Abuse*, *16*(4), 466–475. 10.1177/1524838014557287

Nuttman-Shwartz, O., & Sternberg, R. (2017). Social work in the context of an ongoing security threat: Role description, personal experiences and conceptualisation. *British Journal of Social Work*, *47*(3), 903–918. (2017-30604-013).

Pair, J. M. (2018). A qualitative inquiry into the phenomenon of vicarious resilience in law enforcement officers [Walden University]. https://scholarworks.waldenu.edu/dissertations/5244/.

Pearlman, L., & Saakvitne, K. (1995). *Trauma and the therapist: Countertransference and vicarious traumatization in psychotherapy with incest survivors*. Norton.

Pearlman, L. A., & Mac Ian, P. S. (1995). Vicarious traumatization: An empirical study of the effects of trauma work on trauma therapists. *Professional Psychology: Research and Practice*, *26*(6), 558–565. 10.1037/0735-7028.26.6.558

Puvimanasinghe, T., Denson, L. A., Augoustinos, M., & Somasundaram, D. (2015). Vicarious resilience and vicarious traumatisation: Experiences of working with refugees and asylum seekers in South Australia. *Transcultural Psychiatry*, *52*(6), 743–765. 10.1177/1363461515577289

Reynolds, A. (2019). Exploring vicarious resilience among practitioners working with clients who have experienced traumatic events [City University of New York (CUNY)]. https://academicworks.cuny.edu/gc_etds/3529/

Roepke, A. M. (2015). Psychosocial interventions and posttraumatic growth: A meta-analysis. *Journal of Consulting and Clinical Psychology*, *83*(1), 129–142. 10.1037/a0036872

Silveira, F. S., & Boyer, W. (2015). Vicarious resilience in counselor of child and youth victims of interpersonal trauma. *Qualitative Health Research*, *25*(4), 513–526. 10.1177/1049732314552284

Tassie, A. K. (2015). Vicarious resilience from attachment trauma: Reflections of long-term therapy with marginalized young people. *Journal of Social Work Practice*, *29*(2), 191–204. 10.1080/02650533.2014.933406

Tedeschi, R. G., & Calhoun, L. (2004) Posttraumatic growth: Conceptual foundations and empirical evidence. *Psychological Inquiry*, *15*(1), 1–18. 10.1207/s15327965pli1501_01

Tosone, C. (2011). The legacy of September 11: Shared trauma, therapeutic intimacy, and professional posttraumatic growth. *Traumatology*, *17*(3), 25–29. 10.1177/1534765611421963

Tosone, C., Nuttmann-Shwartz, O., & Stephens, S. (2012). Shared trauma: When the professional is personal. *Clinical Social Work Journal*, *40*, 231–239. 10.1007/s10615-012-0395-0

Trivedi, S. E. (2017). Vicarious resilience: Psychotherapists' experiences working with survivors of trauma [Smith College]. https://scholarworks.smith.edu/theses/1947/.

Ungar, M. (2015). Varied patterns of family resilience in challenging contexts. *Journal of Marital and Family Therapy*, 42(1), 19–31. 10.1111/jmft.12124

Ungar M. (2019). *Change your world: The science of resilience and the true path to success.* Sutherland House.

Ungar, M., & Theron, L. (2019). Resilience and mental health: How multisystemic processes contribute to positive outcomes. *Lancet Psychiatry*, 7(5), 441–448. 10.1016/S2215-0366(19)30434-1

Varghese, R., Quiros, L., & Berger, R. (2018). Reflective practices for engaging in trauma-informed culturally competent supervision. *Smith College Studies in Social Work*. 10.1080/00377317.2018.1439826

Walsh, F. (2021). Family resilience: A dynamic systemic framework. In Ungar, M. (Eds.), *Multisystemic resilience: Adaptation and transformation in contexts of change* (pp. 255–270). New York, NY: Oxford University Press. https://doi.org/10.1093/oso/9780190095888.003.0015

Weingarten, K. (2003). *Common shock: Witnessing violence every day*. Dutton.

Woodwick, I. (2021). Tenacious hope: A grounded theory model of how vicarious resilience develops in clinicians who work with children who have experienced trauma. *Dissertation Abstracts International: Section B: The Sciences and Engineering*, *82*(12–B).

41

VICARIOUS POSTTRAUMATIC GROWTH IN SOCIAL WORKERS

The Israeli Case

Anat Ben-Porat

The Exposure of Israeli Social Workers to Traumatic Content

The practice of social work embodies within it the potential for stress, secondary traumatization, and vicarious traumatization, but also for growth. Social workers serve trauma victims and different populations in crisis or distress. Working in welfare departments, hospitals, crisis centers, and domestic violence centers often exposes social work practitioners to traumatic content as ear-witnesses, and sometimes even as eyewitnesses (Ben-Porat & Itzhaky, 2009; Bride, 2007). The intense responsibility that social workers bear for their clients' well-being, heavy caseloads, lack of resources and, in some situations, lack of ability to affect decision-making or change negative situations contribute to the high degree of stressfulness that characterizes their work (Evans et al., 2006).

Social workers often receive negative treatment from the media, and unfavorable stereotypes of the profession abound in the public in general (Lecroy & Stinson, 2004; Tower, 2000). Consequently, social workers may feel undervalued and see their profession as perceived negatively by others, potentially leading to additional stress and emotional exhaustion (Evans et al., 2006). Furthermore, over the last two decades, social workers have been playing a major role following terrorist attacks and during post-disaster situations, both in and outside of their home communities (Adams et al., 2008; Pulido, 2007), adding yet another stressful dimension to the nature of their job. The worldwide phenomenon of terrorism poses a great number of challenges to individuals, especially those who live under an ongoing threat, as well as to the social workers who serve them. Given that most social workers tend to work and live in the same area, the experience of "double exposure," as private individuals and as professionals, is common (Baum, 2014).

The aforementioned challenges are further exacerbated in Israel due to its unique socio-political and cultural context. Social workers in Israel work in all sectors (especially in public and nonprofit services), and in general, their working conditions (i.e., safety, salary, potential for promotion, and caseload) are thought to be poor. They are tasked with addressing a huge spectrum of needs because of Israel's high poverty rates, aging population (many of the elderly suffer from the consequences of traumas, such as the Holocaust), cultural diversity, conflicts between different cultural and religious groups, and the ongoing Israeli–Palestinian

DOI: 10.4324/9781032208688-51

conflict (Katan, 2013). Because the Israeli-Palestinian conflict exists both between Israel and the Palestinian Authority, as well as between Israel and its many neighboring Arab states (Kimmerling, 2001) it is not contained within Israel's borders, exposing social workers both to cross-border military conflicts and internal terrorist attacks, especially during the two major Palestinian uprisings, known as the first and second Intifada (1987 and 2000–2004, respectively). Working in hospital information centers, municipal facilities, and the army, Israeli social workers provide crisis interventions immediately after a terrorist attack and military conflict as well as long-term assistance. This includes helping families search for missing loved ones, accompanying them to the morgue to identify bodies, determining necessary arrangements when family members are injured or die, and offering assistance to affected communities (Shamai & Ron, 2009)

Indications of Vicarious Posttraumatic Growth (VPTG) in Social Workers

Increased research attention has been paid in recent years to the experience of growth among therapists who treat trauma victims. Pearlman and Saakvitne (1995) suggested that the courage and determination that they see in their clients might serve as an inspiration for therapists in their own continuing journeys of personal growth. In addition, the idealistic aspirations and the wish to change the world, which tend to characterize social workers in particular, especially at the beginning of their careers, may allow for growth alongside their vulnerability to distress (Lev-Wiesel & Amir, 2003). However, research is still lacking in this area, particularly regarding social workers as a unique group of practitioners with distinct professional tasks. Moreover, the positive implications of working with trauma victims for trauma therapists have been addressed mainly as secondary to the negative consequences, such as secondary trauma, compassion fatigue, and vicarious traumatization (Arnold et al., 2005).

The literature indicates that indeed therapists who treat trauma victims such as survivors of family violence, sexual abuse, and incest, as well as refugees, may experience positive changes in their lives, manifested in enhanced sensitivity to and empathy for others. They may also gain awareness of the positive elements in life and a change in values (Arnold et al., 2005; Barrington & Shakespeare-Finch, 2013; Bell, 2003; Brady et al., 1999; Brockhouse et al., 2011; Linley & Joseph, 2007; O'Sullivan & Whelan, 2011; Steed & Downing, 1998). Some have a greater appreciation for family and friends and experience positive changes in their interpersonal relationships (Barrington & Shakespeare-Finch, 2013). Further, they may feel an increased sense of self-worth as professionals, increased self-awareness, empowerment, self-validation, and an appreciation of life (Cohen & Collens, 2013).

Regarding social workers specifically, studies have pointed to the possibility of VPTG among those who work in services for victims of family violence, child protection, and clients contending with substance abuse (Ben-Porat, 2015; Cosden et al., 2016; Gibbons et al., 2011; Weiss-Dagan et al., 2020(. For example, Rinkel and colleagues (2018) found that members of the National Association of Social Workers (NASW) believed that working with trauma victims could serve as a source of new spiritual knowledge, growth, and challenge. Bauwens and Tosone (2010) found that practitioners who worked with victims of the New York City 2001 9/11 terror attack reported enhanced self-care, forging of new skills, and increased compassion and connectedness with clients as a result of the traumatic event.

In Israel, social workers who work with victims of domestic violence reported positive changes in their own interpersonal communications, spousal relations, and parenting (Ben-Porat & Itzhaky, 2009). Menashe et al. (2012) found that the dialogue between the parenting and the professional roles in female child protection social workers contributed to the redefinition of their parental selves and to a new and positive construction of the meaning of their professional role and personal role as mothers. In regard to the double exposure of living and working in the same trauma-exposed place, Lev-Wiesel et al. (2009) found among social workers who shared a war-related reality with their clients during the 2006 second Lebanon-Israel War that posttraumatic symptoms and VPTG co-existed. Shamai and Ron (2009) found that Israeli social workers who provided help to direct and indirect victims of national terror attacks experienced symptoms similar to those of secondary traumatic stress disorder (STSD) for a few days, whereas in the long run, they perceived their experience as leading to personal and professional growth.

Supervision and Academic Training as Facilitators of VPTG

Understanding the factors that foster growth among social workers in general and social work students, in particular, is critical in order to build supervisory and training programs that address the aforementioned stresses and enable opportunities for growth.

Supervision

Social work students are susceptible to high rates of emotional overload. During their field practicums, they must cope with the stress of work placement expectations, direct and indirect encounters with traumatic content due to interactions with people who have been exposed to trauma combined with reading and presenting case studies in class (Ben-Porat et al., 2020, 2021; Butler et al., 2017; Carello & Butler, 2013; Cunningham, 2004). In addition, their lack of experience and skills may put them at greater risk of stress or denial of the high price entailed by working in the social work profession (Lev-Wiesel, 2003; Litvack et al., 2010).

Alongside their academic studies, students working toward a qualifying degree in social work (which in Israel is BSW) must take part in supervised fieldwork. The preparation of field instructors who provide the supervision includes a one-to-two-year weekly course, as well as workshops and study days organized by the universities. Each year, students are assigned to agencies that can be either "primary" (i.e. where social workers are the only or main professionals working, e.g., social service departments) or "secondary" (i.e. social workers are among multiple professionals working in the facility, e.g., the army, hospitals, prisons, schools). Clients who utilize these services include victims of domestic violence, terror attacks, at-risk children and youth, Holocaust survivors, sexual assault victims, and military veterans suffering from PTSD. As such, the question emerges of how encounters with the fragility of life can increase growth among social work students and practitioners.

Supervision is one of the most important components in social workers' professional development (Beddoe, 2015; O'Donoghue & Tsui, 2013) and is critical to helping students cope with the aforementioned challenges and potentially grow from the struggle. Supervision has long been used in various disciplines as a way for experienced practitioners to impart knowledge, values, and skills to students and beginning practitioners (Kadushin & Harkness, 2002). Properly supervised, social work practitioners can receive emotional support as well as an opportunity to review their clinical work in the presence of an experienced practitioner, enhancing their personal and professional growth (Bledsoe, 2012; Cohen, 2004). Specifically, the greater awareness in recent years of the negative and positive implications for practitioners of trauma work has led to the encouragement of trauma-informed supervisory practices (Berger & Quiros, 2014; Sommer, 2008). Such practices use the basic building blocks of supervision in general (Kadushin & Harkness, 2002) but also contain supervisors' specific knowledge about trauma, i.e. supervision in this context includes supervisors' understanding of trauma and its implications for victims and for practitioners. In addition, supervisors must assess supervisees' vulnerabilities and resilience in the face of trauma content, based on their own experiences, as well as help them address job-related stresses and challenges, exercise self-care, and carry a balanced trauma-related caseload.

For supervision to be effective, there must be between supervisor and supervisee a strong supervisory working alliance that creates a physically and emotionally safe space for the supervisee and fosters trust and open communication (Berger & Quiros, 2014). When supervisors can listen without judging, help supervisees reflect on their practice, provide feedback about their work, and remain present (Quiros et al., 2013), supervisees (students as well as practitioners) can experience growth. Building a "growth narrative" in the supervisory framework may enable supervisees to change their self-perceptions and begin to see that through their difficult work, they have become stronger as people, have worthy life priorities, and are fighting for a just society (Zeevi-Selay, 2017).

Training

Sommer (2008) argued that heightening the awareness of practitioners regarding the risks and rewards of working with trauma victims is an essential part of proper training in the field and saw it as the *ethical obligation* of professionals who train workers as well as of the academic institutions where social work students study. This claim is supported by research conducted among social work students pointing to negative implications for them of their trauma-focused field work, such as stress or secondary and vicarious traumatization, alongside the possibility for growth (Ben-Porat et al., 2021; Goldblatt & Buchbinder, 2003).

A review of the academic track for the qualifying BSW degree in Israel indicates that there is no specific model designed for students who are training to work with trauma victims, or for trauma-informed supervision. While the curricula in various programs include a course on trauma or on specific populations of trauma victims, such as children at risk or domestic violence, very few programs are fully devoted to providing students and supervisors with training that includes addressing the potential impacts of trauma work. Additionally, many practitioners who work with trauma victims in all sectors report insufficient supervision frameworks, and those that do exist lack trauma-informed practices (Abu-Bader, 2003). Thus, it is reasonable to suggest that neither the Israeli academic and professional community nor policymakers recognize fully the potential negative and positive consequences of working in the field of trauma for students and practitioners. Further, there is scant awareness of specific issues and challenges relevant to the Israeli context such as the role of being doubly exposed to trauma and the role of a violent political conflict in the supervisor-supervisee relationship, e.g. if the two are on opposing sides of the conflict (Baum, 2012). These are issues of universal importance, as violent political conflicts exist in many parts of the world. Although such situations can lead to growth, they exist alongside strain on social work values and may raise ethical concerns regarding relationships with colleagues and service users who may be perceived as sharing the same cultural or political status or, alternatively, as being the enemy (Guru, 2010).

Implications for Professional Training

The increasing recognition that growth can occur, alongside distress, via social workers' exposure to trauma victims makes it incumbent upon academic institutions to build curricula that, in addition to knowledge on trauma and the possible distress of practitioners in response to traumatized clients, also educate students about their own potential for growth, as a result of working in the field. The students' understanding that the difficult work they will be engaged in as trauma workers can also foster growth may enable them to experience relief and hope as well as have an opportunity to recognize some benefits the profession offers. Such knowledge can be provided in the classroom, where students would learn about factors that can promote growth, self-care strategies, and the importance of receiving help from support systems such as family, peer groups, and classmates. It would also be important to discuss with students how they can use supervision to gain knowledge and skills alongside support.

In addition to educating students, providing training in trauma-informed practice to supervisors by academic institutions can enhance their skills in facilitating supervisees' growth. Such training can be accomplished during study days for supervisors (organized by the academic institutions as well as including this content in the courses for training supervisors).

Finally, at the policy level, it is binding upon us as a society to recognize trauma and its consequences for victims and social workers alike, and to take moral responsibility for assisting those who have chosen to stand on the front lines. To do so, a collaborative effort must be made by academic institutions, supervisors, and practitioners, demanding the appropriate allocation of resources for students and practitioners who work with different populations of trauma victims in order to address the stresses entailed by this work and create opportunities for growth.

References

Abu-Bader, S. H. (2003). Work satisfaction, burnout, and turnover among social workers in Israel: A causal diagram. *International Journal of Social Welfare*, *9*(3), 191–200. 10.1111/1468-2397.00128

Adams, R. E., Figley, C. R., & Boscarino, J. A. (2008). The compassion fatigue scale: Its use with social workers following urban disaster. *Research on social work practice*, *18*(3), 238–250.

Arnold, D., Calhoun, L. G., Tedeschi, R., & Cann, A. (2005). Vicarious posttraumatic growth in psychotherapy. *Journal of Humanistic Psychology*, *45*(2), 239–263. 10.1177/0022167805274729

Barrington, A. J., & Shakespeare-Finch, J. (2013). Working with refugee survivors of torture and trauma: An opportunity for vicarious post-traumatic growth. *Counselling Psychology Quarterly*, *26*(1), 89–105. 10.1080/09515070.2012.727553

Baum, N. (2012). Field supervision in countries ridden by armed conflict. *International Social Work*, *55*(5), 704–719.

Baum, N. (2014). Professionals' double exposure in the shared traumatic reality of wartime: Contributions to professional growth and stress. *The British Journal of Social Work*, *44*(8), 2113–2134. 10.1093/bjsw/bct085

Bauwens, J., & Tosone, C. (2010). Professional posttraumatic growth after a shared traumatic experience: Manhattan clinicians' perspectives on post-9/11 practice. *Journal of Loss and Trauma*, *15*(6), 498–517. 10.1080/15325024.2010.519267

Beddoe, L. (2015) Supervision and developing the profession: One supervision or many?. *China Journal of Social Work*, *8*(2), 150–163. DOI: 10.1080/17525098.2015.1039173

Bell, H. (2003). Strengths and secondary trauma in family violence work. *Social Work*, *48*(4), 513–522. 10.1093/sw/48.4.513

Ben-Porat, A. (2015). Vicarious post-traumatic growth: Domestic violence therapists versus social service department therapists in Israel. *Journal of family violence*, *30*(7), 923–933.

Ben-Porat, A., Gottlieb, S., Refaeli, T., Shemesh, S., & Reuven Even Zahav, R. (2020). Vicarious growth among social work students: What makes the difference?. *Health & social care in the community*, *28*(2), 662–669.

Ben-Porat, A., & Itzhaky, H. (2009). Implications of treating family violence for the therapist: Secondary traumatization, vicarious traumatization, and growth. *Journal of Family Violence*, *24*, 507–515. 10.1007/s10896-009-9249-0

Ben-Porat, A., Shemesh, S., Reuven Even Zahav, R., Gottlieb, S., & Refaeli, T. (2021). Secondary Traumatization among social work students—the contribution of personal, professional, and environmental factors. *The British Journal of Social Work*, *51*(3), 982–998.

Berger, R., & Quiros, L. (2014). Supervision for trauma-informed practice. *Traumatology*, *20*(4), 296–301. 10.1037/h0099835

Bledsoe, D. E. (2012). Trauma and supervision. In L. Lopez Levers (Ed.), *Trauma counseling: Theories and interventions* (pp. 569–578). Springer Publishing Company. 10.1891/9780826106841.0033

Brady, J., Guy, J., Poelstra, P., & Brokaw, B. (1999). Vicarious traumatization, spirituality, and the treatment of sexual abuse survivors. *Professional Psychology*, *30*(4), 386–393. 10.1037/0735-7028.30.4.386

Bride, B. E. (2007). Prevalence of secondary traumatic stress among social workers. *Social Work*, *52*(1), 63–70. 10.1093/sw/52.1.63

Brockhouse, R., Msetfi, R., Cohen, K., & Joseph, S. (2011). Vicarious exposure to trauma and growth in therapists: The moderating effects of sense of coherence, organizational support, and empathy. *Journal of Traumatic Stress*, *24*(6), 735–742. 10.1002/jts.20704

Butler, L. D., Carello, J., & Maguin, E. (2017). Trauma, stress, and self-care in clinical training: Predictors of burnout, decline in health status, secondary traumatic stress symptoms, and compassion satisfaction. *Psychological Trauma: Theory, Research, Practice, and Policy*, *9*(4), 416–424. 10.1037/tra0000187

Carello, J., & Butler, L. D. (2013). Potentially perilous pedagogies: Teaching trauma is not the same as trauma-informed teaching. *Journal of Trauma & Dissociation*, *15*(2), 153–168. 10.1080/15299 732.2014.867571

Cohen, C. S. (2004). Clinical supervision in a learning organization. In M. J. Austin, & K. M. Hopkins (Eds.), *Supervision as Collaboration in the Human Services: Building a Learning* Culture (pp. 71–84). Thousand Oaks, C: SAGE Publications.

Cohen, K., & Collens, P. (2013). The impact of trauma work on trauma workers: A met synthesis on vicarious trauma and vicarious posttraumatic growth. *Psychological Trauma: Theory, Research, Practice, and Policy*, *5*(6), 570–580.

Cosden, M., Sanford, A., Koch, L. M., & Lepore, C. E. (2016). Vicarious trauma and vicarious posttraumatic growth among substance abuse treatment providers. *Substance abuse*, *37*(4), 619–624. 10.1080/08897077.2016.1181695

Cunningham, M. (2004). Teaching social workers about trauma: Reducing the risks of vicarious traumatization in the classroom. *Journal of Social Work Education*, *40*(2), 305–317. 10.1080/10437797.2004.10778495

Evans, S., Huxley, P., Gately, C., Webber, M., Mears, A., Pajak, S., Medina, J., Kendall, K., & Katona, C. (2006). Mental health, burnout and job satisfaction among mental health social workers in England and Wales. *The British Journal of Psychiatry*, *188*(1), 75–80.

Gibbons, S., Murphy, D., & Joseph, S. (2011). Countertransference and positive growth in social workers. *Journal of Social Work Practice*, *25*(1), 17–30. 10.1080/02650530903579246

Goldblatt, H., & Buchbinder, E. (2003). Challenging gender roles. *Journal of Social Work Education, 39*(2), 255–275. 10.1080/10437797.2003.10779135
Guru, S. (2010). Social work and the 'War on Terror'. *British Journal of Social Work, 40*(1), 272–289. 10.1093/bjsw/bcn129
Kadushin, D., & Harkness, D. (2002). *Supervision in social work* (4th ed.). New York, NY: Columbia University Press.
Katan, J. (2013). Personal social services. In J. Katan, E. Lewental, & M. Hovav (Eds.) *Social Work in Israel* (419-438). Tel Aviv: Israel Hakibbutz Hameuchad (Hebrew).
Kimmerling, B. (2001). *The invention and decline of Israeliness*. University of California Press.
LeCroy, C. W., & Stinson, E. L. (2004). The public's perception of social work: Is it what we think it is? *Social Work, 49*(2), 164–174.
Lev-Wiesel, R. (2003). Expectations of costs and rewards: Students versus practicing social workers. *International Social Work, 46*(3), 323–332.
Lev-Wiesel, R., & Amir, A. (2003). Posttraumatic growth among holocaust child survivors. *Journal of Loss and Trauma, 8*(4), 229–237. 10.1080/15325020305884
Lev-Wiesel, R., Goldblatt, H., Eisikovits, Z., & Admi, H. (2009). Growth in the shadow of war: The case of social workers and nurses working in a shared war reality. *British Journal of Social Work, 39*(6), 1154–1174. 10.1093/bjsw/bcn021
Linley, P. A., & Joseph, S. (2007). Therapy work and therapists' positive and negative well- being. *Journal of Social and Clinical Psychology, 26*(93), 385–403. 10.1521/jscp.2007.26.3.385
Litvack, A., Mishna, F., & Bogo, M. (2010). Emotional reactions of students in field education: An exploratory study. *Journal of Social Work Education, 46*(2), 227–243.
Menashe, A., Possick, C., & Buchbinder, E. (2012). Between the maternal and the professional: The impact of being a child welfare officer on motherhood. *Child & Family Social Work, 19*(4), 391–400.
O'Donoghue, K., & Tsui, M.-s. (2013). Social work supervision research (1970-2010): The way we were and the way ahead. *British Journal of Social Work*, 45(2), 616–633. 10.1093/bjsw/bct115
O'Sullivan, J., & Whelan, T. A. (2011). Adversarial growth in telephone counsellors: Psychological and environmental influences. *British Journal of Guidance and Counselling*, 39(4), 307–323. 10.1080/03069885.2011.567326
Pearlman, L. A., & Saakvitne, K. W. (1995). Treating therapists with vicarious traumatization and secondary traumatic stress disorders. In C. R. Figley (Ed.), *Compassion fatigue: Coping with secondary traumatic stress disorder in those who treat the traumatized* (pp. 150–177). Brunner/Mazel.
Pulido, M. L. (2007). In their words: Secondary traumatic stress in social workers responding to the 9/11 terrorist attacks in New York City. *Social Work, 52*(3), 279–281.
Quiros, L., Kay, L., & Montijo, A. M. (2013). Creating emotional safety in the classroom and in the field. *Reflections: Narratives of Professional Healing, 18*(2), 39–44.
Rinkel, M., Larsen, K., Harrington, C., & Chun, C. (2018). Effects of social work practice on practitioners' spirituality. *Journal of Religion & Spirituality in Social Work: Social Thought, 37*(4), 331–350. 10.1080/15426432.2018.1512388
Shamai, M., & Ron, P. (2009). Helping direct and indirect victims of national terror: Experiences of Israeli social workers. *Qualitative health research, 19*(1), 42–54.
Sommer, C. A. (2008). Vicarious traumatization, trauma-sensitive supervision, and counselor preparation. *Counselor Education and Supervision, 48*(1), 61–71.
Steed, L. G., & Downing, R. (1998). A phenomenological study of vicarious traumatization amongst psychologists and professional counselors working in the field of sexual abuse/assault. *The Australasian Journal of Disaster and Trauma Studies, 1998-2*, Retrieved from: http://www.massey.ac.nz/~trauma/issues/1998-2/steed.htm
Tower, K. (2000). In our own image: Shaping attitudes about social work through television production. *Journal of Social Work Education, 36*(3), 575–585.
Weiss-Dagan, S., Ben-Porat, A., & Itzhaky, H. (2020). Secondary traumatic stress and vicarious posttraumatic growth among social workers who have worked with abused children. *Journal of Social Work*. 10.1177%2F1468017320981363
Zeevi-Selay, H. (2017). A training model for therapists dealing with secondary and vicarious traumatization: From struggle to resilience and growth. *Society and welfare, 37*(1), 451–474. (Hebrew)

42

VICARIOUS POSTTRAUMATIC GROWTH (VPTG) IN TRAUMA RESEARCHERS

Roni Berger

The idea of posttraumatic growth (PTG) by affiliation has been gaining recognition in recent years (Dar & Iqbal, 2020; Doherty et al., 2020). It has been acknowledged that following vicarious exposure to highly stressful events, positive psychological outcomes are also likely, though they are less studied than vicarious negative effects (Kalaitzaki et al., 2021). Just like PTSD can have "contagious" effects on people associated with those directly traumatized, PTG can have a similar effect. Benefits and positive changes as a result of vicarious traumatic exposure were conceptualized as vicarious PTG (VPTG) (Berger, 2021) and vicarious resilience (Engstrom et al., 2008; Killian et al., 2017). Subtly different related concepts are vicarious transformation (Pearlman & Caringi, 2009), secondary PTG (Zerach, 2020), compassion satisfaction (Hunter, 2012), and counter resilience (Gartner, 2014).

VPTG has been conceptualized in two ways. Arnold and colleagues (2005), Abel et al. (2014), and Galea (2017) defined VPTG as deriving meaning and developing positive changes through a vicarious traumatic exposure via another source rather than as a result of direct traumatic exposure, i.e. VPTG is growth associated with indirect trauma exposure (Yaakubov et al., 2020). A more limited interpretation of VPTG connotes reporting growth following the interaction with direct survivors of a trauma who report growth (Berger, 2021), i.e. witnessing positive changes in direct survivors of adversity who move past trauma experience and thrive can trigger and inspire the same in others associated with them and with whom they have close relationships (Bartoskova, 2015).

Reported vicarious positive changes are consistent with but not identical to those described by individuals who were directly exposed to the traumatic event and may include transformations in the philosophy of life, goals, and perspectives (Hernandez et al., 2018). In a systematic review of the literature, Manning-Jones and colleagues (2017) identified subtle differences between direct and vicarious growth as well as aspects unique to VPTG. For example, vicarious growth that professionals reported relative to their identity and spiritual growth was more abstract and less integrated with their self-concept than the personal growth reported by direct trauma survivors. Killian and colleagues (2017) developed the Vicarious Resilience Scale (VRS) and administered it to help professionals serving survivors of severe traumas around the globe. The results yielded seven aspects of vicarious resilience: changes in life goals and perspectives, client-inspired hope, increased

DOI: 10.4324/9781032208688-52

recognition of clients' spirituality as a therapeutic resource, increased self-awareness and self-care practices, consciousness about power and privilege relative to clients' social location, increased resourcefulness, and increased capacity to remain present while listening to trauma narratives.

Some studies documented a curvilinear relationship between negative and positive outcomes in individuals indirectly exposed to trauma. For example, Manning-Jones et al. (2017) found an inverted U curvilinear relationship between secondary traumatic stress (STS) and VPTG among psychologists; Colville and Cream (2009) documented the same pattern in parents of children admitted to intensive care; Shiri and colleagues (2008) reported a similar association in physicians and therapists but not in nurses and Dar and Iqbal (2020) reported that moderate levels of STS are most associated with the highest levels of VPTG. A meta-analytic study indicated that STS may be positively associated with VPTG (Cleary et al., 2022).

To date, the discussion and research of VPTG have focused mostly on family members and professionals providing services to those traumatized directly. Research on VPTG in family members included wives of veterans (Dekel & Solomon, 2007; McCormack et al., 2011; Ochoa Arnedo & Casellas-Grau, 2016) and adult offspring of ex-POWs (Zerach, 2020). Among professionals, VPTG was reported in medical personnel (Beck et al., 2017; Ogińska-Bulik, 2018; Shiri et al., 2008), social workers (Gibbons et al., 2011; Shamai & Ron, 2009), mental health practitioners (Hernandez-Wolfe et al., 2015; Hunter, 2012; Weingarten, 2010), teachers (Acevedo & Hernandez-Wolfe, 2014), addiction and human service providers (Arnold et al., 2005; Cieślak et al., 2016; Cosden, 2016), those working in different capacities with refugees (Barrington & Shakespeare-Finch, 2013; Splevins et al., 2010; Puvimanasinghe et al., 2015), counselors (Bartoskova, 2015; Pack, 2013; Silveira & Boyer, 2015), advocates (Frey et al., 2017), clergymen (Juczyński et al., in press) and community leaders (Acevedo & Hernandez-Wolfe, 2017).

Knowledge regarding secondary reactions in trauma researchers has been limited (Nikischer, 2019) and to the degree that it exists, focused on negative effects (Bloor et al., 2007; Coles et al., 2014; Drozdzewski & Dominey-Howes, 2015; Jackson et al., 2013; Kennedy et al., 2014; Kiyimba & O'Reilly, 2016; Lalor et al., 2006; Parker & O'Reilly, 2013). However, recently, some attention to potential secondary positive effects in trauma researchers also began to emerge (Berger, 2021). At this time, no study could be identified that used the VRS or any other strategy to assess VPTG in trauma researchers. This chapter summarizes the currently available knowledge about VPTG in trauma researchers.

Growth in Trauma Researchers

Researchers who study survivors of traumatic exposure may experience, in addition to negative effects, also positive secondary personal and professional outcomes inspired by their interaction with research participants who experienced trauma directly. Available knowledge regarding VPTG in trauma researchers has related to its prevalence, manifestations, correlates, and process.

Prevalence of VPTG in Trauma Researchers

Findings regarding the impact of studying trauma on researchers were inconclusive. Some studies documented vicarious trauma in researchers of victims of violence (Coles et al., 2014) whereas others failed to find such evidence (Coles & Mudaly, 2010; Grundlingh et al., 2017). A handful of studies addressed growth following involvement in exploring trauma survivors. For example, in a study of novice trauma interviewers, Smith and colleagues (2021) reported that participants described positive and negative symptoms. In a study of mental health professionals who researched survivors of a community disaster in Hermosillo, Mexico, participants reported personal growth, changes in self-efficacy and self-concept, increased awareness, and perspective changes (Shannonhouse et al., 2016). McLennan and colleagues (2016) documented, in addition to negative effects, positive effects on researchers who interviewed individuals affected by severe wildfire events in Australia with 63.6% of researchers reporting positive effects of the research on their lives.

Manifestations of VPTG in Trauma Researches

Parallel to PTG in general and extrapolating from knowledge about VPTG in practitioners, it is conceivable that following the study of research participants' stories of resilience, the researcher's growth may manifest in both professional and personal changes. Professionally, changes may include better satisfaction and skills, increased awareness of potential effects of their own and participants' positionality, power, and privilege, an increased capacity for being attentive to participants' narratives, empathic, compassionate, tolerant, and sensitive. Personally, researchers may experiences changes in their life goals and perspectives, have a greater appreciation for their own life and sense of justice, live more fully and meaningfully, improve their interpersonal relationships, become more emotionally expressive with loved ones, increase their appreciation for the resilience of people and become more spiritual (Barrington & Shakespeare-Finch, 2013; Bartoskova, 2015; Goldenberg, 2002). It is plausible that, like PTG, these domains and their specific manifestations would be culture-dependent. To date, no study could be identified that examined this question.

Correlates of Researchers' VPTG

No research could be identified regarding the predictors of VPTG in trauma researchers. Although findings regarding correlates of the secondary transformative impact of those directly traumatized on the lives of practitioners who serve them it inconsistent, extrapolating from it, conceivably both personal and contextual factors may impact on researcher's VPTG (Abel et al., 2014; Arnold et al., 2005; Brockhause et al., 2011; Cohen & Collens, 2013; Froman, 2014, Linley & Joseph, 2007). Potential *personal factors* include researchers' gender, age, and own background, specifically trauma history, professional experience and orientation, training, skills, ability to cope with stress, personality traits of optimism, spirituality, empathy, and sense of coherence as well as involvement in leisure and self-care activities. For example, females reported higher levels of positive psychological changes than men (Linley & Joseph, 2007). Sharing with research participants similar traumatic histories or environments and personal circumstances that mirrored those of the participants, generated similar feelings of PTG, such as hope and optimism and an increased appreciation of their resilience. *Contextual factors* may include the volume and intensity of exposure to research participants' positive transformation in life goals and perspectives, the availability of social and organizational support and models for PTG, availability of trauma-informed supervision, job satisfaction, and attributing high value to work (Hernandez-Wolfe, 2018; Manning-Jones et al., 2017; Ogińska-Bulik et al., 2021).

The Process of VPTG in Researchers

According to the original model of PTG in direct survivors developed by Tedeschi and Calhoun (2004), the process of PTG begins following a major life crisis or traumatic event that challenges or shatters the individual's schemas of themselves, others, and the world. To pave the road to potential PTG, those traumatized need to be involved in intense cognitive processing of the event, making meaning of it, and restructuring narratives. Personality characteristics, the nature of the event, pre-existing schemas, the ability of those impacted to manage distressing emotions and the availability of social support may influence the ensuing PTG.

Studies of VPTG in spouses focused on how growth was experienced and manifested (Dekel & Solomon, 2007; McCormack et al., 2011) whereas an in-depth understanding of the process leading to it is yet to be developed. Several questions arise regarding the process of VPTG in researchers. One question relates to the trigger of VPTG in researchers. Literature about PTG consistently emphasizes that growth is generated by struggling with the event rather than the event itself (e.g. Calhoun et al., 2010). The question is whether in order for researchers to grow, they need to struggle or merely witness their participants struggle. An additional question refers to the mechanism of "transmission" of direct survivors' PTG to researchers who study them. Is the PTG experienced by researchers similar to that of survivors or might it have different characteristics? Two main approaches to the process of VPTG are evident in the literature. One approach explains VPTG as produced through "infection" of the direct survivor's growth while the other approach attributes vicarious PTG to observational, imitating, and contagious learning that the significant other derives from the survivor's growth (Ochoa Arnedo & Casellas-Grau, 2016). The question remains which of these processes applies to trauma researchers? Another question is regarding the duration of VPTG. A longitudinal study over three decades found that VPTG in wives of veterans decreased over time (Bachem et al., 2018) raising the question of how long VPTG in researchers exists. No study was identified that addressed these important questions and future research will need to examine them.

Strategies for Fostering VPTG in Researchers

Trauma researchers and research institutes should be aware of the potential for growth involved in trauma research and exercise contextual and personal measures for acknowledging its importance and facilitating it.

Contextual Measures

Universities and research institutes must ensure that researchers on all levels understand, in addition to the risk involved, also the potential for growth. A non-punitive approach toward secondary trauma reactions needs to be adopted by creating a trauma-informed environment that promotes an organizational culture. Such an environment acknowledges both the potential negative impact and potential for researchers to experience growth from their study of traumatized populations, normalizes it, and gives researchers permission to address those effects in their own work and lives. Strategies to achieve these goals include training, supervision, support groups, and appropriate institutional policies.

Training

Because it has been found that researcher preparedness is a key factor for securing their safety, especially in those who study sensitive topics (Fenge et al., 2019), emphasis should be placed on training prior to and during conducting the research. Such training should educate researchers about the potential impact of researcher exposure to traumatic material including the possibility of growth and guidance for developing skills to achieve it such as keeping a reflexive diary. Such measures are valuable across all stages of the research to create an environment that fosters VPTG.

Supervision

Trauma-informed supervision and mentoring should be employed to create an environment that supports the safety, well-being, and opportunities for the growth of researchers. Gleeson (2021) who reported her own trauma incited by intensive involvement in research of child abuse, advocates incorporating in trauma research principles of trauma-informed care, which realize the impact of trauma, recognize the signs and symptoms of trauma, respond by integrating knowledge about trauma and resist retraumatization (Campbell et al., 2019). This recommendation should be expanded to include also supervision and mentoring that acknowledges and fosters growth.

Support Groups

The PTG model emphasizes the critical role of social support. Mutual support forums should be established as a standard measure for all trauma research to provide appropriate opportunities for researchers to safely reflect upon their experiences, as the importance of debriefing is well recognized in the field of trauma, and rumination, i.e. cognitive processing of the traumatic experience that is deliberate, reflective and constructive, which is a critical element in the PTG model (Tedeschi & Calhoun, 2004). Such forums can also offer modeling of VPTG, eventually enabling researchers to develop resilience when studying challenging topics (Fahie, 2014). However, evidence regarding the effectiveness of groups is not consistent. For example, Grundlingh et al. (2017) found no difference between group debriefings and leisure activities in violence researchers.

Institutional Policies

Gleeson (2021) suggests that trauma-informed care principles be introduced into IRB approvals. This means that IRB requires that all applications for trauma-related research provide, in addition to a discussion of potential risks for study participants and measures designed to protect them, also an assessment of the anticipated level of researchers' vicarious trauma and plans for detecting and addressing it as well as facilitating VPTG (Berger, 2021; Dominey-Howes, 2015;).

Personal Level

Coles and Mudaly (2010) identify effective measures for protecting trauma researchers by exercising a balanced exposure to trauma-heavy content (e.g. by taking breaks as needed), learning stress management techniques, and using one's peers for support and debriefing. To promote resilience and PTG, self-care should be adopted by trauma researchers (Smith et al., 2021) including mindfulness, meditation, relaxation, grounding, deep breathing, physical exercise, hobbies, music, and recreational activities. Recent studies indicate that relationships with pets can also enhance human PTG (Hernandez-Wolfe & Acevedo, 2021).

Summary and Conclusions

This chapter focused on VPTG in trauma researchers. It summarized the scant available knowledge about its prevalence, manifestations, correlates, and process as well as offers systemic and personal strategies to enable and foster it. Future research should examine the mechanisms by which trauma researchers can grow, conditions that may be conducive to such growth and strategies that can enable and foster it. As individual and collective traumas increasingly impact the world, they trigger extensive studies of it as can be manifested by the flood of studies regarding the economic, social, and psychological impact of the Covid-19 pandemic that were published in 2020–2021. A literature review with the search concept "studies about the effects of the Covid-19 pandemic" generated 209,885 results for the year 2020 alone. 698 of these studies addressed PTG and 30 mentioned VPTG. This suggests that trauma researchers encounter traumatized individuals and communities in an unprecedented volume. Understanding their experiences, factors that can help them grow, strategies and policies that can enhance their growth has never before been so important.

References

Abel, L., Walker, C., Samios, C., & Morozow, L. (2014). Vicarious posttraumatic growth: Predictors of growth and relationships with adjustment. *Traumatology*, *20*(1), 9–18. 10.1037/h0099375

Acevedo, V. E., & Hernandez-Wolfe, P. (2014). Vicarious resilience: An exploration of teachers and children's resilience in highly challenging social contexts. *Journal of aggression, Maltreatment & Trauma*, *23*(5), 473–493. 10.1080/10926771.2014.904468

Acevedo, V. E., & Hernandez-Wolfe, P. (2017). Community mothers and vicarious resilience: An exploration in a Colombian community. *Journal of Humanistic Psychology*, *60*(3), 365–383. 10.1177/0022167817717840

Arnold, D., Calhoun, L. G., Tedeschi, R., & Cann, A. (2005). Vicarious posttraumatic growth in psychotherapy. *Journal of Humanistic Psychology*, *45*(2), 239–263.

Bachem, R., Mitreuter, S., Levin, Y., Stein, J. Y., Xiao, Z., & Solomon, Z. (2018). Longitudinal development of primary and secondary posttraumatic growth in aging veterans and their wives: Domain-specific trajectories. *Journal of Traumatic Stress*, *31*(5), 730–741. 10.1002/jts.22331

Barrington, A. G., & Shakespeare-Finch, J. (2013). Working with refugee survivors of torture and trauma: An opportunity for vicarious post-traumatic growth. *Counselling Psychology Quarterly*, *26*(1), 89–105.

Bartoskova, L. (2015). Research into post-traumatic growth in therapists: A critical literature review. *Counselling Psychology Review*, *30*(3), 57–68. 10.5964/pch.v2i1.39

Beck, C. T., Rivera, J., & Gable, R. K. (2017). A mixed-methods study of vicarious posttraumatic growth in certified nurse-midwives. *Journal of midwifery & women's health*, *62*(1), 80–87.

Berger, R. (2021). Studying trauma: Indirect effects on researchers and self-and strategies for addressing them. *European Journal of Trauma & Dissociation*, *5*(1), article 100149. 10.1016/j.ejtd.2020.100149.

Bloor, M., Fincham, B., & Sampson, H. (2007). Qualiti (NCRM) commissioned inquiry into the risk to well-being of researchers in qualitative research. *Cardiff ESRC National Centre for Research Methods: Cardiff University*, URL: http://www.cardiff.ac.uk/socsi/qualiti/CIReport.pdf

Brockhouse, R., Msetfi, R. M., Cohen, K., & Joseph, S. (2011). Vicarious exposure to trauma and growth in therapists: The moderating effects of sense of coherence, organizational support, and empathy. *Journal of Traumatic Stress*, *24*(6), 735–742. 10.1002/jts.20704

Calhoun, L. G., Cann, A., & Tedeschi, R. G. (2010). The posttraumatic growth model: Sociocultural considerations. In T. Weiss, & R. Berger (Eds.) *Posttraumatic growth and culturally competent practice: Lessons learned from around the world* (pp. 1–14). NJ: John Wiley.

Campbell, R., Goodman-Williams, R., & McKenzie, J. (2019). A trauma-informed approach to sexual violence research ethics and open science. *Journal of Interpersonal Violence*, *34*(23-24), 4765–4793. 10.1177/0886260519871530

Cieślak, R., Benight, Ch., Rogala, A., Smoktunowicz, E., Kowalska, M., Żukowska, K., Yeager, C., & Łuszczyńska, A. (2016). Effects on internet-based self-efficacy on secondary traumatic stress and secondary posttraumatic growth among health and human service professionals exposed to indirect trauma. *Frontiers in Psychology*, 7. 10.3389/fpsyg.2016.01009

Cleary, E., Curran, D., Kelly, G., Dorahy, M. J., & Hanna, D. (2022). The meta-analytic relationship between secondary traumatic stress and vicarious posttraumatic growth in adults. *Traumatology*. 10.1037/trm0000373

Cohen, K., & Collens, P. (2013). The impact of trauma work on trauma workers: A meta- synthesis on vicarious trauma and vicarious posttraumatic growth. *Psychological Trauma: Theory, Research, Practice, and Policy*, *5*, 570–580. 10.1037/a0030388

Coles, J., Astbury, J., Dartnall, E., & Limjerwala, S. (2014). A qualitative exploration of researcher trauma and researchers' responses to investigating sexual violence. *Violence against Women*, *20*(1), 95–117. 10.1177/1077801213520578

Coles, J., & Mudaly, N. (2010). Staying safe: Strategies for qualitative child abuse researchers. *Child Abuse Review*, *19*, 56–69. 10.1002/car.1080

Colville, G., & Cream, P. (2009). Post-traumatic growth in parents after a child's admission to intensive care: maybe Nietzsche was right? *Intensive care medicine*, *35*(5), 919–923. 10.1007/s00134-009-1444-1

Cosden, M., Sanford, A., Koch, L. M., & Lepore, C. E. (2016). Vicarious trauma and vicarious posttraumatic growth among substance abuse treatment providers. *Substance Abuse*, *37*(4), 619–624. 10.1080/08897077.2016.1181695

Dar, I. A., & Iqbal, N. (2020). Beyond linear evidence: The curvilinear relationship between secondary traumatic stress and vicarious posttraumatic growth among healthcare professionals. *Stress and Health*, *36*(2), 203–212. 10.1002/smi.2932

Dekel, R., & Solomon, Z. (2007). Secondary traumatization among wives of war veterans with PTSD. In C. Figley, & W. Nash (Eds.), *Combat stress injury: Theory, research, and management* (pp. 137–157). New York: Routledge.

Doherty, M. E., Scannell-Desch, E., & Bready, J. (2020). A positive side of deployment: Vicarious posttraumatic growth in U.S. military nurses who served in the Iraq and Afghanistan wars. *Journal of Nursing Scholarship*, *52*(3), 233–241. 10.1111/jnu.12547

Dominey-Howes, D. (2015). Seeing "the Dark Passenger"- reflections on the emotional trauma of conducting post-disaster research. *Emotion, Space and Society*, *17*, 55–62. 10.1016/j.emospa.2015.06.008

Drozdzewski, D., & Dominey-Howes, D. (2015). Research and trauma: Understanding the impact of traumatic content and places on the researcher. *Emotion, Space and Society*, *100*(17), 17–21.

Engstrom, D., Hernandez, P., & Gangsei, D. (2008). Vicarious resilience: A qualitative investigation into its description. *Traumatology*, *14*(3), 13–21. 10.1177/1534765608319323

Fahie, D. (2014). Doing sensitive research sensitively: Ethical and methodological issues in researching workplace bullying. *International Journal of Qualitative Methods*, *13*(1), 19–36.

Fenge, L. A., Oakley, L., Taylor, B., & Beer, S. (2019). The impact of sensitive research on the researcher: Preparedness and positionality. *International Journal of Qualitative Methods*, *18*, 1–8. 10.1177/1609406919893161

Frey, L. L., Beesley, D., Abbott, D., & Kendrick E. (2017). Vicarious resilience in sexual assault and domestic violence advocates. *Psychological Trauma*, *9*(1), 44–51. 10.1037/tra0000159

Froman, M. (2014). A mixed methods study of the impact of providing therapy to traumatized clients: Vicarious trauma, compassion fatigue, and vicarious posttraumatic growth in mental health therapists. *A Dissertation submitted to the faculty of the University of Minnesota*.

Galea, M. (2017). Vicarious PTG after Fireworks Trauma. *Psychology*, *8*(14), 2496–2515. 10.4236/psych.2017.814158

Gartner, R. B. (2014) Trauma and countertrauma, resilience and counterresilience. *Contemporary Psychoanalysis*, *50*(4), 609–626. 10.1080/00107530.2014.945069

Gibbons, S., Murphy, D., & Joseph, S. (2011). Countertransference and positive growth in social workers. *Journal of Social Work Practice*, *25*(1), 17–30.

Gleeson, J. (2021). Troubling/trouble in the academy: Posttraumatic stress disorder and sexual abuse research. *High Education*, 1–15. 10.1007/s10734-021-00764-x

Goldenberg, J. (2002). The impact on the interviewer of Holocaust survivor narratives: Vicarious traumatization or transformation? *Traumatology*, *8*, 215–231. 10.1177%2F153476560200800405

Grundlingh, H., Knight, L., Naker, D., & Devries, K. (2017). Secondary distress in violence researchers: A randomised trial of the effectiveness of group debriefings. *BMC Psychiatry*, *17*, 1–714. 10.1186/s12888-017-1327-x

Hernandez-Wolfe, P. (2018). Vicarious resilience: A comprehensive review. *Revista de Estudios Sociales*, 66, 9–17. 10.7440/res66.2018.02

Hernandez-Wolfe, P., & Acevedo, V. E. (2021). Helping injured animals helps the helper, too: Vicarious resilience and the animal–human bond. *Ecopsychology*, *13*(1), 19–26.

Hernandez-Wolfe, P., Killian, K., Engstrom, D., & Gangsei, D. (2015). Vicarious resilience, vicarious trauma, and awareness of equity in trauma work. *Journal of Humanistic Psychology*, *55*(2), 153–172. 10.1177/0022167814534322

Hunter, S. (2012). Walking in sacred spaces in the therapeutic bond: Therapists' experiences of compassion satisfaction coupled with the potential for vicarious traumatization. *Family Process*, *51*(2), 179–192. 10.1111/j.1545-5300.2012.01393.x

Jackson, S., Backett-Milburn, K., & Newall, E. (2013). Researching distressing topics: Emotional reflexivity and emotional labor in the secondary analysis of children and young people's narratives of abuse. *SAGE Open*, *3*(2). 10.1177/2158244013490705

Juczyński, Z., Ogińska-Bulik, N., & Binnenbesel, J. (2021). Empathy and cognitive processing as factors determining the consequences of secondary exposure to trauma among Roman Catholic clergymen. *Journal of Religion and Health*, 1–16. https://doi-org.libproxy.adelphi.edu/10.1007/s10943-021-01443-y

Kalaitzaki, A., Tamiolaki, A., & Tsouvelas, G. (2021). From secondary traumatic stress to vicarious posttraumatic growth amid COVID-19 lockdown in Greece: The role of health care workers' coping strategies. *Psychological Trauma: Theory, Research, Practice, and Policy*, *10*. https://doi-org.libproxy.adelphi.edu/10.1037/tra0001078

Kennedy, F., Hicks, B., & Yarker, J. (2014). Work stress and cancer researchers: an exploration of the challenges, experiences and training needs of UK cancer researchers. *European Journal of Cancer Care*, *23*(4), 462–471. 10.1111/ecc.12135

Killian, K., Hernandez-Wolfe, P., Engstrom, D., & Gangsei, D. (2017). Development of the Vicarious Resilience Scale (VRS): A measure of positive effects of working with trauma survivors. *Psychological trauma: Theory, research, practice, and policy*, *9*(1), 23–31.

Kiyimba, K., & O'Reilly, M. (2016). An exploration of the possibility for secondary traumatic stress among transcriptionists: A grounded theory approach. *Qualitative Research in Psychology*, *13*(1), 92–108. 10.1080/14780887.2015.1106630

Lalor, J. G., Begley, C. M., & Devane, D. (2006). Exploring painful experiences: Impact of emotional narratives on members of a qualitative research team. *Journal of Advanced Nursing*, *56*(6), 607–616. 10.1111/j.1365-2648.2006.04039.x. PMID: 17118040.

Linley, P. A., & Joseph, S. (2007). Therapy work and therapists' positive and negative well-being. *Journal of Social and Clinical Psychology*, *26*(3), 385–403.

Manning-Jones, S., de Terte, I., & Stephens, C. (2017). The relationship between vicarious posttraumatic growth and secondary traumatic stress among health professionals. *Journal of Loss and Trauma*, *22*(3), 256–270. http://www.tandfonline.com/loi/upil20

McCormack, L., Hagger, M. S., & Joseph, S. (2011). Vicarious growth in wives of Vietnam veterans: A phenomenological investigation into decades of "lived" experience. *Journal of Humanistic Psychology*, *51*(3), 273–290. 10.1177/0022167810377506

McLennan, J., Evans, L., Cowlishaw, S., Pamment, L., & Wright, L. (2016). Traumatic stress in post-disaster field research interviewers. *Journal of Traumatic Stress*, *29*, 101–105. 10.1002/jts.22072

Nikischer, A. (2019). Vicarious trauma inside the academe: Understanding the impact of teaching, researching and writing violence. *Higher Education*, *77*, 905–916. 10.1007/s10734-018-0308-4
Ochoa Arnedo, C., & Casellas-Grau, A. (2016). Vicarious or secondary post-traumatic growth: How are positive changes transmitted to significant others after experiencing a traumatic event? In C. Martin, V. Preedy, & V. Patel (Eds.) (2016). *Comprehensive guide to post- traumatic stress disorders* (pp. 1767–1782). Springer. 10.1007/978-3-319-08359-9_76
Ogińska-Bulik, N. (2018). Secondary traumatic stress and vicarious posttraumatic growth in nurses working in palliative care – the role of psychological resiliency. *Advances in Psychiatry and Neurology*, *27*(3), 196–210. 10.5114/ppn.2018.78713
Ogińska-Bulik, N., Jerzy Gurowiec, P., Michalska, P., & Kędra, E. (2021). Prevalence and determinants of secondary posttraumatic growth following trauma work among medical personnel: A cross sectional study. *European Journal of Psychotraumatology*, *12*(1), 1876382. 10.1080/20008198.2021.1876382
Pack, M. (2013). Vicarious traumatisation and resilience: An ecological systems approach to sexual abuse counsellors' trauma and stress. *Sexual abuse in Australia and New Zealand*, *5*(2), 69–76.
Parker, N., & O'Reilly, M. (2013). '"We are alone in the house": A case study addressing researcher safety and risk. *Qualitative Research in Psychology*, *10*(4), 341–354. 10.1080/14780887.2011.647261
Pearlman, L. A., & Caringi, J. (2009). Living and working self-reflectively to address vicarious trauma. In C. A. Courtois, & J. D. Ford (Eds.), *Treating complex traumatic stress disorders: An evidence-based guide* (pp. 202–224). The Guilford Press.
Puvimanasinghe, T., Denson, L. A., Augoustinos, M., & Somasundaram, D. (2015). Vicarious resilience and vicarious traumatisation: Experiences of working with refugees and asylum seekers in South Australia. *Transcultural Psychiatry*, *52*(6), 743–765. 10.1177/1363461515577289tps.sagepub.com
Shamai, M., & Ron, P. (2009). Helping direct and indirect victims of national terror: Experiences of Israeli social workers. *Qualitative Health Research*, *19*(1), 42–54.
Shannonhouse, L., Barden, S., Jones, E., Gonzalez, L., & Murphy, A. (2016). Secondary traumatic stress for trauma researchers: A mixed methods research design. *Journal of Mental Health Counseling*, *38*(3), 201–216.
Shiri, S., Wexler, I. D., Alkalay, Y., Meiner, Z., & Kreitler, S. (2008). Positive psychological impact of treating victims of politically motivated violence among hospital-based health care providers. *Psychotherapy and Psychosomatics*, *77*(5), 315–318. 10.1159/000142524
Silveira, F., & Boyer, W. (2015). Vicarious resilience in counselors of child and youth victims of interpersonal trauma. *Qualitative Health Research*, *25*(4), 513–526. 10.1177/1049732314552284
Smith, A. M., Hamilton, A. B., Loeb, T., Pemberton, J., & Wyatt, G. E. (2021). Reactions of novice interviewers conducting trauma research with marginalized communities: A qualitative analysis. *Journal of Interpersonal Violence*, *36*(21-22), NP12176–NP12197. 10.1177/0886260519889925
Splevins, K. A., Cohen, K., Joseph, S. Murray, C., & Bowley, J. (2010). Vicarious posttraumatic growth among interpreters. *Qualitative Health Research*, *20*(12), 1705–1716.
Tedeschi, R. G., & Calhoun, L. G. (2004). Posttraumatic growth: Conceptual foundations and empirical evidence. *Psychological Inquiry*, *15*(1), 1–18. 10.1207/s15327965pli1501_01
Weingarten, K. (2010). Reasonable hope: Construct, clinical applications, and supports. *Family Process*, *49*(1), 5–25. https://doi-org.libproxy.adelphi.edu/10.1111/j.1545-5300.2010.01305.x
Yaakubov, L., Hoffman, Y., & Rosenbloom, T. (2020). Secondary traumatic stress, vicarious posttraumatic growth and their association in emergency room physicians and nurses. *European Journal of Psychotraumatology*, *11*(1), 1830462. 10.1080/20008198.2020.1830462
Zerach, G. (2020). Posttraumatic growth among combat veterans and their siblings: A dyadic approach. *Journal of Clinical Psychology*, *76*(9), 1719–1735. 10.1002/jclp.22949

PART 7

Interventions for Facilitating PTG

43

PHOTOVOICE AS A VEHICLE FOR PROMOTING POSTTRAUMATIC GROWTH

Elizabeth Counselman-Carpenter

The History and Theory of PhotoVoice

PhotoVoice is a form of participatory photography, originally developed in the United Kingdom and first appearing in research and literature in the mid-1990s in a Yunnan, China-based project related to women's health research (Wang & Burris, 1994). Wang and Burris (1997) developed the methodology based on the concept that people can best represent their own realities and tell their own stories as a method of empowering those who often do not hold a lot of social capital or power related to stigma and/or marginalized identities. They initially referred to the process as 'photo-novella' and worked with 62 women in rural China to whom they gave cameras and with whom they facilitated small and large group discussions that explored their similar and diverse views of the world through conversations about the images that they took. Later referred to as Photo Text participant photography, and eventually known as PhotoVoice, this style of documentary photography provided participants with a concrete way in which they could capture their greatest concerns about current health issues and living conditions. While there are many applications of photography that can be used in art therapy and there are exclusive phototherapeutic techniques, such as 'Taking Pictures', PhotoVoice is grounded in a narrative, participatory, and action-based framework (Saita et al., 2019, Wang & Burris, 1994) and is considered a form of social action and research with therapeutic benefits.

PhotoVoice has evolved since its inception nearly thirty years ago. It is considered a form of community-based participatory action research (CBPR or CBPAR), is recognized as a stand-alone data collection tool used in both quantitative and qualitative research as well as considered a form of ethical photography. PhotoVoice's mission is defined as

> "… a world in which everybody has the opportunity to represent themselves and tell their own story. By working in partnership with organisations, communities, and individuals worldwide, we will build the skills and capacity of underrepresented or at-risk communities, creating new tools of self-advocacy and communication."
>
> *(Orton et al., 2016)*

DOI: 10.4324/9781032208688-54

The strongest foundational underpinning of PhotoVoice is centered on the four aspects of participatory action research: participation, action, research, and social change for social justice. At its core, the pedagogy is problem-based and the emerging knowledge is action-directed (Baum et al., 2006; Dobson, 2017). Participatory Action Research (PAR) is about taking action, analyzing power structures, and allowing researchers and participants to share control of the research process (Baum et al., 2006). A loop is created in which stakeholders participate in a research process designed to advance knowledge, which then results in social action and change by these very same stakeholders (Chevalier & Buckles 2013). Research and action work in tandem to create social change. PAR and PhotoVoice are both grounded in the construct of valuing the lived experience of individuals while also addressing mezzo and macro-level change. PAR and PhotoVoice are frequently used for needs assessment in communities with resource disparity and are growing in terms of conducting research in the health sector (Aubeeluck & Buchanan, 2006; Balmer et al., 2015; Dobson, 2017).

PhotoVoice is based on feminist theory, Freire's three levels of consciousness, specifically critical consciousness, the principles of documentary photography, and the experience of clinicians (Freire, 1970; Liebenberg, 2018; Wang & Burris, 1994, 1997). PhotoVoice's core philosophy is based on grassroots principles, as it involves members of a community who are taking photographs, which reflect the community back upon itself and reveal social and political realities. The critical reflection addresses the process, photography, participant-developed captioning to accompany the images, and a subsequent display of the images and text to a group, all of which can serve as agents of social change. As a research modality, PhotoVoice is considered qualitative, although PAR can be both qualitative and quantitative.

PhotoVoice is more than handing someone a camera and asking them to take pictures. Five key concepts at the foundation of PhotoVoice, as defined by Wang (1999), include the idea that images teach, pictures can influence policy changes, community members should be participants in both the creation of and the definition of images that shape positive public policy related to health, plans should be embedded in the project to involve policymakers and other influential stakeholders as an audience to the images and that there are both individual and community levels.

Training for PhotoVoice participants, including basic theory around PAR, comprises the steps for developing a PhotoVoice project and engaging stakeholders as well as the ethics and confidentiality around visual data (Balmer et al., 2015). As it is particularly used with marginalized populations, some of the ethical issues that can arise when using PhotoVoice include protecting the best interests of participants in the project, the privacy of photographed subjects, and addressing the stigma that may be attached to images and activities depicted in the photographs (Barrett, 2004; Drainoni et al., 2019; Prins, 2010). PhotoVoice differs from phototherapy, which has been used in counseling since the 1970s and is rooted solely in individual clinical work. While Phototherapy and PhotoVoice share the common steps of taking photos, viewing, editing, interpreting, and presenting images, phototherapy may include photos taken at a therapist's request, or involve photos from the past and is seen as a clinical tool based on improving well-being, whereas PhotoVoice is a tool facilitation grounded in social action (Sadeghi, 2018, Taminiaux, 2009; Weiser, 2004). PhotoVoice has three primary goals: to enable people to record and reflect on their community's strengths and concerns, to reach policymakers, and to promote critical dialogue (Wang & Burris, 1997).

The Application of PhotoVoice to Trauma Work

Core to the work of PhotoVoice is an analysis and understanding of power. Within the PhotoVoice framework, power is 'flipped' so that the participants are photographers rather than just subjects, and through the process they become engaged in their community and tell the story of their own life (Orton et al., 2016). For trauma survivors, this aspect of regaining control of their narrative can be a powerful healing experience (Evans, 2021b; Levy et al., 2020). As a form of research, it allows trauma survivors to control how their survivorship experience is told versus their story being 'mined' for dissemination purposes (Pearce et al., 2017). PhotoVoice and posttraumatic growth (PTG) naturally intersect through the elements of story-telling, narrative, and transformation. Meichenbaum (2006) states in his model of constructive narratives of posttraumatic reactions that the first premise is that "human beings are storytellers and account makers, especially following trauma experiences" (p. 356) and people " ... offer accounts that are designed to make sense of the world and their place in it" (p. 358). The process of taking images, curating them to share with one's group every week and then narrowing them down to share in a final exhibition contribute to the story-telling process of making sense. The constructive narrative approach, both in terms of self-narrative and group narrative, calls on this narrative as the pathway that determines the level of adjustment and distress following a traumatic event. PhotoVoice allows for the individuals to share their own self-narrative, and each PhotoVoice project also tells the story of a group; participating in the group is just one of the many resilience-building activities that foster PTG.

To keep the fidelity of PhotoVoice, tremendous thought and intention should be put into the project design particularly when related to trauma-informed work. The first step involves securing the trust and support of community stakeholders before the project begins because the collaborative aspect of PhotoVoice is at the core of its success. Groups may already exist or may be assembled exclusively for the purpose of the PhotoVoice project. Once the project is underway, participants must be trained and educated in the use of a camera and the principles of ethical photography. It is important for group members to understand the time involved in taking the images, how to protect those featured in the images, that there may be a cost incurred through the use of a camera, and to ensure participants know that they can share whatever aspect they want or do not want to tell about their stories. Although smartphones can be used, having a device exclusively for image capturing is encouraged (Orton et al., 2016). Typically, images are captured between group sessions rather than during the sessions, and participants may take as many or as few as they like.

Typically, group work is present throughout the entire PhotoVoice project and is an important aspect of the process and of how the factors of PTG may be facilitated. Participants meet as a group, which is often facilitated by a mental health professional and a photographer. Training in the use of the camera and the principles of ethical and documentary photography take place within this group while the actual photographing of images is typically done individually by group members. The group meets with predetermined regularity with the foci on sharing the images with other group members, processing the image-capturing that took place between group meetings, choosing the images that they would like to share, and then the final, critical step is group members/ photographers writing a caption or text for the photograph.

Interacting with others can be a positive, healing experience that allows individuals to process the traumatic events, and participate in emotional disclosure, which can serve to regulate emotion and reduce emotional distress (Devine et al., 2003; Lepore & Revenson, 2006). Further, these discussions allow participants to explore the social conditions that enhance and detract from personal and community well-being (Christensen, 2018; Dobson, 2017). Perhaps the most important step in the process is the viewing of the images by those in the community who hold the space and bear witness to the story being told. Wang (1999) stated the importance of this step, sharing that it is important to understand the " ... influence of images by analysing ... the reception of the images and the meanings attributed to them by audiences. (p. 186)". The community becomes the container to hold, and sometimes facilitate, change based on the stories shared in the exhibit.

Because PTG is grounded in the foundation that life struggles can lead to powerful change, the intersection between PTG and PhotoVoice is a natural one as PhotoVoice is a vehicle to both capture, process one's struggles and share the stories of one's journey with and through the struggles. As PhotoVoice participants take their images, they can capture what some of these difficult life challenges may be, often in a way that words alone cannot describe. Trauma results from the disruption in one's assumptive world, and documentary photography can memorialize the assumptive world both pre and post-disruption (Calhoun & Tedeschi, 2009). Photographs are often used to capture the same 'before' and 'after' that frames the traumatic event but can also capture the struggle with the trauma that Calhoun and Tedeschi emphasize as the catalyst for PTG.

PhotoVoice as a Research Strategy in Populations that have Experienced Trauma

Participatory action research can be powerful in facilitating PTG due to the active role participants take in creating knowledge. It asks participants to become co-researchers and advocates, with the foundational belief that they are experts in their own lives and environment. Another core aspect of CBPR is that participants should guide the actions that create mezzo-level change, which can lead to meaning-making, another core aspect of PTG. PhotoVoice also allows the sampling of different work and social settings that may not be traditionally accessible to researchers (Kutluturkan et al., 2016). In general, PhotoVoice provides a unique perspective in a climate where research is becoming increasingly patient-centered and trauma-informed (Levy et al., 2020).

One significant research area in which PhotoVoice is growing relates to surviving medical trauma including living with chronic and terminal illnesses, such as Huntington's Disease Amyotrophic Lateral Sclerosis (ALS), children and adults living with HIV, and caring for those living with a terminal illness (Adegoke & Steyn, 2017; Aubeeluck & Buchanan, 2006, Gunton et al. 2021). While Aubeeluck and Buchanen (2006) highlight the absence of protective factors that can promote PTG such as loneliness and a sense of powerlessness over one's life, Adegoke and Steyn (2017) and Gunton et al. (2021) found that participating in image-taking and the PhotoVoice research project indicated the presence of protective factors such as instillation of hope, faith and a sense of belonging. Balakrishnan et al. (2017) explored the narrative related to the quality of life of stroke survivors in the process of recovering who identify as urban dwellings with minority identities. The findings of this study, which kept to the fidelity of the PhotoVoice method, reported value in the actual act of taking the photographs as well as sharing them in a group setting as a way for decreasing isolation, empowering deeper participation in own community, and creating new social connections. Research related to the COVID-19 pandemic, factors of PTG, and the expression of these factors through PhotoVoice is also developing (Dell et al., 2021).

PhotoVoice as a Practice Intervention

Participating in a PhotoVoice project can be considered a trauma-informed practice intervention. The process of telling one's story through images has been shown to give participants a sense of control over their past experiences and to explain how they have been transformed through the survival of trauma (Evans, 2021a; Lurie et al., 2020). One of the greatest strengths of PhotoVoice is that it is considered an inclusive intervention that challenges more ableist forms of treatment as projects can provide a vehicle for communication for those who may be otherwise limited in their ability to speak to tell their story and communicate in traditional interviewing techniques, which may be emotionally challenging particularly when recounting aspects of trauma, they have physical limitations, such as survivors of physical trauma and/or terminal illness (Balmer et al., 2015, Gunton et al., 2021).

There is a limited amount of studies that explicitly explore the intersection of PTG and PhotoVoice, which focused on the experiences of survivors of cancer, stroke, or sex trafficking, those living with HIV, survivors of 9/11, natural disasters, and most recently, coping with the COVID-19 pandemic (Dell et al., 2021; Devine et al., 2003; Evans, 2021b; Levy et al., 2020; Teti et al., 2015).

Connections between the Practice of PhotoVoice and the Domains of PTG

PhotoVoice has been found to enhance all five domains of PTG that have been documented in the United States and additional cultures, i.e. personal strength, new possibilities, relating to others, appreciation of life, and spirituality.

Personal Strength

Related to the domain of personal strength, finding one's voice through the actual photography process, reflecting on one's strengths and identity as a survivor, and exhibiting and captioning the images can be a way of tapping into own strength to reclaim their narrative following traumatic experience (Balakrisnan et al., 2017; Evans, 2021a, Teti et al., 2013). PhotoVoice allows for the photographer to learn new skills, use new equipment and demonstrate mastery of a creative and artistic process. As part of the image selection process, participants learn how to select the images that they feel tell their story in the most powerful manner, which respondents in numerous studies have reported increases their feelings of personal strength (Evans, 2021a; Lurie et al., 2020). Further, the skills used to exhibit one's images and connect to the community through the exhibition process taps into both personal strength and new possibilities. For example, Lurie et al. (2020) found that PhotoVoice contributes to increased personal strength in relation to addressing feelings of burnout in those who respond to trauma. Respondents felt that participatory photography helped with coping, alleviated feelings of burnout, and allowed participants to tap back into their own inner strength as they processed their work in trauma-related fields. Evans and colleagues (2021b) also found in their PhotoVoice work with survivors of sex trafficking that group participants reported that the project helped them strengthen their identity development and tap into their personal power. Teti et al. (2013) shared that the women participating in their PhotoVoice project about living with HIV reported that participation helped them feel validated, important, empowered, beautiful, and able to share their feelings as part of the project included taking self-portraits to challenge negative stereotypes about living with HIV.

New Possibilities

New possibilities can include experiences of learning the skills needed to engage in documentary photography as well as expressions of goals and dreams, and the development of new interests and opportunities, some of which may be directly related to the trauma that was experienced. While learning PhotoVoice as a process of self-expression is a new possibility in itself, the steps of the experience have been found to allow for a deepening of possibilities for those who participate in PhotoVoice projects and report that they did not know they had these skills within themselves. For example, Evans (2021b) found that the use of PhotoVoice allowed participants who identified as sex trafficking survivors to express in images some of their new goals and dreams as they went through the post-trafficking healing process. Participants shared that PhotoVoice also allowed them to process aspects of their experience, which had previously gone unnoticed. Lurie et al. (2020) found that participants in their study of volunteer docents from the 9/11 Families Association who traveled to Japan to support survivors of the 3/11 tsunami disaster, felt that in reflecting upon their images, previously un-noticed and/or unappreciated thoughts, feelings and questions could be processed through the photography and exhibit experience in a way that facilitated healing. New possibilities with the identity of the survivor can also be explored through PhotoVoice. Findings from Kabel et al.'s (2016) study on living with an HIV diagnosis showed that participants were able to express through PhotoVoice how they had become 'reacquainted' with themselves after the diagnosis and could work towards a new identity while Teti et al. (2013) found that participants, through both the taking of and the viewing back of their images reported gaining new insights about their survived experiences.

Relating to Others

Relating to others is perhaps the most strongly PTG domain facilitated by PhotoVoice as nearly everything about participating in PhotoVoice can enhance connecting to and processing with others. The benefits of social support in facilitating PTG have been well-documented (Ang et al., 2018; Beaupin et al., 2019; Devine et al., 2003; Evans, 2021a; Kabel et al. 2016) but are particularly present for those who have survived natural disasters. The creation of PhotoVoice groups allows others who have experienced or survived similar traumatic experiences to create a platform for sharing, which allows the processing of the trauma (Lurie et al., 2020) and lets survivors of the experience tell their story in a way that can form a community (Evans, 2021a).

In addition to the group experience of sharing and listening to each other's stories and experiences, there is the added layer of witnessing each other's photos, which also can provide tremendous social support (Budig et al., 2018; Devine et al., 2003; Evans, 2020, Lurie et al., 2020; Rolbiecki et al., 2016; Sadeghi, 2018). Multiple studies documented a particular transformation that occurs by choosing the images, sharing them with others, and having their images witnessed by others (Budig et al., 2018; Evans, 2021b; Lurie et al., 2020; Harley & Hunn, 2015). The weekly sharing of photographs and narratives allows for PhotoVoice participants to feel less alone, particularly when they see similar themes and images related to their own experiences reflected in the images taken by others in the group (Evans, 2020). As one of the participants in Evans' (2021b) study shared, "... the ways that I have found healing in the midst of it and the ways that [PhotoVoice] can really share that narrative and not just share the narrative but also share the future as well. It doesn't just tell the past narrative, it can also share the creation of a future narrative." (pp. 44, 45). Others from this study also reported that sharing images in an exhibition allowed them to feel as if they were helping others by possibly instilling hope in other survivors or by showing that goals and dreams are still possible even after living through such difficult events. Similarly, Balakrishnan et al. (2017) found that stroke survivors, after participating in the PhotoVoice projects felt more empowered to help others and reported an increase in their level of volunteering in the community. The final exhibition creates another layer of social support as community members outside of the group are invited to view a show that is cultivated with specific images in mind by the group participants. This exhibition allows for the story of the struggle experienced by the group members to be witnessed and therefore acknowledged and validated by others (Balakrishnan, 2017; Evans, 2021b).

Appreciation of Life

PhotoVoice participants often mention how the act of photography helps them discover more beauty in the world and see beauty that they had not seen prior to surviving a traumatic event (Balmer et al., 2015; Evans, 2021a). Kabel et al. (2016) found that participants reported after their PhotoVoice experience that they had a new appreciation for what they endured by living with HIV and that while they did not experience a 'restoration' back to their pre-diagnosis selves, they could reflect on themselves as survivors. Teti and colleagues (2015) found that individuals explored through PhotoVoice how their HIV diagnosis led them to make healthier life choices such as entering recovery from substance dependence, practicing safer sex, and addressing mental health issues. The transformative aspects of PhotoVoice have been found to lead to an overall cognitive shift by challenging issues that typically remain unexplored in everyday life and transforming them into topics worthy of critical dialogue (Chonody et al., 2013).

Spirituality

While participating in PhotoVoice does not typically inspire spiritual change as part of the posttraumatic process, themes of spirituality, and one's journey with faith can be processed through the use of imagery and PhotoVoice has been shown to offer a vehicle through which the spiritual change process can be documented and discussed. Levy et al. (2020) found that one theme expressed through PhotoVoice by caregivers to children battling cancer was images that shared how participants coped through prayer. Evans (2021b) shared how survivors of sex trafficking were able to describe how they used prayer to cope with the trauma as it happened, how they grappled with their spiritual identity, even as they were being abused and exploited by those with religious backgrounds and how religion had continued to provide support as they healed.

The images allow for an aesthetic expression of one's faith, faith-based internal change, struggles with faith, or as a vehicle to discuss faith (Ang et al., 2018; Evans, 2021b; Mulder, 2014; Teti et al., 2015). For those living with HIV, images explored what facing death, mortality, and grappling with a terminal illness on a day-to-day basis was like (Teti et al., 2013) and the role that spirituality may have when intersecting with these themes. Harley and Hunn (2015) used PhotoVoice to explore perceptions of hope and spirituality among low-income Black teens, particularly in the face of constant gang violence, and found that more than two-thirds of their participants shared images that described spirituality as a powerful source of hope. Similarly, Ang et al. (2018) recounted how nurses working on trauma units expressed in their imagery the importance that faith and spirituality played in both providing comfort and instilling a sense of resiliency. Pearce et al. (2017) found in their study of South Sudanese refugee women that faith and spirituality were identified as the primary source of instilling a sense of post-trauma resiliency and that PhotoVoice allowed participants to express the process of finding beauty in suffering as a key part of their spirituality journey.

Conclusion

PhotoVoice shows tremendous promise as both a research method and as a channel for promoting overall PTG. Communicating one's journey with trauma and the ensuing changes that occur can be effectively and therapeutically explored and expressed through the use of documentary ethical photography, the captioning process, and the within-group and within-community exhibitions that follow. As a critical vehicle for promoting individual healing and empowerment, community and structural change and as a means for making visible those who are often 'unseen' or socially marginalized, PhotoVoice remains one of the most powerful tools of advocacy, social change, and healing from trauma. Future research should look into how exhibitions have an overall impact on the community. More longitudinal studies to assess the lingering effects of participating in a PhotoVoice project and domains of PTG that may be produced from participating in the project are also needed.

References

Adegoke, C., & Steyn, M. (2017). A photo voice perspective on factors contributing to the \resilience of HIV positive Yoruba adolescent girls in Nigeria. *Journal of Adolescence*, *56*, 1–10. 10.1016/j.adolescence.2017.01.003

Aubeeluck, A., & Buchanan, H. (2006). Capturing the Huntington's disease spousal carer experience: A preliminary investigation using the 'Photovoice' method. *Dementia*, *5*(1), 95–116. 10.1177/1471301206059757

Ang, S., Uthaman, T., Ayre, T., Lim, S., & Lopez, V. (2018). A Photovoice study on nurses' perceptions and experience of resiliency. *Journal of Nursing Management*, *27*(2), 414–422. 10.1111/jonm.12702

Balakrishnan, R., Kaplan, B., Negron, R., Fei, K., Goldfinger, J. Z., & Horowitz, C. R. (2017). Life after stroke in an urban minority population: A photovoice project. *International Journal of Environmental Research and Public Health*, *14*(3), 293–304. 10.3390/ijerph14030293

Balmer, C., Griffiths, F., & Dunn, G. (2015). A 'new' normal: Exploring the disruption of a poor prognostic cancer diagnosis using interviews and participant-produced photographs. *Health*, *19*(5), 451–472. 10.1177/1363459314554319

Barrett, D. (2004). Photo-documenting the needle exchange: Methods and ethics. *Visual Studies*, *19*(4), 145–149. 10.1080/1472586042000301647

Baum, F., MacDougall, C., & Smith, D. (2006). Participatory action research. *Journal of Epidemiology and Community Health*, *60*(10), 854–857. 10.1136/jech.2004/028662

Beaupin, L., Pailler, M., Brewer-Spritzer, E., Kishel, E., Grant, P., Depner, R., Tenzek, K., & Breier, J. (2019). Photographs of meaning: A novel social media intervention for adolescent and young adult cancer patients. *Psychooncology*, *28*(1), 198–200. 10.1002/pon.4896

Budig, K., Diez, J., Conde, P. Sastre, M., Hernán, M., & Franco, M. (2018). Photovoice and empowerment: Evaluating the transformative potential of a participatory action research project. *BMC Public Health*, *18*(432). 10.1186/s12889-018-5335-7

Calhoun, R., & Tedeschi, R. (2009). *Handbook of post-traumatic growth: Research and practice.* NJ: Lawrence Erlbaum.

Chevalier, J. M., & Buckles, D. J. (2013). *Participatory action research: Theory and methods for engaged inquiry.* NY: Routledge.

Chonody, J., Ferman, B., Amitrani-Welsh, J., & Martin, T. (2013). Violence through the eyes of youth: A PhotoVoice exploration. *Journal of Community Psychology*, *41*(1), 84–101.

Christensen, M. C. (2018). Using photovoice to treat trauma resulting from gender-based violence. *Journal of Community Psychology*, *46*(7), 701–714. 10.1002/jcop.21967

Dell, N. A., Brandt-Lubart, K., & Maynard, B. R. (2021). Photovoice, COVID-19, and the possibility of post-traumatic growth. *Reflections: Narratives of Professional Helping*, *27*(2), 63–70.

Devine, D., Parker, P., Fouladi, R., & Cohen, L. (2003). The association between social support, intrusive thoughts, avoidance, and adjustment following an experimental cancer treatment. *Psychooncology*, *12*(5), 453–462. 10.1002/pon.656

Dobson, C. G. (2017). *Using photovoice to understand the meaning of social participation as it impacts transitions for student veterans* (Order No. 10681861). ProQuest Dissertations & Theses Global (1984977558).

Drainoni, M. L., Childs, E., Biello, K. B., Biancarelli, D. L., Edeza, A., Salhaney, P., Mimiaga, M. J., & Bazzi, A. R. (2019). "We don't get much of a voice about anything": Perspectives on photovoice among people who inject drugs. *Harm Reduction Journal*, *16*(1), 1–8. 10.1186/s12954-019-0334-2

Evans, H. (2020). The integral role of relationships in experiences of complex trauma in sex trafficking survivors. *International Journal of Human Rights in Healthcare*, *13*, 109–123. 10.1108/IJHRH-07-2019-0054

Evans, H. (2021a). *From the voices of domestic sex trafficking survivors: Photographic expressions of complex trauma and posttraumatic growth.* Allentown.

Evans, H. (2021b). *Understanding complex trauma and post-traumatic growth in survivors of sex trafficking: Foregrounding women's voices for effective care and prevention.* NY: Routledge.

Freire, P. (1970). *Pedagogy of the oppressed.* NY: Penguin Books.

Gunton, A., Hansen, G., & Schellenberg, K. (2021). Photovoice as a participatory research tool in Amyotrophic Lateral Sclerosis. *Journal of Neuromuscular Diseases*, *8*(1), 91–99. 10.3233/JND-200537

Harley, D., & Hunn, V. (2015). Utilization of Photovoice to explore hope and spirituality among low-income African American adolescents. *Child and Adolescent Social Work Journal*, *32*(1), 3–15. 10.1007/s10560-014-0354-4

Kabel, A., Teti, M., & Zhang, N. (2016). The art of resilience: Photo-stories of inspiration and strength among people with HIV/AIDS. *Visual Studies*, *31*(3), 221–230. 10.1080/1472586X.2016.1210991

Kutluturkan, S., Sozeri, E., Uysal, N., & Bay, F. (2016). Resilience and burnout status among nurses working in oncology. *Annals of General Psychiatry*, *15*(1), 1–9. 10.1186/s12991-016-0121-3

Lepore, S., & Revenson, T. (2006). Resilience and posttraumatic growth: Recovery, resistance and reconfiguration. In R. Calhoun, & R. Tedeschi (Eds.), *Handbook of Posttraumatic Growth: Research and Practice* (pp. 24–46). NJ: Lawrence Erlbaum.

Levy, K.,.Grant, P., Tenzek, K., Depner, R., Pailler, M., & Beaupin, L. (2020). The experience of pediatric palliative caregiving: a qualitative analysis from the photographs of meaning program. *American Journal of Hospice and Palliative Medicine*, *37*(5), 364–370.

Liebenberg, L. (2018). Thinking critically about Photovoice: Achieving empowerment and social change. *International Journal of Qualitative Methods*, *17*(1), 1–9. 10.1177/1609406918757631

Lurie, J. M., Lever, H., Godson, L., Lyons, D. Yanagisama, R., & Katz, C. (2020). Instilling hope and resiliency: A narrative photo-taking intervention during an intercultural exchange involving 9/11 survivors in post 3/11 Japan. *The Journal of Nervous and Mental Disease*, *208*(6), 488–497.

Meichenbaum, D. (2006). Resilience and posttraumatic growth: A constructive narrative perspective. In R. Calhoun, & R. Tedeschi (Eds.), *Handbook of Posttraumatic Growth: Research and Practice* (pp. 355–367). NJ: Lawrence Erlbaum.

Mulder, C. (2014). Unraveling students' experiences with religion and spirituality in the classroom using a PhotoVoice method: Implications for MSW programs. *Social Work and Christianity, 41*(1), 16–44.

Orton, L., Elkins, T., Watson, K., & Warnock, B. (2016). *PhotoVoice Manual.* www.photovoice.org.

Pearce, E., McMurray, K., Walsh, C. A., & Malek, L. (2017). Searching for Tomorrow - South Sudanese women reconstructing resilience through Photovoice. *Journal of International Migration and Integration, 18*(2), 369–389.

Prins, E. (2010). Participatory photography: A tool for empowerment or surveillance? *Action Research, 8*(4), 426–443. 10.1177/1476750310374502

Rolbiecki, A., Anderson, K., Teti, M., & Albright, D. L. (2016). "Waiting for the cold to end": Using Photovoice as a narrative intervention for survivors of sexual assault. *Traumatology, 22*(4), 242–248. 10.1037/trm0000087

Sadeghi, S. (2018). *Photovoice, a long of belonging among Iranian immigrants.* Notre Dame de Namur University. ProQuest Dissertations Publishing, 27544877.

Saita, E., Accordini, M., & Loewenthal, D. (2019). Constructing positive narrative identities in a forensic setting: A single case evaluation of phototherapy. *International Journal of Prisoner Health, 15*(1), 76–90. 10.1108/IJPH-11-2017-0057

Taminiaux, P. (2009). *The paradox of Photography.* Rodopi.

Teti, M., Pichon, L., Kabel, A., Farnan, A. R., & Binson, D. (2013). Taking pictures to take control: Photovoice as a tool to facilitate empowerment among poor and racial/ethnic minority women with HIV. *Journal of the Association of Nurses in AIDS Care, 24*(6), 539–553. 10.1016/j.jana.2013.05.001

Teti, M., French, B., Bonney, L., & Lightfoot, M. (2015). I created something new with something that had died: Photo-narratives of positive transformation among women with HIV. *AIDS Behavior, 19*(7), 1275–1287. 10.1007/s10461-015-1000-7

Wang, C. (1999). Photovoice: A participatory action research strategy applied to women's health. *Journal of Women's Health, 8*(2), 185–192. 10.1089/jwh.1999.8.185

Wang, C., & Burris, M. A. (1994). Empowerment through photo novella: Portraits of participation. *Health Education Quarterly, 21*(2), 171–186. 10.1177/109019819402100204

Wang, C., & Burris, M. A. (1997). Photovoice: Concept, methodology, and use for participatory needs assessment. *Health Education & Behavior, 24*(3), 369–387. 10.1177/109019819702400309

Weiser, J. (2004). PhotoTherapy techniques in counseling and therapy: Using ordinary snapshots and photo-interactions to help clients heal their lives. *Canadian Art Therapy Association Journal, 17*(2), 23–53. 10.1080/08322473.2004.11432263

44

ENHANCING PTG IN A COUPLE'S PTSD INTERVENTION

Clients' and Therapists' Successes and Challenges

Rachel Dekel and Yael Shoval

Posttraumatic stress disorder (PTSD) is one of the most frequently diagnosed disorders following a traumatic event. It includes four symptom clusters: involuntary, intrusive memories and flashbacks; persistent avoidance of trauma-related stimuli; negative alterations in cognitions and mood; and alterations in arousal symptoms (APA, 2013). The frequently chronic nature of PTSD causes many individuals to experience ongoing significant functional and social impairments, affecting many areas of their lives (Bestha et al., 2018; Woodhouse et al., 2018).

The traumatization of an individual can have a "ripple effect" on relationships with close family members, especially spouses (Dekel & Monson, 2010). Partners of loved ones coping with PTSD have been found to suffer from emotional distress (Diehle et al., 2017; Renshaw et al., 2011), anxiety and depression (Murphy et al., 2016; Taft et al., 2017), caregiver burden (Beckham et al., 1996; Caska et al., 2014), overall lower functioning and mental health (Silove et al., 2017; Turgoose & Murphy, 2019), and increased physiological reactivity to couple conflict (Caska et al., 2014).

Given the bidirectional association between PTSD and intimate relationships, several couples-based interventions for PTSD have been created and examined empirically, including behavioral family therapy, emotionally-focused couples' therapy, strategic approach therapy, and cognitive-behavioral conjoint therapy for PTSD (CBCT for PTSD). To date, CBCT for PTSD has accumulated the most supportive evidence among diverse samples (Pukay-Martin et al., 2016). Moreover, this protocol directly addresses posttraumatic growth (PTG) in the last two meetings of the intervention. Indeed, one study that assessed changes in PTG using this protocol found that PTSD severity and PTG scores significantly improved in comparison to these same metrics among the waiting list control group (Wagner et al., 2016).

Although some studies have documented an association between reduced PTSD and increased PTG following individual PTSD interventions (Roepke, 2015), most of these studies have assessed PTG quantitatively via the use of questionnaires. Therefore, we know very little about the factors that promote the effectiveness of PTSD therapies in facilitating PTG and how the idea and implementation of PTG is developed throughout the intervention; e.g., how an intervention that is focused on reducing PTSD distress and increasing

DOI: 10.4324/9781032208688-55

PTG holds both the distress and the PTG simultaneously. Moreover, as these studies have assessed only individual interventions, we do not know enough about the role of the partner in the process. Finally, we have no knowledge about the challenges faced by therapists and clients regarding the implementation of the PTG concept in PTSD interventions.

In this chapter, we review the cognitive processes that underlie the development of PTG and current knowledge regarding changes in PTG in the context of PTSD interventions as well as highlight existing gaps in the knowledge. We describe an intervention that followed the CBCT protocol in the treatment of Israeli couples, in which one partner was diagnosed with PTSD, and our study analyzed videos of two sessions, which focused on PTG in these couples. We report documented manifestations of PTG in couples' reports, unveil the role of significant others in this process, and explore challenges faced by both partners and their therapists in conceptualizing and promoting PTG.

PTG and Cognitive Processing

The PTG process model is based primarily on the work of Janoff-Bulman (1992), with the idea that over the course of their lives, people develop a set of core beliefs about the self and the world, which is influenced by their life circumstances and their culture. In the aftermath of a stressful event, these core beliefs might be challenged, and the previous foundations of a person's assumptive world may become unstable and uncontrollable. In order to manage the distress and reappraise the pre-trauma cognitive schemas, the survivor initiates various cognitive mechanisms, such as using coping strategies, seeking social support, and – importantly – engaging in cognitive processing, specifically rumination, in an attempt to give meaning to the stressful experience (Danhauer et al., 2013).

Rumination encompasses two broad types of repetitive thinking: intrusive rumination and deliberate rumination. *Intrusive rumination* is not totally under a person's control and is more likely to be related to posttraumatic distress. *Deliberate rumination* represents a person's attempt to understand the implications of a traumatic event and to restore or revise their set of core beliefs in the aftermath of trauma. This process can result in PTG (Cann et al., 2011). PTG is considered to be an outcome of cognitive processing and could therefore be part of cognitive behavioral therapy (CBT) for PTSD, even if the goal of this therapy is not specifically PTG. An additional contribution of CBT to PTG could be training people in skills that are found to promote growth such as how to recruit social support, share vulnerable information with others, engage in meaningful activities, and use various coping skills (Bower & Segerstrom, 2004).

PTG Changes during PTSD Therapy

A few studies have reported on the development of PTG during PTSD therapy. Roepke (2015) found in a meta-analysis based on 12 treatment studies that psychosocial interventions increased PTG to a small degree, even though most of the interventions were not specifically designed to target growth. Several different interventions have been shown to promote growth, such as stress management training, skills training, and CBT (Roepke, 2015). Only some of these interventions focused on PTSD (Schubert et al., 2016), and all of them used the PTG inventory. Schubert et al.'s (2019) unique contribution was that they assessed PTG as an outcome of trauma-focused CBT for PTSD by self-report and the report of significant others. During the course of treatment, PTSD severity declined, whereas PTG levels did not change. However, they found a strong association between the PTG of both assessments suggesting that the positive changes in patients were recognizable by significant others. Recent evidence confirmed the longitudinal association between PTG and PTSD severity in clients with a diagnosis of PTSD. Nijdam et al. (2018) investigated PTG during two different trauma-focused psychotherapies, i.e. eye movement desensitization and reprocessing (EMDR) therapy and brief eclectic psychotherapy. Their findings showed that PTG scores increased significantly after trauma-focused psychotherapy, as did the scores in the sub-domains of personal strength, new possibilities, relating to others, and appreciation of life. Additionally, a greater self-reported and clinician-rated PTSD decline was related significantly to a greater increase in PTG. This finding was similar in both types of the abovementioned PTSD interventions.

Although overall, studies suggest that trauma-focused CBT can facilitate growth and that an increase in PTG is associated with a decrease in PTSD, there is a need to better understand PTG as a treatment goal as well as the factors that enhance the effectiveness of PTSD therapies in promoting PTG (Roepke, 2015). The next section presents a study of couples receiving CBCT for PTSD (including its structure, principles, and process) and findings relative to PTG following the intervention.

The Study

Fourteen heterosexual cohabiting dyads participated in a pilot trial, which was conducted at Bar-Ilan University in Israel. One member of each dyad had PTSD (henceforth referred to as the client), while the partner did not. Both partners were between 24 and 71 years old, (with an average age of 42.4) with no current substance use disorder, active suicidal planning or intent, mania, psychosis, or severe partner aggression. Two of the participants with PTSD (i.e., the clients) were women and 12 were men, and all had received prior psychological or pharmacological PTSD treatments. Ten clients had experienced combat-related traumatic events and four had experienced multiple traumatic events (including childhood physical and/or sexual abuse, and car accident). Couples had been together from 1–52 years, with an average of 15.57 years ($SD = 12.81$), and had 2.45 children on average (for a full study description, see Monson et al., 2012).

Participants in the study were treated with CBCT for PTSD. This treatment protocol is a 15-session couples' therapy designed to treat PTSD and enhance relationship functioning (Monson & Fredman, 2012). Each session is designed to last 75 minutes and concludes with between-session assignments designed to facilitate the couple's use of the skills learned outside of therapy sessions. The treatment consists of three phases. *Phase 1* focuses on psychoeducation about the reciprocal influences of PTSD and relationship functioning and uses behavioral strategies to increase positive affect and behaviors. *Phase 2* focuses on the development of communication skills and combating PTSD-related avoidance and emotional numbing so as to increase relationship satisfaction. *Phase 3* focuses on cognitive work to address the meaning-making of the trauma and reduce negative cognitive patterns related to both trauma and relational beliefs that maintain PTSD and relationship problems. This phase (Sessions 8 to 15) capitalizes on the couple's increased satisfaction and skills learned during Phases 1 and 2 by targeting trauma-related cognitions that maintain both PTSD symptoms and relationship problems (e.g., "I have to be in control at all times," "She is too damaged to ever recover from PTSD"). Phase 3 starts with targeting cognitions specific to appraisals of the traumatic event(s) and proceeds to address interpersonal beliefs disrupted or seemingly confirmed by the trauma.

The treatment culminates with Session 14's focus on the potential for individual and couple-level PTG, e.g. inquiring if the couples have noticed any positive aspects that have emerged despite the client's having experienced a traumatic event and its aftereffects, i.e. did they experienced any gains as a result of going through treatment together. The final session (Session 15) starts with a review of the out-of-session assignments regarding PTG with the aim of helping couples consolidate the gains achieved in psychotherapy, anticipate fluctuations in their individual and relationship functioning over time, plans for addressing inevitable lapses and promote ongoing skill use in the future. All the sessions were recorded.

To assess the pilot study, we used the video documentation of meetings 14 and 15 with the couples. The 14 videos that were shown to be of good technical quality were used for the analysis. These videos were analyzed (by the two authors) in three steps. First, we watched individually the entirety of the sessions and documented the main themes that were repeated in the videos and then we compared topics. This analysis yielded three main clusters of PTG (a greater sense of personal strength, changes in personal relationships, and recognition of new possibilities or paths for one's life) as well as clients' and therapists' challenges. In the second step, having now established the general categories, we watched the videos again and inserted any reference that we felt belonged in a particular category. This process allowed for an elaboration of some of the categories; for example, we divided the partner's role into supporting or invalidating the other partner's PTG. Finally, we fine-tuned the main categories and challenges that we had documented. We then looked for additional citations to flesh out some of the categories and checked whether we had enough citations for each category. The aim of this process was to increase the internal validity of each category by having more citations and thus, confirm that the category was indeed reflected by what was revealed in the videos.

Findings

Our study generated four main findings relative to PTG in couples struggling with a spouse's PTSD diagnosis. They included support for domains of PTG, The role of the partner, clients' challenges, and therapists' challenges.

Support for PTG Domains

Our study supported three domains of PTG: a greater sense of personal strength, changes in personal relationships, and recognition of new possibilities or paths for one's life (Tedeschi & Calhoun, 1996).

GREATER SENSE OF PERSONAL STRENGTH

Both partners reported changes in terms of having more positive perceptions of themselves. The verbal expressions they used were in line with expressions that have been documented in previous studies, such as: "I am a survivor" or "What does not kill you makes you stronger." Others said: "I know how to better cope now" or "I know I am strong;

I survived what happened to me." One participant added: "Today, I listen much more to myself, to what my internal self wants." A few (among both partners) added that they had acquired new coping skills, or the ability to cope by themselves.

In relation to the self, there were additional specific references to the way they perceived PTSD and coped with it. For example, Couple 8 said:

> We had a conversation; we talked about how to 'get out of' the PTSD, and how to recover from it. We came to the conclusion that it will always be there, and we simply have to know how to cope with it.

Another couple said: "We have learned that we can live with the PTSD. I feel that I have the tools to cope with PTSD." A female client said:

> I understand that the moments [of fear] are temporary. One thing I used to fear was when I thought something was wrong with me physically. Today, I know that this feeling is PTSD, that it will pass if I give it a second. I do breathing exercises, or I take a shower.

CHANGES IN PERSONAL RELATIONS

Participants mentioned positive changes in their marital/intimate relations. For example: "My partner and I are closer because of having gone through all those difficult events together. Those difficulties strengthened us as a couple to face challenges together." Another shared that his nuclear family became more united and yet another said that thanks to the trauma she realized how important she was to others. One man talked about his choice of a partner:

> The trauma proved to me that I made the right choice in choosing my wife as a life partner. I realized how committed and dedicated my spouse is to me. My wife came to all the meetings with me. I was always afraid to talk about the traumatic thing that happened to me and now we are both united in the treatment and in accepting what happened to me; it enhances my trust in her.

One partner said, "We are back to being a united team, and the level of trust with our children has also improved."; another addressed the partner directly regarding the matter of being more united: "I've always seen that you have difficulties, but now you let me go down into the pit with you and give you a hand so that we can climb back up together." One partner added: "I am not afraid of him anymore. I can tell him things."

In addition, participants talked about their relations with their children and their extended families. For example: "Today I understand that the post-trauma has allowed me to be a better, more sensitive parent, and to be a present dad at home after years of only working all day." Another added: "I feel that the PTSD united my family. Good things happened following my injury; I met my wife, and my children were born." One partner shared that their children said the treatment had helped her and her partner, and that their relationship had gotten better. Such comments were also made in regard to the extended family: "The relationship with my parents and with my siblings has changed;

I had to share the situation with them, in order to help me and my wife, and now we feel closer to each other."

RECOGNITION OF NEW POSSIBILITIES OR PATHS FOR ONE'S LIFE

Individuals and their partners related to changes in preferences and style of living. For example, "I realized that even though something bad had happened to me in the past, my partner and I could decide together how to live the fullest possible life from now on." Another shared: "I discovered the power of motherhood for me; I wanted to be strong for my daughters." One woman shared that the trauma had changed her perspective and led to her wanting to improve her life; therefore, she quit her job and found a place that suited her better. Finally, one woman shared that if this was the path she had to go down, including the trauma, in order for her twins to be born, she would go through it a thousand more times.

The Role of the Partner

Partners had two main roles, i.e. validating the client's PTG, and helping to point out positive changes in the client's PTG. *Validation* occurred in many cases when partners confirmed the client's PTG, reacting to their highlighting a specific change by saying, "Yes, it is true. I can see it.", "Indeed, yes this happened," or "Yes, you are stronger than your friends." However, in a few cases, when an individual talked about and shared positive changes that had taken place, the partner reacted with a non-validating remark, such as: "I do not feel that positive things have happened as a result of the traumatic event", "I do not share the view that good changes have taken place." or, "I see it as a weight, like an iron ball, that makes walking and functioning difficult; everything becomes a war." *Helping to point out positive changes in the client's PTG* became evident especially, though not exclusively when the latter had difficulty in identifying such changes. For example, a partner said: "This thing is horrible, but are there tiny things, maybe, that you can see as positive?" And the client responded: "Like what? I cannot think of an example, can you?" In another attempt to highlight the client's PTG, a partner talked about community activities aimed to prevent and address sexual abuse in which the client was engaged:

Client: To whom does it contribute?
Partner: It contributes to other people, that's who! To other girls who get into trouble. There was a girl on Facebook who you helped for the first two days after the traumatic event she underwent, and that's hardly the only such event. You have a whole page with a lot of followers, a page that deals with how to behave after an attack.

Another individual told her partner (i.e., the client):

> Growth is not about erasing everything you went through, nor is it about ignoring it or branding it as positive. It's about accepting and seeing all the things that have grown in you and changed for the better, and there is an abundance of such things.

Clients' Challenges

One challenge was related to the clients' struggle to hold both the distress and the PTG simultaneously. Clients were still so focused on their distress that they could not find any manifestation of PTG. As part of the effort to document the PTG, one client said:

> I do not feel that this experience is something that has contributed to my personality, except for taking something away from it. I have my partner, but all the rest is awful. I am less successful than I used to be.

In response to the therapist's attempt to identify some PTG, one female client answered:

> I do not see it as meaningful. I was a person with potential, and I was successful in what I used to do. Let's say there is someone who is very successful and could be a prime minister or a basketball player. Now he paints lovely water paintings. Great, but this is not comparable to what he (or me) could be doing; that potential was lost.

As part of the intervention, we attempted to find cognitions that were not helpful and impeded the potential for PTG. Patients shared a few of their cognitions: "If I do find some positive aspects in the traumatic event that happened to me, then does that mean that what I went through was not so traumatic?" "If I see positive things in what happened to me, it might lessen the attacker's guilt and responsibility." "If I am in a better situation today, does that imply that what I have gone through has not been that bad?"

Therapists' Challenges

The analysis suggested that it was challenging for therapists to conceptualize PTG for couples (although psychoeducation on PTG was part of meeting 14). Some therapists phrased things in a cumbersome manner and spent an extensive amount of time focusing on out-of-session assignments rather than moving to the PTG psychoeducation stage. Other therapists began the discussion on PTG with apologetic phrases regarding the necessity of moving on to talking about PTG rather than staying with the challenges of PTSD. For example: "I know it might be difficult for you, but can you think of or identify any positive experiences following the trauma you underwent?" Others exhibited a lack of confidence in the protocol and said regarding the final meetings, which focused on PTG: "You might find this particular meeting less helpful to you compared to the earlier meetings." Finally, although the therapists met the demand to document positive changes that had occurred as well as negative cognitive biases that hindered PTG, the former (i.e., the documentation of positive changes) was shorter than the latter, and the focus was on biases that hindered PTG.

Conclusions and Implications

The findings of the presented study provide evidence of multiple PTG manifestations among clients with PTSD who came to our clinic for CBCT. When focusing on the PTG process, clients and their spouses demonstrated experiences of positive changes in their own perceptions and in how they perceived their intimate relations. Couples talked about acquiring personal strengths, feeling more united, and having the ability to share their emotions with their nuclear and extended family and feeling closer to them. Moreover, although the focus of the protocol is on the couple's relationship, and thus one might expect positive changes in this realm, additional changes were noticed regarding couples' relationships with their children and their extended families. These findings support the notion that whereas PTSD creates circles of vulnerability, couple interventions could create circles of recovery and healing.

Although there is no specific focus within the PTG conceptualization on positive changes in perceptions of the traumatic event, diagnosis, or illness, we found that clients and their spouses did indeed mention specific changes in their perceptions of PTSD. Some clients spoke about learning to live with the disorder; others understood the temporal dynamic of the anxiety symptoms and reported that they had learned to cope with them. These results are consistent with the aims of the CBCT intervention, which focuses on both promoting couple relations and combating PTSD and conveys a message of recovery. Based on this observation, we suggest that changing perceptions of PTSD itself should be an aim for additional PTSD interventions. Moreover, that couples reported changes in multiple aspects of their lives suggests widening the scope of clinical recovery (Yes/No PTSD) to a broader personal recovery. The implication is that recovery is a unique and dynamic process involving changing attitudes, values, emotions, goals, and/or roles, enabling a life of satisfaction, hope, and meaning despite the limitations caused by the disease (Leonhardt et al., 2017).

Our findings support earlier findings that both partners experience and report PTG throughout the process of coping with PTSD (Zwahlen et al., 2010). Moreover, the spouse can be helpful in facilitating PTG in two main roles. Consistent with earlier findings (e.g. Manne, 2004), partners validated patients' reports of PTG. They also learned through the intervention to serve as a possible source of highlighting PTG and indicating where it exists. Spouses tried to help balance the picture and point out "the positive" to their suffering partners. Obtaining information from the spouses helped us distinguish between perceptions of growth, i.e., the ways in which people *think* they have changed, and actual observable growth behaviors as perceived and reported by others (Schubert et al., 2019).

However, we also found that spouses could make invalidating comments about clients' PTG reports. Some partners moved the discussion away from PTG toward distress and suffering or continuously mentioned how they, themselves, did not see any PTG in their partner. Studies regarding the association between partners' perceptions of PTG have yielded mixed findings, with some reporting an association and others not. Moreover, a partner's responsiveness has been found to mediate between mutual perceptions of PTG (Canevello et al., 2016). These findings suggest that although listening, responsiveness, and strengthening of both partners as a dyad were promoted through our intervention process, not every couple achieved these results in relation to PTG.

We were surprised by the therapists' challenges in working with the concept of PTG as reflected in their using cumbersome phrasing with the couples and having difficulty holding together both the distress and the PTG. Although this challenge has been documented theoretically and empirically in the literature, we found relatively little guidance for working with therapists on promoting PTG. Calhoun and Tedeschi (2008) offered advice on working with patients in a clinical setting, advising practitioners to learn about the PTG phenomenon themselves and then "become the expert companion" in patients' potential journey to growth. Reframing patients' perceptions can develop through their own insights, but having a therapist who listens, believes, and is aware of such ideas could strengthen the PTG process (Tedeschi et al., 2015). We would recommend that part of the learning of the protocol and the supervision should focus on PTG and the personal perceptions of the therapists regarding PTG. Moreover, a clearer distinction should be made in the protocol between documenting the different facets of growth and documenting the cognitive challenges to such growth.

The contribution of the findings of the study reported in this chapter should be recognized in light of its limitations. The PTG results might have been different and improved had the therapists been better acquainted with and more experienced at using the protocol as a result of training in applying the protocol. Moreover, because only 14 couples were studied, the findings should be generalized with caution. Despite these limitations, the study offers several practical and theoretical contributions to the field. First, it adds to the understanding of the PTG phenomenon and how it develops through the intervention of CBCT for PTSD, facilitating an understanding of treatment processes rather than exclusively outcomes. The study also highlights changes in clients' perceptions of PTSD, the role of the partners, and the need to work with therapists in order to facilitate and encourage clients' PTG. Finally, our findings strengthen the idea that PTG is a socially dependent process, i.e., it likely emerges with interpersonal, community-based, or societal encouragement (Harvey & Berndt, 2021), thus supporting the inclusion of spouses and therapists in this process.

References

American Psychiatric Association. (2013). *Diagnostic and Statistical Manual of Mental Disorders* (5th ed.). Washington, DC: Author.

Beckham, J. C., Lytle, B. L., & Feldman, M. E. (1996). Caregiver burden in partners of Vietnam. *Journal of Consulting and Clinical Psychology, 64*(5), 1068–1072. 10.1037/0022-006X.64.5.1068

Bestha, D., Soliman, L., Blankenship, K., & Rachal, J. (2018). The walking wounded: Emerging treatments for PTSD established treatments for military. *Current Psychiatry Reports, 20*(94), 1–8. 10.1007/s11920-018-0941-8

Bower, J. E., & Segerstrom, S. C. (2004). Stress management, finding benefit, and immune function: Positive mechanisms for intervention effects on physiology. *Journal of Psychosomatic Research, 56*(1), 9–11.

Calhoun. L. G., & Tedeschi, R. G. (2008). The paradox of struggling with trauma: Guidelines for practice and directions for research. In S. Joseph, & P. A. Linley (Eds.), *Trauma, recovery, and growth: Positive psychological perspectives on posttraumatic stress* (pp. 325–338). New York: John Wiley & Sons.

Canevello, A., Michels, V., & Hilaire, N. (2016). Supporting close others' growth after trauma: The role of responsiveness in romantic partners' mutual posttraumatic growth. *Psychological Trauma: Theory, Research, Practice, and Policy, 8*(3), 334–342.

Cann, A., Calhoun, L. G., Tedeschi, R. G., Triplett, K. N., Vishnevsky, T., & Lindstrom, C. M. (2011). Assessing posttraumatic cognitive processes: The event related rumination inventory. *Anxiety, Stress, & Coping, 24*(2), 137–156.

Caska, C. M., Smith, T. W., Renshaw, K. D., Allen, S. N., Uchino, B. N., Birmingham, W., & Carlisle, M. (2014). Posttraumatic stress disorder and responses to couple conflict: Implications for cardiovascular risk. *Health Psychology, 33*(11), 1273–1280. 10.1037/hea0000133

Dekel, R., & Monson, C. M. (2010). Military-related post-traumatic stress disorder and family relations: Current knowledge and future directions. *Aggression and Violent Behavior, 15*(4), 303–309.

Danhauer, S. C., Case, L. D., Tedeschi, R., Russell, G., Vishnevsky, T., Triplett, K., Ip, E. H., & Avis, N. E. (2013). Predictors of posttraumatic growth in women with breast cancer. *Psycho-oncology, 22*(12), 2676–2683. doi: 10.1002/pon.3298

Diehle, J., Brooks, S. K., & Greenberg, N. (2017). Veterans are not the only ones suffering from posttraumatic stress symptoms: What do we know about dependents' secondary traumatic stress? *Social Psychiatry and Psychiatric Epidemiology, 52*(1), 35–44. 10.1007/s00127-016-1292-6

Harvey, J., & Berndt, M. (2021). Cancer caregiver reports of post-traumatic growth following spousal hematopoietic stem cell transplant. *Anxiety, Stress, & Coping, 34*(4), 397–410.

Janoff-Bulman, R. (1992). *Shattered assumptions: Towards a new psychology of trauma*. Free Press.

Leonhardt, B. L., Huling, K., Hamm, J. A., Roe, D., Hasson-Ohayon, I., McLeod, H. J., & Lysaker, P. H. (2017). Recovery and serious mental illness: a review of current clinical and research paradigms and future directions. *Expert Review of Neurotherapeutics*, *17*(11), 1117–1130. 10.1080/14737175.2017.1378099

Manne, S., Ostroff, J., Winkel, G., Goldstein, L., Fox, K., & Grana, G. (2004). Posttraumatic growth after breast cancer: Patient, partner, and couple perspectives. *Psychosomatic Medicine*, *66*(3), 442–454. 10.1097/01.psy.0000127689.38525.7d

Monson, C. M., & Fredman, S. J. (2012). *Cognitive-behavioral conjoint therapy for PTSD: Harnessing the healing power of relationships*. Guilford Press.

Murphy, D., Palmer, E., & Busuttil, W. (2016). Mental health difficulties and help-seeking beliefs within a sample of female partners of UK veterans diagnosed with post-traumatic stress disorder. *Journal of Clinical Medicine*, *5*(8), 68–81. 10.3390/jcm5080068

Nijdam, M. J., van der Meer, C. A., van Zuiden, M., Dashtgard, P., Medema, D., Qing, Y., Zhutovsky P., Bakker A., & Olff, M. (2018). Turning wounds into wisdom: Posttraumatic growth over the course of two types of trauma-focused psychotherapy in patients with PTSD. *Journal of Affective Disorders*, *227*, 424–431. 10.1016/j.jad.2017.11.031

Pukay-Martin, N. D., Macdonald, A., Fredman, S. J., & Monson, C. M. (2016). Couple therapy for PTSD. *Current Treatment Options in Psychiatry*, *3*(1), 37–47.

Renshaw, K. D., Allen, E. S., Rhoades, G. K., Blais, R. K., Markman, J., & Stanley, S. M. (2011). Distress in spouses of service members with symptoms of combat-related PTSD: Secondary traumatic stress or general psychological distress? *Journal of Family Psychology*, *25*(4), 461–469. 10.1037/a0023994

Roepke, A. M. (2015). Psychosocial interventions and posttraumatic growth: A meta-analysis. *Journal of Consulting and Clinical Psychology*, *83*(1), 129–142. 10.1037/a0036872

Silove, D. M., Tay, A. K., Steel, Z., Tam, N., Soares, Z., Soares, C., Dos Reis, N., Alves, A., & Rees, S. (2017). Symptoms of post-traumatic stress disorder, severe psychological distress, explosive anger and grief amongst partners of survivors of high levels of trauma in post-conflict Timor-Leste. *Psychological Medicine*, *47*(1), 149–159. 10.1017/S0033291716002233

Schubert, C. F., Schmidt, U., & Rosner, R. (2016). Posttraumatic growth in populations with posttraumatic stress disorder—A systematic review on growth-related psychological constructs and biological variables. *Clinical psychology & psychotherapy*, *23*(6), 469–486.

Schubert, C. F., Schmidt, U., Comtesse, H., Gall-Kleebach, D., & Rosner, R. (2019). Posttraumatic growth during cognitive behavioural therapy for posttraumatic stress disorder: Relationship to symptom change and introduction of significant other assessment. *Stress and Health*, *35*(5), 617–625.

Taft, C. T., Creech, S. K., & Murphy, C. M. (2017). Anger and aggression in PTSD. *Current Opinion in Psychology*, *14*, 67–71. 10.1016/j.copsyc.2016.11.008

Tedeschi, R. G., & Calhoun, L. G. (1996). The Posttraumatic Growth Inventory: Measuring the positive legacy of trauma. *Journal of Traumatic Stress*, *9*(3), 455–471. 10.1007/BF02103658

Tedeschi, R. G., Calhoun, L. G., & Groleau, J. M. (2015). Clinical applications of posttraumatic growth. In S. Joseph (Ed.), *Positive psychology in practice: Promoting human flourishing in work, health, education, and everyday life* (pp. 503–518), NJ: John Wiley & Sons.

Turgoose, D., & Murphy, D. (2019). A systematic review of interventions for supporting partners of military veterans with PTSD. *Journal of Military, Veteran and Family Health*, *5*(2), 195–208. 10.3138/jmvfh.2018-0035

Wagner, A. C., Torbit, L., Jenzer, T., Landy, M. S., Pukay-Martin, N. D., Macdonald, A., Fredman, S. J., & Monson, C. M. (2016). The role of posttraumatic growth in a randomized controlled trial of cognitive–behavioral conjoint therapy for PTSD. *Journal of Traumatic Stress*, *29*(4), 379–383.

Woodhouse, S., Brown, R., Ayers, S., Woodhouse, S., Brown, R., & Ayers, S. (2018). A social model of posttraumatic stress disorder (PTSD): Interpersonal trauma, attachment, group identification, disclosure, social acknowledgement and negative cognitions. *Journal of Theoretical Social Psychology*, *2*(2), 35–48. 10.1002/jts5.17

Zwahlen, D., Hagenbuch, N., Carley, M. I., Jenewein, J., & Buchi, S. (2010). Posttraumatic growth in cancer patients and partners—effects of role, gender and the dyad on couples' posttraumatic growth experience. *Psycho-Oncology*, *19*(1), 12–20. 10.1002/pon.1486

45

INTERVENTIONS FOR ENHANCING POSTTRAUMATIC GROWTH FOLLOWING A PHYSICAL DISEASE

Catarina Ramos, Romina Nunes, and Margarida Almeida

Chronic diseases are long-term health conditions that require continuous medical attention and/or cause disability (Centers for Disease Control and Prevention [CDC], 2022). More than 70% of all deaths worldwide are attributed to chronic conditions, such as cardiovascular diseases, respiratory diseases, cancer, diabetes, or mental illnesses. Cancer alone was responsible for approximately 10 million deaths in 2020 (World Health Organization [WHO], 2020). The existence of multimorbidity is common (Australian Institute of Health and Welfare, 2021). In developed countries between 16% to 57% of adults suffer from more than one chronic disease at the same time (Hajat & Stein, 2018).

The Impact of Chronic Illness

Scientific evidence has described the diagnosis of a severe illness as a possible traumatic event. Unlike acute diseases, a chronic illness is long-lasting and requires an adaptation and change in behavior for both the individual and the family (Larsen, 2013). The majority of chronic diseases disrupt the functionality and daily life of those afflicted due to their severity and the level of treatment required. Chronic diseases can therefore have an impact on the individual's overall quality of life and mental health (Megari, 2013; Siboni et al., 2019). Research has shown a higher prevalence of depression and anxiety in patients diagnosed with a chronic disease (DeJean et al., 2013), particularly in cases where there are comorbidities (Yan et al., 2019).

Cancer is considered a chronic illness, as it often involves a long process that goes through different stages, from diagnosis and treatment to survivorship (Holland, 2002, 2003). It is perceived as a serious life threat, which can cause a significant amount of distress and a feeling of being overwhelmed in recently diagnosed patients (Ramos, 2021; Rodin, 2018). Due to the complexity of the cancer experience, the process of adjustment frequently causes anxiety, depression, fear, or guilt (Costa et al., 2016; Moorey & Greer, 2012). Consequently, there is a higher risk for cancer patients to develop mental disorders (Singer et al., 2010), ultimately affecting the quality of life and cancer-specific mortality (Kuhnt et al., 2016; Zhu et al., 2017).

DOI: 10.4324/9781032208688-56

Research on the psychological effects of cancer has focused primarily on anxiety and depression, due to their prevalence (e.g., Kuhnt et al., 2016; Michel et al., 2019: Singer et al., 2010; Zhu et al., 2017). There has been however, a shift in focus to coping mechanisms and positive emotional outcomes (Johansson et al., 2011), such as psychological adjustment and posttraumatic growth (PTG) (Costa et al., 2016; Singer, 2018).

PTG in Oncological and Chronic Illness

The diagnosis of a chronic illness can represent an extremely stressful experience and even a traumatic one, possibly resulting in psychological suffering and emotional distress. In this context, both the diagnosis and the progression of the disease can be perceived as unexpected, requiring a constant need for adjustment to different stages and treatments, which can lead to high levels of depression and posttraumatic stress (Purc-Stephenson, 2014). On the other hand, it can also encourage the recognition of positive cognitive changes that result from struggling with the diagnosis of a severe illness, i.e., PTG (Calhoun & Tedeschi, 1998), and are caused by the (re)interpretation and meaning that the patient gives to the traumatic event, and the way they (try to) deal with its consequences (Tedeschi et al., 2018).

The literature has demonstrated the relationship between PTG and different medical conditions, such as chronic diseases (Purc-Stephenson, 2014), brain damage (Rogan et al., 2013), transplant patients (Battaglia et al., 2021; Pérez-San-Gregorio et al., 2017; Scrignaro et al., 2016; Sheerazi & Kamran, 2020), cancer (Ramos et al., 2017; Yastıbaş & Karaman, 2021), HIV (Lau et al., 2018), Parkinson (Vescovelli et al., 2021), multiple sclerosis (Gil-González et al., 2022), inflammatory bowel disease (Hamama-Raz et al., 2021; Wu et al., 2022), and patients in hemodialysis (Arjeini et al., 2020; Li et al., 2018).

The Path to PTG in the Context of Serious Illness

PTG is an extremely complex construct, considered both a process and an outcome, which can occur in different domains of life. Tedeschi et al. (2018) identified five domains where changes can become perceptible: personal strength, relating to others, new possibilities, appreciation of life, and spiritual and existential change. Considering that the definition of trauma is relative to an individual's perception of the event's impact as devastating, their core beliefs regarding self and the world can be challenged (Tedeschi & Calhoun, 2004). Metaphorically compared to an earthquake, a traumatic event can "shake" the perception that the individual has of their assumptive world (Janoff-Bulman, 2004, 2006). It is at this point that the PTG process begins, i.e., when the distress and suffering inherent to the diagnosis (traumatic event) result in the challenge to core beliefs, which are the basis of the assumptive world, the PTG process can be triggered (Calhoun & Tedeschi, 2013; Janoff-Bulman, 2004). The core beliefs about the world and others, prevalent until that moment, no longer make sense and become meaningless, while the individual is challenged by a combination of automatic and intrusive thoughts, referred to as intrusive rumination. In the effort to manage the situation cognitively and emotionally, through an attempt to find an explanation for the event, while seeking to understand its impact on life, the individual starts a cognitive process, in which intrusive rumination gives way to deliberate rumination; it is this stage that the individual begins to reflect on what has occurred (Tedeschi & Calhoun, 2004). By entering this state of reflection, seeking answers and new meanings, the individual becomes able to reconstruct their assumptive world by integrating the traumatic event. In the earthquake metaphor, this stage is equivalent to the structural reconstruction of the buildings damaged by seismic activity (Calhoun & Tedeschi, 2013; Tedeschi & Calhoun, 2004).

The road to PTG is not linear. A constructive perspective underlining PTG describes how the process is more than just overcoming the diagnosis and the experience of the illness: rather, PTG also encompasses building new cognitive schemes to interpret and provide new meaning to the experience, self, others, and the world, as well as modifying the life narrative through the integration of the experience (Tedeschi et al., 2018). These changes are neither easy nor simple. They are highly transformative and imply change and growth in life (Tedeschi & Calhoun, 2004). It is when trying to assess and address the consequences, and attach meaning to the event, that the chance for PTG arises (Hamama-Raz et al., 2021; Lau et al., 2018). PTG is a complex process, mediated and influenced by mutual interaction among several aspects. Empirical research has shown that personality characteristics, illness representation, coping, emotional regulation and expression, and sociocultural context influence PTG in chronic or oncology patients (Hegarty et al., 2021; Henson et al., 2021; Tedeschi et al., 2018).

Personality Characteristics

The role of personality features in PTG endorsement has been thoroughly researched and studies have shown that certain characteristics significantly predict the use of adaptive coping strategies and consequently encourage PTG. Characteristics such as agreeableness, extraversion, openness, and conscientiousness are positively correlated with PTG (Henson et al., 2021). Recent studies have demonstrated that openness and extraversion best predict PTG, possibly because individuals who are more open to the experience are also more likely to adapt to unexpected life events (Hegarty et al., 2021; Henson et al., 2021; Lee et al., 2022; Linley & Joseph, 2004; Tedeschi & Calhoun, 1996, 2004). Spirituality, optimism and resilience, and hope are of special importance.

Spirituality

It is important to consider spirituality in the context of a serious illness since there is a constant threat to life, which may lead the patient to question the meaning of life and to face his or her own mortality (Paredes & Pereira, 2018). Individuals with a higher sense of spirituality can consider their experience as a whole, accept inherent difficulties as part of the system of religious and existential beliefs, and focus on the positive aspects of the event (Danhauer et al., 2013; Lee et al., 2022). In a study with cancer patients, religiousness was positively correlated with PTG as a coping strategy; i.e., individuals who perceived a higher sense of spirituality and religiousness felt a stronger connection with an existence bigger than themselves, which facilitated the search for new meaning in life through such as prayer and additional strategies (Abdullah et al., 2019).

Optimism and Resilience

Optimism and resilience are often explored in the context of cancer (Abdullah et al., 2019; Zhang et al., 2019) and HIV (Rzeszutek & Gruszczyńska, 2018), and the results display a positive correlation with PTG. A systematic review in the context of cancer in children and adolescents has shown that optimism facilitated PTG, promoting the use of coping strategies directed towards a positive assessment of the diagnosis and experience of the illness (Turner et al., 2018).

Hope

Hopefulness is a cognitive process that determines the motivation and perception of an individual's ability to achieve goals. A high level of hope can be associated with a cognitive reevaluation of traumatic events, enabling a positive reflection on such events. By accommodating new information (e.g., new beliefs) related to the trauma, individuals restructure their assumptive world (Abdullah et al., 2019). A recent study found that hopefulness played a determining role in PTG as it helped participants rethink the discrepancies within their assumptive world before and after the trauma (Abdullah et al., 2019).

Illness Representation

An illness representation is the set of beliefs and expectations that patients have of a disease and its symptoms. It can include two forms of representation – cognitive and emotional – which are integrant and decisive components of the self-regulation model (Leventhal et al., 1984, 1997). When there is a stimulus related to the illness, such as the diagnosis of a severe illness (e.g., chronic, oncological), this stimulus will induce cognitive (related to the identity, consequences, cause, duration, and capacity of cure/control of the illness) and emotional (related to fears and worries associated with expected consequences of the illness) representations. Recent studies have shown a noteworthy association between positive cognitive and emotional illness representations and PTG in chronic illnesses, such as HIV (Lau et al., 2018), cardiovascular disease (Hegarty et al., 2021; Lee et al., 2022), inflammatory bowel disease (Hamama-Raz et al., 2021), and cancer (Abdullah et al., 2019).

Coping

Coping can be perceived as the way through which individuals dealing with the experience and consequences of a severe illness adapt and integrate new information into their pre-existing belief schemes. Coping reconstructs the assumptive world, i.e., the inner world where the individual feels comfortable and safe, by integrating the traumatic experience (Danhauer et al., 2013; Janoff-Bulman, 2004, 2006). A recent systematic review has reported that problem-focused coping is an important predictor of PTG in survivors of breast cancer as this coping strategy enables cognitive processing and can promote the recognition of positive changes by assigning a positive new meaning to the diagnosis (Yastıbaş & Karaman, 2021). Another study demonstrated that in patients with inflammatory bowel disease, acting upon the discomfort and confusion inherent to the illness, there was a higher perception of control and well-being (through cognitive restructuring), and consequently PTG occurred (Wu et al., 2022). A growing body of literature has demonstrated that emotion-focused coping plays an important role in PTG, as the ability to express emotions favors their recognition and understanding, helping the attribution of meaning to a traumatic event (Darabos et al., 2021; Linley & Joseph, 2004; Taku et al., 2009; Tedeschi & Calhoun, 2004).

Emotional Regulation and Expression

Emotional regulation, i.e., the individual's ability to assess, regulate and disclose emotions, has a protective role, induces distress reduction, and facilitates PTG (Arjeini et al., 2020; Darabos et al., 2021; Tedeschi et al., 2018). In the context of cancer, emotional regulation and disclosure in response to traumatic situations, are emotion-focused strategies with an important role in the adjustment to the illness and in promoting PTG (Darabos et al., 2021), possibly leading to improved personal strength and changes in life priorities (Baziliansky & Cohen, 2021).

Sociocultural Context

Recent studies have corroborated the notion that social support is directly and positively related to PTG (Tedeschi & Calhoun, 2004; Wang et al., 2021). In the context of chronic and oncological disease, the dimension "Relating to Others" is often a major manifestation of PTG, through relationships with family members and/or caregivers, healthcare professionals, and others. For example, patients' feeling of gratitude to donors or to the medical team, as they perceive a transplant as epitomizing the beginning of a new life (Pérez-San-Gregorio et al., 2017; Scrignaro et al., 2016). A recent qualitative study of individuals with inflammatory bowel disease found that more than 50% of the participants searched for social support in their family circle or in the context of hospitalization, as the first response to their diagnosis (Wu et al., 2022). The positive association between social support and PTG was also observed in studies with cardiac patients (Lee et al., 2022). Studies have shown that women with breast cancer who described increased perception of social support from a specific person (such as a friend or family member), also reported higher levels of PTG (Abdullah et al., 2019; Yastıbaş & Karaman, 2021).

Sharing the experience and talking about emotions inherent in the illness process (e.g., emotional expression) with someone who is receptive and empathetic, reduces the risk of developing psychopathology and promotes the reinterpretation of the event, stimulating cognitive processing and the search for meaning (Calhoun & Tedeschi, 2013; Henson et al., 2021; Quiroga et al., 2018; Turner et al., 2018).

Interventions to Promote PTG

To facilitate the emergence of PTG after a traumatic event, an intervention based on the model of PTG was developed (Calhoun & Tedeschi, 2013; Tedeschi et al., 2018). This intervention consists of five steps that can be adapted according to the problem, the individual, socio-economic status, and/or human resources (Calhoun & Tedeschi, 2013; Tedeschi et al., 2018).

Step 1 Psychoeducation consists of a set of techniques designed to promote an understanding of the broad spectrum of individual reactions to trauma, which can vary in intensity, duration, or frequency, according to the disease's progression. Through psychoeducation, intense physiologic, cognitive, and emotional responses are normalized, which allows individuals to realize that there is nothing wrong with them and that their reactions are expectable considering the stage of the disease. This awareness and normalization allow the individual to perceive having control over their reactions and feel confident about recovery.

Step 2 Emotional distress management consists of a reduction in anxiety and frequency of intrusive ruminant thoughts related to the illness experience, which is crucial to enable becoming involved in the process of assigning meaning to the trauma and consequently developing PTG. At this stage, the psychotherapist can use cognitive-behavioral strategies such as relaxation exercises, guided imagination, physical exercise, or activities for artistic expression.

Step 3 Constructive emotional disclosure promotes the expression of feelings and reactions inherent to the illness experience. The exploration of intrusive ruminant thoughts through emotional disclosure enables a sense of control over intrusive thoughts, which in turn allows a cognitive reconstruction of the traumatic experience through more deliberate thoughts. The psychotherapist can encourage emotional disclosure to relatives or members of one's social circle. Participation in psychotherapeutic or mutual help groups makes emotional expression and the validation and integration of the illness experience easier. Narrative writing (Pennebaker, 2010) can also be used in this step.

Step 4 (Re)construction of the life narrative, which implies the development of a coherent life narrative that can integrate life before the diagnosis, the experience of illness and respective treatments, and life after the traumatic event, including eventual restrictions and illness-related changes. In this stage, there can be a recognition of the positive changes, representing one or more of the PTG domains, which must be validated and recognized by the therapist. Dialectical and paradoxical thinking (e.g., "The illness brought suffering but also allowed me to appreciate more the interactions with my family.") is encouraged.

Step 5 Redefinition of new life goals. Following the reconstruction of the life narrative, the individual is encouraged to review their pre-diagnosis life goals, and reconstruct new ones, more in line with the present life narrative and worldview. For example, consolidation of PTG in daily life may include greater compassion for others who are experiencing trauma, or increased selflessness towards others. This intervention, recently defined as integrative, includes elements of cognitive-behavioral, narrative, existential, and interpersonal therapy, while emphasizing the relevance of the therapeutic relationship conceptualized as "Expert Companionship" (Tedeschi & Moore, 2021).

Cognitive-behavior elements are reflected in the change of cognitive schemes (Janoff-Bulman, 2006) and in aspects of cognitive-behavioral therapy (Calhoun & Tedeschi, 2013). Following a traumatic event disruptive enough to "rattle" the individual's assumptive world, questioning core beliefs and the guiding principles that help individuals to interpret the self, others, and the world (Janoff-Bulman, 2004, 2006), a process of cognitive reconstruction of the shattered core beliefs takes place. Psychoeducation about reactions to trauma and training in cognitive and/or behavioral strategies for emotional regulation is key to re-establishing homeostatic balance and preparing for deliberate rumination.

Narrative elements, i.e., the change of core beliefs that arises from experiencing a traumatic event, based on perception before and after the trauma, generates feeling a need to reconstruct own beliefs and assign meaning to the traumatic event via integrating it into the reconstructed life narrative. Reconstruction of the core belief system implies a revision of the future and one's life goals. The development of the chronological life narrative, which integrates negative and positive aspects of the traumatic experience and incorporates its physiologic, cognitive, and affective effects in the newly reconstructed belief schemes and new life goals, promotes the development of PTG (Tedeschi & Moore, 2021).

Existential elements result from confronting the trauma and lead the individual to confront other questions related to one's existence, such as uncertainty, freedom and responsibility, meaning of life, and finitude. In the process of reconstructing one's core beliefs system, trauma survivors can be pushed to confront complex existential dilemmas and thus, feel a need to reconsider and opt for life goals that have meaning for them (Tedeschi & Moore, 2021; Tedeschi & Riffle, 2016).

Interpersonal elements, i.e., relationships with others play a significant role in maintaining the psychological symptoms. Group psychotherapy significantly promotes the perception of support and social support from the survivor's standpoint. In individual psychotherapy, the therapist should encourage the expansion of the survivor's social network by identifying the people who are closest and can support the process of managing and understanding the trauma experience as an expert companion (Tedeschi & Moore, 2021). An expert companion is a person, such as a spouse, relative, friend, clinician, nurse, or psychologist, who may encourage the discussion of uncomfortable emotions as well as help the survivor to look at things in a different and more hopeful or adaptive way and also a person who is able to understand and explain the common physiological and psychological responses to a traumatic event and validate the process of PTG, which comes naturally in response to the individual process of reconstruction after the trauma (Calhoun & Tedeschi, 2006). The psychotherapist, in assuming the role of "expert companion" and being aware of how the whole process unfolds, recognizes the individual's struggles that are part of the path of surviving the trauma and developing PTG (Tedeschi & Moore, 2021). This way the psychotherapist – as an expert companion – facilitates the acceptance of positive changes in everyday life and the assumption of an active role in structuring a (re) constructed identity.

Effects of Interventions on PTG in Patients with Chronic Diseases

Studies documented the effectiveness of interventions in facilitating PTG. Roepke (2015) conducted a meta-analysis of 12 studies that assessed the efficacy of group and couple interventions in reducing psychological symptoms (e.g., depression, distress, posttraumatic stress) across a variety of traumas, including cancer, and measured the impact on PTG as a secondary outcome. Despite some methodological limitations, it was concluded that participants in intervention groups reported higher levels of PTG than those in the control no-intervention group. Averill's (2007) study applied an emotional expression intervention to 48 patients with amyotrophic lateral sclerosis and reported statistically significant differences in PTG between the intervention group and the control group when assessed at 3 and 6 months. Wolever et al. (2010) evaluated the effectiveness of a 6-month integrative health (IH) telephone-based coaching intervention on psychosocial and other health factors in 56 patients with type 2 diabetes. The results showed that the intervention group reported more perceived benefits when compared to the control group. Zoellner et al. (2011) evaluated the effects of cognitive-behavioral therapy in 40 motor vehicle accident survivors with PTSD and found that the intervention was effective in reducing PTSD symptomatology but not in promoting an increase in PTG, although increases were reported in two domains of PTG, namely New Possibilities and Personal Strength.

A pilot study of eight weekly sessions of mindfulness-based cognitive therapy in 64 adolescents and young adults with inflammatory bowel disease found that the intervention was effective in reducing depressive symptoms but there were no significant differences between groups in PTG either after 8 or 20 weeks (Ewais et al., 2021). Manzoni et al. (2011) evaluated the physical and psychological effects of a four-week-long disease-related expressive writing procedure on 64 patients with coronary heart disease who were randomly assigned to write thoughts and emotions (intervention group) or facts (control group) about heart disease and treatment. PTG showed a significant improvement only within the intervention group. Sarizadeh et al. (2019) evaluated the effectiveness of acceptance and commitment therapy (ACT), provided in eight 90 minutes individual sessions to patients who were undergoing hemodialysis and found an increase in PTG in the ACT group (n = 18) compared to the control group (n = 18). Despite the aforementioned evidence that PTG can be enhanced in patients with a chronic disease by interventions that assess PTG as a secondary outcome, further RCTS studies with larger sample sizes are needed to evaluate the effectiveness of different types of interventions in enhancing PTG in the long term, especially considering the different levels of disease severity, treatment phases, and the social support received.

A recent systematic review and meta-analysis (Zhang et al., 2022) evaluated the effects of physical activity interventions on PTG after a traumatic event (including cancer, spinal cord injury, and other conditions). Of the 12 selected articles, five interventions included yoga, four were health coaching interventions, and three were sports-related interventions. The authors found that the effects of physical activity interventions on posttraumatic growth are somewhat smaller than those of psychosocial interventions.

Psychological interventions for cancer patients are mostly based on the cognitive-behavioral model, which implies the use of a variety of strategies of psychoeducation, abdominal breathing, relaxation, and mindfulness with the goal of modifying reactions, thoughts, behaviors, and/or social interactions (Li et al., 2020). Group psychosocial interventions for cancer patients, irrespective of whether they include the specific goal of promoting PTG, facilitate the expression of emotions related to the cancer experience, the learning of cognitive-behavioral strategies for self-regulation, the attribution of meaning, and the reintegration of the traumatic event into the life narrative. This enhances the probability of developing or increasing PTG, even though the main goal was to reduce psychological symptoms (e.g., depression and anxiety) and pain or fatigue (Li et al., 2020).

Studies have shown an increase in PTG as a secondary outcome of group interventions specific to cancer patients, including cognitive-behavioral therapy for stress management (e.g., Antoni et al., 2001), peers support therapy (Morris et al., 2014), cognitive-existential therapy (Kissane et al., 2003), psycho-spiritual therapy (Garlick et al., 2011), build-resilience group therapy (Pat-Horenczyk et al., 2015), a group therapy based on behavior change (Hawkes et al., 2014), or mindfulness-based interventions (Victorson et al., 2017). However, some studies have not identified significant differences between the intervention and control group (Kenne Sarenmalm et al., 2017; Kubo et al., 2019; Van Der Spek et al., 2017; Zernicke et al., 2014; Zhang et al., 2017).

A recent meta-analysis by Li et al. (2020) assessed the effectiveness of 15 randomized controlled trials (RCT) that included psychosocial interventions for PTG in cancer patients and concluded that psychosocial interventions are effective in promoting PTG in cancer patients, as there was an improvement in the levels of PTG in all the studies. However, not all studies demonstrate a significant difference between the intervention and control groups (Li et al., 2020). The subgroup analysis regarding the type of cancer showed that the intervention's effect in increasing PTG was higher in studies where the sample was comprised of breast cancer patients, in comparison with studies that assessed other types of cancer, which yielded a smaller effect size.

The interventions more commonly tested and effective were mindfulness-based interventions, which allow individuals to maintain awareness of the present moment, acquire an acceptance judgmental-free attitude, free themselves of beliefs, thoughts, and emotions that cause psychological suffering, be more open to the experience, increase self-control and emotional self-regulation over the cancer experience (Kabat-Zinn, 2005). Mindfulness-based interventions most often used are Mindfulness-Based Stress Reduction (MBSR), Mindfulness-Based Stress Reduction for Breast Cancer (MBSR(BC), Mindfulness-Based Care Recovery (MBCR), Mindfulness-Based Cognitive Therapy (MBCT), Mindfulness-Based Art Therapy (MBAT), and Acceptance and Commitment Therapy (ACT) (Xunlin et al., 2020). In a systematic review and meta-analysis study, Shiyko and colleagues (2017) aimed to verify the effects of mindfulness intervention on PTG. Of the 11 studies selected, 10 included samples of cancer patients and conducted interventions for an average of 8 weeks. The results demonstrated a small positive effect, reporting an increase in PTG following mindfulness training.

A recent systematic review and meta-analysis (Xunlin et al., 2020) assessed the effect of mindfulness-based interventions on PTG and other psychological variables among adult cancer patients and survivors. From the selected 29 RCT studies, only eight assessed PTG as a secondary outcome. The results confirmed that mindfulness-based interventions are effective (with a large effect size [0.58]) for the development of PTG, showing a post-intervention increase in PTG. Another systematic review on eHealth and Mobile Health Mindfulness-Based Programs for cancer patients showed that from the three articles (Hawkes et al., 2014; Kubo et al., 2019; Zernicke et al., 2014) that assessed the effects of the interventions on PTG, only one (Hawkes et al., 2014) revealed statistically significant improvements in PTG after the group intervention (Matis et al. 2020). A narrative review also concluded that mindfulness-based interventions may be promising for enhancing PTG and spirituality in cancer patients and survivors (Abdullah & Mohamad, 2018).

Two interventions were developed and adapted for women with breast cancer, with the purpose of facilitating the perception of PTG (e.g., primary outcome) and enhancing psychosocial adjustment. In South Korea, a group intervention was developed to facilitate PTG in 74 breast cancer female survivors. The six-weekly-session program was constructed by applying the self-analysis, self-disclosure, and socio-cultural influence mentioned in the PTG model. The results showed a statistically significant difference between groups regarding PTG; specifically for patients in the intervention group who presented higher levels of PTG (Choi et al., 2022).

In Portugal, a group intervention program for women with breast cancer (Ramos et al., 2016, 2017) has been developed. This program includes eight 90 minutes weekly sessions, where 58 participants of the intervention group were divided into small groups and assessed longitudinally. The results revealed that the program is very promising for generating PTG and that it plays a moderator role in the change of core beliefs and intrusive rumination (Ramos et al., 2017). The results of this research highlight the importance of integrating PTG assessment in current intervention programs with oncology patients, favoring the intergroup context, the identification among participants, and consequently, the sharing of experiences and emotions, cognitive processing, and attribution of meaning to the traumatic experience.

In sum, recent years have witnessed an increase in the empirical study of PTG and the different interventions that evaluate PTG as a result of the effectiveness of these interventions in patients with chronic disease, particularly in cancer patients. The results of these interventions and of the different systematic reviews conducted reinforce the importance of challenging core beliefs, cognitive processing, and assigning meaning to the traumatic event for the development of PTG, which is in line with the theoretical model of PTG (Tedeschi & Calhoun, 2004; Tedeschi et al., 2018). Cognitive-behavioral interventions and expressive therapies may influence more direct cognitive processing concerning the traumatic experience and thus foster PTG.

References

Abdullah, M. F. I., Hami, R., Appalanaido, G. K., Azman, N., Mohd Shariff, N., & Md Sharif, S. S. (2019). Diagnosis of cancer is not a death sentence: Examining posttraumatic growth and its associated factors in cancer patients. *Journal of Psychosocial Oncology*, *37*(5), 636–651. 10.1080/07347332.2019.1574946

Abdullah, M. F. I. L. B., & Mohamad, M. A. B. (2018). Does psychosocial interventions enhance posttraumatic growth and spirituality in cancer patients and survivors? A narrative review of the literature. *Malaysian Journal of Medicine and Health Sciences*, *14*, 164–172.

Antoni, M. H., Lehman, J. M., Klibourn, K. M., Boyers, A. E., Culver, J. L., Alferi, S. M., Yount, S. E., McGregor, B. A., Arena, P. L., Harris, S. D., Price, A. A., Carver, C. S. (2001). Cognitive-behavioral stress management intervention decreases the prevalence of depression and enhances benefit finding among women under treatment for early-stage breast cancer. *Health Psychology*, *20*(1), 20–32. 10.1037/0278-6133.20.1.20

Arjeini, Z., Zeabadi, S., Hefzabad, F., & Shahsavari, S. (2020). The relationship between post-traumatic growth and cognitive emotion regulation strategies in hemodialysis patients. *Journal of Education and Health Promotion*, *9*(January), 1–6. 10.4103/jehp.jehp_673_19

Australian Institute of Health and Welfare. (2021). *Chronic condition multimorbidity*. AIHW, Australian Government. accessed 16 March 2022.

Averill, A. J. (2007). Emotional disclosure in patients with amyotrophic lateral sclerosis: A randomized, controlled trial. *Dissertation Abstracts International: Section B: The Sciences and Engineering*, *68*(4-B), 2636.

Battaglia, Y., Zerbinati, L., Belvederi Murri, M., Provenzano, M., Esposito, P., Andreucci, M., Storari A., & Grassi, L. (2021). Exploring the level of post traumatic growth in kidney transplant recipients via network analysis. *Journal of Clinical Medicine*, *10*(20), 4747. 10.3390/jcm10204747

Baziliansky, S., & Cohen, M. (2021). Emotion regulation and psychological distress in cancer survivors: A systematic review and meta-analysis. *Stress and Health*, *37*(1), 3–18. 10.1002/smi.2972

Calhoun, L. G., & Tedeschi, R. G. (1998). Posttraumatic growth: Future directions. In R. G. Tedeschi, C. L. Park, & L. G. Calhoun (Eds.), *Posttraumatic growth: Positive changes in the aftermath of crises* (pp. 215–238). Mahwah, NJ: Lawrence Erlbaum Associates.

Calhoun, L. G., & Tedeschi, R. G. (2006). The foundations of posttraumatic growth: An expanded framework. In L. G. Calhoun, & R. G. Tedeschi (Eds.). *The handbook of posttraumatic growth: Research and practice* (pp. 1–23). Mahwah, NJ: Lawrence Erlbaum Associates, Publishers.

Calhoun, L. G., & Tedeschi, R. G. (2013). *Posttraumatic growth in clinical practice*. New York, NY, US: Routledge/Taylor & Francis Group.

Centers for Disease Control and Prevention. (2022). About chronic diseases. https://www.cdc.gov/chronicdisease/about/index.htm. Accessed September 26, 2022.
Choi, S. H., Lee, Y. W., Kim, H. S., Kim, S. H., Lee, E. H., Park, E. Y., & Cho, Y. U. (2022). Development and effects of a post-traumatic growth program for patients with breast cancer. *European Journal of Oncology Nursing*, *57*(February), 102100. 10.1016/j.ejon.2022.102100
Costa, D. S. J., Mercieca-Bebber, R., Rutherford, C., Gabb, L., & King, M. T. (2016). The impact of cancer on psychological and social outcomes. *Australian Psychologist*, *51*(2), 89–99. 10.1111/ap.12165
Danhauer, S. C., Case, L. D., Tedeschi, R., Russell, G., Vishnevsky, T., Triplett, K., Ip, E. H., & Avis, N. E. (2013). Predictors of posttraumatic growth in women with breast cancer. *Psycho-Oncology*, *22*(12), 2676–2683. 10.1002/pon.3298
Darabos, K., Renna, M. E., Wang, A. W., Zimmermann, C. F., & Hoyt, M. A. (2021). Emotional approach coping among young adults with cancer: Relationships with psychological distress, posttraumatic growth, and resilience. *Psycho-Oncology*, *30*(5), 728–735. 10.1002/pon.5621
DeJean, D., Giacomini, M., Vanstone, M., & Brundisini, F. (2013). Patient experiences of depression and anxiety with chronic disease: A systematic review and qualitative meta-synthesis. *Ontario Health Technology Assessment Series*, *13*(16), 1–33.
Ewais, T., Begun, J., Kenny, M., Hay, K., Houldin, E., Chuang, K. H., Tefay, M., & Kisely, S. (2021). Mindfulness based cognitive therapy for youth with inflammatory bowel disease and depression - findings from a pilot randomised controlled trial. *Journal of Psychosomatic Research*, *149*(October), 110594. 10.1016/j.jpsychores.2021.110594
Garlick, M., Wall, K., Corwin, D., & Koopman, C. (2011). Psycho-spiritual integrative therapy for women with primary breast cancer. *Journal of Clinical Psychology in Medical Settings*, *18*, 78–90. 10.1007/s10880-011-9224-9
Gil-González, I., Pérez-San-Gregorio, M. Á., Conrad, R., & Martín-Rodríguez, A. (2022). Beyond the boundaries of disease—significant post-traumatic growth in multiple sclerosis patients and caregivers. *Frontiers in Psychology*, *13*(June). 10.3389/fpsyg.2022.903508
Hajat, C., & Stein, E. (2018). The global burden of multiple chronic conditions: A narrative review. *Preventive Medicine Reports*, *12*, 284–293. 10.1016/j.pmedr.2018.10.008
Hamama-Raz, Y., Nativ, S., & Hamama, L. (2021). Post-traumatic growth in inflammatory bowel disease patients: the role of illness cognitions and physical quality of life. *Journal of Crohn's and Colitis*, *15*(6), 1060–1067. 10.1093/ecco-jcc/jjaa247
Hawkes, A. L., Pakenham, K. I., Chambers, S. K., Patrao, T. A., & Courneya, K. S. (2014). Effects of a multiple health behavior change intervention for colorectal cancer survivors on psychosocial outcomes and quality of life: a randomized controlled trial. *Annals of Behavioral Medicine*, *48*(3), 359–370. 10.1007/s12160-014-9610-2
Hegarty, G., Storey, L., Dempster, M., & Rogers, D. (2021). Correlates of post-traumatic growth following a myocardial infarction: A systematic review. *Journal of Clinical Psychology in Medical Settings*, *28*(2), 394–404. 10.1007/s10880-020-09727-3
Henson, C., Truchot, D., & Canevello, A. (2021). What promotes post traumatic growth? A systematic review. *European Journal of Trauma and Dissociation*, *5*(4), 100195. 10.1016/j.ejtd.2020.100195
Holland, J. C. (2002). History of psycho-oncology: overcoming attitudinal and conceptual barriers. *Psychosomatic Medicine*, *64*(2), 206–221. 10.1097/00006842-200203000-00004
Holland, J. C. (2003). American Cancer Society Award lecture. Psychological care of patients: Psycho-oncology's contribution. *Journal of Clinical Oncology*, *21*(23 Suppl), 253s–265s. 10.1200/JCO.2003.09.133
Janoff-Bulman, R. (2004). Posttraumatic growth: Three explanatory models. *Psychological Inquiry*, *15*(1), 130–134.
Janoff-Bulman, R. (2006). Schema-change perspectives on posttraumatic growth. In L. G. Calhoun, & R. G. Tedeschi (Eds.), *Handbook of posttraumatic growth: Research and practice* (pp. 81–99). Mahwah, NJ: Lawrence Erlbaum.
Johansson, M., Rydén, A., & Finizia, C. (2011). Mental adjustment to cancer and its relation to anxiety, depression, HRQL and survival in patients with laryngeal cancer - A longitudinal study. *BMC cancer*, *11*, 283. 10.1186/1471-2407-11-283

Kabat-Zinn, J. (2005). *Full catastrophe living: Using the wisdom of your body and mind to face stress, pain, and illness.* Delta Trade Paperback.
Kenne Sarenmalm, E., Mårtensson, L. B., Andersson, B. A., Karlsson, P., & Bergh, I. (2017). Mindfulness and its efficacy for psychological and biological responses in women with breast cancer. *Cancer medicine*, *6*(5), 1108–1122. 10.1002/cam4.1052
Kissane, D. W., Bloch, S., Smith, G. C., Miach, P., Clarke, D. M., Ikin, J., Love A., Ranieri, N., McKenzie, D. (2003). Cognitive-existential group psychotherapy for women with primary breast cancer: A randomized controlled trial. *Psycho-Oncology*, *12*, 532–546. 10.1002/pon.683
Kubo, A., Kurtovich, E., McGinnis, M. A., Aghaee, S., Altschuler, A., Quesenberry, C., Kolevska, T., & Avins, A. L. (2019). A randomized controlled trial of health mindfulness intervention for cancer patients and informal cancer caregivers: A feasibility study within an integrated health care delivery system. *Integrative Cancer Therapies*, *18*. 10.1177/1534735419850634
Kuhnt, S., Brähler, E., Faller, H., Härter, M., Keller, M., Schulz, H., Wegscheider, K., Weis, J., Boehncke, A., Hund, B., Reuter, K., Richard, M., Sehner, S., Wittchen, H. U., Koch, U., & Mehnert, A. (2016). Twelve-month and lifetime prevalence of mental disorders in cancer patients. *Psychotherapy and Psychosomatics*, *85*(5), 289–296. 10.1159/000446991
Larsen, P. D. (2013). The illness experience. In I. M. Lubkin, & P. D. Larsen (Eds.) *Chronic illness: Impact and intervention* (8th Ed., pp. 23–46). Jones & Bartlett Learning.
Lau, J. T. F., Wu, X., Wu, A. M. S., Wang, Z., & Mo, P. K. H. (2018). Relationships between illness perception and post-traumatic growth among newly diagnosed hiv-positive men who have sex with men in China. *AIDS and Behavior*, *22*(6), 1885–1898. 10.1007/s10461-017-1874-7
Lee, S. Y., Park, C. L., & Laflash, S. (2022). Perceived posttraumatic growth in cardiac patients: A systematic scoping review. *Journal of Traumatic Stress*, *35*(3), 791–803. 10.1002/jts.22799
Leventhal, H., Benyamini, Y., Brownlee, S., Diefenbach, M., Leventhal, E. A., Patrick-Miller, L., & Robitaille, C. (1997). Illness representations: Theoretical foundations. In K. J. Petrie, & J. Weinman (Eds.), *Perceptions of health and illness* (pp. 19–45). London: Harwood Aca- demic Publishers.
Leventhal, H., Nerenz, D. R., & Steele, D. J. (1984). Illness representations and coping with health threats. In Baum, A., Taylor, S. E., & Singer, J. E. (Eds.), *Handbook of Psychology and Health* (pp. 219–252). Hillsdale, NJ: Erlbaum.
Li, J., Peng, X., Su, Y., He, Y., Zhang, S., & Hu, X. (2020). Effectiveness of psychosocial interventions for posttraumatic growth in patients with cancer: A meta-analysis of randomized controlled trials. *European Journal of Oncology Nursing*, *48*(May), 101798. 10.1016/j.ejon.2020.101798
Li, T., Liu, T., Han, J., Zhang, M., Li, Z., Zhu, Q., & Wang, A. (2018). The relationship among resilience, rumination and posttraumatic growth in hemodialysis patients in North China. *Psychology, Health and Medicine*, *23*(4), 442–453. 10.1080/13548506.2017.1384553
Linley, P. A., & Joseph, S. (2004). Positive change following trauma and adversity: A review. *Journal of Traumatic Stress*, *17*(1), 11–21. 10.1023/B:JOTS.0000014671.27856.7e
Manzoni, G. M., Castelnuovo, G., & Molinari, E. (2011). The WRITTEN-HEART study (expressive writing for heart healing): rationale and design of a randomized controlled clinical trial of expressive writing in coronary patients referred to residential cardiac rehabilitation. *Health and quality of life outcomes*, *9*(1), 1–8. 10.1186/1477-7525-9-51
Matis, J., Svetlak, M., Slezackova, A., Svoboda, M., & Šumec, R. (2020). Mindfulness-Based Programs for patients with cancer via ehealth and mobile health: Systematic review and synthesis of quantitative research. *Journal of Medical Internet Research*, *22*(11), 1–21. 10.2196/20709
Megari K. (2013). Quality of life in chronic disease patients. *Health Psychology Research*, *1*(3), e27. 10.4081/hpr.2013.e27
Michel, G., François, C., Harju, E., Dehler, S., & Roser, K. (2019). The long-term impact of cancer: Evaluating psychological distress in adolescent and young adult cancer survivors in Switzerland. *Psycho-Oncology*, *28*(3), 577–585. 10.1002/pon.4981
Moorey, S., & Greer, S. (2012). *Oxford guide to CBT for people with cancer* (2nd ed.). Oxford University Press.
Morris, B. A., Lepore, S. J., Wilson, B., Lieberman, M. A., Dunn, J., & Chambers, S. K. (2014). Adopting a survivor identity after cancer in a peer support context. *Journal of Cancer Survivorship*, *8*(3), 427–436. 10.1007/s11764-014-0355-5

Paredes, A. C., & Pereira, M. G. (2018). Spirituality, distress and posttraumatic growth in breast cancer patients. *Journal of Religion and Health*, *57*(5), 1606–1617. 10.1007/s10943-017-0452-7
Pat-Horenczyk, R., Perry, S., Hamama-Ray, Y., Yuval, Z., Schramm-Yavin, S., & Stemmer, S. M. (2015). Posttraumatic Growth in breast cancer survivors: Constructive and illusory aspects. *Journal of Traumatic Stress*, *28*, 214–222. 10.1002/jts.22014
Pennebaker, J. W. (2010). An expressive writing in a clinical setting. *The Independent Practicioner*, *30*, 23–25.
Pérez-San-Gregorio, M. Á., Martín-Rodríguez, A., Borda-Mas, M., Avargues-Navarro, M. L., Pérez-Bernal, J., Conrad, R., & Gómez-Bravo, M. Á. (2017). Post-traumatic growth and its relationship to quality of life up to 9 years after liver transplantation: A crosssectional study in Spain. *BMJ Open*, *7*(9), 1–9. 10.1136/bmjopen-2017-017455
Purc-Stephenson, R. J. (2014). The posttraumatic growth inventory: Factor structure and invariance among persons with chronic diseases. *Rehabilitation Psychology*, *59*(1), 10–18. 10.1037/a0035353
Quiroga, C., Binfaré, L., Rudnicki, T., & Argimon, I. (2018). Rumination and social support as predictors of posttraumatic growth in women with breast cancer: A systematic review. *Psicooncologia*, *15*(2), 301–314. 10.5209/ PSIC.61437
Ramos, C. (2021). Cancro. In I. Leal, & J. P. Ribeiro (Coord.), *Manual de Psicologia da Saúde* (pp. 227–233). Pactor.
Ramos, C., Leal, I., & Tedeschi, R. G. (2016). Protocol of a randomized controlled trial of a psychotherapeutic intervention for facilitating Posttraumatic Growth in nonmetastatic breast cancer patients. *BMC Women's Health*, *16*, 22–30. 10.1186/s12905-016-0302-x
Ramos, C., Costa, P. A., Rudnicki, T., Marôco, A. L., Leal, I., Guimarães, R., Fougo, J. L., & Tedeschi, R. G. (2017). The effectiveness of a group intervention to facilitate Posttraumatic Growth among women with breast cancer. *Psycho-Oncology*, *27*(1), 258–264. 10.1002/pon.4501
Roepke, A. M. (2015). Psychosocial interventions and posttraumatic growth: A meta-analysis. *Journal of Consulting and Clinical Psychology*, *83*(1), 129–142. 10.1037/a0036872
Rodin, G. (2018). From evidence to implementation: The global challenge for psychosocial oncology. *Psycho-Oncology*, *27*(10), 2310–2316. 10.1002/pon.4837
Rogan, C., Fortune, D. G., & Prentice, G. (2013). Post-traumatic growth, illness perceptions and coping in people with acquired brain injury. *Neuropsychological Rehabilitation*, *23*(5), 639–657. 10.1080/09602011.2013.799076
Rzeszutek, M., & Gruszczyńska, E. (2018). Posttraumatic growth among people living with HIV: A systematic review. *Journal of Psychosomatic Research*, *114*(June), 81–91. 10.1016/j.jpsychores.2018.09.006
Sarizadeh, M. S., Rafieinia, P., Sabahi, P., & Tamaddon, M. R. (2019). Effectiveness of acceptance and commitment therapy on subjective well-being among hemodialysis patients: A randomized clinical trial study. *Koomesh*, *21*(1), 61–66.
Scrignaro, M., Sani, F., Wakefield, J. R. H., Bianchi, E., Magrin, M. E., & Gangeri, L. (2016). Posttraumatic growth enhances social identification in liver transplant patients: A longitudinal study. *Journal of Psychosomatic Research*, *88*, 28–32. 10.1016/j.jpsychores.2016.07.004
Sheerazi, S., & Kamran, F. (2020). Resilience and posttraumatic growth in renal transplant recipients. *Journal of Behavioural Sciences*, *30*(1), 9–25.
Shiyko, M. P., Hallinan, S., & Naito, T. (2017). Effects of mindfulness training on posttraumatic growth: A systematic review and meta-analysis. *Mindfulness*, *8*(4), 848–858. 10.1007/s12671-017-0684-3
Siboni, F. S., Alimoradi, Z., Atashi, V., Alipour, M., & Khatooni, M. (2019). Quality of life in different chronic diseases and its related factors. *International Journal of Preventive Medicine*, *10*, 65. 10.4103/ijpvm.IJPVM_429_17
Singer, S. (2018). Psychosocial impact of cancer. In A. Mehnert, & U. Goerling (Eds.), *Psycho-Oncology* (2nd ed., pp. 1–11). Springer. 10.1007/978-3-319-64310-6_1
Singer, S., Das-Munshi, J., & Brähler, E. (2010). Prevalence of mental health conditions in cancer patients in acute care – A meta-analysis. *Annals of Oncology*, *21*(5), 925–930. 10.1093/annonc/mdp515
Taku, K., Cann, A., Tedeschi, R. G., & Calhoun, L. G. (2009). Intrusive versus deliberate rumination in posttraumatic growth across US and Japanese samples. *Anxiety, Stress and Coping*, *22*(2), 129–136. 10.1080/10615800802317841

Tedeschi, R., & Calhoun, L. (1996). The Posttraumatic Growth Inventory: Measuring the positive legacy of trauma. *Journal of Traumatic Stress*, *9*(3), 455–471. 10.1002/jts.2490090305

Tedeschi, R., & Calhoun, L. (2004). Posttraumatic growth: Conceptual foundations and empirical evidence. *Psychological Inquiry*, *15*(1), 1–18. 10.1207/s15327965pli1501_01

Tedeschi, R. G., & Moore, B. A. (2021). Posttraumatic growth as an integrative therapeutic philosophy. *Journal of Psychotherapy Integration*, *31*(2), 180–194. 10.1037/int0000250

Tedeschi, R. G., & Riffle, O. M. (2016). Posttraumatic growth and logotherapy: Finding meaning in trauma. *International Forum for Logotherapy*, *39*(1), 40–47.

Tedeschi, R. G., Shakespeare-Finch, J., Taku, K., & Calhoun, L. G. (2018). *Posttraumatic growth: Theory, research, and applications*. New York, US: Routledge.

Turner, J. K., Hutchinson, A., & Wilson, C. (2018). Correlates of post-traumatic growth following childhood and adolescent cancer: A systematic review and meta-analysis. *Psycho-Oncology*, 27(4), 1100–1109. 10.1002/pon.4577

Van Der Spek, N., Vos, J., Van Uden-Kraan, C. F., Breitbart, W., Cuijpers, P., Holtmaat, K., Witte, B. I., Tollenaar, R. A. E. M., & Verdonck-De Leeuw, I. M. (2017). Efficacy of meaning-centered group psychotherapy for cancer survivors: A randomized controlled trial. *Psychological Medicine*, 47(11), 1990–2001. 10.1017/S0033291717000447

Vescovelli, F., Minotti, S., & Ruini, C. (2021). Exploring post-traumatic growth in parkinson's disease: A mixed method study. *Journal of Clinical Psychology in Medical Settings*, *28*(2), 267–278. 10.1007/s10880-020-09713-9

Victorson, D., Hankin, V., Burns, J., Weiland, R., Maletich, C., Sufrin, N., Schuette, S., Gutierrez, B., & Brendler, C. (2017). Feasibility, acceptability and preliminary psychological benefits of mindfulness meditation training in a sample of men diagnosed with prostate cancer on active surveillance: results from a randomized controlled pilot trial. *Psycho-oncology*, *26*(8), 1155–1163. 10.1002/pon.4135

Wang, J., She, Y., Wang, M., Zhang, Y., Lin, Y., & Zhu, X. (2021). Relationships among hope, meaning in life, and post-traumatic growth in patients with chronic obstructive pulmonary disease: A cross-sectional study. *Journal of Advanced Nursing*, *77*(1), 244–254. 10.1111/jan.14605

Wolever, R. Q., Dreusicke, M., Fikkan, J., Hawkins, T. V., Yeung, S., Wakefield, J., Duda, L., Flowers, P., Cook, C., & Skinner, E. (2010). Integrative health coaching for patients with type 2 diabetes: A randomized clinical trial. *Diabetes Educator*, *36*(4), 629–639. 10.1177/0145721710371523

World Health Organization. (2020). *Noncommunicable diseases progress monitor 2020*. Geneva: World Health Organization. https://www.who.int/publications/i/item/9789240000490

Wu, Q., Zhu, P., Liu, X., Ji, Q., & Qian, M. (2022). Nirvana: A qualitative study of posttraumatic growth in adolescents and young adults with inflammatory bowel disease. *Children*, *9*(6), 879. 10.3390/children9060879

Xunlin, N., Lau, Y., & Klainin-Yobas, P. (2020). The effectiveness of mindfulness-based interventions among cancer patients and survivors: A systematic review and meta-analysis. *Supportive Care in Cancer*, *28*(4), 1563–1578. 10.1007/s00520-019-05219-9

Yan, R., Xia, J., Yang, R., Lv, B., Wu, P., Chen, W., Zhang, Y., Lu, X., Che, B., Wang, J., & Yu, J. (2019). Association between anxiety, depression, and comorbid chronic diseases among cancer survivors. *Psycho-oncology*, *28*(6), 1269–1277. 10.1002/pon.5078

Yastıbaş, C., & Karaman, İ. G. (2021). Breast cancer and post-traumatic growth: A systematic Review. *Psikiyatride Guncel Yaklasimlar - Current Approaches in Psychiatry*, *13*(3), 490–510. 10.18863/pgy.817760

Zernicke, K. A., Campbell, T. S., Speca, M., McCabe-Ruff, K., Flowers, S., & Carlson, L. E. (2014). A randomized wait-list controlled trial of feasibility and efficacy of an online mindfulness–based cancer recovery program: The eTherapy for cancer applying mindfulness trial. *Psychosomatic medicine*, 76(4), 257–267. 10.1097/PSY.0000000000000053

Zhang, C., Gao, R., Tai, J., Li, Y., Chen, S., Chen, L., Cao, X., Wang, L., Jia, M., & Li, F. (2019). The relationship between self-perceived burden and posttraumatic growth among colorectal cancer patients: The mediating effects of resilience. *BioMed Research International*, Article ID 6840743 10.1155/2019/6840743

Zhang, J. Y., Zhou, Y. Q., Feng, Z. W., Fan, Y. N., Zeng, G. C., & Wei, L. (2017). Randomized controlled trial of mindfulness-based stress reduction (MBSR) on posttraumatic growth of Chinese breast cancer survivors. *Psychology, Health & Medicine*, 22(1), 94–109. 10.1080/13548506.2016.1146405

Zhang, N., Xiang, X., Zhou, S., Liu, H., He, Y., & Chen, J. (2022). Physical activity intervention and posttraumatic growth: A systematic review and meta-analysis. *Journal of Psychosomatic Research*, *152*(November 2021), 110675. 10.1016/j.jpsychores.2021.110675

Zhu, J., Fang, F., Sjölander, A., Fall, K., Adami, H. O., & Valdimarsdóttir, U. (2017). First-onset mental disorders after cancer diagnosis and cancer-specific mortality: A nationwide cohort study. *Annals of Oncology*, *28*(8), 1964–1969. 10.1093/annonc/mdx265

Zoellner, T., Rabe, S., Karl, A., & Maercker, A. (2011). Post-traumatic growth as outcome of a cognitive-behavioural therapy trial for motor vehicle accident survivors with PTSD. *Psychology and Psychotherapy: Theory, Research and Practice*, *84*(2), 201–213. 10.1348/147608310X520157

46

A COMMUNITY-BASED INTERVENTION TO ENHANCE POSTTRAUMATIC GROWTH AMONG REFUGEES IN RECEIVING SOCIETIES

Virginia Paloma, Sara M. Martínez-Damia, Irene de la Morena, Clara López-Torres, and Isabel Berbel

Introduction

The past years have been characterized by an ever-increasing influx of forcibly displaced people all over the world. The United Nations High Commissioner for Refugees estimates that global forced displacement has surpassed 84 million people in mid-2021, with 85% of them being hosted by developing countries including Turkey, Colombia, Uganda, and Pakistan (UNHCR, 2021a). More than two-thirds of forcibly displaced people are coming from five countries: the Syrian Arab Republic, Venezuela, Afghanistan, South Sudan, and Myanmar (UNHCR, 2021a). In this context, a refugee is someone "who is unable or unwilling to return to their country of origin owing to a well-founded fear of being persecuted for reasons of race, religion, nationality, membership of a particular social group, or political opinion" (United Nations General Assembly, 1951, p. 3). An asylum seeker is someone "who has applied for refugee status [...] and has not yet received a final decision on their claim" (UNHCR, 2021b). Although these terms are different, in the interest of simplification, in this chapter, "refugees" is used to refer both to "refugees" and "asylum seekers."

We can conceptualize forced migration as a traumatic event or as an extremely painful experience that challenges the psychological stability of any individual. Forced migration involves "separations, losses, changes, conflicts, and demands that severely challenge or shatter individuals' past ways of making meaning and defining themselves" (Berger & Weiss, 2003, p. 22). Under certain circumstances, the adverse experiences suffered by refugees during the pre-migration (e.g., witnessing some atrocities), transit (e.g., living in refugee camps), and settlement stages (e.g., social isolation) may lead to pathological conditions such as depression, anxiety, posttraumatic stress disorder, or psychosomatic disorders (Fazel et al., 2005; Slobodin & Jong, 2015). However, research on refugees has suggested that in addition to being a traumatic event with negative consequences, forced migration may also represent an opportunity for posttraumatic growth (PTG; e.g., Abraham et al., 2018; Ferriss &

 DOI: 10.4324/9781032208688-57

Forrest-Bank, 2018; Gökalp et al., 2021; Matos et al., 2021; Shakespeare-Finch et al., 2014; Taylor et al., 2020).

PTG refers to an individual's perceptions of significant positive changes resulting from the struggle with trauma and involves a cognitive processing of the losses and a rebuilding of one's assumptive world and views of self, relationship with others, and philosophy of life (Tedeschi & Calhoun, 2004). Thus, PTG is a positive mental health indicator that, far from negating the suffering of forced displacement for refugees, views it as a potential learning experience and a personal strengthening source for them (Paloma et al., 2020a). This can imply appreciating life more, becoming more aware of one's strengths, experiencing the value of significant relationships more, recognizing new opportunities for flourishing in the receiving society, and increasing one's spirituality (Gökalp & Haktanir, 2021; Taher & Allan, 2020; Taku et al., 2008). A systematic review found that PTG predicts the overall quality of life among refugees settled in high-income countries (van der Boor et al., 2020).

Although there is a clear interest in strengthening the mental health of refugees in host societies (WHO, 2018), particularly during the crisis of the COVID-19 pandemic (WHO, 2020), there is still little practice-based evidence that informs how to appropriately enhance refugees' PTG. In this chapter, we offer insights from an intervention designed for that purpose. Going beyond an individualistic perspective of treatment (e.g., psychotherapy, medication), we present a community-based intervention through which refugees are actively involved in peer-mentoring and peer-support-group formats.

This chapter is organized as follows. First, we offer an overview of the main literature about refugees' PTG. Second, we offer a practice-driven applied view by describing a community-based intervention aimed at enhancing refugees' PTG. Finally, based on our experience of implementation of the proposed intervention in southern Spain, we discuss some lessons learned and implications for the promotion of PTG among forcibly displaced individuals.

An Overview of PTG among Refugees

Berger and Weiss (2003) were the first authors to highlight the "missing link" between migration and PTG. In this section, we offer an overview of the main topics and findings in the literature about refugees' PTG. Rather than intending to be exhaustive, this overview offers a general overview of what has been studied to date regarding the link between "forced migration" and "PTG."

The first line of research has addressed efforts towards the identification of the main factors that fuel the emergence of PTG among refugees. At the individual level, variables such as hope, dispositional optimism, coping strategies, religiosity, and some socio-demographic characteristics have been identified as important facilitators of PTG. *Hope*, a positive emotional state through which refugees are confident about the future, has been found to be related to PTG (Ai et al., 2007; Umer & Elliot, 2021). Apart from being hopeful, people with *dispositional optimism* also have a higher chance of gaining growth after a traumatic event (Acquaye, 2017). Refugees who use adaptive cognitive or emotional *coping strategies*, such as processing, positive refocusing, putting their situation into perspective, emotion regulation, or problem-focused coping, show higher levels of PTG (Acar et al., 2021; Ai et al., 2007; Ersahin, 2020; Gökalp & Haktanir, 2021; Hussain & Bhushan, 2011; Prasetya et al., 2020). On the contrary, maladaptive strategies such as suppression or avoidance were found to be negatively associated with PTG (Ai et al., 2007;

Kira et al., 2019), albeit in some cases, avoidance was found to be a positive tool for surviving (McCormack & Tapp, 2019). *Religiosity* represents a spiritual resource and can be considered a specific coping strategy that refugees often use during difficult times (e.g., praying, attending church), thus promoting their PTG (Abraham et al., 2018; Kim & Lee, 2009). However, Acquaye et al. (2018) noted that when religiosity is high, the effect of trauma on PTG decreases and that a moderate level of religiosity is more adequate. All these individual factors can be conceptualized within the *resilience* term, that is, the process through which refugees are competent to successfully adapt to and/or withstand inevitable adversity (Paloma et al., 2020b). The literature suggests that resilience promotes PTG among displaced people (Cengiz et al., 2019). Regarding *socio-demographic characteristics*, being young, female, educated, and with high income has been related to a stronger PTG (Ai et al., 2007; Hussain & Bhushan, 2011; Powell et al., 2003; Rizkalla & Segal, 2018), although some studies found that these variables were not related to PTG (Berger & Weiss, 2006; Özdemir et al., 2021).

At the relational level, *social support* has been found to be connected to the increase in PTG (Chan et al., 2016; Joseph, 2009). In particular, refugees report a higher degree of personal growth when they feel supported by professionals (Copping et al., 2010; Gökalp & Dilmac, 2021; Rizkalla & Segal, 2018), by people of their countries of origin (Abraham et al., 2018), and by people of the receiving society (Kim & Lee, 2009; Kroo & Nagy, 2011). This suggests that having opportunities to process the trauma by talking about it with others is important to increase PTG (Berger & Weiss, 2006).

At the community level, Matos et al. (2021) highlight how a *welcoming and safe receiving country* may provide the conditions for refugees to reappraise the world and the self in a positive light. Similarly, others have stressed the relevance of enjoying retributive justice and perceiving support from official authorities in the receiving sociopolitical context as factors that facilitate the PTG among refugees (Kira et al., 2006; Taylor et al., 2020).

The *type of trauma* has also been identified as an important variable to take into account when explaining the emergence of PTG among refugees. Trauma that is collective and shared positively predicted personal growth, while personal trauma that is directed toward the self hinders it (Kiliç et al., 2016). Concerning the *severity of trauma*, an inverted-U hypothesis has been observed (Chan et al., 2016), such that moderate levels of trauma promote the highest degree of PTG, while low and high levels block it (Acar et al., 2021; Berger & Weiss, 2006; Powell et al., 2003; Teodorescu et al., 2012; Wen et al., 2020).

The second line of research has addressed the design, implementation, and evaluation of interventions that aim at enhancing the refugees' PTG. Slobodin and Jong (2015) pointed out that the majority of the studies used the improvement of posttraumatic stress disorder symptoms as an indicator of intervention efficacy and stressed the need to include other more positive dimensions. Maybe for this reason, to our knowledge, only four studies addressed the issue focusing on PTG. The first intervention was developed in Liberia with refugees from Côte d'Ivoire (Gregory & Prana, 2013). This intervention was based on the companion recovery model, built on peer-support theory, gestalt therapy, and cognitive behavioral therapy, and was developed through group-based sessions in a six-day period. A second intervention based on brief narrative exposure therapy was developed in the United States with Iraqi refugees (Hijazi et al., 2014) and was run through three individual sessions. The third intervention was developed with young East African refugees in the United States and consisted of eight group therapy sessions (Acquaye et al., 2020). Finally, Paloma et al. (2020a) carried out a community-based intervention with refugees from different countries in conflict who settled in southern Spain. This intervention will be described in depth in the following section. All these interventions were considered to be good practices to enhance refugees' PTG.

As can be seen, practice-based research that describes interventions aimed at enhancing PTG in this population is scarce, especially from a community-based approach. However, "support groups or mentoring schemes may be particularly effective for forced migrants, particularly when involving members of the [...] community who have made a successful transition" (Copping et al., 2010, p. 58). Murray et al. (2010) warn that more practice-based evidence is needed on "community-based interventions that aim to facilitate personal and community growth and change during the refugee resettlement phase" (p. 583). To address this knowledge gap, the following section presents a community-based intervention that has been labeled "best practice" by the Spanish Commission for Refugee Aid. Empirical evidence shows how this intervention generates significant improvements in refugees' PTG while simultaneously showing high intervention acceptability, appropriateness, and feasibility (Paloma et al., 2020a).

A Community-Based Intervention to Enhance Refugees' PTG

The community-based intervention presented in this chapter was designed by the Center for Community Research and Action at the University of Seville (CESPYD; see https://cespyd.es/en/). CESPYD is one of the leading research units in Spain conducting high-quality community-based research projects designed to increase the power, health, and well-being of low-income migrants, refugees, and other unprivileged groups. This intervention has been successfully implemented twice, in 2017 and 2021, thanks to collaboration agreements between CESPYD and the Spanish Commission for Refugee Aid, and the Cepaim Foundation. The implementation manual of this intervention has been published in an open-access format and is freely available in English and Spanish on the CESPYD web page (Paloma et al., 2021).

This intervention is framed within the Comprehensive Mental Health Action Plan (2013–2030), which has among its main objectives: (a) the implementation of strategies for the promotion of mental health and the prevention of mental disorders for those at risk; and (b) the provision of comprehensive mental health services in community-based settings (WHO, 2021). The intervention was designed to be implemented over fifteen weeks and comprises two phases: (1) a peer-mentorship training targeting settled refugees and led by a professional, who uses a peer-support-group format; and (2) cultural peer-support groups comprised of newly arrived refugees and led by the trained settled refugees, which follows a peer-mentoring format (an overview of the intervention's structure can be seen in Figure 46.1).

During the first phase, the sessions follow a peer-support group format and are facilitated by a researcher or professional who aims to train settled refugees as mentors. Settled refugees are understood in this intervention as meeting three criteria: (a) residing in the receiving country for at least one year; (b) being proficient in the dominant language of the receiving country; and (c) having leadership skills and a high degree of social awareness that enable them to help others in a situation of vulnerability (e.g., experience leading groups, volunteering in social projects). During the sessions, settled refugees meet twice weekly in a safe environment of equitable, reciprocal, and supportive interpersonal relationships (Paloma et al., 2020b). Each session lasts two to three hours, depending on the

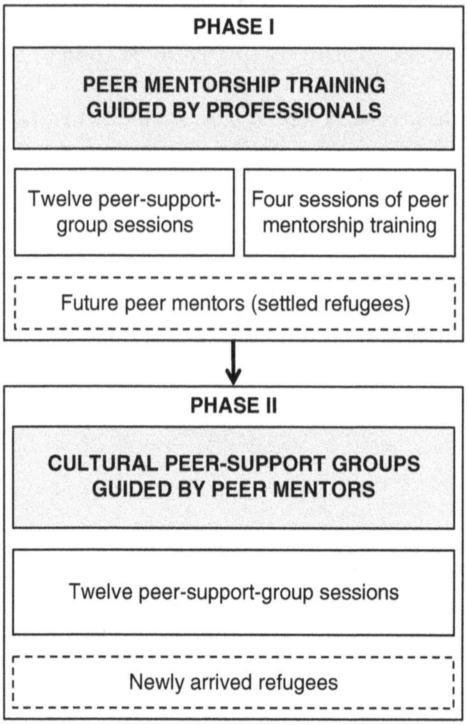

Figure 46.1 A community-based intervention to enhance PTG among refugees.

planned activity, the time participants need to express their thoughts and feelings, and group dynamics.

The first twelve sessions (six weeks) are designed to acknowledge the types of mourning participants experienced after trauma, identify personal strengths, and share community resources. These sessions aim to help participants to effectively manage their mourning thanks to building a more positive narrative alongside peers in the same situation. During the first session, the project is explained in detail, participants and staff introduce themselves, and a brief analysis of the main difficulties that refugees find in the new society is performed as a first task stimulus. The second session explores participants' sociopolitical and personal reasons for migration. From the third to the ninth session, the content is structured around the seven "migratory mournings" identified in the literature, i.e., social network, language, culture, land, status, discrimination, and health (Atxotegui, 2000). The last three sessions explicitly focus on participants' identifying their own strengths, acknowledging positive changes following migration, increasing self-confidence for taking action to enhance their own well-being and that of their community, and envisioning the future. As Berger and Weiss (2003) indicate, "after the losses have been recognized and cognitively processed, perceptions of benefits from the immigration experience might be evident" (p. 26). All twelve sessions follow a similar structure including a guided relaxation, individual reflection or activity about a question or task stimulus related to the session content, sharing of migratory stories based on the previous individual reflection or activity, and presentation by participants and staff of community resources available in the receiving society related

Table 46.1 Session Content of the Community-Based Intervention to Enhance Refugees' PTG

Session	*Content*	*Sample Activity Carried Out in the Session*
1	Introduction	Writing the negative and positive aspects of the migratory experience (i.e., the balance of migration).
2	Reasons for migration	Writing one's reasons for migration and asylum and sharing with the group.
3	Social network	Writing the current social network and the extent of support that participants feel they can count on.
4	Language	Writing down a difficult account that happened as a consequence of the language barrier and describing how participants overcame these situations.
5	Culture	Creation of a cultural collage to express the feelings about one's own culture and the new one.
6	Land	Painting a landscape that reminds participants of their homeland.
7	Social Status	Drawing a river that represents the timeline of the three life stages: the past, the present, and the future.
8	Discrimination	Sharing experiences of discrimination and possible actions to combat it.
9	Health	Writing down on post-its words or phrases that participants link to the concept of health, creating a network of concepts.
10	Strengths and self-esteem	Describing each other's use of positive adjectives and then assessing themselves according to the descriptions given by others.
11	Taking action	Writing a letter to a refugee who has recently arrived in the country and suggesting some useful recommendations at this initial stage.
12	Expectations for the future	Imagining a day like any other in 5 years, describing what participants' life would be like.

to the session content. Table 46.1 lists an overview of the twelve sessions' contents as well as a sample of individual reflections or activities carried out in each session. The following four sessions (two weeks) are destined to offer future mentors clear mentoring guidelines that can help them during the implementation of the second phase (e.g., the process of group revitalization, leadership, or the creation of material adapted to each cultural group, among others).

During the second phase, aimed to accompany a group of newly arrived refugees, the sessions follow a peer-mentoring format facilitated by one or a pair of settled refugees, trained as mentors in the first phase. Newly arrived refugees are understood in this intervention as meeting three criteria: (a) residing in the receiving country for less than six months, (b) having their basic needs addressed, and (c) lacking a social support network and/or showing little knowledge of the main community resources available in the receiving society. The groups of newly arrived refugees created in this phase are called "cultural peer-support groups," because they are made up of culturally similar people who share a common language. Consequently, the number of cultural peer-support groups that can be created in this phase depends on the correspondence of language and cultural origins among newly arrived refugees and mentors. During these sessions, the groups work in parallel, and the mentors recreate in their native language the previous twelve peer-support sessions such that the duration, frequency, and content of the sessions are the same as the corresponding first six weeks of the first phase.

During the final fifteenth week of the intervention, it is recommended to finish the project with a closing ceremony involving all participants (i.e., researchers, community-partner professionals, mentors, and newly arrived refugees). During this event, awards related to the project are given to refugees (e.g., certificates, letters of recommendation) and it can be accompanied by an informal meeting such as an intercultural luncheon.

Lessons Learned for Promoting PTG in Forced Migration

Results obtained after the implementation in southern Spain of the community-based intervention presented above suggest that it is a useful format to increase the PTG of refugees in receiving societies (for an in-depth discussion, please see Paloma et al., 2020a). Quantitative and qualitative data collected in a pretest-posttest evaluation design have shown that refugees appreciated life more, felt stronger, developed deeper connections with others, and discovered new possibilities in their lives (Paloma et al., 2020a). Specifically relative to mentors, besides the increase in PTG, there is evidence that their involvement as key agents of change in the intervention increased their levels of resilience and empowerment, which are indicators of their positive and active adaptation in the receiving society (Paloma et al., 2020b). Beyond the program's effectiveness, the implementation outcomes revealed high levels of acceptability, appropriateness, and feasibility (Paloma et al., 2020a). Participants perceived the intervention as satisfactory, useful, tailored to their needs and values, and easily implementable. This intervention reveals "the decisive role that host communities can play in promoting adaptive adjustment when refugees are provided with safe opportunities for self-realization" (Matos et al., 2021, p. 15).

The peer-support-group format allows refugees to develop an inner strength that includes hope regarding their future, optimism, and self-confidence in using an active coping strategy to face adversity. These individual factors that positively influence the increase of PTG are fueled by the social support achieved and the knowledge of community resources shared during the sessions. Participants can enjoy social connectedness with peers in an empathy-based setting where they can freely express suffering and be listened to by others in a similar situation. Peers can assist in fostering the PTG of each member by offering new perspectives that help participants rebuild the meaning of the trauma and integrate it more positively into their life narrative. It is important to note that the building of this inner strength is equally relevant for settled and newly arrived refugees. For settled refugees who later become mentors, the peer mentorship training is mostly experiential and fuels self-reflection on their own life, which is considered a necessary first step before taking action as mentors of others in a situation of more vulnerability. For newly arrived refugees who participate as peers, being in this psychologically comfortable setting where they can manage their personal struggles is expected to create a solid base that helps them to progressively open up towards the receiving society.

The peer-mentoring format allows overcoming language barriers and establishing more equitable power relationships between providers and participants, which is often in the hands of the former to the detriment of the latter. Indeed, mentors use their mother tongue to accompany their cultural peer-support groups so that the intervention can reach newly arrived refugees who may not yet know the receiving society's dominant language. Because this accompaniment is carried out by people who have already undergone similar experiences as those of the participants, they can act as models and potential sources of inspiration for newly arrived refugees who must "rebuild a life and start from scratch, both logistically and psychologically" (Gökalp & Haktanir, 2021, p. 12). Settled refugees receive and experience the same intervention that they will later implement with newly arrived refugees. This makes possible a "butterfly effect", i.e., those who have been supported have the tools to support in the future others who later will have the competencies to do the same with others, and so on. This format helps to offer culturally sensitive services and to overcome barriers that most refugees encounter in accessing mental health services in receiving societies (WHO, 2018). At the same time, this approach enables settled refugees "to contribute to society, rather than being excluded and stigmatized" (Taylor et al., 2020, p. 28).

Among the lessons learned during the implementation of the aforementioned community-based intervention, is the importance of facilitating participants' engagement over time. Due to the high degree of mobility and uncertainty linked to the administrative status and labor conditions that characterize this population, we have learned that it is important to carry out an intensive intervention (with two sessions weekly) like the one shown herein. This, together with great schedule flexibility to adjust the program to participants' availability, improves adherence and helps guarantee that participants can benefit from the complete intervention. In addition, it is crucial to provide some forms of gratification (e.g., certificates, letters of recommendation, intercultural celebrations, access to university facilities). Although our experience is that mentors show (and should show) high intrinsic motivation and commitment to engage in the program, it would be practical to offer some kind of gratuity to them to reward their efforts. Finally, it is recommended to stress the importance for participants to view the sessions as a flexible collective-building process. Thus, refugees can perceive the intervention as relevant, useful, and tailored to their needs, promoting their involvement throughout the process.

The second noteworthy lesson learned relates to the selection of participants. Combined with considering the inclusion criteria presented above, ideally, participants would not know each other in order to maximize positive outcomes of the intervention as prior knowledge, common contacts, and social desirability may hinder an honest opening during group sessions. However, this recommendation cannot be always followed when refugees meet in language classes or in other activities offered by the community partner, or even when they live in the same shelter. In this case, it is important to be careful about the process of setting up the groups and pay specific attention to this aspect, so that prior knowledge could benefit sharing rather than blocking openness.

A third lesson is the need to support the mentors throughout the second phase when they are expected to play a more active and autonomous role with their cultural peer-support groups. We can offer them both emotional (e.g., how to manage sensitive psychological processes emerging in the group) and pragmatic support (e.g., how to prepare material adapted to their group). We can accompany them through (a) individual meetings of monitoring after each session or weekly; (b) group sessions for the exchange of views among all the mentors involved in the program; and (c) a communication channel, such as a Whatsapp group, available for discussing doubts, help, or emotional support.

A fourth lesson relates to the evaluation of the intervention. Given the importance of evaluating the effectiveness of our endeavors and guaranteeing the accuracy of the data collected, mentors must be trained (during the peer mentorship training) in the formative and summative evaluation process. Depending on the decisions taken regarding the measurement instruments to be used in the program (see Paloma et al., 2021, for a suggestion), it is necessary to train mentors in filling out their own scales and field notes, reporting the progress of their cultural peer-support groups using structured observational grids, and/or administering scales or conducting focus groups with open questions to participants. To avoid participants' fatigue, we recommend using only a few well-selected short scales together with several minimally invasive sources of evaluation (e.g., open questions at the end of each session, field notes, and observational data from mentors). Moreover, for cultural peer-support groups where participants are struggling with the language or with a limited educational background, it is recommended to set aside two extra sessions for evaluation, before and after the second phase. In these sessions, mentors can support newly arrived refugees in filling out the scales, explaining the meaning of challenging items, and thus guarantee successful completion of the assessment.

Finally, we have learned some lessons that allow us to envision directions for future action for this community-based intervention in its promotion of refugees' PTG. In order to refine it, we found that art-based sessions were powerful in eliciting intimate feelings, especially when participants had a very heterogeneous educational background. Although this format is quite present in the existing proposal for group dynamics (Paloma et al., 2021), we need to advance this line of work. In addition, the training sessions in peer mentorship should be fortified by providing more specific content about leadership, group processes, emotional management, and evaluation. Lastly, we think it would be useful to stress an intercultural and gender approach to this intervention. For example, carrying out joint sessions between different cultural peer-support groups, adding a third phase where members of the receiving society are matched with participants, or offering child care for women who intend to participate in the sessions and be sensitive to their specific feminine view.

The aforementioned program points to directions for future research. For example, future research should advance evaluating the consequences of this community-based intervention in the whole field of refugees' mental health. Some studies found a positive correlation between PTG and posttraumatic stress disorder (Acquaye, 2017; Cengiz et al., 2019; Hussain & Bhushan, 2011; Kiliç et al., 2016) whereas others found a negative correlation (Davey et al., 2015; Teodorescu et al., 2012) or no correlation (Ai et al. 2007; Powell et al., 2003; Sleijpen et al., 2016). This suggests that PTG may coexist with symptoms of suffering in refugees. Therefore, together with PTG, we need to evaluate also negative mental health outcomes to be able to establish which specific aspects of mental health this intervention can impact. As Roepke (2005) concluded, "more research is needed to uncover the relationship between growth and distress during intervention programs" (p. 139). In addition, our findings suggest that active participation and social connectedness play an important role in the development of PTG, which seems to be encouraged by others and fueled when one feels valued within a group of people in a similar situation. Future research could analyze the role of the evolution of the psychological sense of community throughout the program in PTG. As Gökalp and Dilmac (2021) argue, "social support systems can be made use of to speed up refugees' posttraumatic growth processes" (p. 107). Finally, this intervention is currently limited to its implementation with refugees. However, it is expected that economic migrants and other unprivileged groups on the move may also benefit from the program. Future practice-based research should verify this.

Summary and Conclusions

This chapter presents an intervention that offers a way to increase PTG beyond individual-oriented treatments, by creating supportive community-based scenarios as well as valuing the refugees' own capabilities as the main resources for the program's success. Through peer-mentoring and peer-support-group formats, this intervention offers refugees the possibility of playing an active and significant role within the program for their own growth and that of their community. Thus, our intervention adheres to the guidelines proposed by the UNHCR (2017), as it: (a) strengthens refugees' capacity to support each other through community-based activities, and (b) promotes the meaningful engagement of refugees, who are not experts, as agents of change within their communities. Moreover, as our program aligns with the Comprehensive Mental Health Action Plan (WHO, 2021), we expect it to contribute to the advancement towards the consolidation of a community-based mental health approach (Baumann, 2018; Hamza & Clancy, 2020). This approach allows to avoid pathologization of the refugees' condition by understanding suffering as the normal reaction in those who have experienced social injustices such as forced migration. It also allows to broaden the pool of potential beneficiaries of the intervention beyond those with severe psychological distress, strengthening and building capacities within the refugee community as a whole. As Hussain and Bhushan (2011) stated, "refugee trauma is a collective phenomenon. Therefore, psychosocial intervention at the community level should be integrated for promoting mental health and psychological and social growth of the community" (p. 733).

References

Abraham, R., Lien, L., & Hanssen, I. (2018). Coping, resilience and posttraumatic growth among Eritrean female refugees living in Norwegian asylum reception centres: A qualitative study. *International Journal of Social Psychiatry*, *64*(4), 359–366. 10.1177/0020764018765237

Acar, B., Acar, İ.H., Alhiraki, O. A., Fahham, O., Erim, Y., & Acarturk, C. (2021). The role of coping strategies in post-traumatic growth among Syrian refugees: A structural equation model. *International Journal of Environmental Research and Public Health*, *18*(16), 8829. 10.3390/ijerph18168829

Acquaye, H. E. (2017). PTSD, optimism, religious commitment, and growth as post-trauma trajectories: A structural equation modeling of former refugees. *Professional Counselor*, *7*(4), 330–348. 10.15241/hea.7.4.330

Acquaye, H. E., John, C. M., Bloomquist, L. A., & Milne, N. M. (2020). Using the post-traumatic growth model to explore trauma narratives in group work with African refugee youth. *The Journal for Specialists in Group Work*, *45*(3), 185–199. 10.1080/01933922.2020.1789791

Acquaye, H. E., Sivo, S. A., & Jones, K. D. (2018). Religious commitment's moderating effect on refugee trauma and growth. *Counseling and Values*, *63*(1), 57–75. 10.1002/cvj.12073

Ai, A. L., Tice, T. N., Whitsett, D. D., Ishisaka, T., & Chim, M. (2007). Posttraumatic symptoms and growth of Kosovar war refugees: The influence of hope and cognitive coping. *The Journal of Positive Psychology*, *2*(1), 55–65. 10.1080/17439760601069341

Atxotegui, J. (2000). Los duelos de la migración: Una aproximación psicopatológica y psicosocial. In E. Perdiguero, & J. Comelles (Eds.), *Medicina y cultura: Estudios entre la antropología y la medicina* (pp. 83–100). Edicions Bellaterra.

Baumann, S. L. (2018). From posttraumatic stress disorder to posttraumatic growth: A paradigm shift or paradox? *Nursing Science Quarterly*, *31*(3), 287–290. 10.1177/0894318418774923

Berger, R., & Weiss, T. (2003). Immigration and posttraumatic growth: A missing link. *Journal of Immigrant & Refugee Services*, *1*(2), 21–39. 10.1300/J191v01n02_02

Berger, R., & Weiss, T. (2006). Posttraumatic growth in Latina immigrants. *Journal of Immigrant & Refugee Studies*, *4*(3), 55–72. 10.1300/J500v04n03_03

Cengiz, I., Ergün, D., & Cakici, E. (2019). Posttraumatic stress disorder, posttraumatic growth and psychological resilience in Syrian refugees: Hatay, Turkey. *Anadolu Psikiyatri Dergisi*, *20*(3), 269–276. 10.5455/apd.4862

Chan, K. J., Young, M. Y., & Sharif, N. (2016). Well-being after trauma: A review of posttraumatic growth among refugees. *Canadian Psychology*, *57*(4), 291. 10.1037/cap0000065

Copping, A., Shakespeare-Finch, J., & Paton, D. (2010). Towards a culturally appropriate mental health system: Sudanese-Australians' experiences with trauma. *Journal of Pacific Rim Psychology*, *4*(1), 53–60. 10.1375/prp.4.1.53

Davey, C., Heard, R., & Lennings, C. (2015). Development of the Arabic versions of the Impact of Events Scale-Revised and the Posttraumatic Growth Inventory to assess trauma and growth in Middle Eastern refugees in Australia. *Clinical Psychologist*, *19*(3), 131–139. 10.1111/cp.12043

Ersahin, Z. (2020). Post-traumatic growth among Syrian refugees in Turkey: The role of coping strategies and religiosity. *Current Psychology*, 1–10. 10.1007/s12144-020-00763-8

Fazel, M., Wheeler, J., & Danesh, J. (2005). Prevalence of serious mental disorder in 7000 refugees resettled in western countries: A systematic review. *The Lancet*, *365*, 1309–1314. 10.1016/S0140-6736(05)61027-6

Ferriss, S. S., & Forrest-Bank, S. S. (2018). Perspectives of Somali refugees on post-traumatic growth after resettlement. *Journal of Refugee Studies*, *31*(4), 626–646. 10.1093/jrs/fey006

Gökalp, Z. S., & Dilmac, B. (2021). Predictive relationship between war posttraumatic growth, values, and perceived social support. *Illness, Crisis & Loss*, *29*(2), 95–111. 10.1177/1054137318788655

Gökalp, Z. S., & Haktanir, A. (2021). A posttraumatic growth experiences of refugees: A meta-synthesis of qualitative studies. *Journal of Community Psychology*, 1–16. 10.1002/jcop.22723

Gökalp, Z. S., Dilmaç, B., & Özteke-Kozan, H.İ. (2021). Posttraumatic growth experiences of Syrian refugees after war. *Journal of Humanistic Psychology*, *61*(1), 55–72. 10.1177/002216781 8801090

Gregory, J. L., & Prana, H. (2013). Posttraumatic growth in Côte d'Ivoire refugees using the companion recovery model. *Traumatology*, *19*(3), 223–232. 10.1177/1534765612471146

Hamza, M. K., & Clancy, K. (2020). Building mental health and resilience: Regional and global perspectives from the inaugural Syrian American Medical Society Mental Health Mission Trip. *Avicenna Journal of Medicine*, *10*(1), 54–59. 10.4103/ajm.ajm_157_19

Hijazi, A. M., Lumley, M. A., Ziadni, M. S., Haddad, L., Rapport, L. J., & Arnetz, B. B. (2014). Brief narrative exposure therapy for posttraumatic stress in Iraqi refugees: A preliminary randomized clinical trial. *Journal of Traumatic Stress*, *27*(3), 314–322. 10.1002/jts.21922

Hussain, D., & Bhushan, B. (2011). Posttraumatic stress and growth among Tibetan refugees: The mediating role of cognitive-emotional regulation strategies. *Journal of Clinical Psychology*, *67*(7), 720–735. 10.1002/jclp.20801

Joseph, S. (2009). Growth following adversity: Positive psychological perspectives on posttraumatic stress. *Psychological Topics*, *18*(2), 335–344. https://hrcak.srce.hr/48217

Kiliç, C., Magruder, K. M., & Koryürek, M. M. (2016). Does trauma type relate to posttraumatic growth after war? A pilot study of young Iraqi war survivors living in Turkey. *Transcultural Psychiatry*, *53*(1), 110–123. 10.1177/1363461515612963

Kim, H. K., & Lee, O. J. (2009). A phenomenological study on the experience of North Korean refugees. *Nursing Science Quarterly*, *22*(1), 85–88. 10.1177/0894318408329242

Kira, I. A., Lewandowski, L., Templin, T., Ramaswamy, V., Ozkan, B., Hammad, A., & Mohanesh, J. (2006). The mental health effects of retributive justice: The case of Iraqi refugees. *Journal of Muslim Mental Health*, *1*(2), 145–169. 10.1080/15564900600980756

Kira, I. A., Shuwiekh, H., Al Ibraheem, B., & Aljakoub, J. (2019). Appraisals and emotion regulation mediate the effects of identity salience and cumulative stressors and traumas, on PTG and mental health: The case of Syrian's IDPs and refugees. *Self and Identity*, *18*(3), 284–305. 10.1080/152 98868.2018.1451361

Kroo, A., & Nagy, H. (2011). Posttraumatic growth among traumatized Somali refugees in Hungary. *Journal of Loss and Trauma*, *16*(5), 440–458. 10.1080/15325024.2011.575705

Matos, L., Costa, P. A., Park, C. L., Indart, M. J., & Leal, I. (2021). 'The war made me a better person': Syrian refugees' meaning-making trajectories in the aftermath of collective trauma. *International Journal of Environmental Research and Public Health*, *18*(16), 8481. 10.3390/ijerph18168481

McCormack, L., & Tapp, B. (2019). Violation and hope: Refugee survival in childhood and beyond. *International Journal of Social Psychiatry*, *65*(2), 169–179. 10.1177/0020764019831314

Murray, K. E., Davidson, G. R., & Schweitzer, R. D. (2010). Review of refugee mental health interventions following resettlement: Best practices and recommendations. *American Journal of Orthopsychiatry*, *80*(4), 576–585. 10.1111/j.1939-0025.2010.01062.x

Özdemir, P. G., Kırlı, U., & Asoglu, M. (2021). Investigation of the associations between post-traumatic growth, sleep quality and depression symptoms in Syrian refugees. *Eastern Journal of Medicine*, *26*(2), 265–272. 10.5505/ejm.2021.48108

Paloma, V., de la Morena, I., & Busche, V. (2021). Posttraumatic Growth Intervention for Refugees: Implementation Manual. *Center for Community Research and Action at the Universidad de Sevilla*. Available at https://cespyd.es/a/wp-content/uploads/2021/10/Implementation-Manual.pdf [English version]; https://cespyd.es/a/wp-content/uploads/2021/09/Manual-de-Implementacion.pdf [Spanish version].

Paloma, V., de la Morena, I., & López-Torres, C. (2020a). Promoting posttraumatic growth among the refugee population in Spain: A community-based pilot intervention. *Health & Social Care in the Community*, *28*(1), 127–136. 10.1111/hsc.12847

Paloma, V., de la Morena, I., Sladkova, J., & López-Torres, C. (2020b). A peer support and peer mentoring approach to enhancing resilience and empowerment among refugees settled in southern Spain. *Journal of Community Psychology*, *48*(5), 1438–1451. 10.1002/jcop.22338

Powell, S., Rosner, R., Butollo, W., Tedeschi, R. G., & Calhoun, L. G. (2003). Posttraumatic growth after war: A study with former refugees and displaced people in Sarajevo. *Journal of Clinical Psychology*, *59*(1), 71–83. 10.1002/jclp.10117

Prasetya, E. C., Muhdi, N., & Atika, A. (2020). Relationship between previous traumatic experience, post-traumatic growth, coping strategy to mental health state on refugees in Sidoarjo Camp. *Systematic Reviews in Pharmacy*, *11*(5), 750–754. 10.31838/srp.2020.5.108

Rizkalla, N., & Segal, S. P. (2018). Well-being and posttraumatic growth among Syrian refugees in Jordan. *Journal of Traumatic Stress*, *31*(2), 213–222. 10.1002/jts.22281

Roepke, A. M. (2005). Psychosocial interventions and posttraumatic growth: A meta-analysis. *Journal of Consulting and Clinical Psychology*, *83*(1), 129–142. 10.1037/a0036872

Shakespeare-Finch, J., Schweitzer, R. D., King, J., & Brough, M. (2014). Distress, coping, and posttraumatic growth in refugees from Burma. *Journal of Immigrant & Refugee Studies*, *12*(3), 311–330. 10.1080/15562948.2013.844876

Sleijpen, M., Haagen, J., Mooren, T., & Kleber, R. J. (2016). Growing from experience: An exploratory study of posttraumatic growth in adolescent refugees. *European Journal of Psychotraumatology*, *7*(1), 28698. 10.3402/ejpt.v7.28698

Slobodin, O., & Jong, J. T. (2015). Mental health interventions for traumatized asylum seekers and refugees: What do we know about their efficacy? *International Journal of Social Psychiatry*, *61*(1), 17–26. 10.1177/0020764014535752

Taher, R., & Allan, T. (2020). Posttraumatic growth in displaced Syrians in the UK: A mixed-methods approach. *Journal of Loss and Trauma*, *25*(4), 333–347. 10.1080/15325024.2019.1688022

Taku, K., Cann, A., Calhoun, L. G., & Tedeschi, R. G. (2008). The factor structure of the Posttraumatic Growth Inventory: A comparison of five models using confirmatory factor analysis. *Journal of Traumatic Stress*, *21*(2), 158–164. 10.1002/jts.20305

Taylor, S., Charura, D., Williams, G., Shaw, M., Allan, J., Cohen, E., Meth, F., & O'Dwyer, L. (2020). Loss, grief, and growth: An interpretative phenomenological analysis of experiences of trauma in asylum seekers and refugees. *Traumatology*. 10.1037/trm0000250

Tedeschi, R. G., & Calhoun, L. G. (2004). Posttraumatic growth: Conceptual foundations and empirical evidence. *Psychological Inquiry*, *15*(1), 1–18. 10.1207/s15327965pli1501_01

Teodorescu, D. S., Heir, T., Hauff, E., Wentzel-Larsen, T. O. R. E., & Lien, L. (2012). Mental health problems and post-migration stress among multi-traumatized refugees attending outpatient clinics upon resettlement to Norway. *Scandinavian Journal of Psychology*, *53*(4), 316–332. 10.1111/j.1467-9450.2012.00954.x

Umer, M., & Elliot, D. L. (2021). Being hopeful: Exploring the dynamics of post-traumatic growth and hope in refugees. *Journal of Refugee Studies*, *34*(1), 953–975. 10.1093/jrs/fez002

UNHCR (2017). *Community-based protection & Mental health & Psychosocial support*. Switzerland: United Nations High Commissioner for Refugees. https://www.refworld.org/docid/593ab6add.html

UNHCR (2021a). *Refugee Data Finder*. United Nations High Commissioner for Refugees. https://www.unhcr.org/refugee-statistics/

UNHCR (2021b). *UNHCR Master Glossary of Terms*. United Nations High Commissioner for Refugees. https://www.unhcr.org/glossary/

United Nations General Assembly (1951). *Convention relating to the status of refugees*. United Nations General Assembly. https://www.unhcr.org/3b66c2aa10

van der Boor, C. F., Amos, R., Nevitt, S., Dowrick, C., & White, R. G. (2020). Systematic review of factors associated with quality of life of asylum seekers and refugees in high-income countries. *Conflict and Health*, *14*(1), 1–25. 10.1186/s13031-020-00292-y

Wen, K., McGrath, M., Acarturk, C., Ilkkursun, Z., Fuhr, D. C., Sondorp, E., Cuijpers, P., Sijbrandij, M., Roberts, B., & STRENGTHS consortium (2020). Post-traumatic growth and its predictors among Syrian refugees in Istanbul: A mental health population survey. *Journal of Migration and Health*, *1*, 100010. 10.1016/j.jmh.2020.100010

WHO (2018). *Mental health promotion and mental health care in refugees and migrants*. Copenhagen: WHO Regional Office for Europe. https://www.euro.who.int/__data/assets/pdf_file/0004/386563/mental-health-eng.pdf

WHO (2020). *ApartTogether survey: Preliminary overview of refugees and migrants self-reported impact of COVID-19*. Geneva: World Health Organization. https://apps.who.int/iris/handle/10665/337931

WHO (2021). *Comprehensive mental health action plan 2013–2030*. Geneva: World Health Organization. https://www.who.int/publications/i/item/9789240031029

INDEX

For Product Safety Concerns and Information please contact our EU
representative GPSR@taylorandfrancis.com
Taylor & Francis Verlag GmbH, Kaufingerstraße 24, 80331 München, Germany

www.ingramcontent.com/pod-product-compliance
Lightning Source LLC
Chambersburg PA
CBHW081212220326
41598CB00037B/6761

* 9 7 8 1 0 3 2 2 0 8 6 6 4 *